Clinical Pharmacology for Anesthesiology

Ken B. Johnson, MD
Professor
Director, Center for Patient Simulation
Carter M. Ballinger Presidential Chair in Anesthesiology
Department of Anesthesiology
University of Utah
Salt Lake City, Utah

Mc Graw Hill Education | Medical

New York Chicago San Francisco Athens London Madrid Mexico City
Milan New Delhi Singapore Sydney Toronto

Clinical Pharmacology for Anesthesiology

1 2 3 4 5 6 7 8 9 0 CTP/CTP 19 18 17 16 15 14

ISBN 978-0-07-173616-9
MHID 0-07-173616-6

Notice

Medicine is an ever-changing science. As new research and clinical experience broaden our knowledge, changes in treatment and drug therapy are required. The authors and the publisher of this work have checked with sources believed to be reliable in their efforts to provide information that is complete and generally in accord with the standards accepted at the time of publication. However, in view of the possibility of human error or changes in medical sciences, neither the authors nor the publisher nor any other party who has been involved in the preparation or publication of this work warrants that the information contained herein is in every respect accurate or complete, and they disclaim all responsibility for any errors or omissions or for the results obtained from use of the information contained in this work. Readers are encouraged to confirm the information contained herein with other sources. For example and in particular, readers are advised to check the product information sheet included in the package of each drug they plan to administer to be certain that the information contained in this work is accurate and that changes have not been made in the recommended dose or in the contraindications for administration. This recommendation is of particular importance in connection with new or infrequently used drugs.

This book was set in Minion pro by Cenveo® Publisher Services.
The editors were Brian Belval and Christina M. Thomas.
The production supervisor was Catherine Saggese.
Project management was provided by Anupriya Tyagi, Cenveo Publisher Services.
The cover designer was Thomas De Pierro.
Cover Image Credit: © Aeriform/Ikon Images/Corbis.
China Translation & Printing Services, Ltd. was printer and binder.

This book is printed on acid-free paper.

Library of Congress Cataloging-in-Publication Data

Johnson, Ken (Ken B.), author.
Clinical pharmacology for anesthesiology / Ken Johnson.
p. ; cm.
Includes bibliographical references and index.
ISBN 978-0-07-173616-9 (pbk. : alk. paper)—ISBN 0-07-173616-6 (alk. paper)
I. Title.
[DNLM: 1. Anesthetics—pharmacology. 2. Anesthesia. QV 81]
RD82.2
615.781—dc 3

2014003875

To my wife Jenifer, and our children, Cathryn, Ryan, Rachel, and Andria for their gifts of time and encouragement.

Contents

SECTION IV Special Populations

SECTION V Perioperative Dosing Considerations

SECTION VI Dosing Considerations for Selected Cases

Contributors

Stephen Aniskevich, MD
Instructor of Anesthesiology
Mayo Clinic
Jacksonville, Florida

Byron Bankhead, MD
Associate Professor
Department of Anesthesiology
University of Utah
Salt Lake City, Utah

Michael Behrens, MD
Department of Anesthesiology
University of Utah
Salt Lake City, Utah

Nathan Birgenheier, MD
Assistant Professor
Department of Anesthesiology
University of Utah
Salt Lake City, Utah

Lara Brewer, PhD
Assistant Professor
Department of Bioengineering
University of Utah
Salt Lake City, Utah

Sorin J. Brull, MD, FCARCSI (Hon)
Professor of Anesthesiology
Mayo Clinic
Jacksonville, Florida

Tyler Call, MD
Assistant Professor
Department of Anesthesiology
University of Utah
Salt Lake City, Utah

Clint Christensen, MD
Assistant Professor
Department of Anesthesiology
University of Utah
Salt Lake City, Utah

Dustin E. Coyle, MD
Assistant Professor
Department of Anesthesiology
University of Utah
Salt Lake City, Utah

Jennifer J. Davis, MD
Professor
Department of Anesthesiology
University of Utah
Salt Lake City, Utah

Jennifer DeCou, MD
Assistant Professor
Department of Anesthesiology
University of Utah
Salt Lake City, Utah

Marcel E. Durieux, MD, PhD
Professor
Departments of Anesthesiology and Neurological Surgery
University of Virginia
Charlottesville, Virginia

Talmage D. Egan, MD
Professor
Department of Anesthesiology
K.C. Wong Presidential Chair
University of Utah
Salt Lake City, Utah

Douglas J. Eleveld, PhD
Research Engineer
Department of Anesthesiology
University Medical Center Groningen
University of Groningen
Groningen, The Netherlands

John Farr, MD
Department of Anesthesiology
University of Utah
Salt Lake City, Utah

Aaron Freeman, BS
Department of Anesthesiology
University of Utah
Salt Lake City, Utah

Charles Galaviz, MD
Assistant Professor (Clinical)
Department of Anesthesiology
University of Utah
Salt Lake City, Utah

Daniel Gammon, MD
Assistant Professor
Department of Anesthesiology
University of Utah
Salt Lake City, Utah

Tong J. Gan, MD
Professor
Department of Anesthesiology
Duke University Medical Center
Durham, North Carolina

Ben Gmelch, MD
Assistant Professor
Department of Anesthesiology
University of Utah
Salt Lake City, Utah

Philip N. Gnadinger, MD, MPH
Assistant Clinical Professor
Department of Anesthesiology
University of Utah School of Medicine
Salt Lake City, Utah

Austin Healy, BS
Department of Anesthesiology
University of Utah
Salt Lake City, Utah

Elise Heath, MD
Department of Anesthesiology
University of Utah
Salt Lake City, Utah

John Hille, MD
Department of Anesthesiology
Intermountain Healthcare
Salt Lake City, Utah

Ken B. Johnson, MD
Professor
Director, Center for Patient Simulation
Carter M. Ballinger Presidential Chair in Anesthesiology
Department of Anesthesiology
University of Utah
Salt Lake City, Utah

Cristen D. Lapierre, PhD
Department of Radiology, Massachusetts General Hospital
Department of Physics, Harvard University
Charlestown, Massachusetts

Jeffrey K. Lu, MD
Professor
Department of Anesthesiology
University of Utah
Salt Lake City, Utah

Amy K. Manchester, MD
Assistant Professor
Department of Anesthesiology
Duke University Medical Center
Durham, North Carolina

Jeff E. Mandel, MD, MS
Assistant Professor of Anesthesiology & Critical Care
Perelman School of Medicine
University of Pennsylvania
Philadelphia, Pennsylvania

David N. Morgan, MD
Assistant Professor
Department of Bioengineering
University of Utah
Salt Lake City, Utah

Mohamed Naguib, MB, BCh, MSc, FFARCSI, MD
Professor of Anesthesiology
Cleveland Clinic
Cleveland, Ohio

James H. Philip, MEE, MD, CCE
Anesthesiologist and Director of Bioengineering
Department of Anesthesiology, Perioperative and Pain Medicine
Brigham and Women's Hospital
Medical Liaison for Anesthesia
Department of Biomedical Engineering
Partners HealthCare System
Professor of Anaesthesia
Harvard Medical School
Boston, Massachusetts

L. Lazarre Ogden, MD
Professor and Vice Chair
Residency Director
Department of Anesthesiology
University of Utah
Salt Lake City, Utah

Paola Pinzón, MD
Assistant Professor
Fundación Universitaria de Ciencias de la Salud
Facultad de Medicina
Hospital de San José
Bogotá, Colombia

Johannes H. Proost, PharmD, PhD
Associate Professor
Department of Anesthesiology
University Medical Center Groningen
University of Groningen
Groningen, The Netherlands

Sean Runnels, MD
Assistant Professor
Department of Anesthesiology
University of Utah
Salt Lake City, Utah

Sonal Sharma, MD
Fellow, Neurosurgical Anesthesia
Northwestern University Feinberg School of Medicine
Chicago, Illinois

Warner Smith, MD
Assistant Clinical Professor
Department of Anesthesiology
University of Utah
Salt Lake City, Utah

Brian St. George, MD
Staff Anesthesiologist
Northwest Anesthesia Physicians
Springfield, Oregon

Zuzana Stehlikova, MD
Associate Professor
Department of Anesthesiology
University of Utah
Salt Lake City, Utah

Michel M.R.F. Struys, MD, PhD
Professor and Chairman, Department of Anesthesiology
University Medical Center Groningen
University of Groningen
Groningen, The Netherlands
Professor in Anesthesia
Ghent University
Gent, Belgium

Jeffrey Swenson, MD
Professor
University of Utah
Salt Lake City, Utah

Carl Tams, BS
Department of Biomedical Engineering
University of Utah
Salt Lake City, Utah

Elizabeth M. Thackeray, MD, MPH
Assistant Professor
Department of Anesthesiology
University of Utah
Salt Lake City, Utah

Hugo EM Vereecke, MD, PhD
Anesthesiologist
Assistent Professor Anesthesiology
University Medical Center Groningen
University of Groningen
Groningen, The Netherlands

Austin Wallace, MD
Assistant Professor
Department of Anesthesiology
University of Utah
Salt Lake City, Utah

Gregory Wallace, MD
Department of Anesthesiology
University of Utah
Salt Lake City, Utah

Natalie Winter, MD
Department of Anesthesiology
University of Utah
Salt Lake City, Utah

Preface

The intent of this book is to provide a succinct resource for anesthesiologists to use when formulating an anesthetic regimen for both routine and complex cases based on expert opinion and referenced literature. The book leverages from recent advances in clinical pharmacology to describe how anesthetics behave and aims to present this information in such a way that practicing clinicians find it useful.

Clinical pharmacologists have devoted years of research to describing drug behavior. Some of their work is interesting, and certainly relevant to medical practice in general, but not to an anesthesiologist. For example, anesthesiologists rarely, if ever, consider the half-life of propofol when formulating an induction dose. Half-life offers no insight into the onset and duration of loss of consciousness. Much of their research, however, is relevant to anesthetic practice, but uses complex math models to predict drug concentrations and their associated effects. Unfortunately, these models are too complicated to use during patient care. Anesthesiologists, for example, never use tri-exponential equations to determine the optimal dose of fentanyl.

A significant advance in anesthetic drug pharmacology is the use of computers to simulate drug behavior. Where appropriate and supported by published models, simulations will be used throughout this book to illustrate drug concentrations that result from various dosing regimens, predictions of selected drug effects, and interactions between various classes of anesthetic drugs.

Although simulations offer a power tool to visualize drug behavior, readers should be aware of their limitations. The science behind modeling techniques is evolving. Creating a robust pharmacologic model is an expensive and tedious process. Because of these reasons, many anesthetic drugs remain poorly characterized while others have been characterized with relatively simple models. Selected newer anesthetic drugs, developed in an era of sophisticated modeling techniques, have been characterized with more complex models. They may account for patient age, body habitus, or other patient demographics. Simulations presented in the book utilize the best available models at the time of its writing, but newer models are certainly on the horizon. As newer models become available, regular updates to this book will be provided.

It is important to recognize that all simulations are inherently wrong. They use population models to predict how drugs will behave in an individual. Many models were developed from observations in healthy volunteers, not patients. Other models were developed from observations in patients with unique demographics. Given the extensive interindividual variability, it is nearly impossible for models to consistently make accurate predictions. Thus, as with any simulation, these limitations should be considered when interpreting the simulations presented in this book.

The book is divided into six sections. The first section provides an overview of basic principles of clinical pharmacology and how they can be adapted to patient care. The second and third sections address anesthetic and other types of drugs (ie, antiemetics, antiseizure medications, etc) anesthesiologists routinely use. The fourth section will explore how patient demographics, described as covariates such as age and weight, influence anesthetic drug behavior. The fifth section will rely on simulation to illustrate various anesthetic techniques for premedication, induction and maintenance of anesthesia, moderate sedation, and postoperative pain control. This section will briefly explore how various anesthetic techniques compare with one another. The sixth section will provide a selection of sample cases associated with challenging considerations when dosing an anesthetic.

I wish to thank the many contributors to this book, whose expertise in clinical pharmacology have made **Clinical Pharmacology for Anesthesiology,** a distinctive addition to the anesthesia literature. Many of the contributing authors are thought leaders on topics covered in this text and have published numerous manuscripts on topics related to anesthetic drug behavior. Specifically, I wish to thank Noah Syroid, whose programming expertise and creative rendering of anesthetic drug pharmacology was instrumental in developing many of the figures used in this book. I also wish to thank the editors at McGraw Hill for their commitment and consistent support in preparing and editing this text. Finally I am grateful to my wife and family for their enduring support and encouragement, without which this book would not have come to fruition.

Ken B. Johnson, MD

SECTION I

Core Concepts in Clinical Pharmacology

CHAPTER 1

Pharmacokinetics, Biophase, and Pharmacodynamics and the Importance of Simulation

Ken B. Johnson, MD, and Talmage D. Egan, MD

ANESTHETIC CONSIDERATIONS IN FINDING THE CORRECT DOSE

When selecting an anesthetic, anesthetists often consider, among others, the questions presented in Table 1–1. To answer these questions, anesthetists turn to textbooks, journal articles, and drug package inserts. These resources provide dosing recommendations (ie, bolus doses and infusion rates) and important features of anesthetic drugs but often fall short of providing useful answers. Anesthetists therefore rely on years of training and experience to formulate the correct dose and safely administer it. Experienced anesthetists develop a sense of how individual drugs behave and can easily tailor them to meet the needs of their patients. For example, anesthetists have a good "feel" for what a 3-mL (150 mcg) intravenous bolus of fentanyl will accomplish in a healthy adult and can accurately predict the onset and duration of analgesic effect.

Most anesthetics, however, are neither single agents nor are they consistently administered to healthy patients. Suppose an anesthetist has to answer the same questions posed in Table 1–1 for that 3-mL bolus of fentanyl in the presence of 2% sevoflurane. How are the onset and duration changed? For a morbidly obese patient, how does the difference in body habitus influence the onset and duration of effect? With unanticipated severe blood loss, how will fentanyl behave?

The most widely used predictor of anesthetic effect is the minimum alveolar concentration (MAC), the concentration of inhalation agent in the alveoli necessary to keep 50% patients from moving when exposed to a noxious stimulus. Originally used in laboratory investigations to differentiate the potency of inhalation agents from one another, MAC has become a well-known clinical descriptor of drug effect. In fact, modern physiologic monitors display estimates of anesthetic effect as percentages of MAC based on expired concentrations of inhalation agents.

MAC and its derivatives (the concentration of inhalation agent in the alveoli necessary to block an autonomic response in 50% patients when exposed a noxious stimulus [MACbar] and the concentration of inhalation agent in the alveoli in which 50% patients are awake [MACawake]) are by design not reflective of what anesthetists aim to achieve—why blunt the response to a noxious stimulus in only 50% of patients? Why not 99% or 100%? In practice, clinicians use percentage multiples of MAC along with opioids and other anesthetics to ensure that *all* of their patients are adequately anesthetized. Although this approach works, it remains somewhat vague. For example, what multiple of MAC (or MACbar) combined with what dose of opioid are required

TABLE 1–1 Common questions when formulating an anesthetic.

What drug or drug combination will work best for the patient?
What are the adverse effects?
After giving a dose, when will it start to have an effect and how long will it last?
When using a combined technique, how do different anesthetics interact with one another to prolong various drug effects?
How do age, body habitus, blood loss, gender, organ function, medications, health supplements, and so on, influence the onset and duration of anesthetic effects?
Once turned off, how long will it take for the patient to emerge from anesthesia?
In procedures associated with moderate to severe postoperative pain, what dose of analgesic will be safe but still provide adequate pain control?

to ensure 99% of patients do not move during skin incision or are unconscious?

THE IMPORTANCE OF SIMULATION

A more refined approach is to consider an anesthetic as a composite of effects. This is consistent with how anesthesia is delivered—a combination of sedative hypnotics, analgesics, and neuromuscular blockers. An ideal anesthetic technique would tailor doses to achieve a 95% or 99% probability of each effect. An ideal monitor system would have an easily measured parameter for each effect. Such capability would likely help avoid overdosing, minimize hemodynamic disturbances, and plan for rapid emergence while ensuring adequate analgesia. Unfortunately, with the exception of neuromuscular blockade monitors and to some extent processed electroencephalograph (EEG) monitors, such devices do not yet exist.

With advances in clinical pharmacology and through the use of simulation, sophisticated tools have been developed that predict the onset and duration of sedation, unresponsiveness, analgesia, and neuromuscular blockade. Although not a direct measurement, simulation provides real-time visualization of the time course of anesthetic drug concentrations and their effects both for individual drugs and drug combinations. Simulations rely on complex models of pharmacokinetics, pharmacodynamics, and drug interactions to predict drug behavior. Until recently, these models have been too mathematically cumbersome and difficult to display. With advances in computer technology, they are now being introduced as educational supplements and as drug displays at the point of care (Figure 1–1). These displays create pictures of drug behavior that are useful when considering some of the questions listed in Table 1–1.

As an example, consider the simulation of an induction with propofol and fentanyl. This simulation provides predictions of propofol and fentanyl concentrations over time and a prediction of response to laryngoscopy (Figure 1–2). With this picture, several points of interest are easily appreciated. One, fentanyl takes longer to reach peak effect than propofol. Administration should be offset by 3 to 4 minutes if it is desirable to have them reach peak effect simultaneously. Two, by itself, fentanyl contributes very little to blunting the response to laryngoscopy (peak probability of < 1%). Three, propofol alone blunts the response to laryngoscopy for more than 2 minutes. Four, fentanyl and propofol combined blunt the response to laryngoscopy for more than 4 minutes. Similar pictures can be drawn for other effects of interest such as loss of responsiveness or onset of ventilatory depression.

For selected anesthetic drugs and combinations of drug, models are well developed, making simulations easy to conduct; for others, models are not as well established. Throughout this book, where supported by high-quality research, simulations will be used to illustrate the time course of anesthetic drug behavior. For common dosing regimens, depending on available models, some or all of the concentrations and effects presented in Table 1–2 will be simulated.

To fully appreciate the value and limitations of simulations in a clinical context, a working knowledge of core concepts in clinical pharmacology is

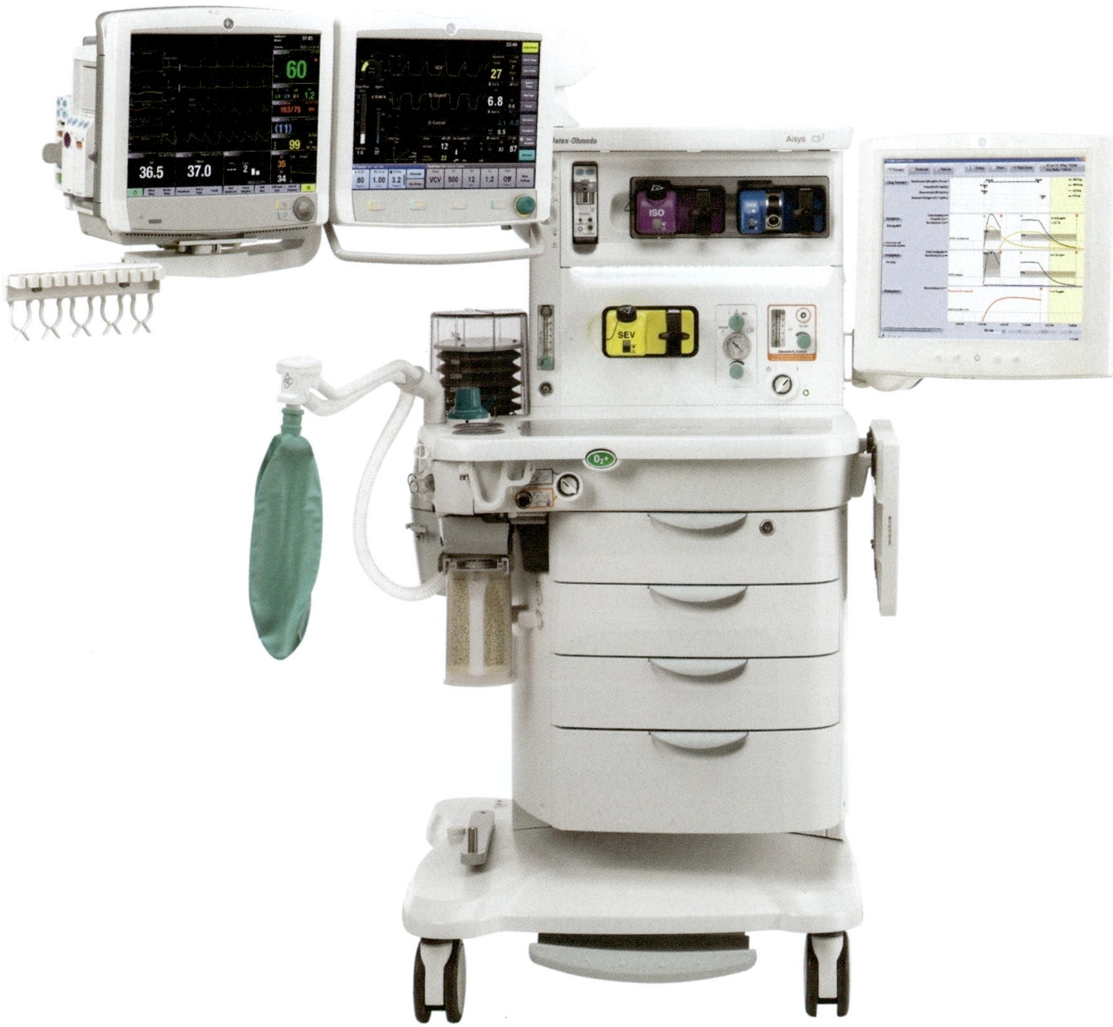

FIGURE 1–1 Example of a drug display system, the Navigator Suite (GE Healthcare, Madison, WI, with permission) as part of an anesthesia work station.

useful. The following sections will review how the basic elements (pharmacokinetics, biophase, and pharmacodynamics) are used to predict and illustrate drug behavior.

PHARMACOKINETICS

Pharmacokinetics describe how the body influences drug behavior; namely how drug concentrations change over time in response to a given dose. Clinical pharmacologists have developed both qualitative descriptors and kinetic models to characterize drug pharmacokinetics. Qualitative descriptors include terms such as volume of distribution, lipid solubility, percent protein binding, among many others. They provide a means of comparing drugs to one another. For example, comparing the lipid solubility of fentanyl to morphine helps explain differences in their kinetic behavior. Kinetic models use mathematical equations to empirically model how

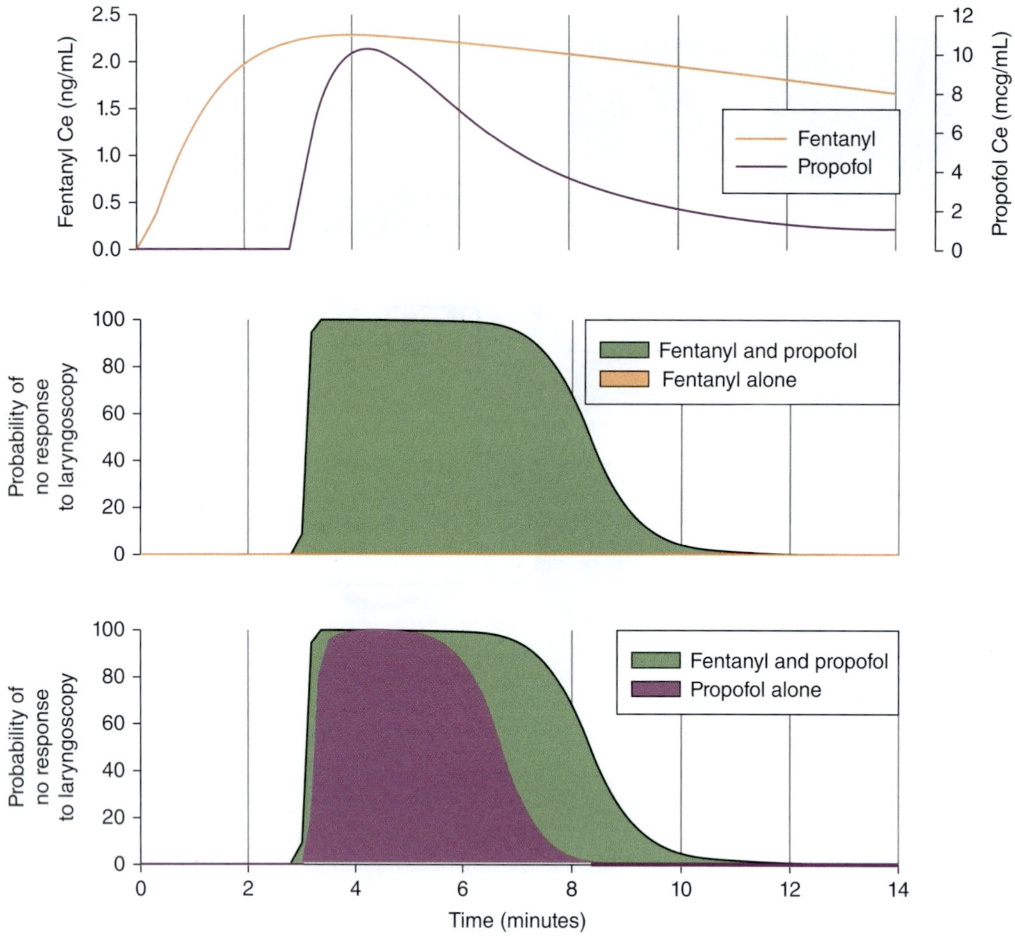

FIGURE 1–2 How simulations are used to create a "picture" of drug effect. In this simulation, published pharmacokinetic[1,2] and pharmacodynamic models[3] are used to predict the loss of response to laryngoscopy following bolus doses of fentanyl (2 mcg/kg) and propofol (2 mg/kg). The top plot presents the effect-site concentrations for each drug over 14 minutes. The fentanyl was administered 3 minutes prior to the propofol, so that they would both peak at the same time. The middle plot presents the probability of no response to laryngoscopy for fentanyl and for the fentanyl and propofol combined. The bottom plot presents the probability of no response to propofol and for the fentanyl and propofol combined.

concentrations change over time. Once built, models are used to predict concentrations over time for various dosing regimens. Kinetic models are based on collecting blood samples from numerous people and compiling them to create a population kinetic model. An important limitation of kinetic models is that they are useful in illustrating the time course of drug concentration over time but do not provide any estimate of drug effect. This chapter will review both aspects of kinetics: definitions of qualitative descriptors and core concepts used in the construction of a pharmacokinetic model.

Qualitative Descriptors of Drug Kinetics

To illustrate important descriptors of drug kinetics, consider an intravenous 2-mcg/kg bolus of fentanyl (Figure 1–3). This simulation illustrates the fentanyl

TABLE 1–2 Drug concentrations and effects illustrated through simulation.

Concentrations
Plasma
End tidal
Effect site
Effects[a] (Onset and Duration)
Sedation and Hypnosis
Mild and moderate sedation
Loss of responsiveness
Electroencephalographic changes[b]
Analgesia
Loss of response to moderately painful stimuli (ie, electrical tetany, pressure)
Loss of response to laryngoscopy and tracheal intubation
Loss of response to esophageal instrumentation
Neuromuscular Blockade
Loss of train-of-four
Ventilatory Depression

[a]Where supported by published models for both single drugs and combined drugs. Drug combinations are limited to potent inhalation agents and selected intravenous opioids and propofol and selected intravenous opioids.
[b]Electroencephalographic (EEG) changes include spectral edge changes and processed EEG (eg, Bispectral Index Scale) changes.

plasma concentration over a 20-minute period. With intravenous administration, the plasma concentration quickly rises and then wanes. During this time period, there are 3 phases.

(1) The distribution phase, where fentanyl moves from the plasma into surrounding tissues. Fentanyl rapidly distributes throughout the vascular compartment and into vascular organs (the heart, brain, kidneys, and liver). At a slower rate, it distributes to muscle and at an even slower rate to adipose tissue, skin, and bone.

(2) The redistribution phase, where fentanyl returns from tissues back into the plasma. The length of drug administration influences duration of the redistribution phase. For example, if fentanyl is administered as a continuous infusion and allowed to accumulate in the muscle and adipose, once the infusion is terminated, fentanyl will continue to move back into the vascular compartment for a prolonged period of time. With fentanyl, this is especially true for infusions of duration longer than 2 hours.

(3) The elimination phase, where fentanyl is removed from the plasma.

Two general terms are used to characterize how the body influences drug behavior: *volume of distribution* and *clearance*. The volume of distribution describes how drug distributes throughout fluid and tissues in the body and is measured in terms of liters per kilogram of body weight (L/kg). Clearance describes drug removal from the body. It includes any process that leads to drug excretion or drug metabolism. The units for clearance are liters per hour (L/h).

Volume of Distribution

The volume of distribution is the volume once the drug has distributed throughout the body. A simplified model of this concept is presented in **Figure 1–4A**. In this example, a 2-mcg/kg fentanyl bolus dose is administered to a 70-kg person with an unknown volume in their vascular compartment. After thorough mixing, the measured plasma concentration will provide an estimate of the volume of distribution using the relationship:

$$\text{Measured concentration} = \text{Fentanyl dose (total mcg)/Volume of distribution} \qquad \text{(Eqn. 1)}$$

Rearranging:

$$\text{Volume of distribution} = \text{Fentanyl dose (total mcg)/Measured concentration} \qquad \text{(Eqn. 2)}$$

If the measured concentration is 28 ng/mL, then the volume of distribution would be 5 L. Unfortunately, this simplified model has significant limitations. As seen in Figure 1–3, the concentration does not stay fixed (as it would in a container) but rather declines over time. To estimate the volume of distribution under these circumstances, clinical pharmacologists extrapolate from the elimination phase of the plasma concentration versus time data as illustrated in Figure 1–3. The place where the dotted line crosses the vertical axis (at time 0) represents the fentanyl concentration (0.5 ng/mL) at

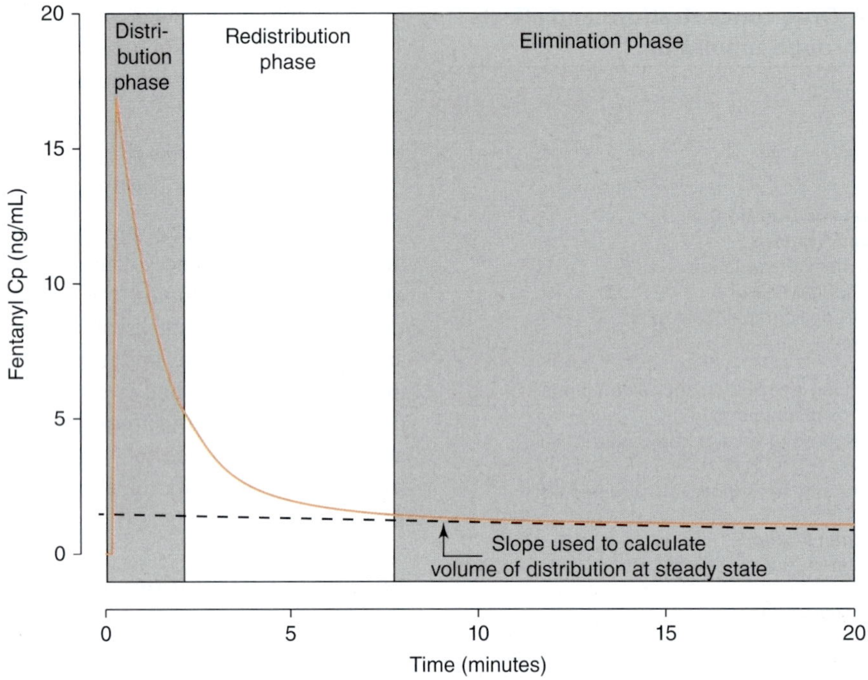

FIGURE 1–3 Plasma concentrations versus time following a 2-mcg/kg bolus of fentanyl. The curve is divided into 3 phases: distribution, redistribution, and elimination. The dashed line represents the slope of the concentration curve during the elimination phase. Where this line crosses the vertical access is used to estimate the volume of distribution at steady state.

which it has distributed through out the entire body and is at steady state with the plasma. Using Eqn. 2, the apparent volume of distribution is 280 L. This is significantly larger than 5 L (or an entire human for that matter)! It is important to recognize that the *apparent* volume of distribution does not have an anatomic correlate; it does *not* represent the vascular volume, the intracellular volume, or the total body water. It is only a mathematical estimate of how much fentanyl is taken up by the body.

To explain this phenomenon, consider Figure 1–4B. The vascular compartment is permeable to small molecules (including fentanyl). Substances (ie, plasma proteins) within the blood and tissues outside of the vascular compartment tightly bind to fentanyl. With much of the fentanyl diffused out of the vascular compartment and bound up in tissue, the vascular compartment fentanyl concentration is much lower, yielding an almost unbelievably large apparent volume of distribution. This phenomenon applies to many anesthetic drugs (Table 1–3).

Protein Binding

Protein binding describes the amount of drug in the plasma that is protein bound. It does not describe how much drug is bound to protein or other tissues outside the vascular compartment, but proteins capable of binding drug are prevalent throughout peripheral tissues. Plasma proteins include albumin (the most abundant), α-1 glycoprotein, and lipoproteins among others. Albumin binds primarily to acidic drugs (eg, fentanyl) whereas α-1 acid glycoprotein binds basic drugs (eg, sufentanil, alfentanil, lidocaine). When bound to protein, anesthetic drugs are pharmacologically inactive. For example, fentanyl is 80% to 85% protein bound, so only 15% is available to diffuse out of the plasma. The fraction of drug not bound to protein in plasma varies significantly for many anesthetic drugs (Table 1–4).

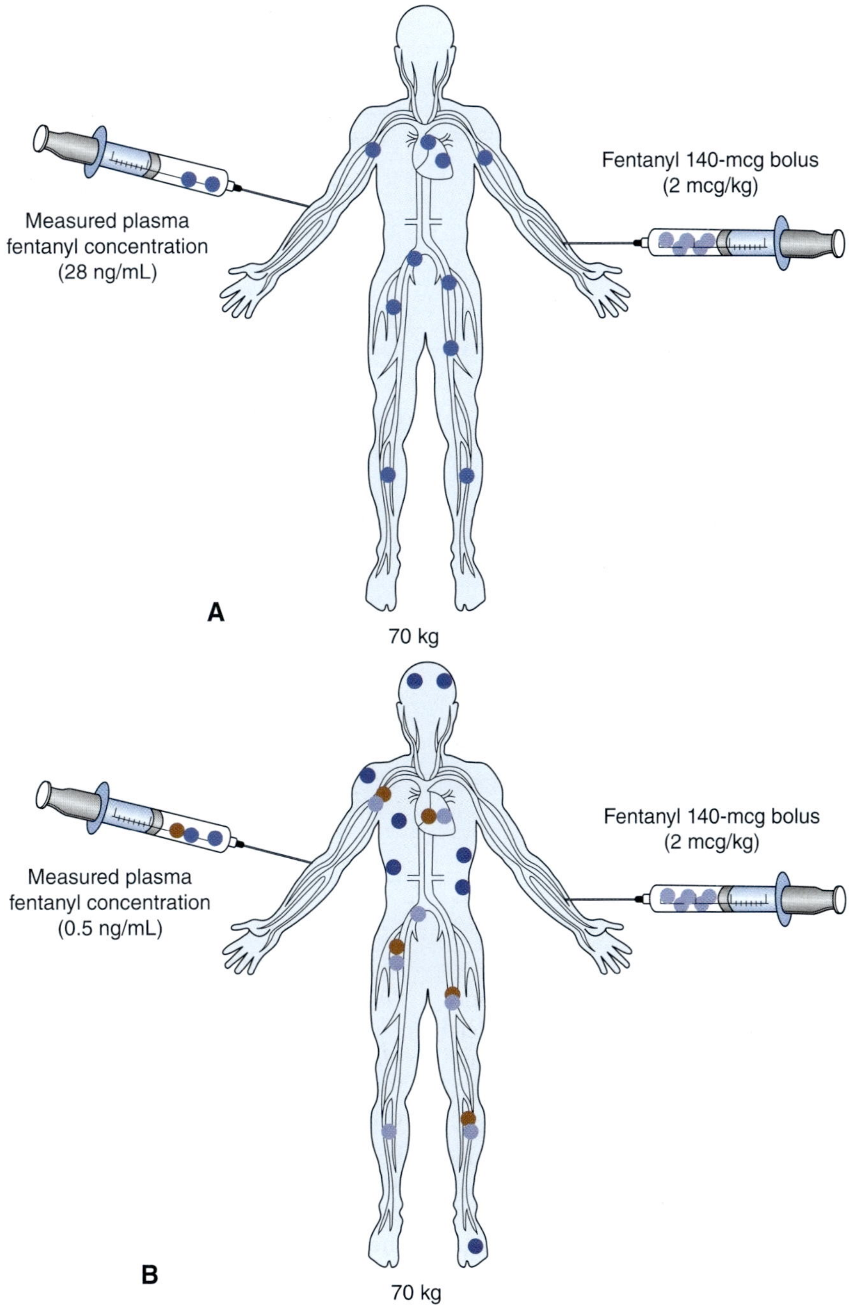

FIGURE 1–4 Schematic illustration of estimating the volume of distribution for fentanyl. A, Simplified model: a known amount of fentanyl (light blue circles indicating 140 mcg in a syringe) is administered to a 70-kg person with an unknown vascular volume. After thorough mixing, the measured concentration is 28 ng/mL, corresponding to a distribution volume of 5 L. B, Sophisticated model: a known amount of fentanyl is administered (light blue circles), and most drug diffuses into tissues outside the vascular compartment (dark blue circles). The majority of the fentanyl that remains in the vascular compartment is protein bound (brown–light blue circles). After thorough mixing, the measured fentanyl concentrations are low (0.5 ng/mL), corresponding to a distribution volume of 280 L.

TABLE 1–3 Volume of distribution for selected intravenous anesthetics.

Anesthetic Drug	Apparent Volume of Distribution
Opioids	
Fentanyl	4.0 L/kg
Sufentanil	5.0 L/kg
Remifentanil	0.4 L/kg
Morphine	1.0–4.7 L/kg
Meperidine	3.7 L/kg
Sedative Hypnotics	
Propofol	2.0 L/kg
Etomidate	4.5 L/kg
Ketamine	4.0 L/kg
Midazolam	1.6.L/kg
Neuromuscular Blockade Agents	
Rocuronium	0.3 L/kg
Vecuronium	0.3 L/kg
Pancuronium	0.1–0.3 L/kg

TABLE 1–4 Percent of protein bound drug in plasma for selected anesthetics.

Anesthetic Drug	% Protein Bound
Opioids	
Morphine	30%–40%
Meperidine	65%–70%
Fentanyl	84%
Sufentanil	92%
Remifentanil	70%
Sedative Hypnotics	
Propofol	95%–99%
Etomidate	76%
Ketamine	60%
Sodium Pentothal	80%
Midazolam	95%
Neuromuscular Blockade Agents	
Rocuronium	50%–75%
Vecuronium	60%
Pancuronium	87%

Clinical Implications

As is appreciated by anesthetists, the onset and duration of effect can be much different than anticipated (eg, prolonged drug effect with intermediate nondepolarizing neuromuscular blockers). Various disease states that influence protein levels can significantly impact the amount of unbound drug. Low protein states (ie, liver disease, nephrotic syndrome) increase the amount of available drug and by contrast high protein states (ie, traumatic injury, surgery) decrease the amount of available drug.

Membrane Permeability

Membrane permeability describes the ability of a drug to move from blood through capillary walls to peripheral tissues. In general, membrane permeability is dependent upon 3 features of an anesthetic drug: lipid solubility, ionization, and molecular size as well as membrane thickness and the integrity of endothelial cell wall junctions.

Lipid Solubility This describes the ability of a drug to move through lipid bilayer membranes. It is characterized by a partition coefficient (also known as a partition constant). It is estimated by mixing a known amount of drug in a container with both octanol (hydrophobic) and water (hydrophilic) and then measuring how much drug is in each solute. The ratio of fentanyl in octanol to fentanyl in water is 860:1. So, it has high lipid solubility and can rapidly move from plasma to peripheral tissues. This explains in part why its apparent volume of distribution is so large; most of the fentanyl has moved out of the vascular compartment. The lipophilic properties of selected anesthetics are presented in Figure 1–5.

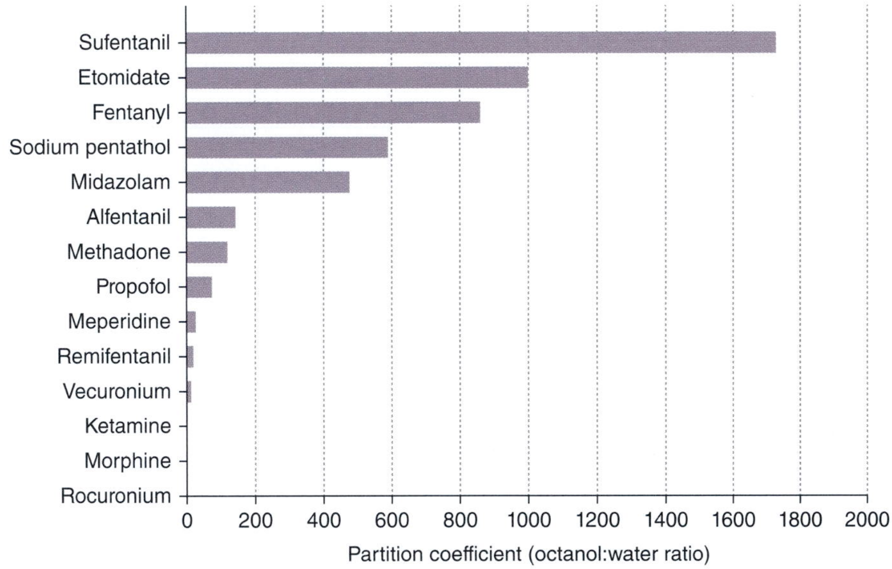

FIGURE 1–5 Lipophilic properties (octanol-to-water ratios) for selected intravenous anesthetics.

Ionization Drugs primarily move through a lipophilic membrane in an un-ionized state. The extent a drug is un-ionized is a function of its pKa at physiologic pH. The pKa values for selected anesthetics are presented in Table 1–5. Drugs that are weak acids with a pKa more than 7.5 are almost entirely un-ionized at a physiologic pH and easily move through membranes. If the pKa is lower, then their movement through membranes becomes pH dependent. Weak bases with a pKa less than 5 are also are almost entirely un-ionized. If the pKa is higher, then movement through membranes is also pH dependent. Fentanyl is a weak base with a pKa of 8.4, so at physiologic pH, most of it exists in a un-ionized state and easily moves through tissue membranes. The amount of unbound ionized drug, depending on the pKa, can change with changes in pH (Table 1–5).

Molecular Size Larger molecules are less likely to move through membranes than smaller ones. Most anesthetic drugs are small molecules and move relatively easily through membranes if un-ionized. Anesthetic drugs bound to plasma protein behave as large molecules and do not easily pass through lipid bilayers.

Membrane Thickness and the Blood-Brain Barrier In general, the thicker the bilipid layer membrane, the lower the permeability. Endothelial cell wall membranes range in thickness from 0.005 to 0.01 μm. In addition to membrane thickness, the integrity of the junction between endothelial cells influences drug diffusion from plasma to peripheral tissues. Endothelial cells in the central nervous system have enhanced "tight junctions" that impede drug movement from plasma to the brain constituting the blood-brain barrier. Tight junctions consist of proteins that tightly glue cell walls together and projections from astrocytes, known as "astrocyte feet," surround the junctions between endothelial cells.

Enantiomers

Enantiomers are assorted structures (isoforms) of a drug. All isoforms have the identical chemical formula. The difference in enantiomers is the orientation of atoms within the drug molecule. Several anesthetic drugs exist as enantiomers. Various schemes have been used to describe how isoforms differ from one another. In some cases, 2 isomers of a molecule exist as mirror image of one another.

TABLE 1–5 pKa values for selected anesthetic drugs over a range of blood ph levels.[a]

Drug Name	pKa	Percent Un-ionized			
		pH			
		7.0	7.2	7.4	7.6
Acids					
ASA	3.0	0	0	0	0
Thiopental	7.4	72	61	50	39
Bases					
Meperidine	8.6	2	4	6	9
Fentanyl	8.4	4	6	9	14
Bupivacaine	8.1	7	11	17	24
Sufentanil	8.0	9	14	20	28
Morphine	7.9	11	17	24	33
Lidocaine	7.9	11	17	24	33
Ketamine	7.5	24	33	44	56
Remifentanil	7.1	44	56	67	76
Midazolam	6.1	89	93	95	97
Etomidate	4.5	100	100	100	100
Diazepam	3.3	100	100	100	100

ASA, acetylsalicylic acid.
[a]Cells colored with gray represent percentages with minimal change over the this pH range

These isoforms are characterized by their ability to rotate polarized light: clockwise (*dextro*, abbreviated D) versus counterclockwise (*levo*, abbreviated L).

More recently, drugs with several isoforms are characterized by their chirality. Chirality refers to the orientation of atoms or groups of atoms (known as substituents) about a single atom, such as carbon, that has 4 potentially asymmetric bonding sites. Substituents are prioritized based on their anatomic number (eg, size). If the smallest substituent is pointed away, the orientation of the remaining 3 substituents from smallest to largest determines the chirality as either clockwise (R for *rectus*) or counterclockwise (S for *sinister*). A given molecule may have more than 1 chiral center and more than 2 isomers. In some instances, these 2 classifications are mixed together. S(–) bupivacaine has a "S" chiral center that polarizes light in a "–" counterclockwise direction. A third method used to describe different isomers is *cis* and *trans*. This nomenclature is primarily used to describe the orientation of substituents about a double carbon bond that is unable to rotate. Table 1–6 presents a list of selected enantiomers of common anesthetic agents.

Isoforms of the same drug can have different effects. For selected drugs, isoforms are separated to take advantage of desirable features of one isoform while avoiding unwanted features of the other isoform (eg, cis-atracurium). Separating out isomers is costly and so many anesthetic drugs are distributed as a mixture of isomers known as racemic mixtures.

TABLE 1–6 Types of enantiomers for selected anesthetics.

Anesthetic Drug	Enantiomer Types
Atropine	D and L
Bupivacaine	R and S
Ropivacaine	R and S
Etomidate	R and S, potency R > S
Ketamine	R and S, potency S > R
Methohexital	R and S, potency S > R
Atricurium	Cis and Trans among 10 different isomers

D, dextro; L, levo; R, rectus; S, sinister.

Clearance

Clearance is a constant used to describe how much drug is removed from the body for a given concentration. It is typically presented as a volume rate (mL/min) or a volume rate normalized to weight (mL/kg/min). It can be used to estimate the rate of elimination according to the following relationship:

$$\text{Rate of elimination} = \text{Clearance} \times \text{concentration}$$

The actual rate of drug removed (ie, mcg/min) is a function of the clearance and the drug concentration. For example, if the clearance of fentanyl is 21 mL/kg/min and the plasma concentration is 3 ng/mL,[4] the rate of elimination is 63 ng/kg/min (or 264 mcg/hour for a 70-kg patient).

Mechanisms of drug clearance include metabolic processes and/or excretion of drug unchanged from its form when first administered. Several anesthetics are excreted in large part in their original form. Drug excretion occurs primarily via the kidneys but can be via the lungs or bile.

Metabolic processes occur primarily in the liver but can also occur in the plasma, lung, kidney, and gut. Metabolic processes, also known as *biotransformation*, include hydrolysis, oxidation or reduction, and conjugation. Many drugs undergo a sequence of metabolic events referred to as phase I and phase II reactions. Phase I reactions include oxidation, reduction, or hydrolysis, and they occur primarily in hepatocytes via microsomal enzymes. Microsomal enzymes are located along the endoplasmic reticulum, a network of membranes within the hepatocyte cytoplasm. Phase II reactions include conjugation, oxidation, reduction, or hydrolysis, and they typically involve nonmicrosomal enzymes.[5]

Hydrolysis Hydrolysis refers to the break down of water to catalyze an enzymatic reaction that metabolizes a drug. Esterases are a class of enzymes that hydrolyze many substrates including selected anesthetic drugs. Common esterases include cholinesterases. There are 2 major types: acetylcholinesterases, which are primarily in blood and nerve endings, and pseudocholinesterases, which are primarily in the liver. Other esterases exist throughout tissues and blood, such as carboxyesterases, among many others. Ester—based anesthetics (eg, succinylcholine, atracurium, esmolol, or remifentanil) are quickly metabolized by esterases, leading to a kinetic profile where these drugs have a rapid decline in plasma concentrations when compared to other anesthetics that require hepatic metabolism.

Many esterase drugs are classified as "soft." This refers to drugs that are designed to be safer with an increased therapeutic index and a rapid predictable metabolism to inactive metabolites.[6] "Soft" is not to be confused with psychoactive agents without addictive properties (ie, cannabis, mescaline, lysergic acid diethylamide) that carry the same label (ie, soft versus hard). Aspects of "soft" that are of particular interest to anesthesiologist include rapid onset of effect and quick recovery.[7]

In the realm of intravenous agents, remifentanil and esmolol have an ester moiety that yields rapid predictable drug metabolism. It is important to recognize that not all ester-type drugs are the same. Depending on neighboring molecular structures, metabolism rates may vary. Some esters may metabolize too quickly, requiring rapid infusions to achieve a desired effect at the same time, creating excessive metabolites. Others may metabolize too slowly and accumulate with continuous infusions. Clinical pharmacologists often evaluate numerous analogs to find a structure with a favorable ester metabolism yet maintains a desirable drug effect.

Oxidation/Reduction This process changes the molecular configuration of an anesthetic by removing or adding an electron (oxidation or reduction, respectively). In some instances, this makes the drug more polar (hydrophilic). In a more polar state, drugs are rendered inactive and excreted in the urine. In other instances, as with prodrugs, this process renders the drug pharmacologically active (eg, codeine metabolized to morphine). These reactions are catalyzed by the cytochrome (CYP) P450 system, a large family of metabolic enzymes (> 50 human isoforms), officially labeled CYP, in the endoplasmic reticulum of hepatocytes and to a lesser extent outside the liver in other organs such as the small intestine. Microsomal enzymes responsible for metabolizing several anesthetics agents include CYP3A4, CYP3A3, and CYP2B6.

Enzymes within this family are influenced by many factors. Hepatocyte function can be impaired with advanced age, cirrhosis, cancer, or viral infection. CYP enzymes are dependent on adequate blood flow to the liver for substrate (drug) delivery and oxygen delivery. Of major importance is the influence of various drugs that either inhibit or induce CYP activity. For example, drugs such as the proton pump inhibitor omeprazole inhibit CYP activity, reducing drug metabolism. Others induce CYP activity, such as the anticonvulsant and mood-stabilizing drug carbamazepine.

Clinical Implications

The impact of drugs that induce or inhibit CYP enzymes can be significant. Consider a patient on a selective serotonin reuptake inhibitor (SSRIs) that receives codeine. SSRIs inhibit the CYP isoform (CYP2D6) that converts codeine to morphine. The result is poor analgesia with conventional dosing. As another example, consider the popular herbal treatment for depression, St. John's wort, (an extract from a flowering plant, *Hypericum perforatum*). It induces selected CYP isoforms (eg, CYP2C9, CYP34A) that metabolizes several drugs of interest to an anesthetist, including fentanyl, midazolam, nifedipine, and selected statins among others.[8,9] Patients can require higher than normal doses of these medications to achieve a therapeutic effect whereas withdrawal of St. John's wort without adjustment in dosing to other drugs may lead to toxicity, such as liver toxicity with chronic consumptions of statins.

Conjugation is a process where various moieties are attached to a parent drug. Examples include sulfates, glutathione, and glucuronic acid. Conjugation generally renders a drug inactive and more polar, making it more easily extracted by the kidney via urine. For some drugs, however, conjugation creates active metabolites, as with morphine when conjugated with glucuronic acid to form morphine-3-glucuronate. When lipid soluble drugs are conjugated with glucuronic acid, the resultant compound retains its lipophilic properties, but is also more water soluble making it favorable for excretion in the urine or bile.

Hepatic Clearance

The liver is the largest metabolic organ and therefore responsible for most of drug metabolism. The hepatic extraction ratio is a term used to define hepatic drug clearance as a function of blood flow to the liver. Hepatic extraction is a function of (1) the amount of drug that is not bound to plasma proteins or is able to disassociate from plasma proteins and pass through hepatocyte cell walls and (2) the ability of hepatocytes to pass drug onto bile, metabolize drug, or both.

Drugs that have a high extraction ratio (eg, morphine, meperidine, lidocaine, nitroglycerin) are easily removed from blood passing through the liver. The difference in drug content between hepatic arterial and venous blood is large, and drug metabolism becomes a function of hepatic blood flow. Drugs that have a low extraction ratio (eg, warfarin and naproxen) undergo relatively little hepatic metabolism. The difference in drug content between hepatic arterial and venous blood is small, and drug metabolism becomes independent of hepatic blood flow. Differences in hepatic extraction ratios can be related to how well drugs are bound to plasma proteins or circulating cells within blood.

Renal Clearance

Drug clearance from this organ is a function of renal blood flow, plasma protein binding, urine pH, and urine flow. Renal blood flow consists of approximately 20% of the cardiac output (ie, 1 L/min). Of that flow, approximately 10% is filtered through the glomerulus. Large molecules (eg, albumin, α-acid glycoproteins, hetastarches) do not pass through this filter. Drugs bound to large proteins also do not pass through the glomerulus whereas unbound drugs do.

Once past the glomerulus, the filtrate is processed by the collecting tubules at a rate of 100-120 mL/min in a healthy 70-kg adult. This is known as the *glomerular filtration rate*. Drug excretion is dependent on the amount of drug that is reabsorbed as it passes through the collecting tubules. The ionic state and polarity play a role in how much drug is reabsorbed. Urine pH influences percentage of drug that is in an un-ionized state and can be reabsorbed and in an ionized state and can be excreted in the urine (urine pH varies between 4.4 and 8). Weak acids and weak bases with pKa values near physiologic pH are especially sensitive to urine pH. For example, a weak base (eg, midazolam) with a pKa of 6.1 will be 99% un-ionized at a pH of 4.4 but 2% un-ionized at a pH of 7.9. Drugs with large pKa (eg, atropine) or small pKa (eg, diazepam) are less sensitive to this phenomenon.

Blood flow near the proximal tubules also contributes to renal drug clearance. Drugs are actively transported from plasma through the proximal tubules into the collecting duct system. This process is a function of how quickly bound drug can disassociate from plasma proteins in time to be transported into the collecting duct system.

Pharmacokinetic Modeling

Model Construction

Pharmacokinetic models are based on data where a known amount of drug is administered and then blood or plasma concentrations are measured over time until drug levels become undetected. Plasma concentrations are more routinely measured than whole blood even though many drugs have significant uptake by red blood cells. To illustrate how models are built, consider a 2 mcg/kg fentanyl bolus. Plasma concentrations are measured every 1 to 2 minutes to capture the rapid rise and then slow decline in fentanyl levels. A computer adapts an exponential equation to the time versus plasma fentanyl concentration data. The equation includes coefficients and exponents that are adjusted to best fit the data (Figure 1–6). The parameters that make

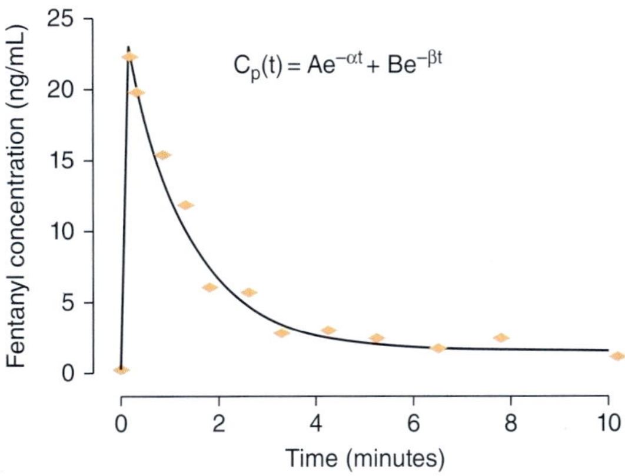

FIGURE 1–6 Sample data used to build a pharmacokinetic model for fentanyl. Following a 2 mcg/kg bolus, plasma concentrations in ng/mL are measured over time. An exponential curve that best approximates the plasma concentrations. The equations contain coefficients (A and B) and exponentials (α and β) that are used to predict the plasma concentration $C_p(t)$ as a function of time.

up this equation are the pharmacokinetic parameters. As can be appreciated, when just considering the parameters, they are not very useful when formulating an appropriate dose for a patient.

For many drugs, 2 to 3 exponents are adequate, but some drugs may require more. Since coefficients and exponents are difficult to interpret or implement in patient care, they are often converted into more recognizable terms, such as volumes and clearances, and used to describe compartment models (Figure 1–7). Although the compartments have no anatomic correlate, they do provide a schematic framework for clinical discussion. For example, in a 3-compartment model, drug enters into and is eliminated from the central compartment and moves from the central compartment to the peripheral slow and fast compartments using rate constants derived from exponential equations. By combining data from numerous subjects, population pharmacokinetic models can be built that estimate drug concentrations and give some estimate of variability between people.

The main purpose of a pharmacokinetic model is to explore how plasma concentrations will change in response to various dosing regimens. Models can

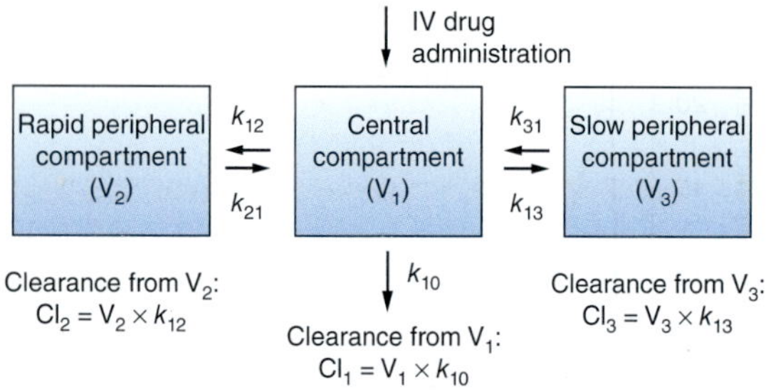

FIGURE 1–7 The 3-compartment pharmacokinetic model. The terms in the exponential equation (Figure 1–6) are rearranged as compartment volumes and rate constants between compartments. A 3-compartment model is used to describe an exponential equation with 3 terms. Rate constants are converted into clearance rates. Compartment volumes and clearances are used to generate predictions of drug concentration for various dosing regimens. IV, intravenous.

visually express the kinetic behavior of a drug. This can be a complex endeavor. An analogy would be to estimate the balance in principle owed on a car loan 30 months after purchase without the use of a calculator. Advances in computer technology have largely eliminated this limitation. Model predictions of drug levels can be made real time and at the point of care in a format that is potentially useful to an anesthetist.

Half-Life A popular kinetic parameter, *half-life or half-time*, is used to characterize drug behavior. By definition, it is the amount of time required for the plasma concentration to decrease by 50% (Figure 1–8). Assuming a linear decay, half-life can be useful in predicting the time required for drug concentrations to decline to negligible levels. For example, after waiting 5 half-lives, plasma concentrations will drop by 97% (1/32nd) of the original concentration.

Half-life is perhaps most useful to an anesthesiologist when considering drugs that are consumed on a chronic basis that have important perioperative clinical implications. Drugs such as oral anticoagulants, antihypertensives, or cholesterol-lowering agents fit into this group. A working knowledge of how long these agents will remain in the body once patients have stopped taking them can impact the anesthetic and perioperative care plans.

For most drugs in an anesthesiologist's drug box, however, half-life is not that useful and may even be misleading.[10,11] Anesthetists rarely ask, "What is the half-life of the induction agent or opioid I am about to give?" The problem is that half-life does not offer much help in predicting the onset and duration of effect. For example, when dosing intermittent boluses of fentanyl throughout a long anesthetic, half-life provides little insight into identifying the time between doses that is required to maintain plasma concentrations near therapeutic levels.

Another challenge with using half-life, especially with boluses of anesthetic agents, is that the rate of decline in plasma concentrations is not linear. In fact, the rate of decline is rarely best described by just 1 slope but rather by 2 or more different slopes. Researchers often provide multiple half-lives, one for each slope. It quickly becomes confusing as to which half-life best describes drug behavior that is of interest to an anesthetist. For example, the after an intravenous fentanyl bolus, the profile of fentanyl plasma concentration decline is characterized by 3 different slopes.[12] The first slope, or distribution half-life, is 1 minute, the second slope, or redistribution half-life, is 17 minutes, and the third slope, or terminal half-life, ranges from 2 to 6 hours (Figure 1–8). Without the aid of a computer to create predictions of how various fentanyl doses can behave, individual half-lives are of little value when identifying the appropriate dose.

Context Sensitive Half-Time A more refined approach to half-life is the *context sensitive half-time*, or *50% decrement time*. Context refers to the dosing history (how much for how long) and estimates how long it will take for the plasma concentration to decrease by 50%.[13,14] For a continuous infusion, the context sensitive half-time changes as a function of the infusion duration. This approach accounts for the accumulation of drug into tissues (modeled using the rapid and slow compartments in the compartment model described above) and how that accumulation impacts the rate of drug level decline once an infusion is terminated. Drugs that are likely to move from the blood into peripheral tissues and organs and accumulate have slow decrement times. Drugs that have a rapid metabolism have rapid decrement times. Fentanyl, because of its

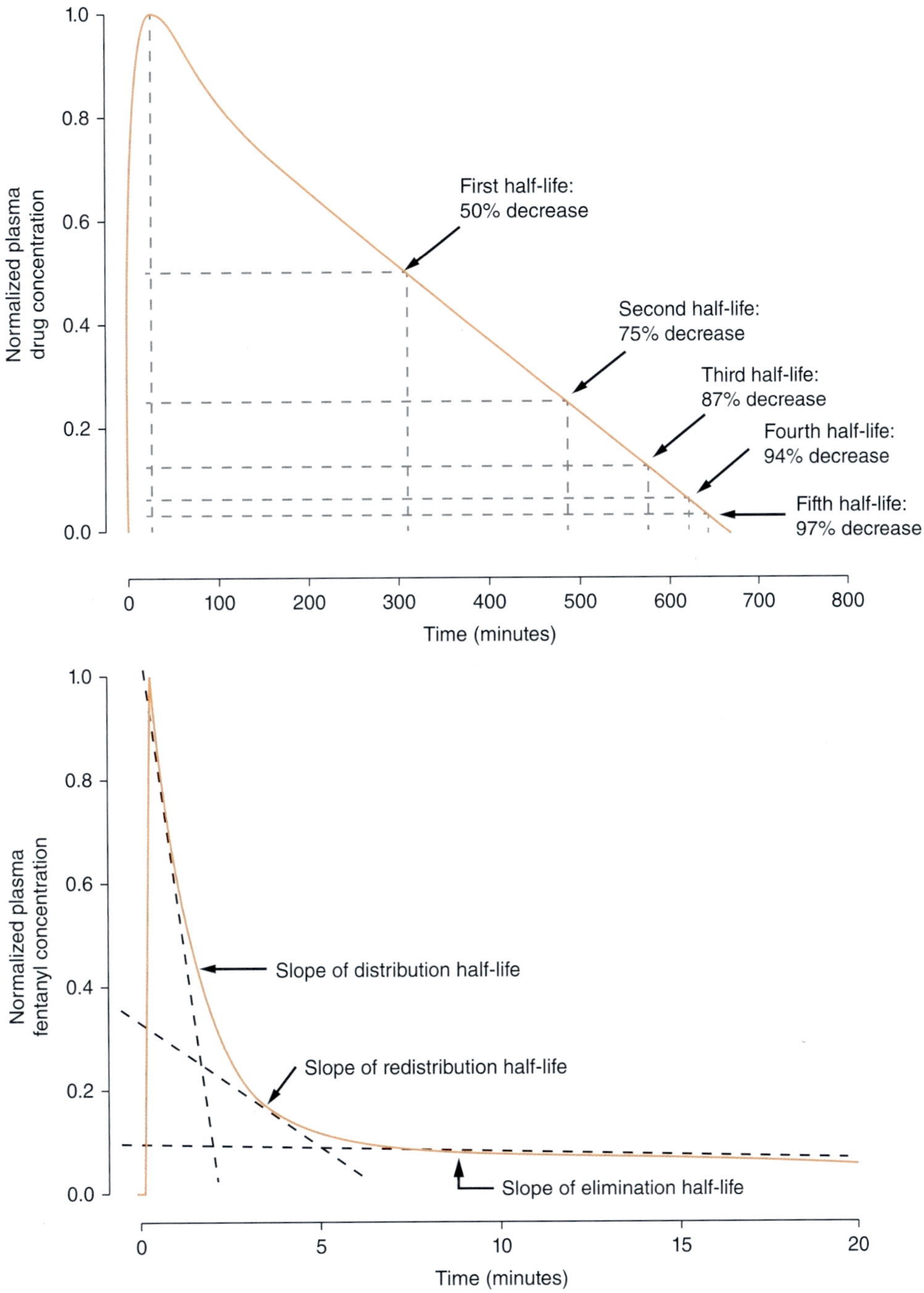

FIGURE 1–8 Illustration of half-life estimates. For drugs that have a steady decline in plasma concentrations once drug administration is terminated, a single half-life can be used to describe the slope of the plasma concentration versus time curve (top plot). For drugs that have a variable decline in plasma concentrations once drug administration is terminated, multiple half-lives are used to describe the various slopes of the plasma concentration versus time curve (bottom plot).

highly lipophilic profile, is an example of a drug that quickly moves out of the blood into peripheral tissues. With short infusions, not much fentanyl accumulates in peripheral tissues, and once an infusion is terminated, it is quickly eliminated from the plasma. With longer infusions, more fentanyl accumulates in peripheral tissues and when the infusion is terminated, fentanyl from peripheral tissues moves back into the vascular system and slows the rate of elimination from the plasma.

The context sensitive half-time is primarily used as a qualitative comparison of drugs within a given drug class. For example, the context sensitive half-time for selected opioids can be used to estimate the rate of drug decline following a long infusion (Figure 1–9) using parameters from the literature.[1,12,14,16] In this example, fentanyl has a long context sensitive half-time when compared to sufentanil and remifentanil especially for infusions longer than 2 hours.

Clinical Implications

The qualitative comparison between opioids can be used to select an analgesic drug that will meet the anesthetic demands of a given procedure. One advantage of fentanyl infusion for procedures associated with postoperative tracheal intubation is that the long decrement time provides prolonged analgesia and a gradual emergence from anesthesia. By contrast, remifentanil, because of its rapid metabolism, has a fast decrement time that is independent of infusion duration. This feature is attractive for procedures associated with noxious stimuli followed by minimal discomfort after the procedure is completed. This may be especially useful in patients where prolonged opioid effect may lead to unwanted respiratory depression. For long infusions (ie, > 4 hours), sufentanil's kinetic profile is different from fentanyl's. With fentanyl, the decrement times continue to rise, but with sufentanil, they plateau. This may be useful in procedures where the duration of the procedure is unpredictable and a long decrement time is not ideal. Sufentanil's decrement time plateaus to 45 to 60 minutes even after a long infusion. Sufentanil has a large peripheral compartment that continues to fill even after the termination of an infusion. This feature, in addition to its metabolism and elimination, results in a steady decline in drug concentration.

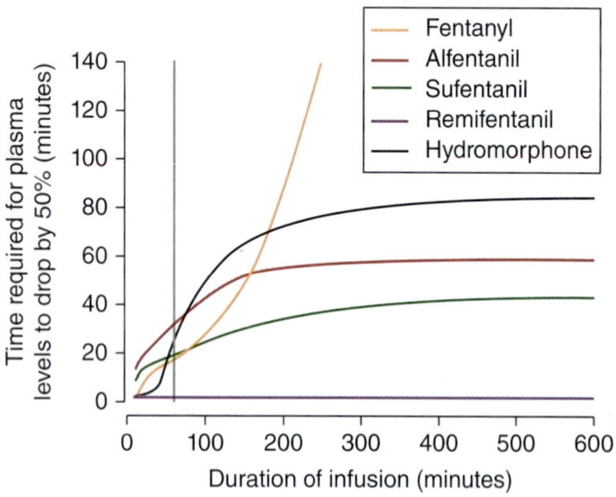

FIGURE 1–9 Context-sensitive half-times for commonly used opioids. The vertical line at 60 minutes represents the infusion duration at which the context-sensitive half-times for each opioid begin to vary. For shorter infusions, the decrement time is very similar between drugs. For longer infusions, the decrement times become substantially different.

Special Populations

As any anesthetist knows, the pharmacokinetic behavior of anesthetic drugs is not consistent for all patients under all conditions. An important aspect of an anesthetist's job is to adjust the anesthetic dose when accommodating for a unique feature of a special population. Clinical pharmacologists have devoted considerable effort in identifying how differences in various patient groups influence anesthetic drugs. Variables used to describe these special populations are called *covariates*. Researchers have used covariates to adapt pharmacokinetic models to some special populations but not others. Many pharmacokinetic models account for age (both pediatric and geriatric populations) and weight. Research is ongoing to improve model predictions by replacing weight with metrics of body habitus. Work has also explored how gender, cardiac output, blood loss, prolonged exposure to opioids, and liver function influence drug kinetics. Although this is a blossoming area of research, at present, many of the models used do not account for special populations. This may explain why model predictions based on pharmacokinetic models can be associated with large inter patient variability.

BIOPHASE

An important observation when measuring drug concentrations over time is that unless a drug exerts an effect in the plasma, changes in drug effect lag behind changes in plasma concentration. This lag time is known as biophase. The lag time is a function of all processes required to exert an effect. Some of these may include diffusion of drug to the site of action, binding of drug to a target protein in the effect site (eg, membrane receptor or ion channel), and the target cell response time to an activated receptor.

Diffusion from the plasma to the site of action usually involves transport of drug through lipid bilayers (eg, vascular endothelium) to reach its target. Drug permeability, as was described above, is a function of drug pKa and the associated amount of un-ionized drug, molecular size, membrane thickness, and the lipophilic properties of the drug. For drugs that exert their effect inside a target cell (eg, local anesthetics), biophase also includes the time required to go from plasma to neurons, diffuse into the cytoplasm, undergo ionization, and then block sodium channels. As described with pharmacokinetics, extremes in plasma pH, temperature, and tissue oxygenation can all influence biophase.

Modeling Biophase

To model biophase, clinical pharmacologist simultaneously capture drug concentration and effect data. With bolus dosing or a change in infusion rates, the lag time is easily appreciated. As an example, in Figure 1–10, consider a simulation of a large bolus of opioid administered to one individual and its associated effect on spectral edge, a common measure of EEG behavior. In this figure, changes in the spectral edge lag behind changes in plasma concentrations.

To characterize a *population* lag time, opioid concentrations and spectral edge responses collected from several individuals are combined and plotted as concentration versus effect (see the simulation in Figure 1–11). Of note, as concentrations rise, the drug effect increases at higher concentrations when compared to when concentrations drop, where drug effect persists at lower concentrations. This phenomenon represents hysteresis in the concentration versus effect. A sigmoid curve is fit to the data that collapses the hysteresis loop to form a pharmacodynamic model.

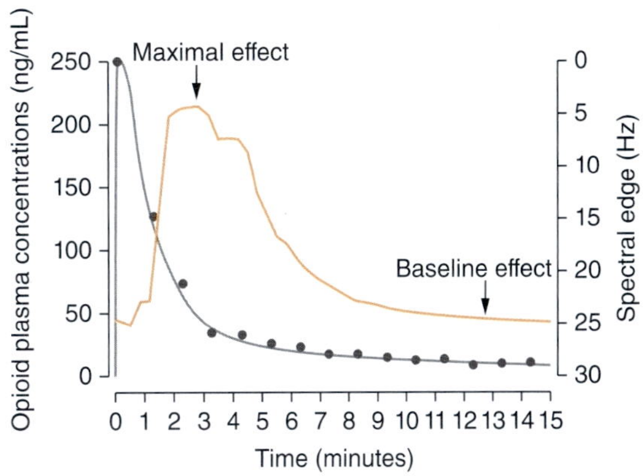

FIGURE 1–10 Illustration of biophase. Schematic representation of drug plasma concentrations (black circles) following a bolus and the associated changes in the electroencephalogram's spectral edge (orange line) measured in one individual. The electroencephalograph (EEG) is characterized as a sum of numerous sine waves. Each sine wave has amplitude and frequency. The spectral edge frequency (in hertz) is the 95th percentile of all the sine wave frequencies. Spectral edge frequencies become smaller in the presence of anesthetic drug concentrations that reduce EEG activity.

The mathematical expression that characterizes biophase is a single exponential equation describing drug movement from the central compartment to a theoretical effect-site compartment. This additional compartment is very small and is known as the *effect site* (Figure 1–12). Like other compartments, it has no anatomic correlate but is a model representation of an exponential equation. A common parameter used to describe biophase is k_{e0}. It represents the elimination rate from the effect site.

Clinical Implications

The main purpose of adding an effect-site compartment to a pharmacokinetic model is to predict effect-site concentrations. This provides a context for comparing drugs in terms of the time required to reach peak effect. For example, consider the time

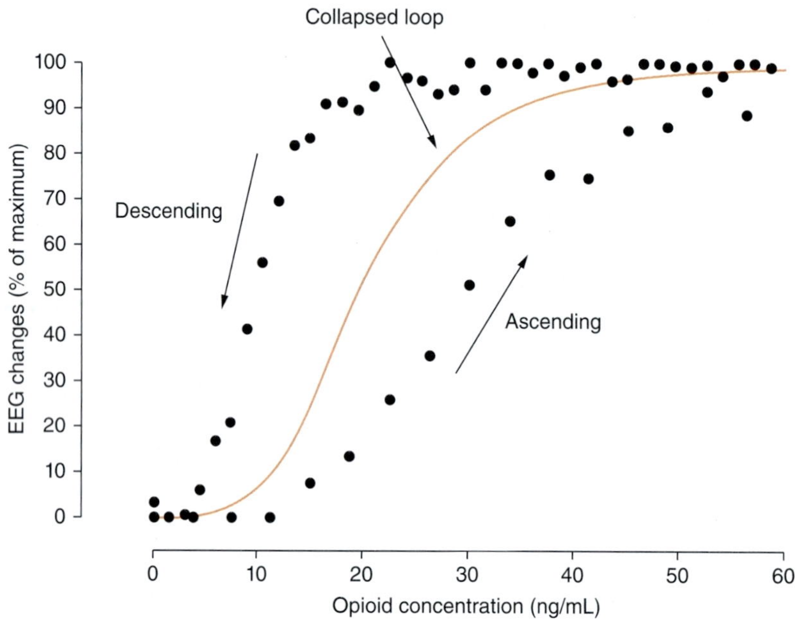

FIGURE 1–11 Schematic representation of plasma concentrations versus normalized spectral edge measurements (presented as a percentage of maximal effect) from several individuals (black circles). The black arrows indicate the ascending and descending arms of a hysteresis loop that coincide with increasing and decreasing drug concentrations. The orange line represents the pharmacodynamic model developed from collapsing the hysteresis loop.

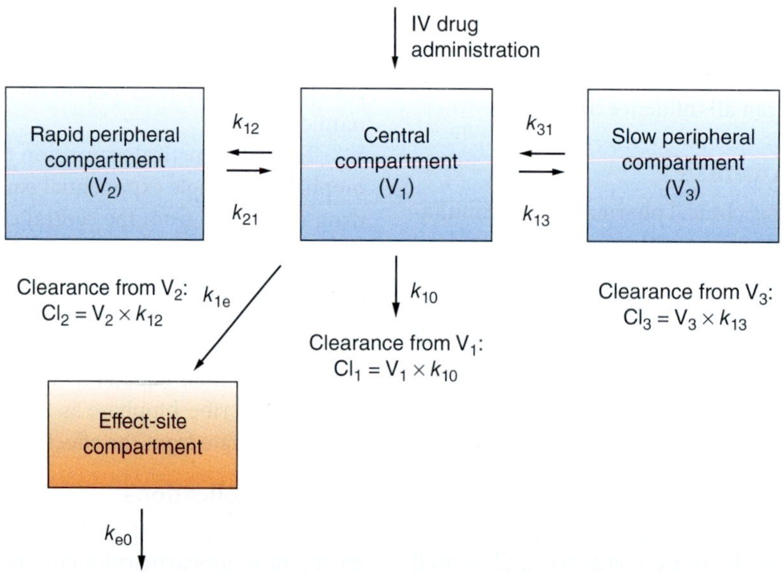

FIGURE 1–12 An additional compartment is added to the 3-compartment model to estimate the concentration at the *effect site*. An additional parameter, k_{e0}, is added to the compartment model. With the k_{e0}, simulations of the effect-site concentration are performed to explore the behavior of various dosing regimens. IV, intravenous.

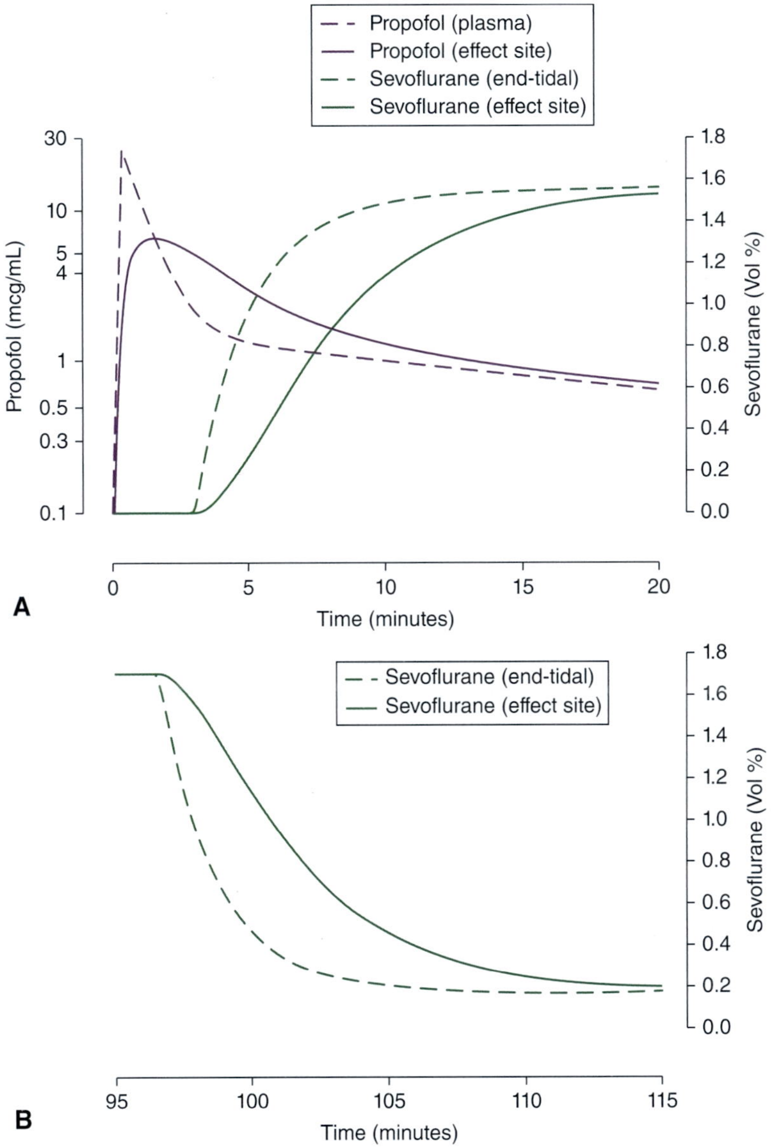

FIGURE 1–13 Simulations of propofol bolus (2 mg/kg) shortly followed by a sevoflurane vaporizer set to 2%. The solid lines represent the propofol plasma and sevoflurane end-tidal concentrations respectively. The dashed lines represent the effect-site concentrations for both drugs. These simulations assume a normal minute volume (6 L/min); normal cardiac output; an intubated, mechanically ventilated patient; and a fresh gas flow of 2 L/min. Panel A presents drug concentrations during the initial 20 minutes following induction with propofol. Panel B presents drug concentrations for 20 minutes once the vaporizer has been turned off.

course of effect-site concentrations following an induction dose of propofol followed by sevoflurane (Figure 1–13). For both drugs, the lag of effect-site concentration changes behind plasma or end-tidal changes is substantial (up to 2 minutes for propofol and 10 minutes for sevoflurane assuming normal ventilation and 2 L/min fresh gas flow).

By visualizing effect-site concentrations, the real power of simulation begins to emerge. With these tools, clinicians can explore various dosing strategies of multiple drugs to optimize drug delivery.

PHARMACODYNAMICS

Pharmacodynamics describe how a drug exerts an effect—namely, drug–concentration relationships. Available drug interacts with receptors on cell membranes that when occupied generate or

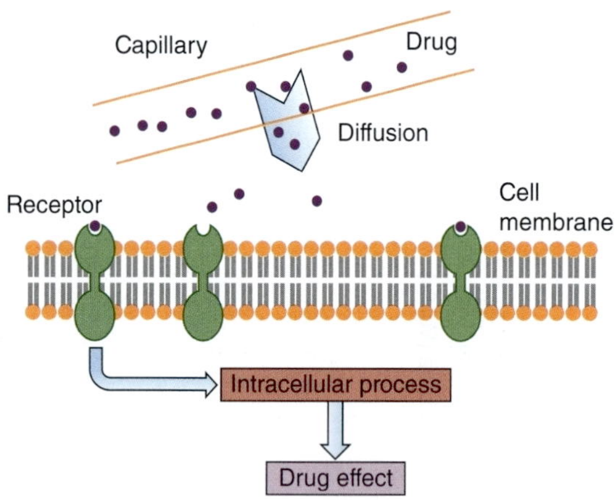

FIGURE 1–14 Simplified schematic representation of pharmacodynamic effect. Drug diffuses from the vascular compartment (capillary) to a receptor site and interacts with a receptor. In this example, the receptor is membrane bound and once activated, it produces an intracellular process that produces a drug effect.

block a process within a cell that results in an effect (Figure 1–14). Drug effect increases as the number of receptors occupied with drug increases. Once all the receptors are occupied, additional drug does not provide additional effect. Other factors that influence the ability drug to exert an effect include the number of receptors available on a cell membrane and the presence of substances that may compete with or block drug occupation of membrane receptors.

Modeling Pharmacodynamics

To study pharmacodynamics, researchers administer escalating doses of a drug and monitor for a drug effect. Pharmacokinetic models (including biophase) are used to predict effect-site concentrations that correspond with observed drug effects. Most effects are characterized as "absent" versus "present," but some are characterized using a continuous variable, such as the bispectral index scale (BIS). Pharmacodynamic models are based on responses from numerous individuals to build a probability of effect versus concentration curve.

The profile of concentration versus drug effect typically follows a sigmoid curve. Low concentrations exert no effect. The dynamic range maps the concentration effect from baseline to maximal effect. The dynamic range is of particular interest to anesthetists. Small changes in effect-site concentrations lead to changes in drug effect. Increasing the effect-site concentration to levels above the dynamic range provide no additional effect. An example of maximal effect is a 0 on the BIS monitor. Concentrations above those required for maximal effect do not provide any additional effect (ie, BIS does not become negative).

The equation used to describe the sigmoid curve has terms that describe the baseline effect when the concentration is 0, the maximal effect, the slope of the curve in the dynamic range, and a term that represents the concentration associated with a 50% probability of effect (Figure 1–15). For effects characterized as "absent" versus "present," the sigmoid curve is based on observations from numerous individuals. The curve is fit to the range of concentrations where individuals transition from no effect to effect. Not every individual transitions at exactly the same concentration.

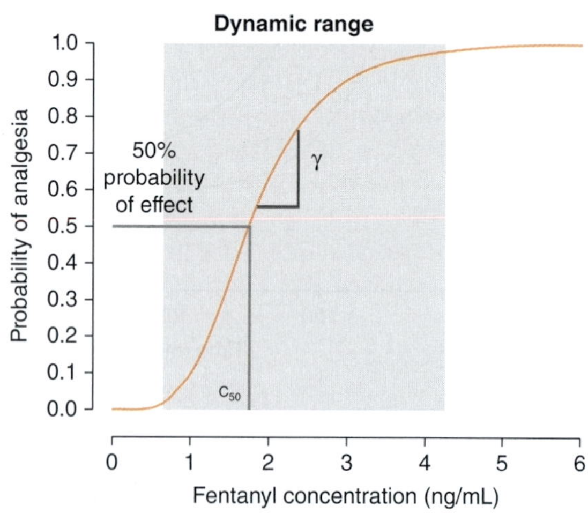

FIGURE 1–15 A pharmacodynamic model for the analgesic effect of fentanyl. The grey area represents the dynamic range where changes in concentration lead to a change in effect. Concentrations above or below the dynamic range do not lead to changes in drug effect. The C_{50} represents the concentration associate with 50% probability of analgesia. The γ represents the slope of the curve in the dynamic range.

Clinical Implications

With the aid of pharmacodynamic models, it is possible to identify concentration ranges that are ineffective, adequate, or excessive for a given drug effect. An ideal dosing regimen would yield effect-site concentrations that are near the shoulder of the sigmoid curve. Maintaining the concentration at that point, known as surfing the concentration effect wave,[17] provides near maximal effect with a rapid decline in drug effect at the end of an anesthetic. Additional advantages with "surfing" include avoiding higher concentrations associated with adverse side effects (eg, respiratory depression with high concentrations of opioids) or prolonged duration of effect as it takes more time for concentrations to decline to those on the slope of the concentration effect curve.

As an example, consider 3 different bolus doses of fentanyl (0.5, 2, or 10 mcg/kg). Using a pharmacodynamic model for fentanyl, the effect site concentrations from these boluses are plotted on a sigmoid curve (**Figure 1–16**). The C_{50} for this curve is 1.5 ng/mL and represents the effect-site concentration at which there is a 50% probability of loss of response to a moderately noxious stimulus.[18] Dosing regimens that maintain drug concentrations along the lower left portion of the sigmoid curve are ineffective as demonstrated by the low-dose fentanyl bolus (0.5 mcg/kg). Dosing regimens that maintain drug concentrations within the dynamic range are ideal (2 mcg/kg). Targeting the crest of the sigmoid curve provide near maximal effect yet a rapid decline in effect once drug levels drop. Dosing regimens that maintain drug concentrations along the upper right portion of the sigmoid curve are excessive as demonstrated by the high-dose fentanyl bolus (10 mcg/kg).

Anesthetic drugs can have multiple effects. For selected drugs, multiple models have been built to describe each effect. Pharmacodynamic models of

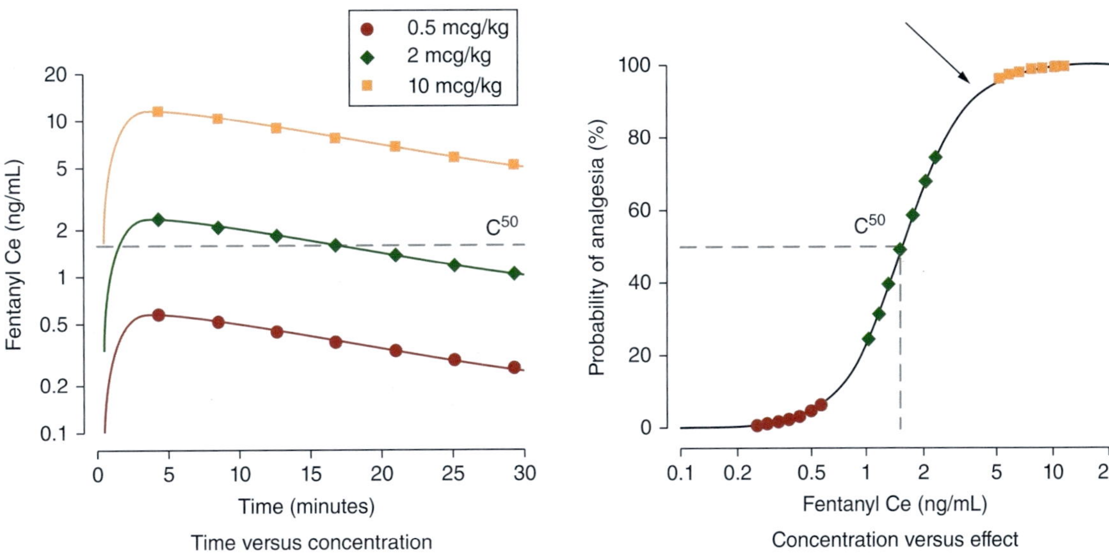

FIGURE 1–16 The effect-site concentration versus time is presented for 3 different fentanyl boluses: 0.5, 2, and 10 mcg/kg (left plot). The effect-site concentrations are plotted on a pharmacodynamic model of loss of response to a moderately painful stimulus (right plot). The gray lines represent the C_{50} for analgesia (1.5 ng/mL). The arrow marks the upper shoulder of the sigmoid curve where effect-site concentrations provide a 99% probability of effect, an ideal location to achieve when dosing an anesthetic. The 0.5 mcg/kg dose only makes it to the start of the dynamic range of the dose response curve. The 10 mcg/kg dose goes beyond the upper shoulder, providing more drug than is necessary to achieve maximal effect. With this dose, effect-site concentrations exceed those needed to surf the wave for more than 25 minutes. The 2 mcg/kg dose is about right. It quickly approaches the upper shoulder of the curve and lingers in this vicinity of the dynamic range for 30 minutes.

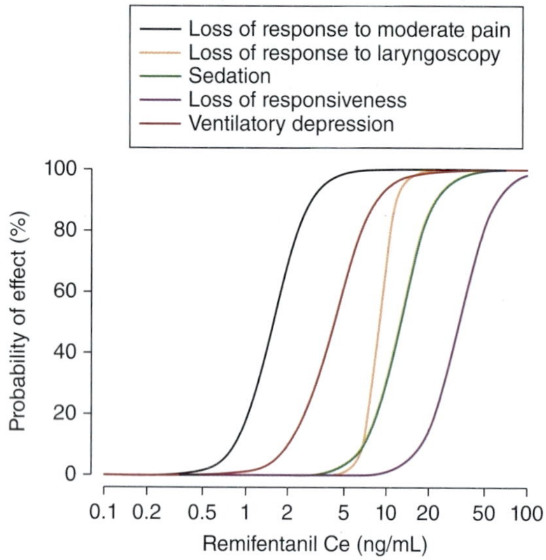

FIGURE 1–17 Concentration effect relationships for various effects of remifentanil. Pharmacodynamic models of probability of loss of response to a moderately painful stimulus, loss of response to laryngoscopy, development of ventilatory depression, sedation, and loss of responsiveness are presented on the same concentration versus effect plot. The vertical lines represent the C_{50} for each drug effect. Sedation is defined as an Observer's Assessment of Alertness and Sedation Score of 3 or less. This score indicates that a person at rest with their eyes closes responds by opening their eyes only after their loudly and/or repeatedly calling out their name.[26] Loss of responsiveness is defined as no response to calling out their name, prodding, and/or shaking. Ventilatory depression is defined as a respiratory rate less than 4 breaths per minute. Loss of response to moderate pain is defined as a loss of response to 30 PSI of tibial pressure.[22]

opioids have been developed for loss of response to moderately painful stimuli, ventilatory depression, loss of response to laryngoscopy, and suppression of EEG activity.[3,18-25]. When compared side by side (Figure 1–17), the concentration effect relationship for each effect is similar—a sigmoid curve. Each curve is separated out by their respective C_{50}s. For example, the C_{50} for loss of response to a moderately painful stimulus is approximately 30% of the C_{50} for ventilatory depression,[18,27] representing a therapeutic window of analgesia that avoids unwanted respiratory depression. This may be important to consider during emergence from anesthesia. By contrast, the C_{50} for blocking the response to laryngoscopy is much higher than other effects, including respiratory depression, and may require large doses to completely block the response to laryngoscopy and tracheal intubation.

COMBINED PHARMACOKINETIC PHARMACODYNAMIC MODELS

The real value of pharmacokinetic and pharmacodynamic models comes when they are combined to explore how drugs behave through simulation. Linking effect-site concentrations from pharmacokinetic models to drug concentration effect relationships from pharmacodynamic models provides a means of visualizing the onset and duration of various effects and exploring different dosing regimens to optimize dosing. Two approaches to simulating drug effects over time are reviewed below: the horizontal line approach and the probability over time approach.

Simulations Using Combined Models

Horizontal Line Approach

One approach to visualizing drug effect over time is to plot the effect-site concentration over time and superimpose horizontal lines that represent concentrations needed for a desired drug effect. As an example, consider the sedative midazolam whose effects of midazolam have been well studied using a variety of metrics. One scale is the modified Ramsay Sedation Scale (RSS).[28] It measures the level of sedation ranging from 1 (anxious) to 6 (unresponsive). Effect-site concentrations for each RSS score have been established in postoperative intubated surgical patients (Table 1–7).[29]

Pharmacokinetics Using a published pharmacokinetic model,[30] effect-site concentrations over time are plotted for various doses of midazolam as a bolus or as a continuous infusion (Figure 1–18). The bolus doses are 2, 3, 5, 7, and 10 mg and the continuous infusion doses are 10, 25, 50, and 75 mcg/kg/hour delivered to a 75-kg patient. Following a bolus dose, effect-site concentrations quickly rise

TABLE 1–7 Modified Ramsay Sedation Scale[28] and Midazolam effect-site concentrations associated with each sedation scale score.[29]

Definition	Awake/ Asleep	Score	Midazolam C_{50} (ng/mL)
Anxious, agitated, or restless	Awake	1	
Cooperative, oriented, and tranquil	Awake	2	68
Responds to command only	Awake	3	101
Brisk response to light glabellar tap[a] or loud auditory stimulus	Asleep	4	208
Sluggish response to light glabellar tap[a] or loud auditory stimulus	Asleep	5	304
No response to light glabellar tap[a] or loud auditory stimulus	Asleep	6	375

[a]A glabellar tap is repetitive tapping on the forehead to illicit a blinking response.

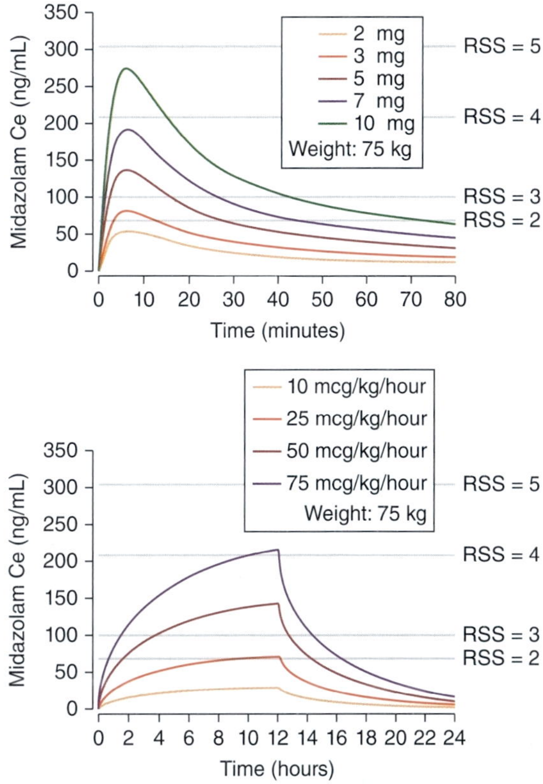

FIGURE 1–18 Simulation of midazolam effect-site concentrations following various intravenous bolus doses (top plot) and continuous infusion rates (bottom plot) administered to a 75-kg patient. The horizontal lines represent the concentrations at which 50% of intubated patients will achieve various levels of sedation according to the Ramsay Sedation Scale (RSS) (Table 1–7).

but then require a relatively long time (6 to 9 minutes) to reach their peak. After the peak, the drop in concentration, by comparison to the quick ascent, is rather slow. For continuous infusions, even after 12 hours at a set rate, plasma concentrations continue to rise slowly. Once terminated, the rate of decline is slow. Although midazolam is known for its rapid onset of effect, from a kinetic standpoint, it is slow to peak and slow to dissipate.

Pharmacodynamics Superimposing horizontal lines associated with each sedation scale score provide an excellent framework from which to explore the behavior of various doses of midazolam. Using the RSS, the onset and duration of effect for these doses are easily visualized (Figure 1–18). For the 2-mg bolus dose, the resultant effect-site concentration does not exceed the C_{50} for a RSS of 2, suggesting that this dose may be inadequate by itself to sedate most postoperative intubated patients. The higher bolus doses do, and the duration of the effect is dose dependent. For the continuous infusions, after 12 hours, the 10-mcg/kg/h infusion rate never achieves an effect-site concentration that exceeds the C_{50} for a RSS of 2. The 25- mcg/kg/h infusion rate does but not until 8 hours of infusion. By contrast, the higher infusion rates achieve this threshold within 1 hour. Once the 12-hour infusion is turned off, effect-site concentrations for the 50- and 75-mcg/kg/h infusion rates persist above the C_{50} for a RSS of 2 for 2 to 5 hours. The prolonged offset of effect once the infusion is turned off represents a significant drawback to this drug when a rapid cessation of effect is desired.

Probability Over Time Approach

Another approach is to present the probability of drug effect over time as a companion plot to the concentration over time plot. Consider a set of simulations that compare analgesic[22] and respiratory depressant effects[18] for a series of repeated boluses of fentanyl versus an infusion of remifentanil over 30 minutes (Figure 1–19). Fentanyl is dosed as three 2 mcg/kg boluses every 10 minutes and the remifentanil is dosed as a continuous infusion at 0.2 mcg/kg/min. Simulations used published pharmacokinetic models for both fentanyl[12] and remifentanil.[1]

Pharmacokinetics With repeated boluses, there is a concentration-stacking phenomenon. Fentanyl concentrations rapidly rise to reach their peak within 5 minutes and slowly decline. Right before the next 10-minute bolus, the fentanyl concentration from the previous bolus has decreased by 16% from the peak (2.3 ng/mL). For the second bolus, the peak

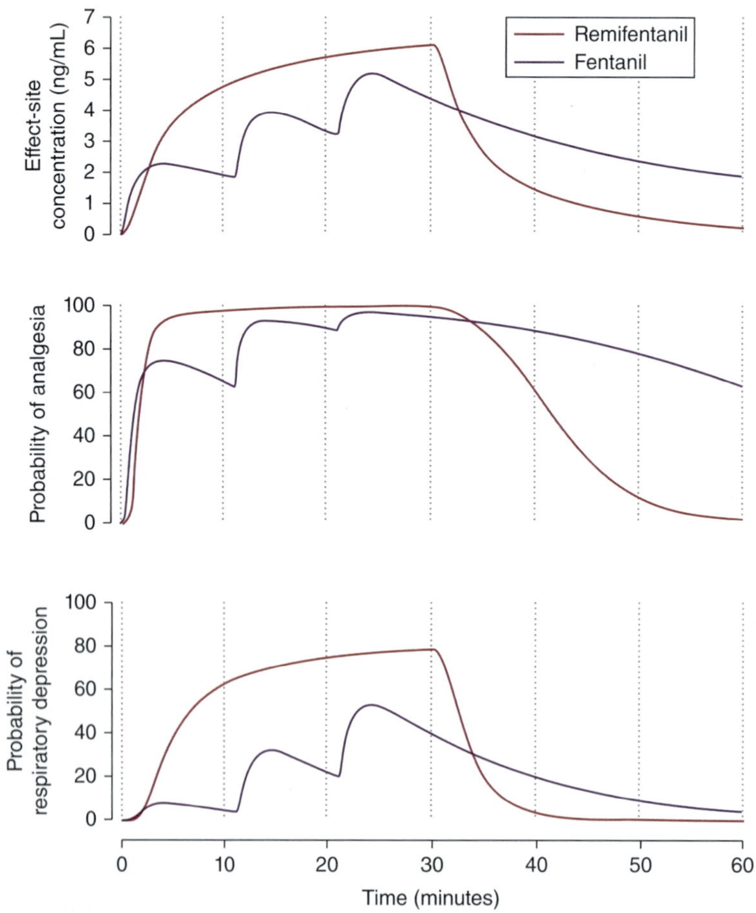

FIGURE 1–19 Comparison of analgesic and ventilatory depressant effects of fentanyl boluses versus a remifentanil infusion. The top plot presents the simulated effect-site concentrations over time for 3 sequential fentanyl boluses (2 mcg/kg) every 10 minutes and a remifentanil continuous infusion (0.2 mcg/kg/min) that runs for 30 minutes. The middle plot presents the probability of loss of response to a moderately painful stimulus. The bottom plot presents the probability of ventilatory depression (respiratory rate < 4 breaths/min) for each drug and dosing scheme.

fentanyl concentration is 174% higher than the previous peak. Following the third dose, fentanyl concentrations slowly decline. For example, it requires over 6 hours to drop by 90% of the peak concentration after the third bolus. With the remifentanil, for the first 15 minutes of the infusion, effect-site concentrations rise fairly quickly and then go into slower rate of rise. Of note, the effect-site concentration never plateaus during the infusion. Once turned off, concentrations quickly drop by 90% of its peak concentration within 20 minutes.

Pharmacodynamics Fentanyl boluses provide a rapid onset of analgesia. With peak fentanyl concentrations, the probabilities of analgesic effect range from 75% to 96%. The probability of significant ventilatory depression (defined as a respiratory rate < 4 breaths/min) rises with each bolus (8% for the first, 32% for the second, and 54% for the third bolus respectively). The probability of ventilatory depression drops below 5% within 40 minutes from the last bolus dose. The remifentanil infusion also provides a rapid onset of analgesic effect (95% probability within 5 minutes) and remains above 95% until 3 minutes after the infusion is terminated. The probability of ventilatory depression with this infusion rate of remifentanil is significant. The probability rises above 50% within 6 minutes and reaches 78% when the infusion is turned off. This effect quickly dissipates reaching less than a 5% probability within 9 minutes after the infusion is turned off. In summary, the repeated fentanyl boluses provide a reasonable analgesia effect that lasted long after the 30-minute time window. With the doses so close together, ventilatory depression may become an issue. The remifentanil infusion quickly achieved an analgesic effect, but it quickly dissipated once the infusion was terminated. Ventilatory depression was significant throughout the infusion.

Clinical Applications

Pharmacokinetic models have been integrated into infusion pumps and are commonly used to deliver anesthetics using target-controlled infusions (TCIs). With TCIs, users enter demographic data (age, weight, height) and set the desired concentration and a microcomputer within the pump uses a pharmacokinetic model to set the infusion rate to achieve and maintain the target concentration. Although widely used throughout the world for decades, this technology has not been approved for use in the United States.[17]

TCI allows anesthesia care providers to administer intravenous drugs in much the same fashion as inhalation agents. As an estimate of drug effect, MAC is used to titrate inhaled agents. Anesthesia care providers use end-tidal inhaled agent levels as a surrogate measure of brain concentrations (a reasonable assumption when end-tidal concentrations are relatively constant). Hence titration of drug delivery is driven by estimates of drug concentrations at the target organ. Titration of simple infusion rates (eg, mcg/kg/min), by contrast, is not as sophisticated. Clinicians make adjustments with no direct conceptualization of how infusion rate changes will influence concentrations at the target organ(s). TCI provides clinicians a means of dosing intravenous drugs in terms of target effect-site concentrations.

To illustrate the difference between TCI and continuous infusions, consider the simulations presented in Figure 1–20. This figure compares the infusion profile of a TCI set to maintain the propofol concentration at 4 mcg/mL with a bolus (2 mg/kg) followed by a continuous infusion of propofol administered at a rate of 150 mcg/kg/min. Both the target effect-site concentration and the infusion rate are associated with a high probability of rendering a person unresponsive. In terms of pharmacokinetics, the TCI infusion quickly achieves and then maintains the target concentration. It is interesting to note the infusion pump profile for the TCI infusion. The initial rate is fast to rapidly achieve the target concentration, but as drug accumulates in peripheral tissues, the rate slows. The propofol bolus mimics the TCI dosing regimen to achieve an effect-site concentration greater than 4 mcg/mL as quickly as the TCI pump did. Upon terminating both infusions, effect-site concentrations with either technique rapidly dissipate with the continuous infusion taking slightly longer than the TCI.

In terms of drug effect, the 2 dosing techniques provide a high probability of keeping a patient unresponsive. The bolus and continuous infusion rate achieve a probability of greater than 95% loss of responsiveness at approximately the same times as the TCI. After the 1-hour infusion is terminated,

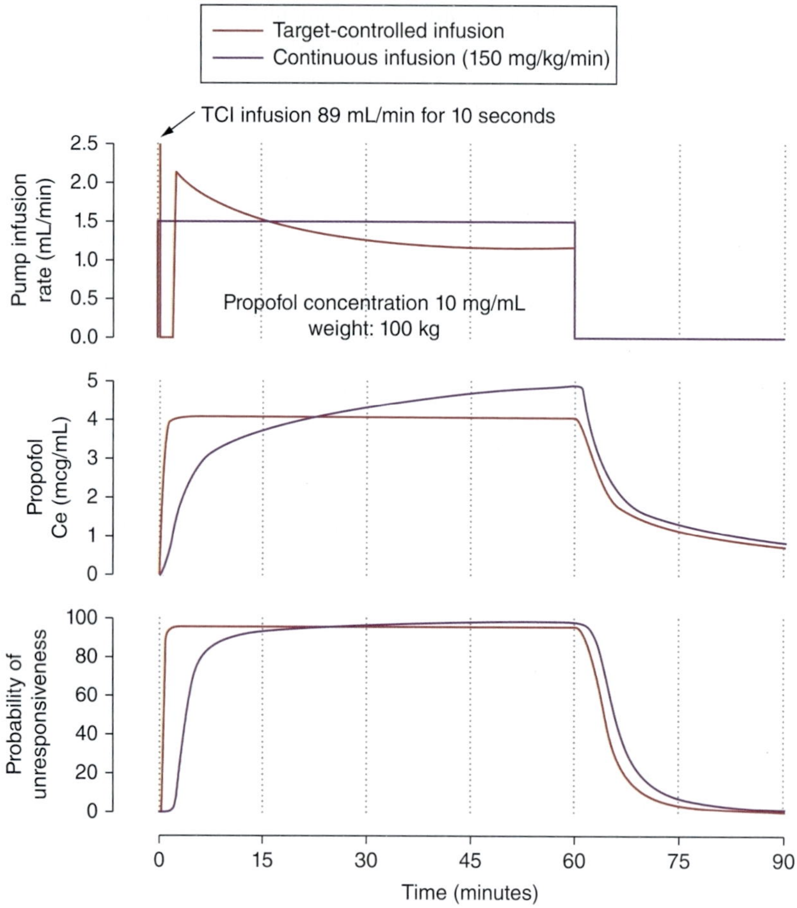

FIGURE 1–20 Comparison of a propofol target-controlled infusion (TCI) a bolus followed by a continuous propofol infusion. The top plot presents the infusion pump rates (mL/hour) for the TCI and continuous infusions. The target effect-site concentration is set to 4 mcg/mL and the continuous infusion rate is set at 150 mcg/kg/min for 60 minutes. The propofol concentration is 10 mg/mL and the weight is 100 kg. The middle plot presents the propofol effect-site concentrations for each infusion. The bottom plot presents the probability of unresponsiveness.

the time required to reach a 95% probability of being awake is slightly longer when using a continuous infusion (18 minutes versus 13 minutes with TCI). This small difference is primarily due to the accumulation of propofol in peripheral tissues that is difficult to account for when running a continuous infusion.

REFERENCES

1. Minto CF, Schnider TW, Egan TD, et al. Influence of age and gender on the pharmacokinetics and pharmacodynamics of remifentanil. I. Model development. *Anesthesiology*. 1997;86(1):10-23.
2. Schnider TW, Minto CF, Gambus PL, et al. The influence of method of administration and covariates on the pharmacokinetics of propofol in adult volunteers. *Anesthesiology*. 1998;88(5):1170-1182.
3. Bouillon TW, Bruhn J, Radulescu L, et al. Pharmacodynamic interaction between propofol and remifentanil regarding hypnosis, tolerance of laryngoscopy, bispectral index, and electroencephalographic approximate entropy. *Anesthesiology*. 2004;100(6):1353-1372.
4. Han T, Harmatz JS, Greenblatt DJ, Martyn JA. Fentanyl clearance and volume of distribution are increased in patients with major burns. *J Clin Pharmacol*. 2007;47(6):674-680. Epub 2007/04/13.

5. Rowland M, Tozer TN. *Clinical Pharmacokinetics and Pharmacodynamics: Concepts and Applications.* Philadelphia: Lippincott Williams & Wilkins; 2011.
6. Bodor N, Buchwald P. Soft drug design: general principles and recent applications. i. Rev. 2000;20(1):58-101.
7. Johnson KB. New horizons in sedative hypnotic drug development: fast, clean, and soft. *Anesth Analg.* 2012;115(2):220-222. Epub 2012/07/25.
8. Hammerness P, Basch E, Ulbricht C, et al. St John's wort: a systematic review of adverse effects and drug interactions for the consultation psychiatrist. *Psychosomatics.* 2003;44(4): 271-282.
9. Martin JH. Cytochrome P450 drug interactions: are they clinically relevant. *Aust Prescr.* 2001;24(1):10-12.
10. Fisher DM. (Almost) everything you learned about pharmacokinetics was (somewhat) wrong! *Anesth Analg.* 1996;83(5):901-903.
11. Shafer SL, Stanski DR. Improving the clinical utility of anesthetic drug pharmacokinetics. *Anesthesiology.* 1992;76(3):327-330.
12. Shafer SL, Varvel JR, Aziz N, Scott JC. Pharmacokinetics of fentanyl administered by computer-controlled infusion pump. *Anesthesiology.* 1990;73(6):1091-1102.
13. Hughes MA, Glass PS, Jacobs JR. Context-sensitive half-time in multicompartment pharmacokinetic models for intravenous anesthetic drugs. *Anesthesiology.* 1992;76(3):334-341.
14. Youngs EJ, Shafer SL. Pharmacokinetic parameters relevant to recovery from opioids. *Anesthesiology.* 1994;81(4):833-842.
15. Boer F, Olofsen E, Bovill JG, et al. Pulmonary uptake of sufentanil during and after constant rate infusion. *Br J Anaesth.* 1996;76(2):203-208.
16. Egan TD, Minto CF, Hermann DJ, Barr J, Muir KT, Shafer SL. Remifentanil versus alfentanil: comparative pharmacokinetics and pharmacodynamics in healthy adult male volunteers. *Anesthesiology.* 1996;84(4):821-833.
17. Egan TD, Shafer SL. Target-controlled infusions for intravenous anesthetics: surfing USA not! *Anesthesiology.* 2003;99(5):1039-1041.
18. Johnson KB, Syroid ND, Gupta DK, et al. An evaluation of remifentanil-sevoflurane response surface models in patients emerging from anesthesia: model improvement using effect-site sevoflurane concentrations. *Anesth Analg.* 2010;111(2):387-394.
19. Egan TD, Muir KT, Hermann DJ, Stanski DR, Shafer SL. The electroencephalogram (EEG) and clinical measures of opioid potency: defining the EEG-clinical potency relationship ('fingerprint') with application to remifentanil. *Int J Pharm Med.* 2001;15(1):1-8.
20. Ausems ME, Vuyk J, Hug CC Jr, Stanski DR. Comparison of a computer-assisted infusion versus intermittent bolus administration of alfentanil as a supplement to nitrous oxide for lower abdominal surgery. *Anesthesiology.* 1988;68(6):851-861.
21. Ausems ME, Hug CC Jr, Stanski DR, Burm AG. Plasma concentrations of alfentanil required to supplement nitrous oxide anesthesia for general surgery. *Anesthesiology.* 1986;65(4):362-373.
22. Johnson KB, Syroid ND, Gupta DK, et al. An evaluation of remifentanil propofol response surfaces for loss of responsiveness, loss of response to surrogates of painful stimuli and laryngoscopy in patients undergoing elective surgery. *Anesth Analg.* 2008;106(2):471-479.
23. Kern SE, Xie G, White JL, Egan TD. A response surface analysis of propofol-remifentanil pharmacodynamic interaction in volunteers. *Anesthesiology.* 2004;100(6): 1373-1381.
24. Nieuwenhuijs DJ, Olofsen E, Romberg RR, et al. Response surface modeling of remifentanil-propofol interaction on cardiorespiratory control and bispectral index. *Anesthesiology.* 2003;98(2):312-322.
25. Fechner J, Hering W, Ihmsen H, Palmaers T, Schuttler J, Albrecht S. Modelling the pharmacodynamic interaction between remifentanil and propofol by EEG-controlled dosing. *Eur J Anaesthesiol.* 2003;20(5): 373-379.
26. Chernick DA, Gillings D, Laine H, Hendler J, Silver JM, Davidson AB. Validity and reliability of the Observer's Assessment of Alertness/Sedation Scale: study with intravenous midazolam. *J Clin Psychopharmacol.* 1990;10(4):244-251.
27. LaPierre CD, Johnson KB, Randall BR, White JL, Egan TD. An exploration of remifentanil-propofol combinations that lead to a loss of response to esophageal instrumentation, a loss of responsiveness, and/or onset of intolerable ventilatory depression. *Anesth Analg.* 2011;113(3):490-499.
28. Ramsay MA, Savege TM, Simpson BR, Goodwin R. Controlled sedation with alphaxalone-alphadolone. *Br Med J.* 1974;2(5920):656-659.
29. Barr J, Zomorodi K, Bertaccini EJ, Shafer SL, Geller E. A double-blind, randomized comparison of i.v. lorazepam versus midazolam for sedation of ICU patients via a pharmacologic model. *Anesthesiology.* 2001;95(2):286-298.
30. Albrecht S, Ihmsen H, Hering W, et al. The effect of age on the pharmacokinetics and pharmacodynamics of midazolam. *Clin Pharmacol Ther.* 1999;65(6): 630-639.

CHAPTER 2

Pharmacokinetics of Inhalational Agents

James H. Philip, MEE, MD, CCE

The kinetics of inhaled anesthetics is fundamental to the clinical practice of anesthesia.[1] This subject is often called uptake and distribution of anesthetics.[2] It explains the time course of anesthetic movement from the delivery system to the site of action, the patient's central nervous system. Although the site of action of inhaled anesthetic agents includes the brain and spinal cord, "brain" will be used alone in the remainder of this chapter. See Chapter 1 for further discussion of anesthesia site of action.

Inhaled agents are either gases or vapors, depending on their physical state at room temperature and pressure. Nitrous oxide, cyclopropane, and xenon are gases. For these agents, the anesthetic source is a flow controller with flow meter. Halothane, isoflurane, sevoflurane, and desflurane, as well as the historical agents diethyl ether, methoxyflurane, fluroxene, and enflurane are vapors. In this chapter, the agent source for all of these will be called a vaporizer. The physical properties of most of these agents are listed in Table 2–1.

DEFINITIONS

The measure of anesthetic level in a compartment or location is the partial pressure. Partial pressure is also called tension. Tension is a generic term that applies to variables that equalize in connected locations. Examples are hydrostatic tension (water height) and electrical tension (voltage). The interchangeable terms "high-tension wires" and "high-voltage wires" are familiar examples.

Anesthetic partial pressure or tension could be expressed in common pressure units such as mm Hg, Pa, or kPa. However, the most commonly used unit for anesthetic partial pressure is % atm (percent of one sea level atmosphere). One percent partial pressure represents 1% × 760 mm Hg = 7.6 mm Hg. The anesthetic tension is then said to be 1%. Commercial vaporizers state their delivered tension in percent and thus are consistent with this description.

Equilibrium is achieved when the tensions in compartments are equal. The locations or compartments of interest for inhaled agents are breathing circuit (inspired gas), lungs (alveolar gas), arterial blood, and the idealized body compartments: vessel-rich group (spinal cord, brain, heart, kidneys [VRG]), muscle, fat, and mixed venous blood. Figure 2–1 shows the Gas Man[3,4] model that shows the compartments and their partial pressures. The model has been validated for induction and emergence of anesthesia[5] and has been used to elucidate fine points of inhalation kinetics.[6]

Although equilibrium is achieved when the anesthetic tensions in compartments are equal, anesthetic concentrations in connected compartments differ at this equilibrium according to agent solubility (λ) in each location. For blood and gas in equilibrium, the ratio of concentration in blood to concentration in gas is the blood-to-gas (blood/gas) solubility ratio or blood/gas solubility, expressed as $\lambda_{b/g}$. The following example explains this.

A 10-mL syringe is filled with 5 mL blood and 5 mL air. A small amount of liquid or vapor anesthetic is added to the syringe, which is then capped and shaken. In the syringe, the tension of anesthetic in the blood and gas compartments equalize while the concentrations equilibrate. At equilibrium, the ratio of concentration in the blood to concentration in the gas is the blood-to-gas solubility ratio or blood/gas solubility. The ratio of drug quantity in these 2 equally sized compartments also equals the blood/gas solubility, $\lambda_{b/g}$. When the term *solubility* is used by itself, it usually refers to blood/gas solubility or blood/gas solubility ratio.

TABLE 2–1 Physical and kinetic properties of anesthetic agents.

	Ether	Halothane	Enflurane	Isoflurane	Sevoflurane	Desflurane	N_2O	Xenon
MAC (%)	1.9	0.8	1.7	1.1	2.1	6.0	110	70
Blood/gas solubility	12.1	2.47	1.90	1.30	0.65	0.42	0.47	0.13
VRG/blood solubility	1.10	1.94	1.47	1.62	1.69	1.29	0.89	1.30
Mus/blood solubility	0.90	4.01	2.42	3.46	3.69	2.31	1.15	2.00
Fat/blood solubility	5.00	60.7	33.2	53.8	52.3	31.0	2.30	10.0
Alveolar plateau height	0.06	0.24	0.30	0.38	0.55	0.66	0.63	0.86
VRG (brain) Tau (minutes)	1.7	3.1	2.3	2.6	2.7	2.0	1.4	2.1
Muscle Tau (hours)	0.6	2.4	1.5	2.1	2.3	1.4	0.7	1.2
Fat Tau (hours)	4	49	27	43	42	25	2	8

Mus, muscle; VRG, spinal cord, brain, heart, kidneys.

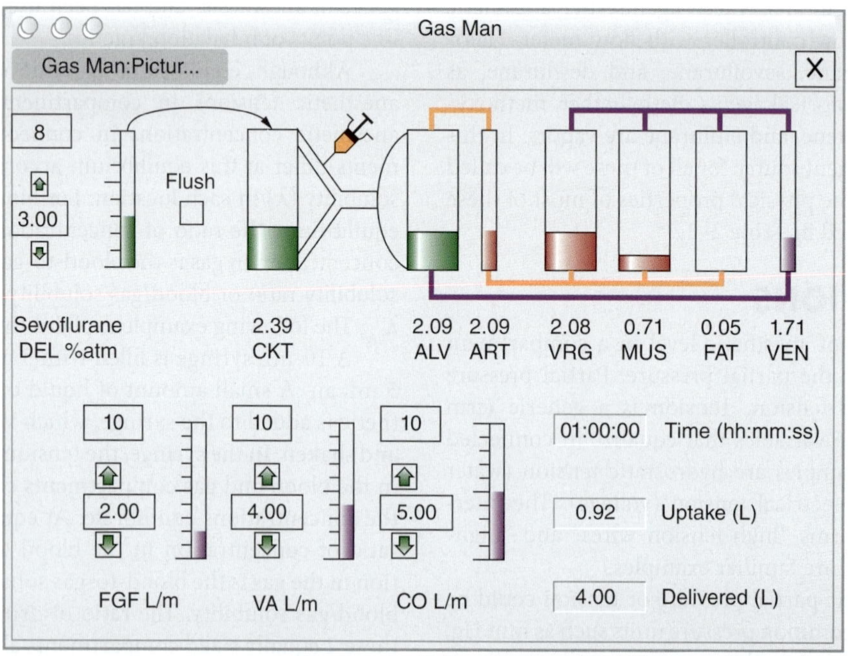

FIGURE 2–1 Gas Man apparatus. The illustration shows a schematic representation of the model for inhalation kinetics. The upper part shows compartments in which anesthetic partial pressure will rise from left to right. The lower part shows the flows that link the compartments. ALV, alveolar tension; ART, arterial tension; CKT, circuit; CO, cardiac output; DEL, tension delivered; FAT, fat; FGF, fresh gas flow; MUS, muscle; VA, alveolar ventilation; VEN, venous; VRG, spinal cord, brain heart, kidneys.

MOVEMENT OF ANESTHETIC

As blood passes through the capillaries of the lungs, anesthetic equilibrium is achieved across the alveolar-capillary membrane. Thus, arterial tension equals alveolar tension. The concentration of anesthetic in blood is equal to the product of the partial pressure and the solubility.

Arterial blood perfuses each tissue and tissue tension rises toward arterial tension. During this period, anesthetic tension in venous blood leaving each tissue equals the partial pressure in that tissue, itself. Eventually, anesthetic tension in the tissue equals that in arterial blood. At this time, venous tension equals arterial tension and there is no longer anesthetic uptake into that tissue. The tissue is in equilibrium with blood. All tissues reach equilibrium, some after a few minutes and some after many hours. When final equilibrium is reached, anesthetic tensions in all gas, liquid, and tissue compartments are equal. This takes many days.

The Alveolar Tension Curve

To understand the kinetics of inhaled agents, we analyze the time course of anesthetic tension in the patient's lungs or alveoli (alveolar tension [PA]) in response to a step change in inspired tension (PI). This was first described by Kety in 1950. This is called the alveolar step response or the alveolar tension curve. The alveolar tension curve describes the time course of PA in response to a step change in PI.

Initial Rise of the Alveolar Tension Curve

The alveolar tension curve has the same general shape for all inhaled agents because they share the same physiology of drug delivery and removal. The alveolar tension curve components are named in accordance to their shape as described by Kety. They are the initial rise, plateau, knee, and tail. The alveolar tension curve for isoflurane is shown in Figure 2–2.

The first portion of the curve is called the initial rise. See Figure 2–3. This is how the shape would look if there were no removal of anesthetic from the alveoli by blood. This would happen in the following imaginary situations: cardiac output is zero, lungs were not connected to the cardiovascular system, and agent solubility in blood ($\lambda_{b/g}$) is zero.

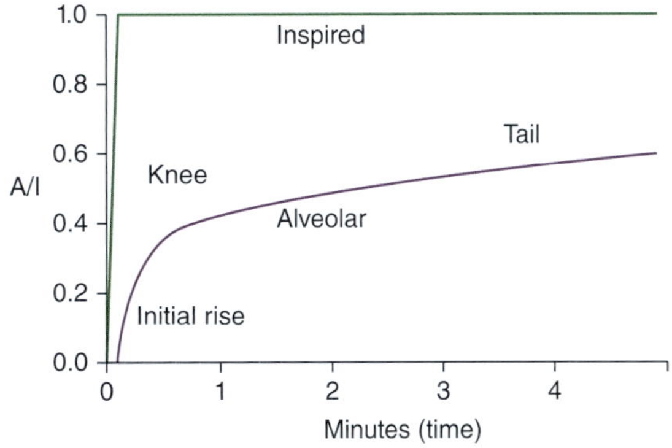

FIGURE 2–2 The alveolar tension curve for isoflurane. The vertical axis labeled A/I reflects the alveolar over inspired ratio of concentration, fraction, partial pressure, or tension. The curve shows the characteristic initial rise, knee, and tail described in the text.

The initial portion of the alveolar tension curve follows this shape for all agents. The curve shape of the initial rise is an exponential curve that is shown in Figure 2–3 and expressed mathematically as

$$P_A/P_I = 1 - e^{-t/\tau} \quad \text{(Eqn. 1)}$$

where τ (tau) is called the time constant. Because of the physics and mathematics of gas mixing, the time constant can be computed as the ratio of volume to flow in the alveolar compartment. The time constant is the time it would take for flow to completely fill

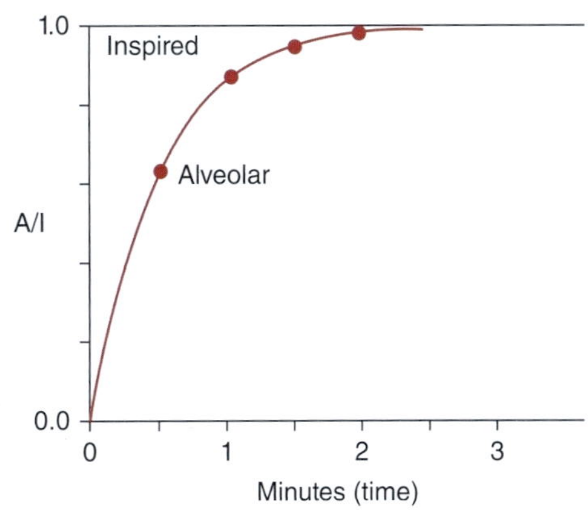

FIGURE 2–3 The rise in alveolar tension in response to a step change in inspired tension in the absence of uptake into blood. Small circles represent values at 1, 2, 3, and 4 time constants. See text for details.

the compartment if it is empty at the beginning. In this example, the volume (V) is the functional residual capacity (FRC), or resting volume, of the lung and the flow (F) is the alveolar ventilation (VA), equal to the effective average minute ventilation of the alveoli.

$$\tau = V/F = FRC/VA \qquad \text{(Eqn. 2)}$$

For the average adult, FRC = 2 L and VA = 4 L/min. So

$$\tau = FRC/VA = (2\text{ L}) / (4\text{ L/min}) = (2/4)\text{ min} = \tfrac{1}{2}\text{ minute} \qquad \text{(Eqn. 3)}$$

The mathematics and shape of the exponential curve of Eqn. 1 and Figure 2–3 can be understood as follows. In Eqn. 1 initially t = 0 and $e^0 = 1$, like any number raised to the zero power. Thus $P_A/P_I = 0$ initially. As time passes, t eventually reaches the value of tau, or ½ minute in this example. At this time, the exponent of e is −1 and $e^{-1} = 1/e = 1/2.718... = 0.37$. Subtracting this value from 1 results in 0.63. Thus, when $t = \tau$, $P_A/P_I = 0.63$. After a second time constant of time has passed (2 × ½ = 1 minute in this example), P_A/P_I has reached 0.86 of the final value. The value at 3 τ = 0.95, 4 τ = 0.98, and 5 τ = 0.99. Thus, at the end of 4 time constants, the curve has reached 0.98 of its way toward 1.0. It will reach *exactly* 1.0 after infinite time has elapsed. It is interesting to note that from any point in the course of the exponential curve, its value will reach 0.63 of the remainder of its course in one time constant.

An exponential curve depicts the input-output relationship for any fully mixed single compartment that is subjected to a step change in the tension entering it. This applies to tissue compartments as well. For a tissue compartment, the effective volume is the actual volume multiplied by the tissue/gas solubility. The effective flow is the actual blood flow times the blood/gas solubility. Solubilities of successive areas relate to each other such that tissue/gas solubility ($\lambda_{t/g}$) equals tissue/blood solubility ($\lambda_{t/b}$) multiplied by the blood/gas solubility ($\lambda_{b/g}$).

$$\lambda_{t/g} = \lambda_{t/b} \cdot \lambda_{b/g} \qquad \text{(Eqn 4)}$$

Plateau of the Alveolar Tension Curve

The next portion of the alveolar tension curve is called the plateau. See Figure 2–4. This portion of the alveolar tension curve is created by the offsetting effects of delivery of anesthetic by VA and the removal of anesthetic by the product of CO and blood/gas solubility ($\lambda_{b/g}$, here called λ). The alveolar plateau height is computed as:

$$P_A/P_I \big|_{plateau} = 1/(1 + CO \cdot \lambda/VA) \qquad \text{(Eqn. 5)}$$

The equation and plateau height can be understood by the following example. Imagine a drug with solubility = 1 and call it unithane. Further, consider the patient in whom CO equals VA. In this situation, $CO \cdot \lambda/VA = 1$ and the alveolar plateau height is calculated to equal 1/(1 + 1) = ½. Thus, the height of the plateau is half the height of the inspired tension. This shows the balance of delivery exactly offset by removal. This establishes an equilibrium where alveolar tension is halfway between zero and inspired tension. If ventilation is higher, the plateau is higher. If the CO is higher or if solubility is higher, the plateau is lower.

The presence in the plateau equation of the mathematical term $CO \cdot \lambda/VA$ is clinically very significant. A change in any one of these parameters can be offset by a proportional or inverse change in another term in determining the plateau height. Thus, halving the ventilation is the same as doubling the solubility. Moreover, doubling the ventilation is the same as halving the solubility. Tripling the ventilation is the same as reducing the solubility by

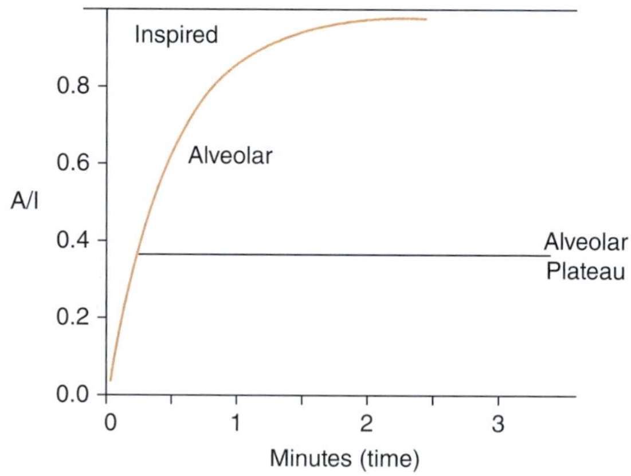

FIGURE 2–4 The alveolar plateau is formed as alveolar ventilation delivers agent to the alveoli while blood flow removes it. Removal rate equals cardiac output times blood/gas solubility.

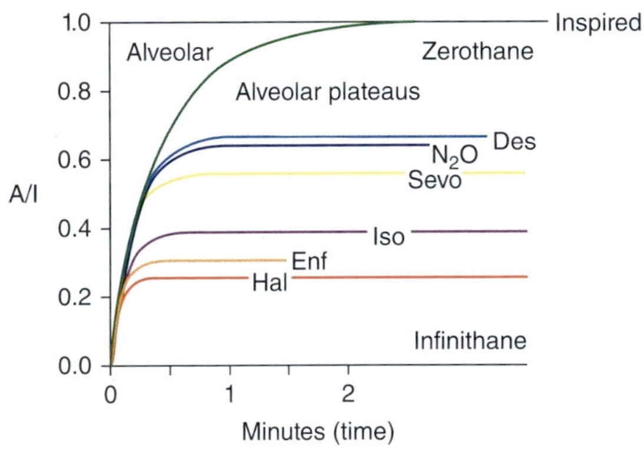

FIGURE 2–5 Alveolar plateaus for real anesthetics and the imaginary zerothane (solubility zero) and infinithane (solubility infinity) anesthetics. Des, desflurane; Enf, enflurane; Hal, halothane; Iso, isoflurane; N_2O, nitrous oxide; Sevo, sevoflurane.

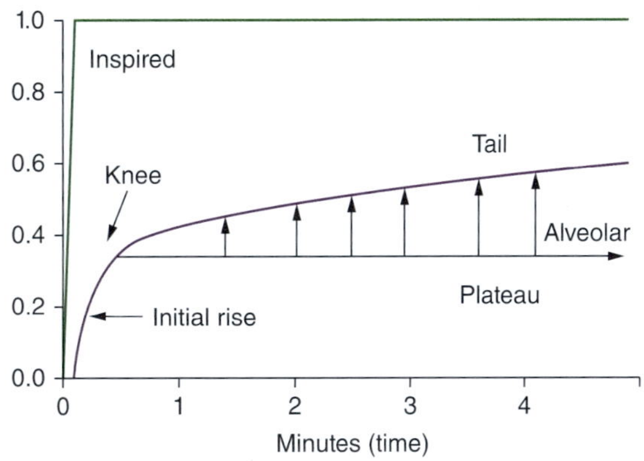

FIGURE 2–6 Tail of the alveolar tension curve. The rise in alveolar tension is produced by venous return of anesthetic-laden blood to the lungs.

a factor of 3. This is significant in that desflurane, sevoflurane, and isoflurane have relative solubilities of approximately 1:2:3. Each time inspired concentration is changed, expired changes according to this relationship within 0.5 minutes. This half-minute is the time it takes for lung wash-in to reach the new plateau. Table 2–1 shows solubilities and plateau heights and Figure 2–5 shows the plateaus.

Knee and Tail of the Alveolar Tension Curve

The final portion of the alveolar tension curve is called the tail. It is formed physically as a result of venous blood from tissues returning anesthetic to the alveoli, thereby causing alveolar tension to rise further. The curve transition from flat theoretical plateau to curved actual tail is called the knee, named by Kety. Alveolar tension rise causes arterial tension to rise. As anesthetic tension in fast tissues (VRG) rises in the first few minutes after the alveolar plateau begins, the plateau is transformed upward into the knee of the curve. See Figure 2–6. The plateau exists in theory while the knee and tail exist in reality. The first portion of the tail is formed by anesthetic-laden blood from VRG. The next, much flatter, portion is formed by anesthetic-laden blood from muscle, culminating a few hours later. The final portion is formed by anesthetic-laden blood from fat, more than 10 hours later. The alveolar tension curve for many agents[7] is shown in Figure 2–7 along with short lines depicting the plateaus. Actual plateau heights and values are shown in Table 2–1.

Fine Points of Expired, Alveolar, and Arterial Tension

Lung Shunt

Arterial blood anesthetic tension follows alveolar gas tension very closely. Blood that passes through

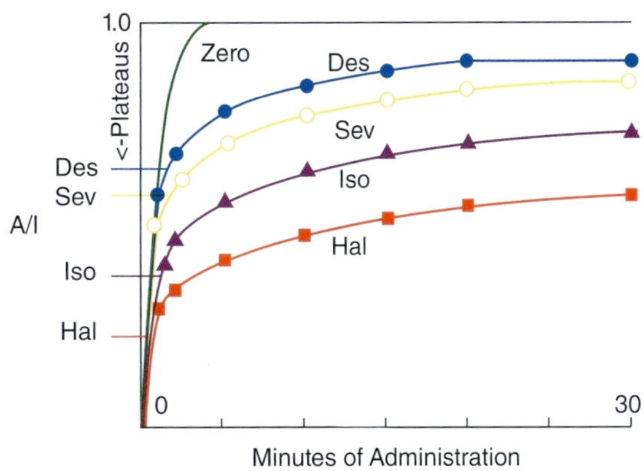

FIGURE 2–7 Alveolar tension curves of several anesthetics. Des, desflurane; Hal, halothane; Iso, isoflurane; Sevo, sevoflurane. Graphs are redrawn from the data of Yasuda M, Lockhart SL, Eger EI, et al. with the plateau height lines of Figs. 2-5 and 2-6 added. (Graphs are redrawn from the data of Yasuda M, Lockhart SL, Eger EI, Weiskopf RB, Liu J, Laster M, Taheri S, Peterson NA. Comparison of kinetics of sevoflurane and isoflurane in humans. *Anesth Analg* 1991;72:316-324.)

alveolar capillaries attains an anesthetic tension equal to that in alveolar gas. However, some blood flow does not pass through alveolar capillaries. This blood is called lung shunt, more precisely right-to-left lung shunt. Lung shunt adds mixed venous blood to the perfect alveolar-equilibrated blood to form arterial blood. Thus, arterial tension has been slightly diluted by mixed venous blood. The impact of this is that during induction, arterial anesthetic tension is lower than alveolar tension. During emergence or anesthetic lightening, arterial tension is higher than alveolar tension once arterial tension falls below venous tension.

Alveolar Dead Space

Agent monitors measure end-tidal (ET) gas tension as an estimate of alveolar tension. In reality, end-tidal gas is comprised of alveolar gas diluted by a small amount of inspired gas. The fraction of inspired gas mixed into the expired gas is the alveolar dead space fraction. This is approximately 10% in normal lungs during anesthesia. The alveolar dead space effect is seen with carbon dioxide, where the end-tidal PCO_2 is typically 10% less than the arterial $PaCO_2$, 36 mm Hg and 40 mm Hg, respectively.

End-Expired Gas Errors

Because there are alveolar-arterial tension differences and alveolar-ET tension differences, the end-tidal agent tension measured by agent monitors differs from arterial tension by 2 effects—lung shunt and alveolar dead space. The total ET-arterial error with isoflurane is approximately 20%.[8]

End-Expired Gas Misinterpretations—Ignoring Brain Delay

At all times during anesthesia, anesthetic tension in the brain lags behind that in the arterial blood. The brain is a compartment that is perfused by blood and takes time to equilibrate with it. For all inhaled anesthetic agents, brain/blood solubility is 0.9 to 1.9 or approximately 1.5 (Table 2–1). Because of this, the brain time constant is between 1.5 and 3 minutes for all anesthetic agents. Recognizing that there is this time delay during clinical care is crucial to effective use of ET agent monitors. The ET agent monitor predicts the level in the brain in approximately 3 minutes, and the value 3 minutes ago on the trend graph estimates the level in the brain now.

Clinical Kinetics—Control of Anesthetic Depth

The goal of administering inhaled anesthetics is to bring the anesthetic tension in the brain to the level desired, manipulate it as clinical conditions dictate, and reduce the brain level to as close to zero as possible at the end of anesthesia. During anesthesia, brain tension is held at or above 1 minimum alveolar concentration (MAC) with pure inhalation anesthesia and less than 1 MAC when other agents form a significant part of the patient's anesthetic. Even if inspired agent tension could be controlled accurately, alveolar and VRG tension would be lower and delayed according to the alveolar tension curve and brain delay described above.

In clinical care, the vaporizer dial is set and fresh gas flow (FGF) with the delivered tension enters the breathing circuit. The FGF mixes with the patient's exhaled gas flow producing an inspired tension that is an average of exhaled and delivered tensions, each weighted by its relative flow and possibly affected by uneven breathing circuit gas mixing. Dilution of the delivered tension occurs unless FGF greatly exceeds minute ventilation. This occurs rarely in clinical practice where such excess is considered wasteful. The limit of low FGF is closed-circuit anesthesia, where FGF is set to exactly mimic the patient's uptake of oxygen and inhaled anesthetic agent. Closed-circuit anesthesia is not addressed in this chapter.

Careful adjustment of vaporizer setting combined with consideration of FGF, ventilation, CO, and blood/gas solubility of the chosen anesthetic are required to achieve and maintain the desired brain anesthetic tension. Fresh gas flow, vaporizer setting, inspired tension, and expired tension should all be observed and preferably recorded for good control, prediction, and understanding of brain anesthetic tension. This is important since changing FGF or patient ventilation often requires changes in vaporizer setting. The need for these changes might not otherwise be appreciated if only expired tension is observed.

Emergence From Anesthesia

Emergence from anesthesia of very long duration is the inverse of anesthesia induction. The alveolar tension curve is inverted. The shape could be described as comprised of the initial fall, plateau, knee, and tail of the curve.

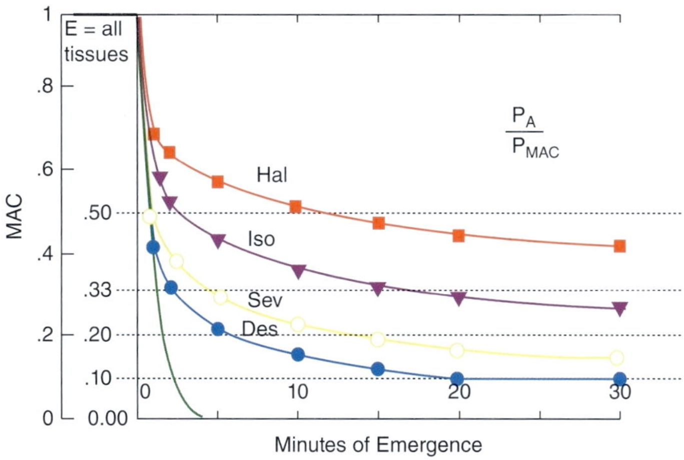

FIGURE 2–8 Alveolar tension fall for various anesthetic agents after an infinitely long 1 MAC anesthetic. These curves are created by inverting the curves of Figure 2–7. Dotted lines are shown at reduction from 1 MAC to 0.50, 0.33, 0.20, and 0.10 MAC reflecting fractional reductions of 0.50, 0.67, 0.80, and 0.90 MAC. Des, desflurane; Hal, halothane; Iso, isoflurane; MAC, minimum alveolar concentration; Sevo, sevoflurane.

The level of anesthesia in the VRG below which 50% of patients follow commands is termed MAC-awake. For all agents, MACawake is approximately 0.33 MAC. A more complete set of benchmarks is 0.75 MAC, 0.5 MAC, 0.33 MAC, 0.2 MAC, and 0.1 MAC. Figure 2–8 shows a graph of emergence after very long anesthesia created by inverting the anesthesia induction curves of Figure 2–7. It can be seen that for most agents, even in the context of a very long anesthetic at 1.0 MAC, the 0.75 MAC level is reached immediately and the 0.5 MAC level is attained in just a few minutes. The time to reach one-half the steady-state initial value is called the half-time. This value is commonly used as a benchmark for drugs. All of the intravenous drugs except remifentanil take much longer than inhaled drugs to reach all benchmarks. More sensitive differentiation among drugs is achieved by observing the 0.67, 0.80, and 0.90 reduction, which represent the 0.33, 0.2, and 0.1 fractions remaining. These are shown as dotted lines in Figure 2–8.

Emergence is faster after short-duration anesthetics than after long-duration anesthetic administrations. This is because very slow body compartments like fat remain empty enough to remove anesthetic *from* blood during emergence. The effect of the muscle compartment changes within clinical durations of anesthesia. As muscle fills with anesthetic, it is transformed from a compartment that augments awakening to one that retards it. Any compartment with a tension lower than that in the blood helps emergence while any compartment with a tension above that in blood hinders emergence.

SUBTLE KINETIC EFFECTS

The Concentration Effect and the Second Gas Effect

The concentration effect and the second gas effect describe the effect of gas uptake on the gas volume and concentration that remains in the alveolar compartment. The concentration effect describes the kinetic impact of breathing a gas in high concentration or fraction. When a high concentration is breathed, most of the gas taken up from the lung is that gas. When alveolar volume is reduced by uptake into blood during one breath, inspired tidal volume is increased in the next breath to offset the missing volume.

This phenomenon increases alveolar ventilation during the period of rapid uptake into blood. The high concentration effect is usually described regarding nitrous oxide because it is the only current agent safe to breathe in high concentration. Figure 2–5 shows that the plateau height for nitrous oxide is lower than that for desflurane. In Figure 2–5, the line is drawn as if nitrous oxide was breathed in a low concentration like the other gases. To avoid confusion Figure 2–7 omits the curve for nitrous oxide since in the actual experiment depicted, nitrous oxide was breathed in high concentration (65%–70%) and the concentration effect displaced the nitrous oxide curve above that of desflurane. Figure 2–9 demonstrates the impact of concentration by overlaying simulated alveolar tension curves when breathing high concentration (70%) and low concentration (7%) nitrous oxide.

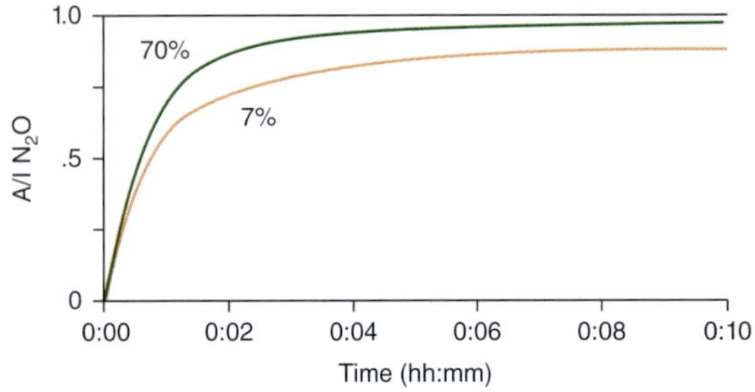

FIGURE 2–9 The concentration effect.

The second gas effect describes the impact of the presence of a high-concentration first gas, such as nitrous oxide, on the alveolar tension curve of a second lower-concentration gas, such as isoflurane. The absorption of the high-concentration, high-volume nitrous oxide concentrates the isoflurane remaining in the alveoli (Figure 2–10). This absorption also augments all ventilation into the lungs by the increased inspired ventilation from the concentration effect. Because alveolar isoflurane concentration is low compared with inspired concentration, alveolar concentration of the second gas can be raised by the uptake of the first gas. For the less soluble drugs sevoflurane and desflurane, the second gas effect has less clinical impact since alveolar concentrations approaches inspired concentration quickly and closely.

The Effect of Tissue Solubilities and Blood Flows

The clinical impact of tissue/blood solubility and the shape of the tail of the alveolar tension curve are subtle. Simulation provides insights. When anesthetic tension in a tissue compartment exceeds MACawake, or any other specified threshold, that tissue compartment delays blood and brain tension from reaching the threshold level. Early in the course of anesthesia, low muscle and fat anesthetic tensions will speed emergence while later, high anesthetic tension in muscle will delay it. The subtleties of tissue solubility, unknown tissue volume and blood flow, and intertissue diffusion make this even more complex.

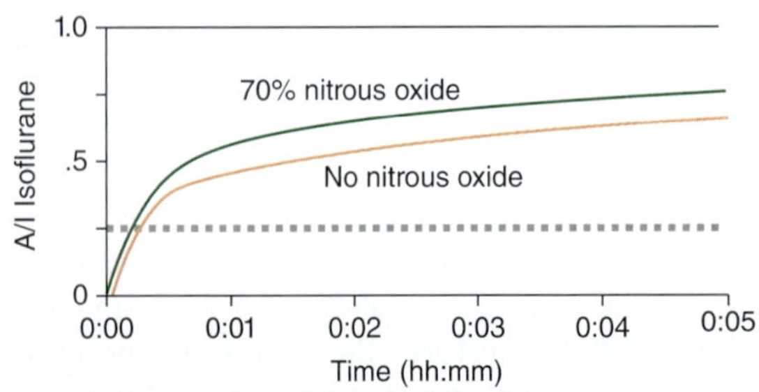

FIGURE 2–10 The second gas effect.

SUMMARY

Inhalation anesthesia kinetics is a key concept in anesthesia practice. The alveolar tension curve in response to a step change in inspired tension unveils the kinetic relationship created by the interconnection of the inspired gas with the alveolar gas, blood, and key body compartments. End-tidal (ET) anesthetic monitors provide good insight into arterial anesthetic tension, but the ET to brain delay of approximately 3 minutes must be appreciated.

REFERENCES

1. Kety SS. The physiological and physical factors governing the uptake of anesthetic gases by the body. *Anesthesiology*. 1950:11:517.
2. Eger EI II. *Anesthetic Uptake and Action*. Baltimore: Williams & Wilkins, 1974.
3. Philip JH. *GAS MAN®—Understanding Anesthesia Uptake and Distribution*. 5th ed. www.gsmanweb.com. Chestnut Hill, MA: Med Man Simulations; 2008.
4. H Philip JH. Gas Man®- An example of goal oriented computer-assisted teaching which results in learning. *Int J Clin Monit & Comp*. 1986;3:165-173.
5. Bouillon T, Shafer S. Editorial: Hot air or full steam ahead? An empirical pharmacokinetic model of potent inhaled agents. *Brit J Anaes*. 2000;84:429-431.
6. Eger EI, Shafer SL. Context-sensitive decrement times for inhaled anesthetics. *Anesth Analg*. 2005;101:688-696.
7. Yasuda M, Lockhart SL, Eger EI, et al. Comparison of kinetics of sevoflurane and isoflurane in humans. *Anesth Analg*. 1991;72:316-324.
8. Frei FJ, Zbinden AM, Thomson DA, Reider HU. Is the end-tidal partial pressure of isoflurane a good predictor of its arterial partial pressure? *Brit J Anaes*. 1991;66:331-339.

C H A P T E R

3

Drug Interactions in Anesthesia

Hugo E.M. Vereecke, MD, PhD, Johannes H. Proost, PharmD, PhD, Douglas J. Eleveld, PhD, and Michel M.R.F. Struys, MD, PhD

INTRODUCTION

Anesthetic drug interactions exist when one anesthetic influences the behavior of another anesthetic. The combined effects can be enhanced or diminished, or a new effect may occur. New effects can be therapeutic, or they can be unwanted side effects. During anesthesia, clinicians make therapeutic decisions routinely involving multiple drugs and as such, anesthesiologists are confronted with anesthetic drug–drug interactions on a daily basis.

Anesthetic effects are achieved using either a single drug or combinations of drugs. Drugs in combination all contribute to the overall effect; most combinations decrease the dose of each individual anesthetic when compared to doses of individual drugs required to achieve an equivalent effect. Taking advantage of interaction may decrease the severity or incidence of adverse effects without hampering desired effects.

Despite years of training, clinicians may not appreciate the magnitude of drug interactions, and they may administer excessive doses of anesthetics, hamper recovery, or increase the risk of adverse effects. Recent work has described several anesthetic interactions, and new display technology has been developed to visualize these interactions at the bedside of the patient. These recent innovations may provide a more evidence-based approach to anesthetic drug administration.

This chapter consists of 3 sections and an appendix. The first section will review basic principles of drug interactions. The second section will review the available models for vapor–opioid, hypnotic–opioid, and hypnotic–hypnotic interactions. The third section will discuss methods for applying interaction models in clinical practice. The appendix will present the methodology used to develop interaction models for interested readers.

Two topics concerning interaction will not be covered in this chapter. First, anesthetic drugs are known to influence the pharmacokinetic profile of one another by altering distribution volumes or clearance. Although many studies have demonstrated the importance of such interactions, the ultimate goal in anesthesia practice is to control effect rather than concentration. Pharmacokinetic interactions eventually result in pharmacodynamic changes. Hence, this chapter will focus on the clinical observable expression of interactions rather than on the (more obscure) changes in plasma concentration. Second, the interaction between paralytic and anesthetic agents is not well defined. This is primarily because the interactions have not been well modeled.

BASIC PRINCIPLES OF ANESTHETIC DRUG–DRUG INTERACTIONS

Additivity, Synergism, and Infra-additivity

One of the main questions concerning interactions between drugs is the nature of the interaction. Three concepts of drug interaction can be distinguished: (1) additivity, (2) supra-additivity (or synergism), and (3) infra-additivity (or antagonism). For additive drugs with equal potency, the sum of the effects evoked by respectively doses (a) and (b) for drug A and drug B is equal to the effect obtained with a solitary administration of either drug A or B given in a dose (a) + (b). For synergistic interactions, the

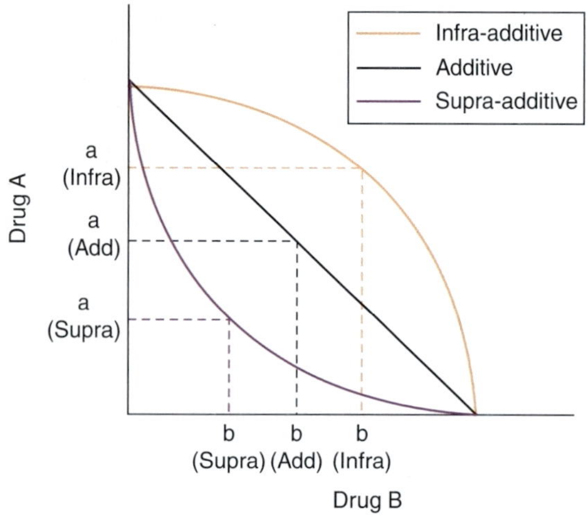

FIGURE 3–1 Schematic of drug interaction types. For drugs A and B, the black, blue, and red lines represent additive, supra-additive (synergistic), and infra-additive (antagonistic) interactions respectively. For synergistic interactions, the amount of each drug, a_{supra} and b_{supra}, required to achieve an effect is lower than the amount of drug, a_{add} and b_{add}, required in an additive interaction. The opposite holds true for the amount of each drug, a_{infra} and b_{infra}, in an antagonistic interaction.

combination of drugs A and B will result in a more pronounced effect compared to additivity. For infra-additive interactions, the combination of drugs will result in a less pronounced effect compared to additivity conditions (Figure 3–1).

In general, the mechanism behind additive interactions is thought to be activation of effect through a single pathway (ie, an identical receptor). In contrast, the mechanism behind synergistic interactions is thought to be activation of effect through multiple pathways (eg, through simultaneous *N*-methyl-D-aspartic acid [NMDA] and type A γ-aminobutyric acid [$GABA_A$] receptor inhibition). The possible advantage of synergism is that a desired effect can be targeted using lower doses of drugs with lower incidence or severity of side effects.

An important descriptor of drug interactions is the term *isobole*. Isobole refers to an isoeffect line on plots that compare effects between 2 drugs (as presented in Figure 3–1). Similar to the way a single drug pharmacodynamic model characterizes the concentration–effect relations, isoboles characterize concentration pairs with an equivalent effect over a range of drug concentrations for drug A and B. For a single drug, a common point of interest is the concentration associated with 50% of the maximal effect (C_{50}). For multiple interacting drugs, the 50% isobole is commonly used as the reference for potency of the drug combination. It represents the concentration pairs where there is a 50% probability of a given maximum effect. Studying one isobole of the interaction spectrum indirectly provides insight in the underlying mechanism of interactions.

For clinical practice, a wider range of probabilities of response should be available to improve dose-finding during ongoing surgery. For example, other isoboles of interest are the 5% and 95% isoboles that represent the concentration pairs where there is likely to be no effect (ie, < 5%) and there is likely to be a high probability of effect (> 95%), respectively. When dosing an anesthetic, it makes sense to administer anesthetics such that pairs of effect-site concentrations are just above, but not way beyond, the 95% isobole. Administering anesthetics that go far above the 95% isobole do not yield substantially more effect but may unnecessarily prolong the duration of effect and increase the risk of adverse side effects. Therefore, readily available advisory information—at the bedside of our patient—on the spectrum of interactions between major anesthetic drugs, may assist in optimizing the titration of multiple drugs throughout an anesthesia case. It would allow to target drug concentrations in a "just enough to do the job" approach.

Researchers have measured various anesthetic effects over a large range of anesthetic drug combinations. They used this information to build complex mathematical models of drug interactions. These models include a term that describes drug interactions (ie, extent of synergism) and a term that characterizes the transition from no effect to maximal effect. To render these complex model predictions in a form that may be used in clinical practice, researchers have developed a 3-dimensional representation of model predictions called *response surfaces*. Response surfaces describe the relation between combined drug concentrations (typically on the horizontal x and y axis of a graph) and the clinical effect (plotted in the vertical z axis). As an example, Figure 3–2 presents the propofol–remifentanil

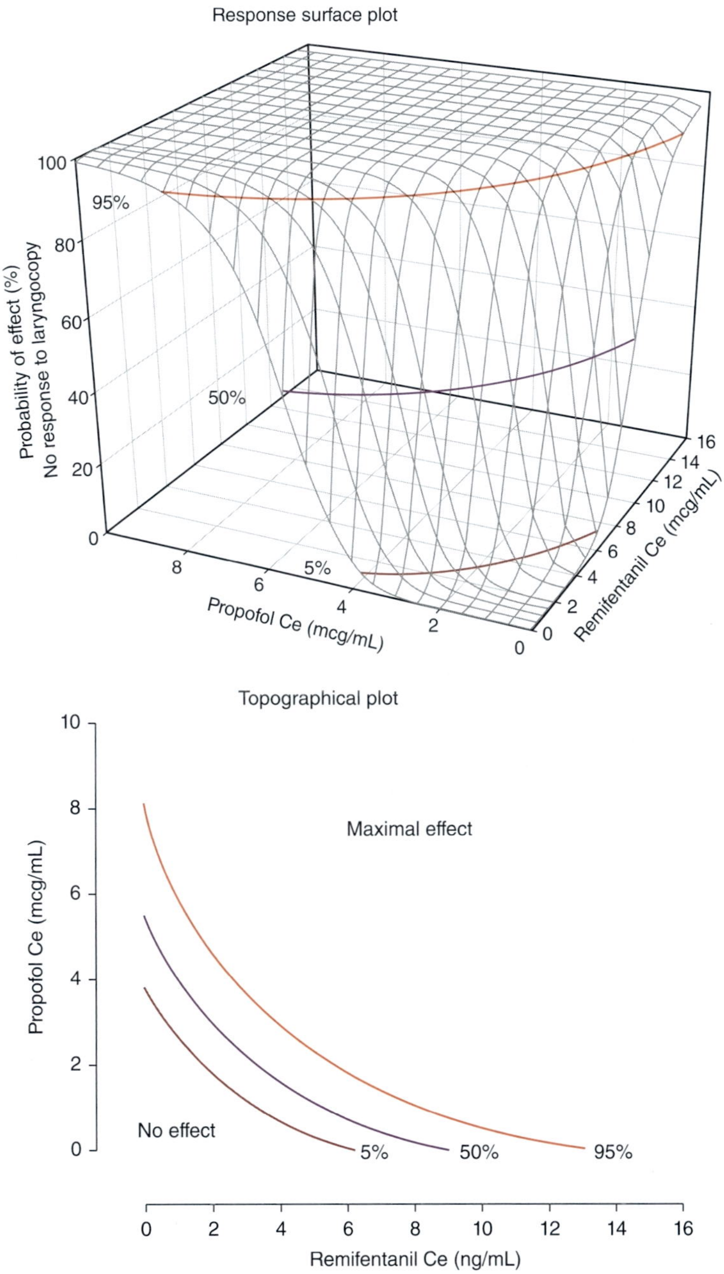

FIGURE 3–2 Example of a 2-drug pharmacodynamic interaction model for loss of response to laryngoscopy.[1] The model predicts the probability of effect (0 to 100% probability of no response to laryngoscopy) over a range of remifentanil and propofol effect-site concentrations (Ce). Two plots are used to illustrate the model: a response surface plot (top) and a topographical plot (bottom). The pink, blue, and red lines represent the 5%, 50%, and 95% isoboles. Each isobole presents the propofol–remifentanil concentration pairs that yield the same probability of effect. The topographical plot presents a top-down view of the response surface plot. Close examination of the isoboles reveals that the interaction between remifentanil and propofol is synergistic for this effect. Also of note is the difference in drug concentrations between the 5%, 50%, and 95% isoboles. The isoboles are in close proximity indicating the transition from no effect to maximal effect is fairly steep as propofol and remifentanil concentrations increase.

interaction surface for tolerance to laryngoscopy as published by Bouillon et al.[1] The response surface describes the complete range of isoboles between 0% and 100% of probability of tolerance to a stimulus with respective drug concentrations as input. As illustrated in this figure, 2 common presentations of response surfaces are used: the 3-dimensional plot described above and a simplified 2-dimensional topographical version of this plot. The topographical version presents drug concentrations on the vertical and horizontal axes with the probability of drug effect as selected isoboles (ie, 5%, 50%, and 95%).

Multiple mathematical approaches have been used to construct response surfaces for combinations of anesthetic drugs, each with specific advantages and disadvantages.[2] More details on the model building technology can be found in the Appendix.

When using response surfaces to optimize an anesthetic dose, it becomes apparent that it is best to titrate to target effect-site concentrations (ie, concentration pairs that provide a 95% probability of effect) rather than simply starting an infusion or turning on a vaporizer. An easy way to titrate individual effect-site concentration is to use target-controlled infusion (TCI) pumps, programmed with the pharmacokinetic models for each drug. Using TCI and response surfaces provides a means of fine-tuning anesthetic delivery.

Consider the simulations presented in Figure 3–3. It presents 2 response surfaces (in the topographical view): the probability of unresponsiveness and the probability of tolerance to laryngoscopy for combinations of remifentanil and sevoflurane.[3,4] Sevoflurane dosing requirements necessary to achieve a 95% probability of effect for 2 different remifentanil TCIs (2 and 4 ng/mL) are presented on each response surface.

A key point of this simulation is that the interaction models for tolerance to laryngoscopy and loss of responsiveness are not identical. The model of tolerance to laryngoscopy has a more pronounced synergistic interaction, as visualized by a larger bow toward the origin of the plot, and the model of loss of responsiveness has synergistic interactions but to a lesser extent. An example of this phenomenon is the difference in sevoflurane effect-site requirements for each target remifentanil infusion (4 versus 2 ng/mL). Vol% sevoflurane of 1.1 and 1.9 are required to achieve a 95% probability of tolerance to laryngoscopy for the remifentanil TCI set to 4 and 2 ng/mL, respectively (a difference of 0.8%). By contrast, vol% sevoflurane of 0.7 and 0.9 are required to achieve a 95% probability of loss of responsiveness for each remifentanil TCI (a difference of 0.2%).

A second key point is that the probability of effect for each drug alone is ineffective. For example, assuming steady-state conditions, the probability of tolerance to laryngoscopy for the sevoflurane (with no remifentanil) at 1.9 and 1.2 vol% is less than 5% and less than 1%, respectively. Similarly, the probability of loss of responsiveness for sevoflurane at 0.9 and 0.7 vol% is 77% and 48%, respectively. For remifentanil (with no sevoflurane) targeted to 2 and 4 ng/mL, the probability of either effect is zero.

Interaction Models in Anesthesia

For several intravenous anesthetic drugs (ie, propofol, remifentanil, sufentanil, alfentanil), pharmacokinetic models have been developed and used in clinical practice to titrate anesthetic delivery (eg, through TCI pumps) in a more individualized and reproducible way compared to classical dosing schemes (eg, weight-based boluses or continuous infusions). However, when combining anesthetic drugs, clinical responses may be substantially altered. As such, models developed for a single drug may have a large prediction error when used in combination with other anesthetics.

Since anesthesiologists rarely use just one drug, clinical pharmacologists have sought to characterize various responses in the presence of hypnotic–opioid and hypnotic–hypnotic drug combinations. Some of these responses include verbal, tactile stimuli, or painful stimuli; hemodynamic or respiratory effects; and changes in cerebral electrical activity during anesthesia. This line of research has led to the development of numerous interaction models for a variety of anesthetic effects. A summary of selected published interaction models of interest to anesthesiologists for various drug combinations is presented in Table 3–1.

Opioid–Inhaled Anesthetic Interactions

The interactions between potent inhaled agents and opioids have been well characterized. For analgesic effects, there is a pronounced synergistic interaction,

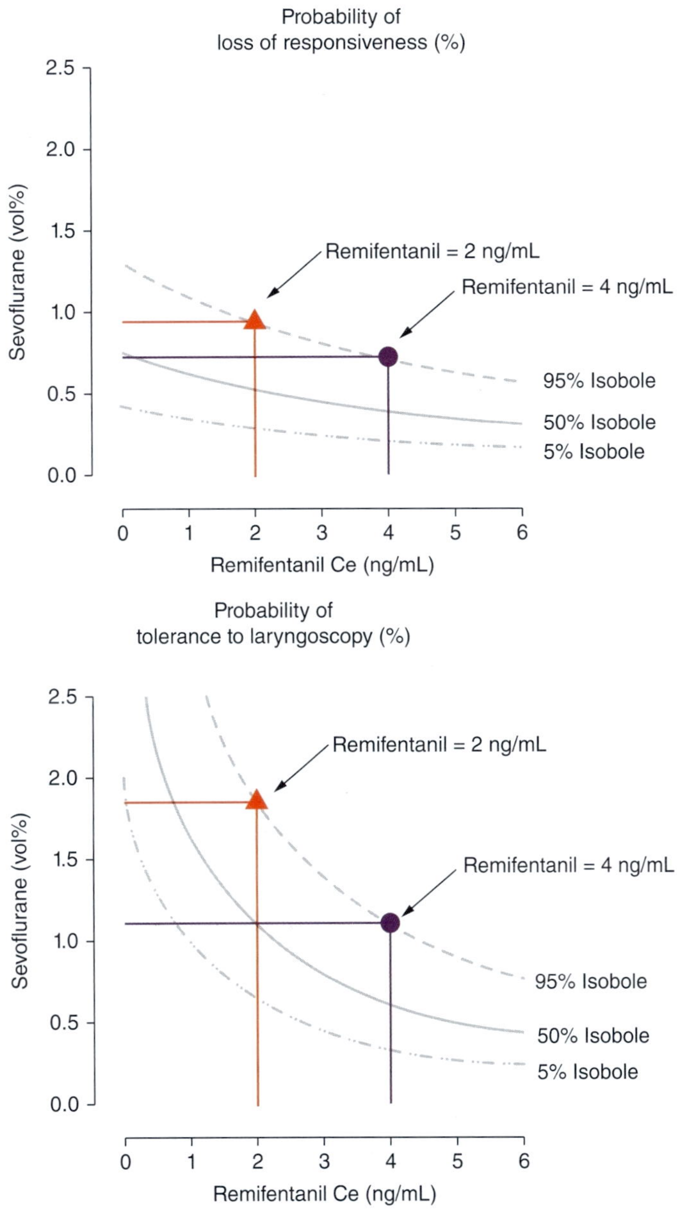

FIGURE 3–3 Response surface (topographical view) of loss of responsiveness (top plot)[3] and tolerance to laryngoscopy[4] (bottom plot) for sevoflurane and remifentanil. The horizontal and vertical axes present effect-site concentrations (Ce) for remifentanil and sevoflurane, respectively. Of note, sevoflurane effect-site concentrations are not equivalent to end-tidal concentrations. Model predictions of effect are represented by 5%, 50%, and 95% isoboles (gray lines). The associated sevoflurane concentrations necessary to achieve a 95% probability of effect for remifentanil target-controlled infusions set to 2 and 4 ng/mL are presented as a red triangle and a blue circle, respectively.

TABLE 3–1 Published anesthetic drug interaction models.

Anesthetic Drug Combinations	Modeled Effects	Reference(s)
Opioid–Inhalation Agent		
Remifentanil–sevoflurane	Loss of responsiveness (OAAS < 2)	2, 14, 12
	Tolerance to shake and shout	2
	Tolerance to laryngoscopy	2, 4
	Tolerance to LMA placement	2
	Tolerance to electrical tetany	2, 4
	Tolerance to pressure algometry	4, 12
Fentanyl–desflurane	Loss of responsiveness	13
	Tolerance to pressure algometry	13
Sevoflurane–opioid–nitrous oxide	MAC and MACbar	17
Opioid–Sedative		
Fentanyl–propofol	Loss of response to verbal command	18
	Loss of response to skin incision	18
Alfentanil–propofol	Loss of response to eyelash reflex	22
	Loss of consciousness	22
	Tolerance to laryngoscopy	22
	Tolerance to intubation	22
	Tolerance to opening the peritoneum	22
Fentanyl congeners–propofol	Recovery times	23
Remifentanil–propofol	Sedation (OAAS < 4)	43
	Loss of responsiveness (OAAS < 2)[1]	
	Tolerance to laryngoscopy and intubation[1, 4a]	
	Esophageal instrumentation	32
	Tolerance to shake and shout	1
	Changes in the Bispectral Index Scale	1
	Return of responsiveness[4a]	
	Tolerance to electrical tetany	43
	Tolerance to pressure algometry	12, 43
	Respiratory depression	31, 32

(Continued)

TABLE 3–1 Published anesthetic drug interaction models. (*Continued*)

Anesthetic Drug Combinations	Modeled Effects	Reference(s)
Sedative–Sedative		
Propofol–midazolam	Loss of responsiveness	37, 38, 39
	Tolerance to electrical tetany	38, 39
Propofol–sevoflurane	Loss of responsiveness	44
	Tolerance to skin incision,	44
	Tolerance to shake and shout	47
	Tolerance to LMA placement	47
	Tolerance to electrical tetany	47
	Tolerance to laryngoscopy	47
	Changes in the Bispectral Index Scale	48

LMA, laryngeal mask airway; MAC, minimum alveolar concentration; MACbar; minimum alveolar concentration required to block autonomic reflexes to noxious stimuli; OAAS, Observer's Assessment of Alertness and Sedation.
Adapted with permission from Chernik, D., D. Gillings, L. Harriet, J. Hnedler, J. Silver, A. Davidson, E. Schawm, and J. Siegel, Validity and reliability of the Observer's Assessment of Alertness/Sedation Scale: study with intravenous midazolam. *J Clin Psychopharmacol* 1990. Aug;10(4):244-51.

for sedation and unresponsiveness, the interaction is synergistic, but to a lesser extent.

Minimum Alveolar Concentration and Minimum Alveolar Concentration Required to Block Hemodynamic Response to Stimuli The first studies that quantified the interaction in anesthesia are the minimum inhibitory concentration (MAC)-reduction studies. MAC is a concept that defines equipotency between inhaled anesthetics with different physicochemical properties. One MAC of inhaled anesthetics represents the minimal alveolar concentration compatible with immobility in 50% of the population after a painful stimulus. Classically, this "standardized" stimulus was an incision at the forearm, but "abdominal" incision has also been used.[5,6] Later, MACbar was defined as the concentration associated with a 50% probability of blocking a hemodynamic response to incision. The MACawake was defined as the concentration associated with a 50% probability of responding to shake and shout during recovery from anesthesia.

If inhaled anesthetics are combined with opioids, MAC, MACbar, and MACawake decrease synergistically with increasing doses of opioids. All opioids appear to produce a comparable level of synergism with inhaled anesthetics provided that they are administered in equipotent dose. Synergism has been shown in clinical trials for isoflurane, sevoflurane, and desflurane using a MAC reduction methodology.[5-11]

Sevoflurane–Remifentanil Expanding on the "one isobole" approach, as used in the MAC reduction studies, Manyam et al explored the interaction between sevoflurane and remifentanil on a wider range of effects.[4] Anesthetic effects included an assessment of sedation and responsiveness using the Observers Assessment of Alertness and Sedation (OAAS) scale (Table 3–2) and several surrogates of surgical pain to include loss of tolerance to electrical tetanic stimulus (up to 50 mA), pressure algometry (reproducible pressure on the anterior tibia), and 50°C hot temperature sensation. Given that this data was collected in volunteers, real surgical stimuli could not be tested. Unfortunately, the end-tidal vapor pressure was used as input for the model instead of effect-site concentrations. Not accounting for the hysteresis between end-tidal and effect-site concentrations of sevoflurane hampers the

TABLE 3–2 Observer's assessment of alertness and sedation score.

	Score
Responds readily to name spoken in normal tone	5
Lethargic response to name spoken in normal tone	4
Responds only after name is called loudly and/or repeatedly	3
Responds only after mild prodding or shaking	2
Does not respond to mild prodding or shaking	1
Does not respond to noxious stimulus	0

From Chernik D, Gillings D, Harriet L, et al. Validity and reliability of the Observer's Assessment of Alertness/Sedation Scale: study with intravenous midazolam. *J Clin Psychopharmacol*. 1990;10:244-251.

interpretation of the results. Follow up work using estimated effect-site concentrations in place of end-tidal concentration substantially improved predictions of drug effects in patients undergoing elective surgery.[3,12,13]

As clinical pharmacology researchers have explored anesthetic interactions between drugs, various approaches (ie, different equations and assumptions) have been developed to predict drug effect. Each approach has advantages and disadvantages. Heyse et al studied several available mathematical approaches to fitting a model to concentration-effect data to identify which approach works best. These researchers studied the interaction of sevoflurane and remifentanil for a number of clinical effects in patients undergoing elective surgery. Effects included a measure of responsiveness using the OAAS scale, tolerance to electrical tetanus, tolerance to laryngeal mask insertion, and tolerance to laryngoscopy.[2] They found that a mathematical approach called "the hierarchical model" fit their observations best.

Expansion to Other Inhalation Agent-Opioid Combinations Given that several other potent inhaled agent–opioid combinations are frequently used in clinical practice, researchers have conducted preliminary studies exploring that adaptability of sevoflurane–remifentanil interaction models to other combinations of potent inhaled agents and opioids. Using MAC equivalencies for potent inhaled agents and selected opioids,[14,15] model predictions from adapted isoflurane–fentanyl interaction models correlated well with observations in patients undergoing elective surgery.[13]

Sevoflurane–Remifentanil–Nitrous Oxide In addition to different opioid–inhalation agent combinations, more than 2 anesthetics are often used. Researchers have developed modeling approaches to estimate the interactions between 3 or more drugs[16] and also have conducted preliminary work to characterize the sevoflurane–remifentanil interaction in the presence of nitrous oxide with reasonable predictions of observed effects.[17] Future work is warranted to fully explore the numerous multidrug combinations frequently used in clinical practice and to explore the ability of model predictions of drug effect to match measures of drug effect with processed electroencephalographic (EEG) values (ie, entropy or bispectral index).

By using models of interactions for inhaled agents and opioids, the concept of "MAC reduction" can be expanded to a variety of more useful clinical end points than MAC. For example, interaction models provide predictions of interest to anesthesiologists such as concentrations necessary to block a given response in 95% of patients or predictions of concentrations where 95% of patients will have a return of response to a stimulus once an anesthetic is terminated. This form of information may be useful in a clinical practice through the use of bedside drug displays. As MAC reduction described how opioids reduced inhalation agent dosing requirements in the previous decades, the next generation of drug displays will provide real-time graphical illustrations of anesthetic drug interactions that may improve clinician's ability to optimize anesthetic dosing.

In summary, sevoflurane–remifentanil interaction models for a variety of sedative–hypnotic and analgesic effects have been published. The analgesic effects are markedly synergistic and the sedative–hypnotic effects are synergistic but to a lesser extent. These models can be expanded to other opioids and inhaled anesthetics using potency-converting factors. Recent work has introduced the addition of nitrous oxide to sevoflurane–opioid models of analgesic effects. Developing modeling techniques to better simulate anesthetics in combination will only improve predictions of overall drug effects.

Hypnotic–Opioid Interaction

In general, the interactions between propofol and opioids are similar to those described for inhalation agents and opioids. For analgesic effects, there is a pronounced synergistic interaction, for sedation and unresponsiveness, the interaction is synergistic, but to a lesser extent.

For total intravenous anesthesia (TIVA), characterizing interactions between propofol and opioids is different from characterizing interactions between inhaled agents and opioids. The main reason is that inhaled anesthetics provide both hypnosis and analgesia, whereas propofol is primarily only a sedative–hypnotic. This is reflected in clinical practice where some anesthetics may consist primarily of a potent inhaled agent and little or no opioid, whereas a TIVA will include a generous dose of opioid (ie, a continuous infusion of remifentanil).

In 1994, Smith et al studied the interaction between fentanyl and propofol on the 50% and 95% probability of loss of consciousness and motor response to incision.[18] They found a moderate synergistic interaction between fentanyl and propofol with a ceiling effect in the reduction of C_{50} for propofol once the fentanyl concentration was equal to or higher than 3 ng/ml. Due to the inconsistency in their methods, these results have remained controversial.

A major contribution to a better understanding of the interaction between propofol and opioids was provided by Vuyk et al.[14,19-23] This study characterized the propofol–alfentanil interaction on loss of response to eyelash reflex, laryngoscopy, intubation, and skin incision in patients undergoing elective surgery.

The propofol alfentanil interaction was synergistic. Alfentanil significantly reduced the propofol C_{50} and C_{95}. Despite the reduction in propofol requirements, hemodynamic stability did not improve. This suggests that the opioid–propofol interaction may be synergistic for potentially adverse hemodynamic effects as well.[22] Thus, dosing an opioid to reduce propofol requirements to improve hemodynamic stability does not appear to be a valid approach. To appreciate the relation between desired and undesired effects during anesthesia, simultaneous response surface modeling for multiple effects is required to untangle the complex coexistence of various clinical responses to stimuli while under anesthesia.[24,25]

Vuyk et al also simulated recovery times after combined administration of propofol and opioids with different context-sensitive half-times (alfentanil, sufentanil, fentanyl, and remifentanil). The researchers defined recovery as a transition time from the isobole of 50% probability of adequate anesthesia to an isobole of 50% probability of return of consciousness.[14] The latter remains a rather arbitrary decision and has not been validated. On the other hand, estimating recovery in this way is innovative and deserves further exploration. These simulations illustrate the advantage of remifentanil kinetic profile compared to other opioids, as it provides a significant reduction of C_{50} of propofol, without slowing recovery times.[14]

Propofol–remifentanil interactions have been extensively studied for a variety of effects. Some authors have presented results for processed and evoked EEG-derived indices, but not full response surface models,[26-29] while others have presented results for metrics of sedation and responsiveness (using OAAS),[1,16] EEG-derived end points,[1] and cardiorespiratory end points.[30-33]

For propofol–remifentanil, Zanderigo et al modeled the relationship between desired and undesired effects simultaneously by defining a new parameter called "well-being."[34] This was defined as a superposition of desired and undesired effects. These researchers characterized the synergistic response for both desired and adverse effects and used it to identify a preferred range of propofol and remifentanil concentrations that provide adequate anesthesia yet have the lowest risk of side effects.[34]

Hypnotic–Hypnotic Interaction

The hypnotic–hypnotic interaction is of interest since multiple sedative–hypnotics are frequently used as part of a combined anesthetic. For example, during induction, it is common to administer propofol followed by an inhaled anesthetic to maintain the hypnotic effect. Another common practice is to administer a benzodiazepine prior to induction. Benzodiazepines, in addition to having a distinct pharmacokinetic interaction with other sedatives, are likely to influence the pharmacodynamic effects of other sedatives.[35] The majority of hypnotic–hypnotic interaction studies focus on triple interactions between midazolam–opioids and propofol or on the propofol–inhaled anesthesia interaction.

Midazolam–Propofol Of particular interest is the interaction between midazolam and propofol. Several researchers have explored this interaction with varied results. Both midazolam and propofol influence each other's kinetics,[19,35,36] and the pharmacodynamic interactions for sedation and loss of responsiveness have been reported as synergistic by some authors[37-39] but additive by others.[40,41]

Short et al examined the triple interaction between midazolam, propofol, and alfentanil in their performance to evoke unresponsiveness to eye opening on verbal command (hypnosis) and anesthesia (defined as unresponsiveness to a short transcutaneous tetanic stimulus). The observations were standardized but were made at non–steady-state conditions (meaning the effect-site concentrations were in flux). The authors focused on differences in the C_{50} and did not explore other concentrations to report a full response surface model (ie, effect over a range of predicted opioid, sedative, or benzodiazepine effect-site concentrations). Combining midazolam with propofol, and alfentanil resulted in smaller-than-expected synergistic effects compared to interactions when given in dual combinations.[39] The interaction between propofol and midazolam appeared not to be attributed to pharmacokinetic shifts in the free fraction of each of the drugs; therefore, a pharmacodynamic mechanism on $GABA_A$ receptor level is suspected.[42]

Vinik et al used isobolographic techniques to determine whether combinations of midazolam–propofol, propofol–alfentanil, midazolam–alfentanil, and midazolam–propofol–alfentanil interacted in a synergistic or additive way. Only the midazolam–propofol interaction was not significantly different from additivity.[41] Fidler et al presented a mathematical approach, called the flexible interaction model, for triple anesthetic interactions.[40] Using data from previously published data,[39,43] they studied the interaction between midazolam and propofol. Their results confirmed the interaction to be additive.

A well-performed assessment of the midazolam–propofol interaction assessed at near steady state, using standardized end points of hypnotic drug effect, is still missing. Although it is clear that midazolam evokes a shift in the response surface between hypnotics and opioids, no full quantification of this interaction can be presented yet.

Sevoflurane–Propofol Concerning the propofol–sevoflurane interaction, both in vivo and in vitro studies indicate additive properties. Harris et al used the Dixon up-and-down method and isobolographic techniques to characterize the propofol–sevoflurane interaction for loss of consciousness and response to skin incision as additive.[44] Similarly, Sebel et al reported the potentiating effects of propofol and sevoflurane on GABA responses[45] and found that both drugs influenced receptor function in an additive manner. The additive properties suggest a single receptor site mechanism. In an accompanying editorial, Hemmings and Antognini[46] suggest that the complexity of neural networks and the involvement of multiple receptor types in vivo do not allow definite conclusions on the underlying molecular mechanism of anesthesia, based on population models only.

Schumacher et al studied the interaction between propofol and sevoflurane for EEG responses, as well as on the probability of response to standardized stimuli[47]; the report also found the interactions to be additive. A similar study by Diz et al confirmed the additive interaction between propofol and sevoflurane on the Bispectral Index Scale. One drawback to this study was the use of midazolam premedication and low-dose opioids.[48]

A Practical Guide for Interaction Model Information in Clinical Practice?

The above review of interaction models is impossible to memorize for later use in clinical care. The final section in the chapter presents methods of implementing this complex information in clinical practice.

DRUG ADVISORY DISPLAYS

Medical device companies have developed drug advisory displays using response surface models.[49] They provide real-time estimates of anesthetic drug effects such as onset and duration of unresponsiveness, analgesia, and muscle relaxation. With manual or automatic input of drug doses and infusion rates, these displays account for anesthetic drug interactions and patient demographics to provide individualized estimates of drug effects at the point of care. This type of information, readily available to clinicians in patient care areas, may lead to more rational, timely, and reproducible drug titration. Commercialized devices using this technology (SmartPilot View, Dräger, Lübeck, Germany; and Navigator Suite, GE Healthcare, Madison, WI) are presented in Figures 3–4 and 3–5, respectively.

These drug advisory displays provide population-based model predictions of drug effects, presented either as isoboles (SmartPilot View) or colored zones of desired effect on the effect-site concentration graphs (Navigator Suite). Proposed doses can be entered before administered to visualize

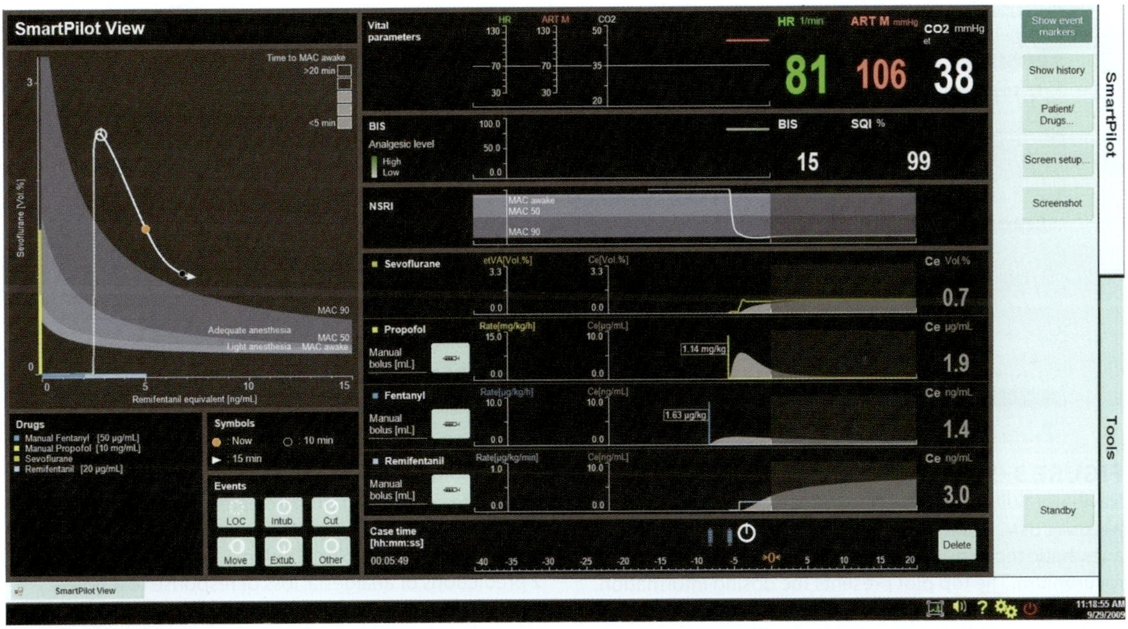

FIGURE 3–4 Example of the drug display system: SmartPilot View (Used with permission from Dräger, Lübeck, Germany). This display presents a general anesthetic using sevoflurane, propofol, remifentanil, and fentanyl. It presents a topographical plot of the interaction between sevoflurane and remifentanil (left plot). It illustrates the synergistic interaction of sevoflurane and remifentanil with gray-scaled isoboles. MACawake, MAC_{50}, and MAC_{90} present model predictions of loss of responsiveness. The estimated time to emergence from anesthesia is presented at the top of the isobole plot. It estimates the time required to reach the MACawake isobole. Fentanyl is converted into remifentanil equivalents and propofol is converted to sevoflurane equivalents so their contributions can be accounted for on the isobole plot. The vital signs, Bispectral Index Scale (BIS), the Noxious Stimulation Response Index (NSRI), and dose and effect over time are shown in the right plots. The series of plots on the lower right present the time course for each drug over the past 30 minutes and 30 minutes into the future. The current predicted effect-site concentrations (Ce) are presented on the far lower right. The time line indicates that induction with fentanyl and propofol occurred 5 minutes in the past. A series of symbols (light green buttons) are used as event markers during a surgical procedure (ie, loss of consciousness, intubation, incision) on both the topographical plot and the dose and effect over time plots. These markers are useful in calibrating the display to individual patients; they allow clinicians to mark the concentration pairs required to meet the anesthetic demands at that event. This display is designed to be used with an anesthesia machine. It collects dosing information either automatically (ie, drug infusion rates and end-tidal potent inhaled agent levels) or manually (ie, intravenous drug bolus doses) to present predictions of drug effect. MAC, minimum alveolar concentration.

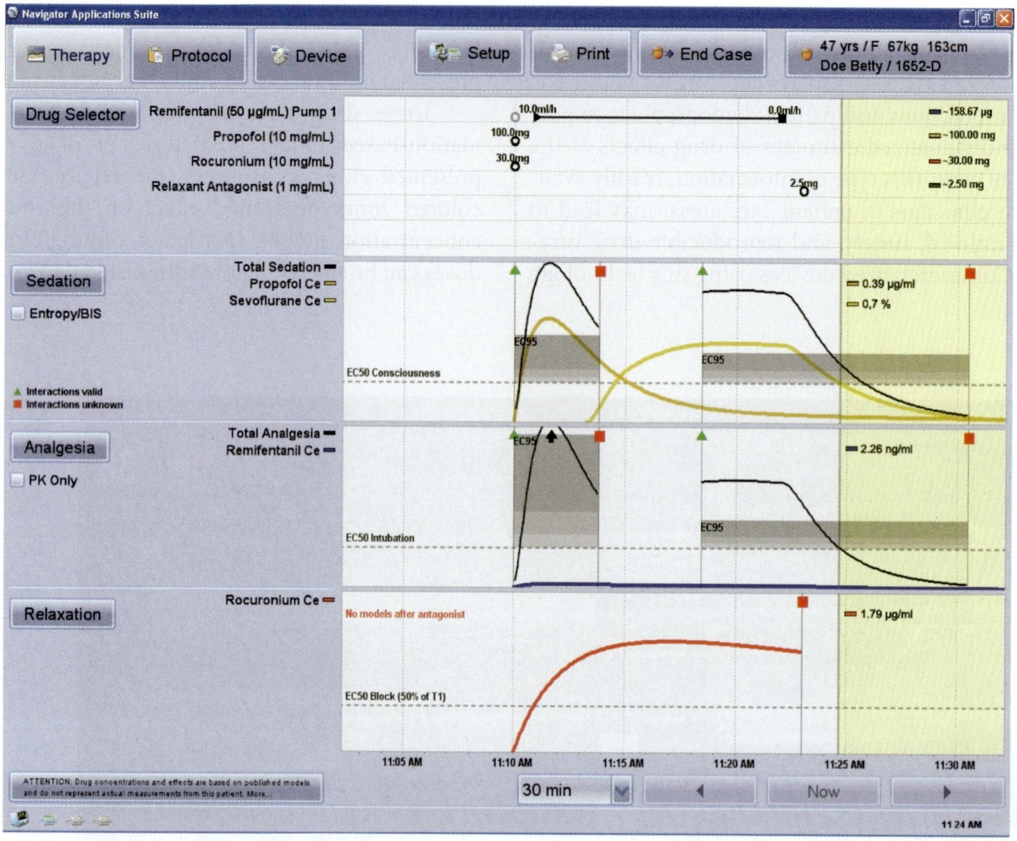

FIGURE 3–5 Example of the drug display system: Navigator Suite (Used with permission from GE Healthcare, Wisconsin, USA). This display presents a total intravenous anesthetic technique with propofol, remifentanil, and rocuronium. The top plot presents the dosing information. Infusion rates and bolus doses are presented as horizontal black lines and black dots, respectively. The cumulative dose for each drug is presented on the right. Beneath the top row, the display presents 3 model predictions over time: the probability of sedation (second plot), analgesia (third plot), and muscle relaxation (bottom plot). Along the horizontal axes of these plots, the solid lines represent the most recent 30 minutes and the dashed lines represent 10 minutes into the future. The vertical axis for each plot is the effect-site concentration (Ce). Individual drug effect-site concentrations are presented as colored lines: yellow for propofol, light blue for remifentanil, and red for rocuronium. The probabilities of unresponsiveness (total sedation) and analgesia from the combined effects of remifentanil and propofol are represented as black lines. EC_{50} and EC_{95} represent the effect-site concentrations associated with a 50% and 95% probability of unresponsiveness (second plot) and analgesia (third plot). The analgesia plot contains 2 predictions of analgesia: loss of response to a severe stimulus (laryngoscopy with intubation) and loss of response to a moderate stimulus (30 pounds per square inch of tibial pressure). This stimulus is used as a surrogate for moderate postoperative pain (postop analgesia). The current effect-site concentrations for each drug are presented on the right of each plot. The synergistic interactions between propofol and remifentanil are easily visualized. For example, the contribution of propofol to the analgesic effects of remifentanil leads to a significant increase in overall analgesia (third row). To a lesser extent, the contribution of remifentanil to the sedating effects of propofol leads to an increase in sedation (second row). EC_{50} block (50% of T1), effect-site concentration associated with a 50% probability of 1 twitch in a train of 4-twitch stimulus, PK/PD, pharmacokinetic/pharmacodynamic.

how drugs will behave. This information may be useful in identifying the appropriate dose for induction of anesthesia. Once the dose is delivered, observed patient responses can be recorded on the drug display and used to calibrate future predictions of drug effect.

SmartPilot View and Navigator Suite displays have similar advisory goals, but differences in predictions of drug effect between the 2 displays are to be expected. The most likely reason for these differences are related to the different models and data sets used as reference in both displays. For interested readers, additional information describing differences between models is presented in the appendix. In order to guarantee optimal performance of this new technology, adequately obtained response surfaces must be available and prospectively validated.

The SmartPilot View advisory screen incorporates an additional tool to assist the clinician in dose finding: the "noxious stimulation response index" (NSRI).[50] NSRI translates the relation between the individual effect-site concentrations and population responsiveness in an index that can be used for quantifying "depth of anesthesia." The NSRI can be used as a measure of potency of the combined anesthetics and therefore, can be used to compare different anesthetic combinations objectively. Using pharmacokinetic characteristics (ie, redistribution and elimination), NSRI predicts the time to recovery (defined as return of response to shake and shout). Currently, the NSRI has only been published for TIVA, but an adapted NSRI for inhalation agent–based anesthesia is being developed. This next version of the NSRI will be able to transition between TIVA and inhaled agent–based anesthetics.

Advantages of Drug Advisory Displays

The introduction of drug advisory displays in clinical practice has several potential advantages. One advantage is they are useful in drug titration. In many studies, including MAC-related studies, interactions are compared to the 50% probability of response isobole. From a practical point of view, this is a "pretty lousy" anesthetic. The 95% isobole is a much more appealing target as this isobole correlates with near-maximal effect while minimizing overdose. When targeting effects above the 95% isobole, the risk of side effects increases with little gain on the desired effect. This approach for drug titration has been lyrically described by Egan and Shafer as "surfing the waves."[51] That is—surfing the 3-dimensional pharmacokinetic/pharmacodynamic interaction waves!

A second advantage is they provide a pharmacologic reference, allowing clinicians to titrate to a more reproducible and predictable anesthetic. For example, consider an elderly patient that is sensitive to anesthetics and loses responsiveness earlier than expected. The display provides predicted effect-site concentration at the time of unresponsiveness. Where these concentrations lie in relation to population isoboles can be used to guide future administration of sedative–hypnotics during surgery. If the patient became unresponsive at concentrations just below the 50% isobole, that information could be used to calibrate anesthetic dosing to achieve a combined effect close to that isobole.

A third advantage is they are a potential surrogate to TCI where TCI is unavailable. TCI enjoys wide spread use throughout Europe and Asia. Extensive clinical experience and several validation studies demonstrate the clinical value of this technology.[52,53] Due to regulatory differences, TCI pumps are not yet allowed in the United States.[51] In the absence of TCI pumps, marking observed responses in relation to population isoboles presented on drug displays makes maintaining steady-state in effect easier to do. Moreover, one may use isoboles to adjust the balance between opioids and hypnotics in such a way that the desired effect is maintained while selecting drug doses that provide shorter recovery times (eg, higher dose of remifentanil and lower dose of propofol). Thus, commercialized drug displays could serve as an alternative to TCI.

A fourth advantage is that drug displays provide a visual confirmation of steady-state conditions. This may be especially helpful when clinicians are tempted to administer additional anesthetic before a previous dose change (ie, a change in vaporizer setting, a change in infusion pump rate, or bolus dose) has had a chance to reach its peak or new steady-state level. This feature improves safety and reproducibility of proposed dosing schemes.

Limitations of Drug Advisory Displays

There are several limitations to these drug display predictions. First, drug displays only provide predictions of drug effects based on population models. As such, even if an anesthetic is dosed to achieve an effect-site concentration at or near the 95% isobole, 5% of patients may have some responses. Second, caution should be used just after bolusing drugs. Predictions of drug effects are less accurate during rapid changes in effect-site concentrations. Third, predictions of sedation and responsiveness may overestimate the level of unresponsiveness in a stimulated state. Fourth, model predictions, although useful for titrating anesthetic dosing, are not perfect. Models used to make predictions are improving with more and more solid observations from methodologically optimal designed studies.

Many drugs, besides opioids and hypnotics, have sedative properties and may affect the accuracy of model predictions when used in combination with the above-mentioned drugs. Dexmedetomidine, clonidine, and ketamine are used regularly as adjuvants in anesthesia. For now, these drugs have not been modeled in such a way that they can be applied in advisory screens. The interpretation of advisory screens should be considered as a reproducible aid to titrate anesthetics, but vigilance must be maintained when adjuncts are used that models do not account for.

Advisory screen drug displays only predict a probability of response, and actual responses may vary. Even if the probability of a response to a standardized stimulus is below 1%, an individual may still respond. That is not in contradiction with the prediction. Based on model predictions, anesthesiologists can conclude that such an event is rare in view of population model predictions for a given drug dose. This type of advisory information may help defend dosing choices during juridical discussions. Additionally, once an unexpected response is observed in a patient, a level of anesthesia with lower probability of response can be maintained throughout the rest of the case, decreasing the chances of a second unexpected event.

Summary

In summary, the theoretical concepts to model anesthetic drug interactions are currently translated to practical tools in the form of drug advisory displays. The displays bring the massive amount of population data to the bedside, in a user friendly way. These displays have large potential to optimize drug titration towards a more reproducible, evidence-based approach in daily clinical practice. They have the potential to increase clinician confidence that their dosing regimen is appropriate, decrease the trainee learning curve in identifying the appropriate dose, and decrease the incidence of under- and/or overdosing. Of course, the real clinical value of this technology will only fully be appreciated once a wider availability has been realized.

REFERENCES

1. Bouillon TW, Bruhn J, Radulescu L, et al. Pharmacodynamic interaction between propofol and remifentanil regarding hypnosis, tolerance of laryngoscopy, bispectral index, and electroencephalographic approximate entropy. *Anesthesiology*. 2004;100(6):1353-1372.
2. Heyse B, Proost JH, Schumacher PM, et al. Sevoflurane remifentanil interaction: comparison of different response surface models. *Anesthesiology*. 2012;116(2):311-323.
3. Johnson KB, Syroid ND, Gupta DK, et al. An evaluation of remifentanil-sevoflurane response surface models in patients emerging from anesthesia: model improvement using effect-site sevoflurane concentrations. *Anesth Analg*. 2010;111(2):387-394.
4. Manyam SC, Gupta DK, Johnson KB, et al. Opioid-volatile anesthetic synergy: a response surface model with remifentanil and sevoflurane as prototypes. *Anesthesiology*. 2006;105(2):267-278.

4a. Mertens MJ, Olofsen E, Engbers FH, Burm AG, Bovill JG, Vuyk J. Propofol reduces perioperative remifentanil requirements in a synergistic manner:response surface modeling of perioperative remifentanil-propofol interactions. *Anesthesiology*. 2003;99(2):347-359.

5. Katoh T, Ikeda K. The effects of fentanyl on sevoflurane requirements for loss of consciousness and skin incision. *Anesthesiology*. 1998;88(1):18-24.
6. Katoh T, Nakajima Y, Moriwaki G, et al. Sevoflurane requirements for tracheal intubation with and without fentanyl. *Br J Anaesth*. 1999;82(4):561-565.
7. Sebel PS, Glass PS, Fletcher JE, Murphy MR, Gallagher C, Quill T. Reduction of the MAC of desflurane with fentanyl. *Anesthesiology*. 1992;76(1):52-59.
8. Albertin A, Casati A, Bergonzi P, Fano G, Torri G. Effects of two target-controlled concentrations (1 and 3 ng/ml) of remifentanil on MAC(BAR) of sevoflurane. *Anesthesiology*. 2004;100(2):255-259.
9. Lang E, Kapila A, Shlugman D, Hoke JF, Sebel PS, Glass PS. Reduction of isoflurane minimal alveolar concentration by remifentanil. *Anesthesiology*. 1996;85(4):721-728.

10. Brunner MD, Braithwaite P, Jhaveri R, et al. MAC reduction of isoflurane by sufentanil. *Br J Anaesth*; 1994; 72(1):42-46.
11. Hall RI, Szlam F, Hug CC Jr.. The enflurane-sparing effect of alfentanil in dogs. *Anesth Analg*. 1987;66(12): 1287-1291.
12. Johnson KB, Syroid ND, Gupta DK, et al. An evaluation of remifentanil propofol response surfaces for loss of responsiveness, loss of response to surrogates of painful stimuli and laryngoscopy in patients undergoing elective surgery. *Anesth Analg*. 2008;106(2):471-479.
13. Syroid ND, Johnson KB, Pace NL, et al. Response surface model predictions of emergence and response to pain in the recovery room: an evaluation of patients emerging from an isoflurane and fentanyl anesthetic. *Anesth Analg*. 2010;111(2):380-386.
14. Vuyk J, Mertens MJ, Olofsen E, Burm AG, Bovill JG. Propofol anesthesia and rational opioid selection: determination of optimal EC50-EC95 propofol-opioid concentrations that assure adequate anesthesia and a rapid return of consciousness. *Anesthesiology*. 1997; 87(6):1549-1562.
15. Eger EI II, Brandstater B, Saidman LJ, Regan MJ, Severinghaus JW, Munson ES. Equipotent alveolar concentrations of methoxyflurane, halothane, diethyl ether, fluroxene, cyclopropane, xenon and nitrous oxide in the dog. *Anesthesiology*. 1965;26(6):771-777.
16. Minto CF, Schnider TW, Short TG, Gregg KM, Gentilini A, Shafer SL. Response surface model for anesthetic drug interactions. *Anesthesiology*. 2000;92(6):1603-1616.
17. Vereecke HEM, Proost JH, Heyse B, et al. Interaction between nitrous oxide, sevoflurane and opioids: A response surface approach. *Anesthesiology* 2013;118(4): 894-902.
18. Smith C, McEwan AI, Jhaveri R, et al. The interaction of fentanyl on the Cp50 of propofol for loss of consciousness and skin incision. *Anesthesiology*. 1994; 81(4): 820-828, discussion 26A.
19. Vuyk J, Hennis PJ, Burm AG, de Voogt JW, Spierdijk J. Comparison of midazolam and propofol in combination with alfentanil for total intravenous anesthesia. *Anesth Analg*. 1990;71(6):645-650.
20. Vuyk J, Lim T, Engbers FH, Burm AG, Vletter AA, Bovill JG. Pharmacodynamics of alfentanil as a supplement to propofol or nitrous oxide for lower abdominal surgery in female patients. *Anesthesiology*. 1993;78(6):1036-1045, discussion 23A.
21. Vuyk J, Lim T, Engbers FH, Burm AG, Vletter AA, Bovill JG. The pharmacodynamic interaction of propofol and alfentanil during lower abdominal surgery in women. *Anesthesiology*. 1995;83(1):8-22.
22. Vuyk J, Engbers FH, Burm AG, et al. Pharmacodynamic interaction between propofol and alfentanil when given for induction of anesthesia. *Anesthesiology*. 1996;84(2):288-299.
23. Vuyk J. Pharmacokinetic and pharmacodynamic interactions between opioids and propofol. *J Clin Anesth*. 1997;9(6 suppl):23S-26S.
24. Billard V, Moulla F, Bourgain JL, Megnigbeto A, Stanski DR. Hemodynamic response to induction and intubation. Propofol/fentanyl interaction. *Anesthesiology*. 1994;81(6):1384-1393.
25. Kazama T, Ikeda K, Morita K. The pharmacodynamic interaction between propofol and fentanyl with respect to the suppression of somatic or hemodynamic responses to skin incision, peritoneum incision, and abdominal wall retraction. *Anesthesiology*. 1998;89(4):894-906.
26. Bruhn J, Bouillon TW, Radulescu L, Hoeft A, Bertaccini E, Shafer SL. Correlation of approximate entropy, bispectral index, and spectral edge frequency 95 (SEF95) with clinical signs of "anesthetic depth" during coadministration of propofol and remifentanil. *Anesthesiology*. 2003;98(3):621-627.
27. Ropcke H, Konen-Bergmann M, Cuhls M, Bouillon T, Hoeft A. Propofol and remifentanil pharmacodynamic interaction during orthopedic surgical procedures as measured by effects on bispectral index. *J Clin Anesth*. 2001;13(3):198-207.
28. Vanluchene AL, Vereecke H, Thas O, Mortier EP, Shafer SL, Struys MM. Spectral entropy as an electroencephalographic measure of anesthetic drug effect: a comparison with bispectral index and processed midlatency auditory evoked response. *Anesthesiology*. 2004;101(1):34-42.
29. Schwilden H, Fechner J, Albrecht S, Hering W, Ihmsen H, Schuttler J. Testing and modelling the interaction of alfentanil and propofol on the EEG. *Eur J Anaesthesiol*. 2003;20(5):363-372.
30. Bouillon T, Schmidt C, Garstka G, et al. Pharmacokinetic-pharmacodynamic modeling of the respiratory depressant effect of alfentanil. *Anesthesiology*. 1999; 91(1): 144-155.
31. Nieuwenhuijs DJ, Olofsen E, Romberg RR, et al. Response surface modeling of remifentanil-propofol interaction on cardiorespiratory control and bispectral index. *Anesthesiology*. 2003;98(2):312-322.
32. LaPierre CD, Johnson KB, Randall BR, White JL, Egan TD. An exploration of remifentanil-propofol combinations that lead to a loss of response to esophageal instrumentation, a loss of responsiveness, and/or onset of intolerable ventilatory depression. *Anesth Analg*. 2011; 113(3):490-499.

33. LaPierre CD, Johnson KB, Randall BR, Egan TD. A simulation study of common propofol and propofol-opioid dosing regimens for upper endoscopy: implications on the time course of recovery. *Anesthesiology*. 2012;117(2):252-262.
34. Zanderigo E, Sartori V, Sveticic G, et al. The well-being model: a new drug interaction model for positive and negative effects. *Anesthesiology*. 2006;104(4):742-753.
35. Lichtenbelt BJ, Olofsen E, Dahan A, van Kleef JW, Struys MM, Vuyk J. Propofol reduces the distribution and clearance of midazolam. *Anesth Analg*. 2010; 110(6):1597-1606.
36. Vuyk J, Lichtenbelt BJ, Olofsen E, van Kleef JW, Dahan A. Mixed-effects modeling of the influence of midazolam on propofol pharmacokinetics. *Anesth Analg*. 2009. 108(5): 1522-1530.
37. McClune S, McKay AC, Wright PM, Patterson CC, Clarke RS. Synergistic interaction between midazolam and propofol. *Br J Anaesth*. 1992;69(3):240-245.
38. Short TG, Chui PT. Propofol and midazolam act synergistically in combination. *Br J Anaesth*. 1991; 67(5):539-545.
39. Short TG, Plummer JL, Chui PT. Hypnotic and anaesthetic interactions between midazolam, propofol and alfentanil. *Br J Anaesth*. 1992;69(2):162-167.
40. Fidler M, Kern SE. Flexible interaction model for complex interactions of multiple anesthetics. *Anesthesiology*. 2006;105(2):286-296.
41. Vinik HR, Bradley EL Jr, Kissin I. Triple anesthetic combination: propofol-midazolam-alfentanil. *Anesth Analg*. 1994;78(2):354-358.
42. Teh J, Short TG, Wong J, Tan P. Pharmacokinetic interactions between midazolam and propofol: an infusion study. *Br J Anaesth*. 1994;72(1):62-65.
43. Kern SE, Xie G, White JL, Egan TD. A response surface analysis of propofol-remifentanil pharmacodynamic interaction in volunteers. *Anesthesiology*. 2004;100(6): 1373-1381.
44. Harris RS, Lazar O, Johansen JW, Sebel PS. Interaction of propofol and sevoflurane on loss of consciousness and movement to skin incision during general anesthesia. *Anesthesiology*. 2006;104(6):1170-1175.
45. Sebel LE, Richardson JE, Singh SP, Bell SV, Jenkins A. Additive effects of sevoflurane and propofol on gamma-aminobutyric acid receptor function. *Anesthesiology*. 2006;104(6):1176-1183.
46. Hemmings HC Jr,. Antognini JF. Do general anesthetics add up? *Anesthesiology*. 2006;104(6):1120-1122.
47. Schumacher PM, Dossche J, Mortier EP, Luginbuehl M, Bouillon TW, Struys MM. Response surface modeling of the interaction between propofol and sevoflurane. *Anesthesiology*. 2009;111(4):790-804.
48. Diz JC, Del Rio R, Lamas A, Mendoza M, Duran M, Ferreira LM. Analysis of pharmacodynamic interaction of sevoflurane and propofol on Bispectral Index during general anaesthesia using a response surface model. *Br J Anaesth*. 2010;104(6):733-739.
49. Short TG. Using response surfaces to expand the utility of MAC. *Anesth Analg*. 2010;111(2):249-251.
50. Luginbuhl M, Schumacher PM, Vuilleumier P, et al. Noxious stimulation response index: a novel anesthetic state index based on hypnotic-opioid interaction. *Anesthesiology*. 2010;112(4):872-880.
51. Egan TD, Shafer SL. Target-controlled infusions for intravenous anesthetics: surfing USA not! *Anesthesiology*. 2003;99(5):1039-1041.
52. Coppens M, van Limmen JG, Schnider T, et al. Study of the time course of the clinical effect of propofol compared with the time course of the predicted effect-site concentration: performance of three pharmacokinetic-dynamic models. *Br J Anaesth*. 2010;104(4):452-458.
53. Struys M, Versichelen L, Thas O, Herregods L, Rolly G. Comparison of computer-controlled administration of propofol with two manually controlled infusion techniques. *Anaesthesia*. 1997;52(1):41-50.

APPENDIX

Origin of Mathematical Models for Anesthetic Drug–Drug Interactions

MODELING CONCEPTS

Modeling is the technique of defining a mathematical equation that fits a data set as accurately as possible. Linear regression could be considered as a rudimentary form of modeling. A linear regression analysis of a data set determines the best-fitting linear correlation between data couples by minimizing the sum of squares of all perpendicular distances from each observation to the proposed line (least-squares principle). As such, the optimal value for parameters a and b in an equation of the form $y = a \cdot x + b$ can be determined from an observational data set. The resulting linear equation describes the correlation of the data couples within the population with the least possible scatter (or residual error). Consequently, the resulting equation can be used to predict prospectively which y can be expected for every known x, with the smallest possible error.

In many pharmacologic processes, the equations that best describe the data are nonlinear in nature. For example, the classical dose- or concentration-response curve is generally described as a sigmoidal E_{max} curve, also called the Hill equation. This equation includes 4 parameters that need to be estimated from data: baseline value of the effect variable (E_0), maximal possible effect obtained at high doses (E_{max}), the effective dose or concentration related to 50% of E_{max} (ED_{50} or EC_{50}), and the slope of the dose or concentration versus effect curve (γ). The ED_{50} or EC_{50} represents potency of the drug, and E_{max} reflects efficacy of the drug.

In order to fit nonlinear equations (also called structural models) on a data set, a statistical approach called *nonlinear mixed effects modeling* (as performed by the software package NONMEM (ICON Development Solutions, Hanover, MD) has become the standard methodology. Several structural models have been applied on anesthesia interaction data. We will review the major differences between structural models later.

In NONMEM, the optimal structural model is selected when it results in the lowest objective function value (OFV), that is, the minimum value of the "−2 log likelihood" function. A low OFV reflects the ability of the model to describe the data with the least amount of scatter. Mixed effects refers to the combination of fixed effects and random effects. Fixed effects are sources of variability in the observation that are the result of covariates that we can measure. For example, we can categorize the studied subjects into relevant groups according to differences in fixed effects (eg, age, weight). If the inclusion of a fixed effect in the structural model improves the fit on the data set significantly, this covariate is considered a relevant improvement for the predictive performance of the model. On the other hand, even after having defined a number of significant fixed effects in the structural model, a residual amount of error will always remain. This is caused by random effects—for example, interindividual variability and residual error. One can only speculate about the causes of these random effects. They are the result of all mechanisms (biological or technical in nature) that evoke the biological variability in individual patients and individual observation. The random effects can therefore never be fully controlled, but they can be quantified as a level of uncertainty in the predictions of the model.

METHODOLOGIC ISSUES

When deciding on which methodology to use for quantifying interactions of drugs on a clinical effect, several well-known sources of variability should be considered (and possibly controlled) in advance. First, a careful definition of the relevant end points of effect needs to be decided. Secondly, maximal reproducibility of the pharmacologic condition during the observations is mandatory.

Defining Relevant End Points of Anesthesia

The therapeutic drug effects from the various components of anesthesia (hypnosis, immobility, analgesia) are commonly measured and expressed as dichotomous clinical end points in the individual patient, or alternatively as a "probability of response" in the population. The dichotomous approach describes the presence or absence of a cognitive, motor, or autonomic response to a verbal, tactile, or painful stimulus. Examples of commonly used stimuli to test responsiveness are loud or repeated name calling, eye lash reflex, shake and shout, a movement to a painful stimulus such as trapezius squeeze, tetanic electrical stimulus or tibial pressure, introduction of a laryngeal mask, laryngoscopy, tracheal intubation, and surgical incision. With these end points, no gradual change in effect can be observed. A response can only be either present or absent. To bypass this shortcoming, stimuli with progressively intensified arousal capacity are applied in consecutive steps, in order to obtain a gradual impression of the clinical onset of anesthetic effect in the individual patient. The observers assessment of alertness and sedation scale (OAAS) is an example of such a gradual intensifying stimulation test.[1,2] A modified version of this scale (see Table 3–2) is commonly used as a reference of clinical effect of anesthesia.

By means of logistic regression, dichotomous individual observations can be translated into a probability of response within the population. The minimal alveolar concentration (MAC) is a well-known example of a population-based measure of drug effect. One MAC of an inhaled anesthetic represents the minimal alveolar concentration needed to evoke a 50% probability of immobility in a population of patients after applying a "standardized" incision.[3]

Continuous measures can also be used to describe anesthetic drug effects. For example, cerebral hypnotic drug effects can be quantified by electroencephalographic-derived indices (such as Bispectral Index [Covidien], M-Entropy [Datex-Ohmeda]).[1,4] Monitoring the cortical activity during anesthesia has contributed largely to a more detailed understanding of the neurophysiologic processes involved in anesthesia and even has triggered a new functional definition of anesthesia.[5]

In contrast to hypnotic effects, the continuous quantification of the balance between nociception and antinociception remains a challenge. A search for new measurements of this complex concept is still ongoing.[6,7] By evaluating the relation between interacting drug combinations and the output of alleged monitors of nociception-antinociception may help differentiating their usefulness for clinical use. Such studies should deal with the fundamental issue concerning how the dose-response curve between interacting drugs and the continuous measures of hypnotic or analgesic effect are influenced by the balance between opioids and hypnotics.

Controlling the Pharmacologic Condition

The observations of anesthetic effect can be performed either in pharmacologic non–steady-state or, preferably, in steady-state conditions. The pharmacologic conditions obtained at the biophase should be as reproducible as possible in order to define interaction models that have direct clinical applicability. Therefore, all methodology developed for studying anesthetic interactions should include a precise description of the method of drug delivery. Currently, modern vaporizers and target-controlled infusion pumps provide excellent tools for the clinician to titrate drugs toward the desired effect-site concentration in a reproducible way.

The end-tidal concentration of an inhaled anesthetic is closely related to the individual plasma concentration of the drug. When kept constant over a sufficiently long equilibration time, a steady-state concentration at the effect site can be assumed. For intravenous anesthetic drugs, there exists no direct individual measurement of plasma or biophase concentration. Therefore, population derived pharmacokinetic-pharmacodynamic (PKPD) models are used to predict the plasma-concentration and effect-site concentration with the least possible error. Much progress has been made in the clinical applicability of contemporary PKPD models, but the use of population estimations—by definition—remains open for prediction errors in the individual patient[8]. Still, as many of the population PKPD models used in interaction studies are commercially available, any anesthesiologist should be able to reproduce the effective drug concentrations described in the model estimations. When studying interactions, computer-controlled drug administration for total intravenous anesthesia is strongly recommended. It standardizes the speed of drug infusion, the timing and magnitude of bolus and maintenance infusions in such a way that the resulting effects reach a higher reproducibility compared to manually administered drug titrations.

Study Design

Studying drug–drug interactions requires a specific study design for optimal data collection. Short et al performed simulations for several study designs in order to determine the most efficient inclusion methodology.[9] The researchers showed that the optimal design for an interaction study (with minimum number of patients and maximal accuracy in prediction of the observed responses) is a so-called "criss-cross" design. In this setting, the study population is randomized to 2 groups. Group 1 receives drug A as a constant pseudo–steady-state effect-site concentration at several predefined targets, while drug B is administered in brief zero-order step-up infusions. Group 2 receives drug B in a constant amount, while drug A varies to maximal effect. This method appears to provide sufficient spread in the data for accurate model building while only including a limited number of patients for the study. However, the exact number of patients as concluded by the study of Short remains open for debate as this number is only valid when all assumptions made by Short are met.[9]

STRUCTURAL MODELS OF INTERACTION

Several mathematical approaches have been proposed to model interaction. A short review of the advantages and disadvantages of currently proposed mathematical equations is therefore discussed here.

Isobolographic Approach

Isoboles are lines that represent conditions of equal effect in relation to the doses (or concentrations) of 2 interacting drugs, respectively, plotted on the x- and y-axes (Figure A3–1). The isobole is the line that connects all drug combinations that evoke an equal effect of interest (eg, the 50% probability of response to incision), including the dose of a solitary administration of drug A or B. Many methods have been proposed to fit isoboles on clinical data sets ranging from drawing by hand to methods that add more statistical rigor. For a thorough review of all these methods, we refer the reader to other publications.[10] In general, a major advantage of the isobolographic approach is the relative simplicity of the statistical method and the availability of software to do so. However, 1 isobole does not contain information on the total spectrum of desired anesthesia effects. For example, a strong synergism between drugs A and B, observed at the 50% probability of response level, does not guarantee a comparable intense synergism at the 95% probability of response. If only the 50% probability of response is targeted during the study,

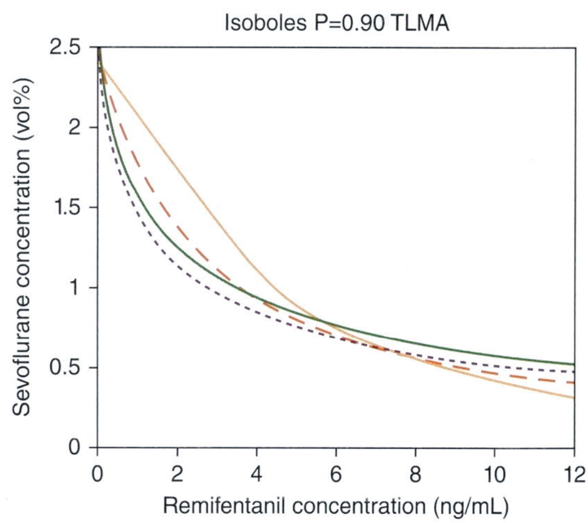

FIGURE A3–1 Comparison of estimations from 4 interaction models using isoboles for 90% probability ($P = 0.90$) of tolerance to laryngeal mask airway placement (TMLA). The thin dashed line represents the reduced Greco model, the thin solid line represents the Minto model, the dotted line represents the scaled C_{500} hierarchical model, and the thick solid line represents the fixed C_{500} hierarchical model.

information on more intense levels of drug effect might not be extractable from the data set.

Logistic Regression Model

For a single drug, the natural logarithm of the odds ratio of drug effect (called the logit) can be expressed in terms of drug concentrations.[11]

$$\text{Logit}(P) = \ln(\text{odds}) = \ln\left(\frac{P}{1-P}\right) = \beta_0 + \beta_1 \times C \quad \text{(Eqn. 1)}$$

where P is probability of response, β_0 and β_1 are estimated parameters, and C is the concentration of the drug. For multiple drugs, this can be expanded by using a linear function of the concentrations of both drugs as shown in Eqn. 2.

$$\text{Logit}(P) = \beta_0 + \beta_1 \times C_A + \beta_2 \times C_B + \beta_3 \times C_A \times C_B \quad \text{(Eqn. 2)}$$

Recalculation allows computing all ranges of probability of response (including EC_{50} and EC_{95}) for 1 drug in relation to different concentrations of the other drug according to Eqn. 3.

$$EC_{P,B} = \frac{\ln\left(\frac{P}{1-P}\right) - \beta_0 - \beta_1 \times C_A}{\beta_2 + \beta_3 \times C_A} \quad \text{(Eqn. 3)}$$

where $EC_{P,B}$ is the effective concentration of drug B to reach a probability of response equal to P, β_0, β_1, β_2, and β_3 are estimated parameters, and C_A is the concentration of drug A. By substituting a value of 0 for C_A in Eqn. 3, the expected effect of a single drug administration of drug B can be solved. Some limitations in this approach remain, such as the presence of a remaining baseline effect estimation, even when no drugs are administered.

Response Surface Interaction Models

Berenbaum[12] and Prichard and Shipman[13,14] pioneered the use of 3-dimensional models of interaction. These models present the dose of drugs A and B on the x and y axes in relation to the studied effect in the z axis. Very rudimentarily explained, their methods extract a primary 3-dimensional model of presumed additivity between drugs A and B, based on the dose-effect curves of the respective solitary administrations of drug A and B. The resulting presumed 3-dimensional additivity model is fitted on the observed data set, and then it is decided whether data points are situated below or above the response surface. Sühnel[15] presented a nonparametric response surface method and Greco et al[16] and Weinstein[17] presented parametric approaches. These models differ with respect to the functional interpretation of the parameters included in the equations. Minto and Bouillon also contributed to the 3-dimensional modeling by providing flexible solutions for anesthesia-related interaction studies. The response surface models used most in anesthesia-related studies are reviewed in depth in the next section. This review is mainly based on the results of the comparative interaction study of Heyse et al.[18]

In general, a response surface needs to define probability of response or probability of no response in relation to an effective drug concentration. The probability of tolerating a stimulus in relation to a drug concentration can be expressed by a sigmoidal equation of the form:

$$P = \frac{U^{\gamma}}{1+U^{\gamma}} \quad \text{(Eqn. 4)}$$

where U represents an effective drug concentration divided by its respective C_{50}. This normalized concentration is advocated as a solution to cope with differences in potency between drugs. γ is the slope factor of the sigmoidal equation that relates drug concentration to probability of response. When P is set at a fixed percentage (eg, 50% or 95% depending on the effect of interest), the corresponding U can be calculated from this equation. In the case of an effect that is evoked by multiple drugs, U can be replaced by one of the interaction equations that we describe later. The final result is a structural model that can be applied for fitting 3-dimensional response surfaces to a data set that contains multiple observations of effect over a wide range of combined drug concentrations.

Greco Model

The Greco model (Eqn. 5) defines U as the total (normalized) effect-site concentration of the interaction between drugs A and B, being a sum of the normalized effect-site concentration of respectively drug A (U_A) and drug B (U_B) plus an additional interaction factor ($\alpha * U_A * U_B$) that is dependent of U_A and U_B. The equation parameters are derived from data revealing the 50% effect isobole and subsequently extrapolated to other levels of effect.[10,16,19,20]

$$U = U_A + U_B + \alpha \cdot U_A \cdot U_B \quad \text{(Eqn. 5)}$$

When the dimensionless interaction parameter $\alpha = 0$, additivity is defined; $\alpha < 0$ indicates infra-additivity, and $\alpha > 0$ supra-additivity. This model implies some assumptions: Both drug A and B are expected to be intrinsically able to evoke the maximal clinical effect. The slope of the dose-response curve is a constant for all combinations of drug A and B. Finally, the single interaction fraction α is considered to be applicable for the total response surface and does not allow any flexibility for adapting the shape of the interaction curve at different levels of drug effect.

Reduced Greco Model

In anesthesia-related studies, involving opioids and hypnotics, these assumptions appear not to be valid at all times. Opioids have a low observed effect on hypnotic end points of anesthesia (eg, the probability of response to a verbal command). As such, unrealistic high C_{50} values are estimated when using the full Greco model as a structural model. In this case, a reduced form of the Greco model is advocated by implementing the assumption that opioids have no direct hypnotic effect at all but rather evoke their hypnotic effect by interacting with the potency of the hypnotic. As such, when U_B is set as the normalized concentration of opioids, it can be considered to have a negligible contribution to the total effect in the formula (U_B is left out). However, U_B remains a cofactor for the interaction fraction $\alpha * U_A * U_B$. Additionally, in order to allow an unambiguous estimation of C_{50B} from data, α is set to 1. The final formula in its reduced form can be solved to

$$U = U_A \cdot (1 + U_B) \quad \text{(Eqn. 6)}$$

where U, U_A, and U_B are the normalized concentrations of respectively the combined drugs A + B, and drug A and drug B separately, respectively. The clinical meaning of this C_{50B} in the reduced Greco formula can be defined as the potency of drug B (opioid) to increase the potency of drug A (hypnotic)—that is, to reduce C_{50A} by 50%.

Minto Model

In contrast to the other models, Minto and colleagues presented an approach to allow a higher flexibility in fitting data sets.[21] In Minto's concept, every combined dosing of drug A and B is considered to be as if it was a new drug C with the potential to have an independent drug response relationship. Therefore, a new parameter, theta, was defined expressed as:

$$\theta = \frac{U_A}{U_A + U_B} \quad \text{(Eqn. 7)}$$

θ is the fraction of normalized effect-site concentration of drug A versus the sum of normalized effect-site concentrations of both drugs A and B. These can be used to develop more complex higher-order structural models for all γ and C_{50} values of the response surface. These models allow U and γ to be variable in relation to the relative contribution of drug A versus drug B. In the original paper of Minto, a quadratic function, using Eqns. 8-10, was presented as an example:

$$U_{50} = 1 - \beta_{U50} \cdot \theta + \beta_{U50} \cdot \theta^2 \quad \text{(Eqn. 8)}$$

$$U = \frac{U_A + U_B}{U_{50}} \quad \text{(Eqn. 9)}$$

$$\gamma = \gamma_A - (\gamma_B - \gamma_A - \beta_\gamma) \cdot \theta + \beta_\gamma \cdot \theta^2 \quad \text{(Eqn. 10)}$$

where U_{50} is the normalized effect-site concentration of 2 drugs in the combination θ yielding half maximal effect, β_{U50} and β_γ are dimensionless interaction coefficients, and γ_A and γ_B are the slope factors (see Eqn. 4) for drug A and B, respectively, when given alone

By implementing these functions into Eqn. 4, the flexibility of the model is increasing and can accommodate more complex deviations in the response surface. In the case that the maximum effect of both drugs is different, the model may be expanded with an interaction term on E_{max}.

This approach was successfully applied to model interactions between multiple drugs also, as demonstrated by Short et al in a combination of propofol, alfentanil, and midazolam.[22] This major improvement of flexibility of the Minto model compared to the Greco model leads to a theoretical advantage. Additionally, although the complexity of the formulas is increased, a simple additive interaction is also defined within the formula. In that specific case, β equals 0 in Eqns. 8 and 10, and U_{50} equals 1 in Eqn. 9 resulting in an additive interaction.

However, the Minto model has some assumptions and limitations. The quadratic function in the estimation of U_{50} (Eqn. 8) appears to result in a consistent "notch" in the estimated isoboles, which is not seen with the other models. A clear example of this is shown in Figure A3–1, where all models are applied on one data set of interactions between remifentanil and sevoflurane. The reduced Greco model results in a smoother shape of the isobole compared to the Minto model during the transition from high opioids–low sevoflurane toward low opioids–high sevoflurane conditions. The notch in the Minto isobole results in differences in the estimation of drug effect compared to the other models. This deviation in steepness of the Minto isobole can be interpreted as the result of "more flexibility" in the model to fit data. But equally, it could be a poor representation of pharmacologic behavior. This issue needs to be confirmed in prospective study.

Hierarchical Model

Bouillon and colleagues presented the sequential or hierarchical model.[23] The hierarchical model is a semimechanistic model that aims to provide a mathematical description of a neurophysiologic definition of anesthesia.[5] A new parameter PAIN IN or preopioid intensity is defined, which represents the intensity of any stimulus in its capacity to cause a response in a patient. The major effect of opioids is considered a decrease in this preopioid intensity to generate a (reduced) postopioid intensity or PAIN OUT. The relation between preopioid and postopioid intensity is affected by the opioid effect-site concentration as shown in Eqn. 11:

$$\text{postopioid\_intensity} = \text{preopioid\_intensity} \cdot \left(1 - \frac{C_O^{\gamma_O}}{(C_{50O} \cdot \text{preopioid\_intensity})^{\gamma_O} + C_O^{\gamma_O}}\right) \qquad \text{(Eqn. 11)}$$

where C_O is the concentration of opioids, C_{50O} is the opioid concentration that results in 50% of the maximal effect, and γ_o is the steepness of the dose-response curve of the opioids.

In the next hierarchical step, the postopioid stimulus intensity is considered to be the trigger that may evoke a response on higher cortical functions. This implies that the normalized potency U is dependent on the post-opioid intensity according to Eqn. 12

$$U = \frac{U_H}{\text{postopioid\_intensity}} \qquad \text{(Eqn. 12)}$$

The postopioid intensity can be eliminated from Eqn. 12 by substitution of Eqn. 11.

$$U = \frac{U_H}{\text{preopioid\_intensity}} \cdot \left(1 + \left(\frac{U_O}{\text{preopioid\_intensity}}\right)^{\gamma_O}\right) \qquad \text{(Eqn. 13)}$$

Equation 13 relates the total normalized effect-site concentration (U) of the interacting drugs to 3 variables: the normalized concentrations of the opioid (U_O) and the hypnotic drug (U_H) on one hand and the preopioid stimulus intensity on the other hand. Again, this model has some assumptions and limitations that need to be taken into account when applying it as a structural model for data fitting. By including the stimulus intensity into the equations, the Bouillon model opens possibilities to quantify and compare the "intensity" of different stimuli in anesthesia according to their respective potency of evoking a response in a patient.

Bouillon presented a first demonstration of the applicability of this model in a data set of propofol–remifentanil interactions.[23] However, the first estimates where characterized by very small standard errors on several parameters suggesting a numerical problem for NONMEM to model the data. This might have been related to the fact that the original model was used in an overparameterized form, since Eqn. 13 does not allow independent estimation of preopioid intensity and C_{50} of the opioids and hypnotics.

In the case of a single stimulus, the preopioid intensity may be fixed to 1, reducing Eqn. 13 to

$$U = U_H \cdot \left(1 + U_O^{\gamma_o}\right) \qquad \text{(Eqn. 14)}$$

Equation 14 is closely related to the reduced Greco model (Eqn. 6), apart from the additional factor γ for the opioid, adding flexibility to describe the response surface.

In the case of multiple stimuli, the overparameterizaton may be solved in various ways, leading to different models, the scaled C_{50} and fixed C_{50} hierarchical models.

Scaled C_{50} Hierarchical Model

By fixing the preopioid intensity from a weak stimulus to 1 and quantifying the relative intensity of other stimuli according to Eqn. 15, both the potency of hypnotics as well as the potency of opioids can be related to the pre-opioid stimulus intensity. For each stimulus i, the C_{50} values are constrained by the following equation:

$$\text{Preopioid\_intensity}_i = C_{50O,\ \text{stimulus\_i}} / C_{50O,\ \text{stimulus\_1}} = C_{50H,\ \text{stimulus\_i}} / C_{50H,\ \text{stimulus\_1}} \qquad \text{(Eqn. 15)}$$

As a consequence, this model will estimate a different C_{50O} for every stimulus, scaled to the intensity of the incoming stimulus. Moreover, this scaling is also affecting the inhibiting potency of the hypnotics (C_{50H}) to the same extent. As this is one of the most unique characteristics of the hierarchical model, it has been named the "scaled C_{50}" model.[18] Equation 15 can be seen as a representation of the decreased capacity of opioids (ie, requiring higher concentrations) to inhibit stronger stimuli (such as incision or laryngoscopy) compared to weak stimuli (such as verbal commands).

Fixed C_{50} Hierarchical Model

A modified hierarchical model was presented by Bouillon to cope with some of the issues discussed above.[20] In contrast with the original hierarchical model ("scaled C_{50} mode"), this modified hierarchical model assumes that C_{50} of the opioids has only one value for all stimuli. Therefore, the model was referred to as the fixed C_{50} model.[18] Even so, the differences in intensity from separate stimuli can still be accounted for by differences in C_{50H}. In this view, the C_{50O} is a reflection of the potency of the opioid to reduce the preopioid intensity by half regardless of the magnitude of this preopioid stimulus, in contrast to the original hierarchical model.[20] Which concept is the best representation of the mechanistic reality remains a subject of speculation at this time.

Comparing Eqns. 6 and 14, the fixed C_{50} hierarchical model may be considered as an extension of the reduced Greco model, apart from the additional factor gamma for the opioid. When the fixed C_{50} hierarchical model (including γ_o) was used on the same data set as the reduced Greco (without γ_o), NONMEM analysis resulted in a significantly better fit compared to the reduced Greco model.[18] Apparently, the extra flexibility in the formula—provided by the additional γ_o—results in lower scatter of data around the response surface compared to the reduced Greco model.

Comparisons Between the Models

The contemporary structural models differ in mathematical and conceptual aspects. However, within certain assumptions, some of these models are mathematically related. This close relationship (eg, between the reduced Greco and fixed C_{50} hierarchical model) can result in very comparable estimations of parameters when applied to a single data set (see Figure A3–1).[18] Still, the fixed C_{50} hierarchical model reached a better population fit compared to the reduced Greco model in the interaction of remifentanil and sevoflurane. With the Minto model, multiple drug interactions can be quantified effectively, but the estimations of the Minto model can deviate compared to the other models.[18] This is probably related to the quadratic function in the estimation of U_{50}. The major question remains which model provides the more realistic and clinically relevant description of the observed population data. According to NONMEM analysis on multiple data sets, it appears that the "ideal" model might vary according to the chosen end points of drug effect (dichotomous versus continuous) or according to the choice of drugs tested. At least we now have the luxury of many mathematical approaches ("Swiss Army Knife of models" according to Bouillon) to explore anesthetic conditions with more validity.

As an example, the next paragraphs review some applications of the above models for propofol–remifentanil interactions and for sevoflurane–remifentanil interactions, studied on a variety of clinical end points.

The Minto model was applied on a data set combining remifentanil and propofol, modeling hypnotic and analgetic end points of anesthesia.[21] As a reflection of adequacy of the model, the synergistic properties found on the C_{50} level were in concordance with formerly published isobolographic-derived values. However, a problem occurred at the sigmoidal E_{max} curve relating remifentanil, administered alone, to hypnotic effect. Unresponsiveness to verbal command was not found in 100% of the patients, and estimation by NONMEM resulted in unrealistic high C_{50} values. The data just did not reveal sufficient information to provide an adequate estimation of the E_{max} curve for hypnotic end points when remifentanil was given alone. Also, the resulting isobole does not reveal a consistent smooth synergism over the wide rage of remifentanil concentrations. For example, for the C_{50} isobole between remifentanil and propofol, a primary almost linear relation is found during initially increasing doses of remifentanil between 0 and 3.8 ng/mL. At higher remifentanil concentration, an inclination point is seen with a less steep synergism above 4 ng/mL of remifentanil effect-site concentration. Additionally, the synergism as reflected by the Minto model never reaches a plateau suggesting that (theoretically) full hypnotic effect can be obtained with high doses of remifentanil and no propofol. Although this possibility is intrinsic to the mathematics of the model, it is not supported by clinical observations.

The Minto model has also been used to model hemodynamic effects of the combination of propofol and remifentanil. Zanderigo et al used historical data to model both the positive (hypnosis) and negative (hypotension) effects in order to create a new end point in anesthesia called "patients well-being." This end point is a subtraction of the negative effects from the positive effects in such a way that the model could be used to identify optimal combinations of remifentanil and propofol that provokes simultaneously adequate hypnotic levels of anesthesia while avoiding negative effects. Not surprisingly, the suggested optimal dosing is within daily used clinical ranges. But additionally, it was shown that the synergism on negative and positive effects is rather comparable. This means that the classical statement that synergism might lead to equal effect while avoiding side effects appears not to be entirely true for anesthesia-related interactions. When the hypnotic effect of propofol is potentiated by remifentanil, the effect on hypotension is comparably affected by the synergistic effect. As such, only limited ranges of optimal well-being can be defined within the spectrum of drug combinations.

Bouillon applied the hierarchical model[23] and later a reduced version of the hierarchical model[20] to estimate a response surface for remifentanil and propofol using both quantal (OAAS) as well as continuous (approximate entropy and bispectral index) end points. Three differences with the Minto estimations are apparent. First, this model revealed a smoother isobole over a wider range of remifentanil and propofol concentrations. Secondly, no hypnotic effect is estimated when only opioids are given, which seems to be a more realistic representation. Third, the synergism between remifentanil and propofol reaches a plateau, indicating that a minimal amount of propofol will always be necessary when aiming for a hypnotic effect. The difference of interpreting solitary opioid drug effect between the Minto and hierarchical model is also reflected in the major difference of the estimated C_{50} for remifentanil alone in its ability to evoke loss of consciousness, which was respectively 54 ng/mL for the Minto model and 19 ng/mL for the hierarchical model. Both values are far out of the clinical scope of use but are a clear reflection of the difference in mathematical approach between models.

For inhaled anesthesia, Figure A3–1 shows isobole estimations using 4 different models. It shows the differences in model estimations of the sevoflurane concentration necessary to evoke a 90% tolerance of laryngeal mask placement. It is apparent that the Minto model estimates a need for higher concentrations to obtain identical effects compared to the other models.

Prospective research will reveal the importance of such differences in estimations between the respective interaction models. Ultimately, they should provide clinicians with a relevant benchmark of evidence based advice on dosing guidelines.[8]

REFERENCES

1. Glass PS, Bloom M, Kearse L, Rosow C, Sebel P, Manberg P. Bispectral analysis measures sedation and memory effects of propofol, midazolam, isoflurane, and alfentanil in healthy volunteers. *Anesthesiology*. 1997;86(4):836-847.
2. Chernik D, Gillings D, Laine H, et al. Validity and reliability of the Observer's Assessment of Alertness/ Sedation Scale: study with intravenous midazolam. *J Clin Psychopharmacol*. 1990;10: 244-251.
3. Eger EI II, Brandstater B, Saidman LJ, Regan MJ, Severinghaus JW, Munson ES. Equipotent alveolar concentrations of methoxyflurane, halothane, diethyl ether, fluroxene, cyclopropane, xenon and nitrous oxide in the dog. *Anesthesiology*. 1965;26(6):771-777.
4. Vanluchene AL, Vereecke H, Thas O, Mortier EP, Shafer SL, Struys MM. Spectral entropy as an electroencephalographic measure of anesthetic drug effect: a comparison with bispectral index and processed midlatency auditory evoked response. *Anesthesiology*. 2004;101(1):34-42.
5. Glass PS. Anesthetic drug interactions: an insight into general anesthesia–its mechanism and dosing strategies. *Anesthesiology*. 1998;88(1):5-6.
6. Luginbuhl M, Schumacher PM, Vuilleumier P, et al. Noxious stimulation response index: a novel anesthetic state index based on hypnotic-opioid interaction. *Anesthesiology*. 2010;112(4):872-880.
7. Ilies C, Gruenewald M, Ludwigs J, et al. Evaluation of the surgical stress index during spinal and general anaesthesia. *Br J Anaesth*. 2010;105(4):533-537.
8. Shafer SL. All models are wrong. *Anesthesiology*. 2012;116(2):240-241.
9. Short TG, Ho TY, Minto CF, Schnider TW, Shafer SL. Efficient trial design for eliciting a pharmacokinetic-pharmacodynamic model-based response surface describing the interaction between two intravenous anesthetic drugs. *Anesthesiology*. 2002;96(2):400-408.
10. Greco WR, Bravo G, Parsons JC. The search for synergy: a critical review from a response surface perspective. *Pharmacol Rev*. 1995;47(2):331-385.
11. Manyam SC, Gupta DK, Johnson KB, et al. Opioid-volatile anesthetic synergy: a response surface model with remifentanil and sevoflurane as prototypes. *Anesthesiology*. 2006;105(2):267-278.
12. Berenbaum MC. The expected effect of a combination of agents: the general solution. *J Theor Biol*. 1985;114(3): 413-431.
13. Suhnel J. Comment on the paper: A three-dimensional model to analyze drug-drug interactions. *Antiviral Res*. 1992;17(1):91-98.
14. Prichard MN, Shipman C Jr. A three-dimensional model to analyze drug-drug interactions. *Antiviral Res*. 1990;14(4-5):181-205.
15. Suhnel J. Evaluation of synergism or antagonism for the combined action of antiviral agents. *Antiviral Res*. 1990;13(1):23-39.
16. Greco WR, Park HS, Rustum YM. Application of a new approach for the quantitation of drug synergism to the combination of cis-diamminedichloroplatinum and 1-beta-D-arabinofuranosylcytosine. *Cancer Res*. 1990;50(17):5318-5327.
17. Weinstein RE, Walker FJ. Enhancement of rabbit protein S anticoagulant cofactor activity in vivo by modulation of the protein S C4B binding protein interaction. *J Clin Invest*. 1990;86(6):1928-1935.
18. Heyse B, Proost JH, Schumacher PM, et al. Sevoflurane remifentanil interaction: comparison of different response surface models. *Anesthesiology*. 2012;116(2): 311-323.
19. Bol CJ, Vogelaar JP, Tang JP, Mandema JW. Quantification of pharmacodynamic interactions between dexmedetomidine and midazolam in the rat. *J Pharmacol Exp Ther*. 2000;294(1): 347-355.
20. Bouillon TW. Hypnotic and opioid anesthetic drug interactions on the CNS, focus on response surface modeling. *Handb Exp Pharmacol*. 2008;182:471-487.
21. Minto CF, Schnider TW, Short TG, Gregg KM, Gentilini A, Shafer SL. Response surface model for anesthetic drug interactions. *Anesthesiology*. 2000;92(6):1603-1616.
22. Short TG, Plummer JL, Chui PT. Hypnotic and anaesthetic interactions between midazolam, propofol and alfentanil. *Br J Anaesth*. 1992;69(2):162-167.
23. Bouillon TW, Bruhn J, Radulescu L, et al. Pharmacodynamic interaction between propofol and remifentanil regarding hypnosis, tolerance of laryngoscopy, bispectral index, and electroencephalographic approximate entropy. *Anesthesiology*. 2004;100(6):1353-1372.

CHAPTER 4

Importance and Limitations of Simulation in Clinical Pharmacology

Ken B. Johnson, MD, and Carl Tams, BS

IMPORTANCE OF SIMULATION

Anesthesiologists use many potent drugs either as single agents or in combination. Each of these drugs has a unique profile in terms of how their concentrations and effects change over time and how they interact with other drugs. Although the basic features of anesthetic drugs are well established, the time course of how the drugs behave, especially in combination with other drugs, is complex and difficult to predict. Anesthesiologists rely on experience and training to formulate dosing regimens, yet they can be confounded by the dynamic changes encountered in the operating room and intensive care unit.

Numerous laboratory investigations have characterized important aspects of drug behavior that are of interest to anesthesiologists. These discoveries often involve complex mathematical formulas and, until recently, have been largely confined to drug package inserts, textbooks, and published manuscripts. With the advent of personal computers and hand-held devices powerful enough to process solutions to these mathematical formulas, models can be used to simulate drug behavior real time and at the point of care.

As a translational tool from laboratory to point of patient care, simulation can be used to visualize drug concentrations and effects over time and how drug combinations influence various drug effects. Figures 4–1 and 4–2 present an example of how simulation illustrates clinical effects of interest. This simulation assumes a 47-year-old, 100-kg, 183-cm male with a history of painful cholelithiasis and anorexia undergoing a laparoscopic cholecystectomy. Propofol, fentanyl, and succinylcholine are used for induction, and sevoflurane, fentanyl, and rocuronium are used for maintenance of anesthesia. Figure 4–1 presents the dosing regimen and the predicted drug effect-site concentrations, and Figure 4–2 presents the predicted drug effects.

This example uses several types of models. Pharmacokinetic models are used to predict both plasma and effect-site concentrations. For intravenous agents, models use weight and in some cases age to make predictions. For inhalation agents, models use weight, minute ventilation, cardiac output, and fresh gas flow to make predictions. Pharmacodynamic interaction models use predicted effect-site concentrations to estimate selected drug effects. There are many drug interaction models available, each with unique drug interactions and dose-response relationships. Some examples include probability of moderate sedation, ventilatory depression, loss of response to esophageal instrumentation, etc. See Chapter 3 for a complete list; only a few are presented in Figure 4–2. These simulations illustrate several important points.

Visualizing Pharmacokinetics

Each anesthetic drug has a unique kinetic profile. This can be appreciated by comparing the rate of drug dissipation following the propofol, fentanyl, succinylcholine, and rocuronium boluses. Of these drugs, fentanyl has the slowest rate of decline whereas propofol has the fastest. It is important to recognize that the rate of drug dissipation does *not* directly correlate to the duration of effect. It is simply a description of anesthetic drug kinetics. Duration of effect is dependent on drug effect-site concentration and interactions with other anesthetic drugs.

Changes in effect-site concentrations lag behind changes in end-tidal concentrations for inhaled

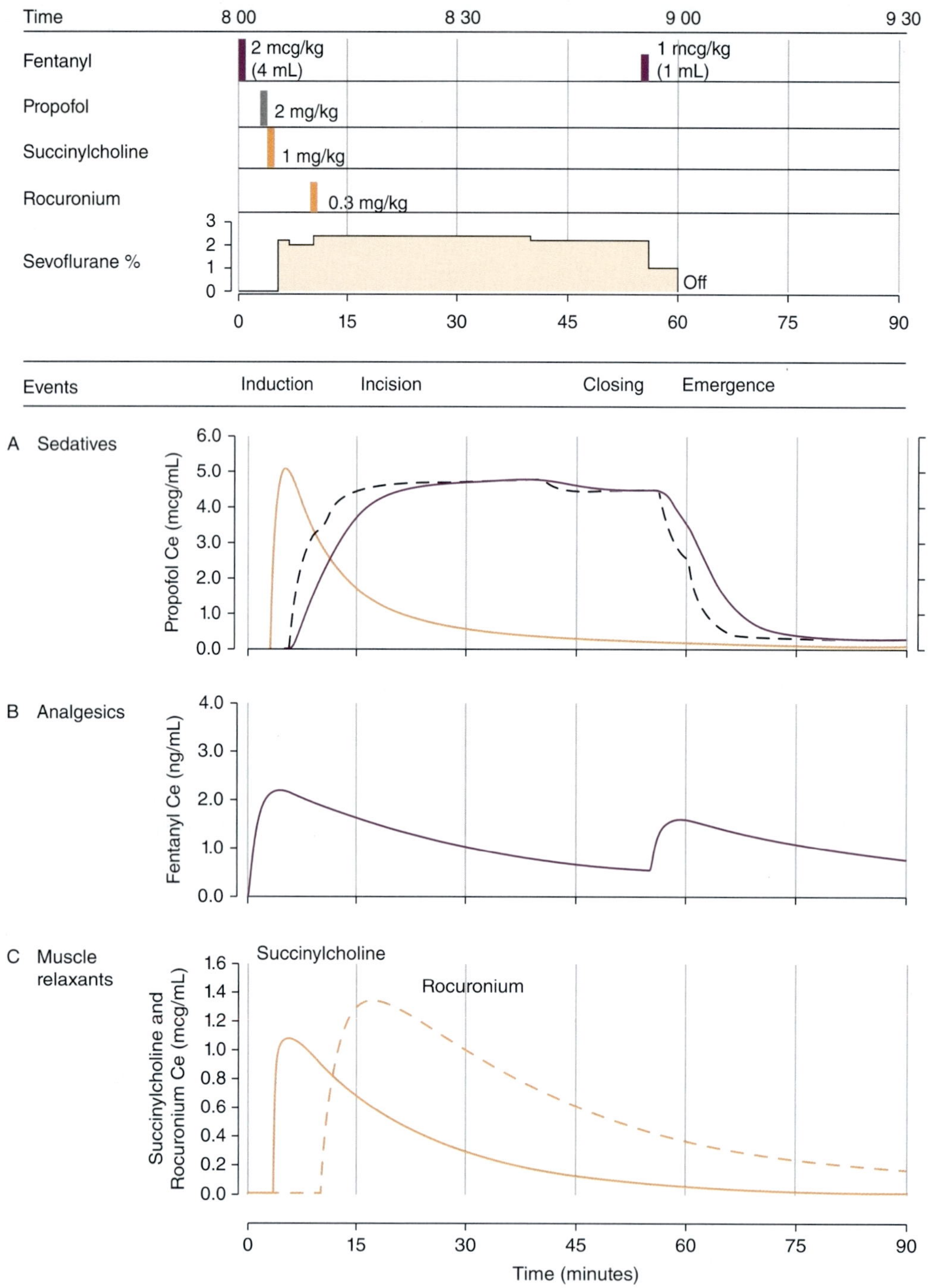

FIGURE 4–1 Simulation of drug effect-site concentrations for a combined anesthetic technique using sevoflurane, fentanyl, succinylcholine, and rocuronium. The top section presents the dosing timeline for a 60-minute procedure. Intravenous bolus doses of fentanyl, propofol, succinylcholine, and rocuronium are presented as colored vertical lines. Sevoflurane vaporizer settings are presented in orange. Using published models,[1-16] predicted effect-site concentrations (Ce) over time were estimated for each drug and are presented in the 3 plots below the dosing time line: A for sedatives, B for analgesics, and C for neuromuscular blockers. The orange, black, and purple lines represent the Ce values for propofol, sevoflurane, and fentanyl. The dashed black line represents the end tidal sevoflurane concentration. The orange solid and dashed lines represent the Ce values for succinylcholine and rocuronium.

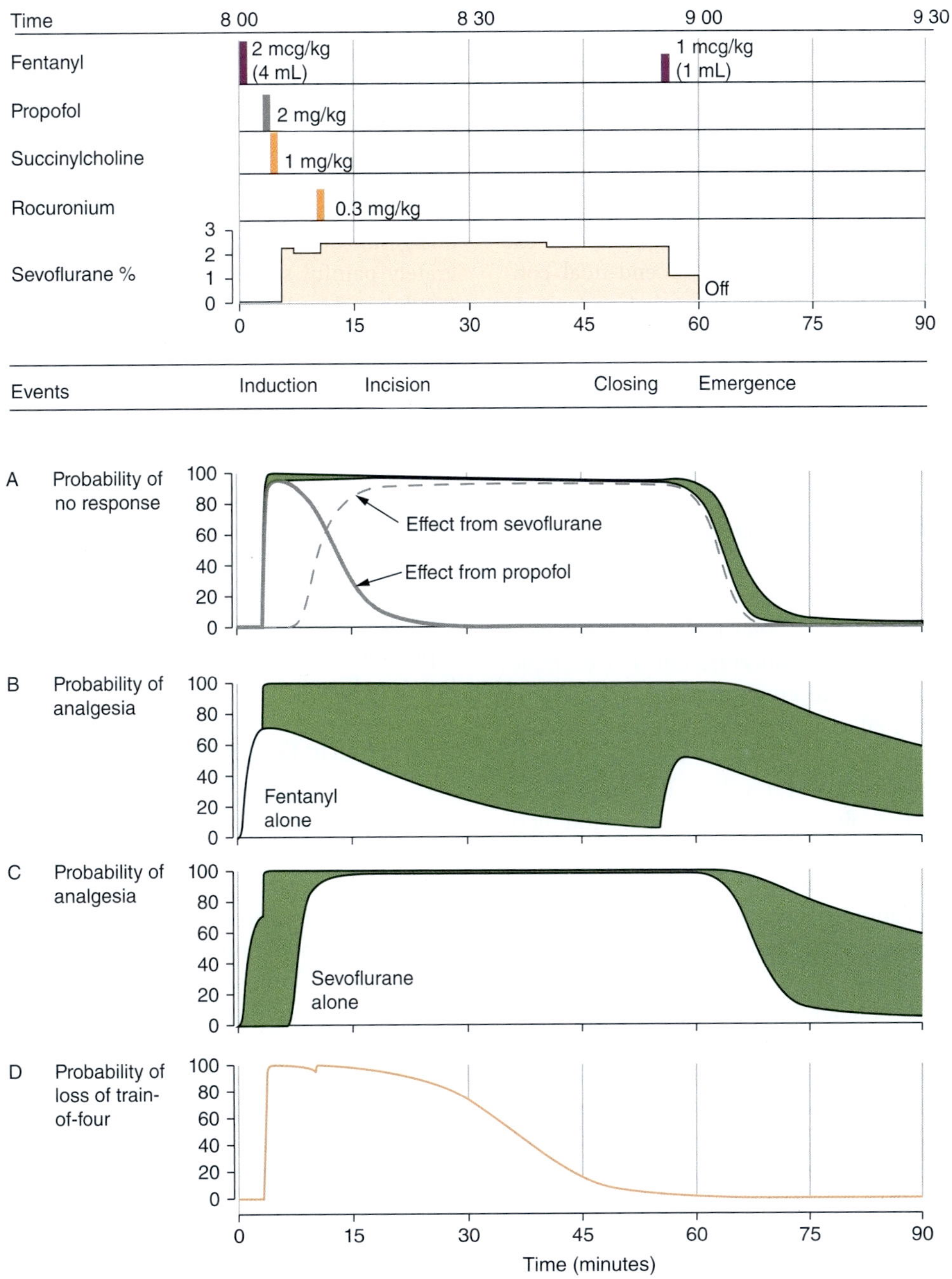

FIGURE 4–2 Predicted drug effects over time. The top section presents the dosing timeline presented in Figure 4–1. Combined effect of propofol, sevoflurane, and fentanyl are presented as a filled-in plot (green), and the effect of individual anesthetics are presented as black lines. Using published interaction models,[17-19] predicted effects include A, loss of responsiveness; B, loss of response to a moderately painful stimulus for fentanyl alone and in combination with sevoflurane; C, loss of response to a moderately painful stimulus for sevoflurane alone and in combination with fentanyl; and D, loss of train-of-four for succinylcholine and rocuronium. Loss of response to a painful stimulus was defined as a loss of response to 30 pounds per square inch of anterior tibial pressure, a surrogate of pain experienced in the recovery room following laparoscopic procedures.[18]

agents and behind changes in plasma concentrations for intravenous agents. This is especially important under non–steady-state conditions (ie, induction and emergence). In this example, after induction, sevoflurane is titrated to maintain unresponsiveness (between 1.5 and 2.5 vol%). The time course of end-tidal and effect-site concentrations is presented as dashed and solid lines in Figure 4–1A. The sevoflurane effect site lags behind end-tidal concentrations. With conventional ventilation (minute volume of 6 L/min), normal cardiac output, and normal fresh gas flow (2 L/min), the time required for effect-site concentration to be near the end-tidal concentration (pseudo–steady-state) can be up to 14 minutes.

Visualizing Pharmacodynamics

Using effect-site concentration models make predictions of effect. For potent inhaled agents, anesthesiologists have a working understanding of drug effect as a function of drug concentration. For example, end-tidal sevoflurane concentrations are used to estimate drug effect in terms of minimum alveolar concentration (MAC) (2.2 vol%), MACbar (3 vol%), and MACawake (0.6–1.0 vol%). For intravenous agents, anesthesiologists' working understanding of drug concentration versus effect is not as well developed. This is because with intravenous agents, there is no presentation of drug concentration to associate with drug effect as there is with potent inhaled agents.

In these simulations, the concentration versus time profile for each drug is presented in graphical form along with a prediction of drug effect. For example, the 2 mg/kg propofol dose led to a predicted peak effect-site concentration of 5 mcg/mL (see Figure 4–1A). This resulted in a high (> 90%) probability of unresponsiveness within 90 seconds that lasted for 3 minutes (see Figure 4–2A).

As dosed, the probability of sedation–hypnosis between the induction with propofol and the administration of sevoflurane remains greater than 95%. As propofol's effect dissipates, the onset of effect from sevoflurane increases (see arrows in Figure 4–2A). This combined effect is dependent upon the time lapse between the administration of propofol and sevoflurane. In this simulation, it is 2.5 minutes. Longer delays may lead to brief gaps in the sedative–hypnotic effect.

The induction dose (2 mcg/kg) of fentanyl reached a peak effect-site concentration of 2.2 ng/mL within 5 minutes and then dissipated over the next 30 to 40 minutes (see Figure 4–1B). This bolus was associated with greater than a 50% probability of analgesia (defined as a loss of response to a moderately painful stimulus) for 15 minutes. The fentanyl dose near the end of the procedure (1 mcg/kg) yielded a peak effect-site concentration of 1.6 ng/mL. This bolus was less effective with only a brief period (2 to 3 minutes) where the probability of analgesia is above 50%.

The induction dose (1 mg/kg) of succinylcholine reached a peak effect-site concentration of 1.1 mcg/mL (see Figure 4–1C). This provided a probability greater than 95% of no train-of-four for 6 minutes. Because of the short procedure time, a small dose of rocuronium (0.3 mg/kg) was administered. It provided an additional 10 minutes of no train-of-four (see Figure 4–2D).

Anesthetic Drug Interactions

Perhaps the most important feature of this simulation is visualization of anesthetic drug interactions. Even with a routine anesthetic, several pharmacodynamic characteristics are not always easy to predict. Experienced anesthesiologists have a sense of onset and duration of action for most, if not all, of these drugs when administered alone and may, at first glance, find drug display technology unnecessary. But even experienced clinicians may find it difficult to predict the onset and duration of a simple bolus of fentanyl when coadministered in the presence of other anesthetic drug. For example, clinicians may find it difficult to predict the duration of analgesia for a 1 mcg/kg fentanyl bolus in the presence of 2 vol% sevoflurane. Or they may have difficulty predicting the duration of unresponsiveness when the same bolus is administered just before adjusting the sevoflurane vaporizer from 2% to 0% at the end of an anesthetic. Low-dose opioids can substantially prolong emergence from an inhalation agent, even at concentrations well below MAC.

Not all drug–drug interactions are alike. For example, sevoflurane provides the majority of the sedative-hypnotic effect with a minor contribution from fentanyl. If no fentanyl were administered, there would likely be no substantial difference in loss of responsiveness during the anesthetic. If no sevoflurane were administered, the patient would likely remain awake. When combined, sevoflurane and fentanyl interact to provide a slightly more pronounced loss of responsiveness. This interaction is best visualized during emergence, where the fentanyl slightly prolongs the return to responsiveness (see Figure 4–2A).

By contrast to loss of responsiveness, both fentanyl and sevoflurane have analgesic properties, and when combined they produce a profound analgesic effect. As dosed, fentanyl alone provides analgesia for a brief period of time (probability > 50% for 15 minutes at induction) but is inadequate to meet the analgesic requirements for the entire procedure (see Figure 4–2B). Sevoflurane at 2 vol% alone provides analgesia for the entire procedure (see Figure 4–2C). When combined, the probability of analgesia to a moderate stimulus is greater than 99% for the entire 60-minute anesthetic. The impact of drug synergism may again be best visualized once the anesthetic is terminated. With both drugs, the duration of analgesia after the anesthetic is terminated is much longer than with either drug alone.

Dose Finding

Simulation allows visualization of a dosing regimen prior to administering it. Figure 4–3 presents a drug display rendition of induction with propofol, and fentanyl followed by maintenance with sevoflurane and intermittent boluses fentanyl. The display provides prediction that span from 30 minutes in the past to 10 minutes into the future. This feature provides the ability to explore various dosing regimens prior to the end of an anesthetic. In this example, the 10-minute time window into the future is labeled Plan A. With that plan, the influence of a 100-mcg fentanyl bolus on analgesia and sedation is well visualized. Other plans might explore the behavior of hydromorphone or sufentanil in a similar fashion and provide additional information before an opioid is selected and administered. Similar explorations of different sevoflurane vaporizer settings can be made to identify doses that account for the addition of an opioid on the time to reach a high probability of return of consciousness. If helpful, time boundaries can also be modified to visualize predicted drug effects into the future longer than 10 minutes. This may be useful for longer acting anesthetics, where accounting for drug accumulation and associated prolonged effect may be difficult to predict.

LIMITATIONS OF SIMULATION

As with other forms of simulation, consistently and accurately predicting reality is difficult. Predictions of drug concentrations and effects have limitations and are important to review. The limitations are primarily a function of prediction variability. Prediction variability is in part due to how data are collected from a population that has substantial inherent variability, assumptions made when building models, and how models are used to make predictions.

Visualizing Prediction Variability

To appreciate the clinical implications of model prediction variability, both kinetic and dynamic variability should be considered simultaneously.[20] Although intuitively straightforward, methods to describe this variability have not been well established. Models consist of a set of model parameters; some published models include a metric of parameter variability (ie, coefficient of variation), while others do not. One approach is to simulate using numerous (ie, 1000) possible modified model parameters randomly selected from within the published range of model variability. This generates a distribution of predictions. A schematic illustrating this process for a remifentanil infusion is presented in Figure 4–4. The kinetic and dynamic variability is expressed as a distribution of predicted effect-site concentrations (top plot) and a distribution of predicted drug effects (bottom plot). These simulations are for illustration purposes only and do not represent real estimates of variability. At this time, none exist.

If considering the variability at 20 minutes into the infusion, the range of variability in effect-site concentrations ranges is large (4–10 ng/mL). Although wide, the impact of this range of concentrations on the concentration-effect plot (bottom plot) is rather small. The infusion is quite effective and providing a high

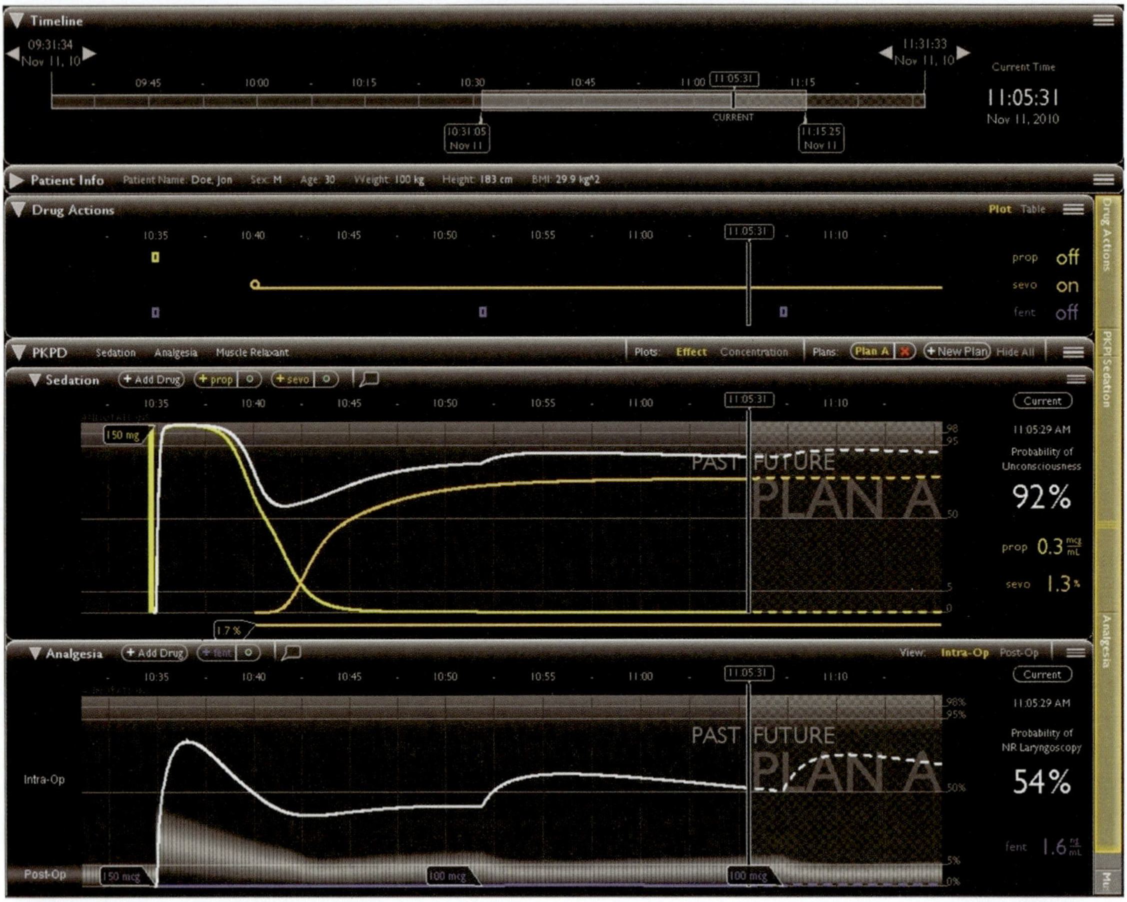

FIGURE 4–3 An example of drug display that presents predictions over the past 30 minutes (solid lines), the present (double vertical line through each plot), and 10 minutes into the future (dashed lines). The top plot is the adjustable timeline. Time–date boxes indicate the past and future time windows. These can be adjusted to expand and/or contract each time window. The second plot is the dosing regimen to a 30-year-old, 100-kg, 183-cm male. The regimen includes a 150-mg propofol bolus, a sevoflurane vaporizer set to 1.7%, and an initial intravenous 150-mcg fentanyl bolus followed by additional 100-mcg boluses. The third and fourth plots are the probability of sedation and analgesia. Prediction probabilities range from 0 to 100%. Bright yellow represents propofol (prop), dark yellow represents sevoflurane (sevo), and blue represents fentanyl (fent). White lines represent combined drug effects. Sedation is defined as the probability of unconsciousness. Analgesia is defined as the probability of no response to laryngoscopy (NR Laryngoscopy). Prediction of drug effects were made using published interaction models for loss of response to laryngoscopy[19] and loss of responsiveness[17]. The values for propofol, sevoflurane, and fentanyl on the right side of the display represent current effect-site concentrations, and the large white numbers represent the current probability of effect.

probability of analgesia (> 90%). This is because the concentrations are near the top of the dynamic range. Despite a large change in concentration, there is little change in effect.

Since an anesthetic rarely consists of a single drug, it is useful to consider the prediction variability for a combined anesthetic. In addition, an anesthetic typically has phases where concentrations are rapidly changing (ie, induction and emergence) and other phases where concentrations are relatively stable. Thus, it is useful to consider the combined kinetic and dynamic prediction variability over time. Figure 4–5 presents a schematic of the kinetic and combined kinetic and dynamic variability for a

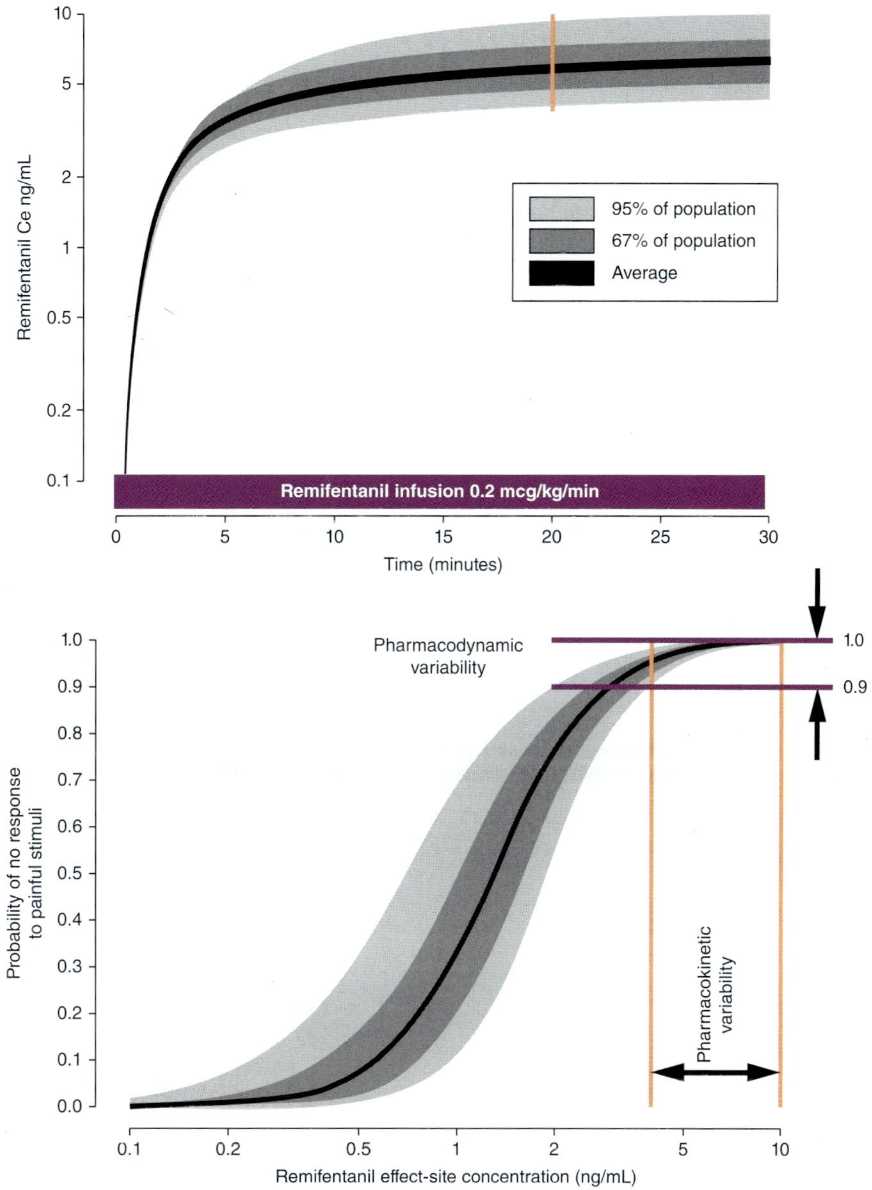

FIGURE 4–4 Schematic of pharmacokinetic-pharmacodynamic variability for a 30-minute remifentanil infusion running at 0.2 mcg/kg/min. Variability is expressed as a distribution of model predictions based on model parameter coefficients of variation.[8,9] The black line represents model predictions using published parameters. The dark and light gray areas represent model predictions that span 67% (± 1 standard deviation) and 95% (± 2 standard deviations) of the population as described by the coefficients of variation. The top plot presents the pharmacokinetic variability. The vertical orange line presents the range of predicted remifentanil effect-site concentrations at 20 minutes into the infusion. Of note, the distribution of remifentanil concentrations at this time point is normally distributed about the model prediction; out of 100 people, 67 would likely have concentrations within the dark gray region (4.7 to 7.3 ng/mL) and 95 would likely have concentrations within the light gray region (4.0 to 10.0 ng/mL). The bottom plot presents a simulation of pharmacodynamic variability. It presents the concentration-effect (probability of analgesia) relationship for remifentanil. The probability of analgesia ranges from 0 for responsive and 1 for unresponsive to a painful stimulus.[21] Over the range of possible remifentanil levels (vertical orange lines), pharmacodynamic model predictions vary from 0.9 to 1.0 (horizontal purple lines) suggesting a high probability of analgesia with this infusion rate. The data presented here are not real. They were created solely for the purpose of illustrating limitation to modeling drug behavior.

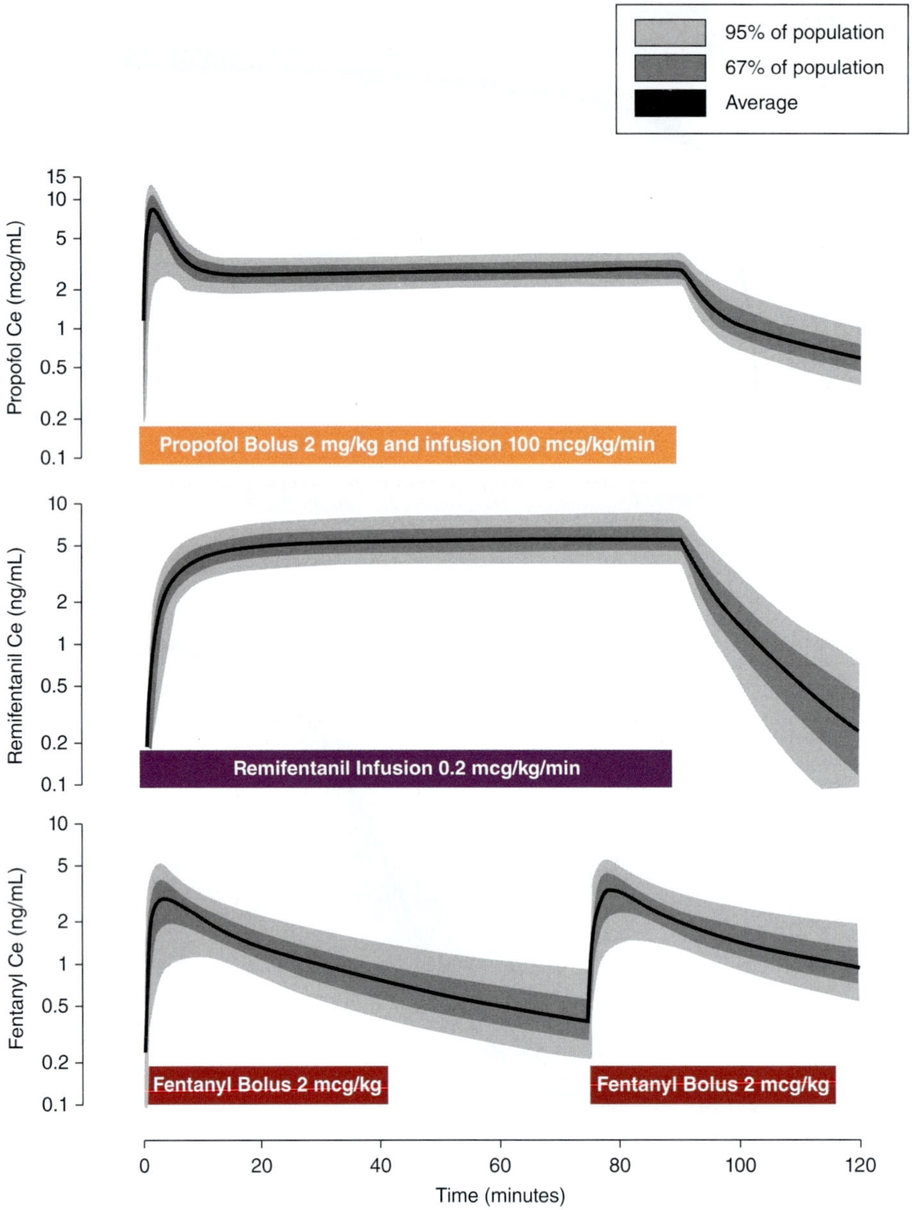

FIGURE 4–5 Schematic of pharmacokinetic and pharmacodynamic variability over time for a total intravenous anesthetic. Simulations included propofol (2 mg/kg bolus followed by an infusion of 100 mcg/kg/min), remifentanil (an infusion of 0.2 mcg/kg/min) and fentanyl (two 2 mcg/kg boluses, one 3 minutes prior to induction and one 15 minutes before terminating the anesthetic). The propofol and remifentanil infusions were terminated at 90 minutes. Panel A: Effect-site concentrations over time for propofol (top plot), remifentanil (middle plot), and fentanyl (bottom plot). Variability is expressed as a distribution of model predictions based on model parameter coefficients of variation for propofol[4,5] and remifentanil.[8,9] Coefficients of variation were not available for fentanyl but assumed to be similar to remifentanil; fentanyl concentrations were predicted using a fentanyl kinetic model.[2] The black line represents model predictions using published parameters. The dark and light gray areas represent model predictions that span 67% (± 1 standard deviation) and 95% (± 2 standard deviations) of the population as described by the coefficients of variation. (Reproduced with permission from Carl Tams* and Ken Johnson: Prediction Variability of Combined Pharmacokinetic Pharmacodynamic Models: A Simulation Study of Propofol in Combination with Remifentanil and Fentanyl, *J Anesth Clin Res* 2014;5(3)393.)

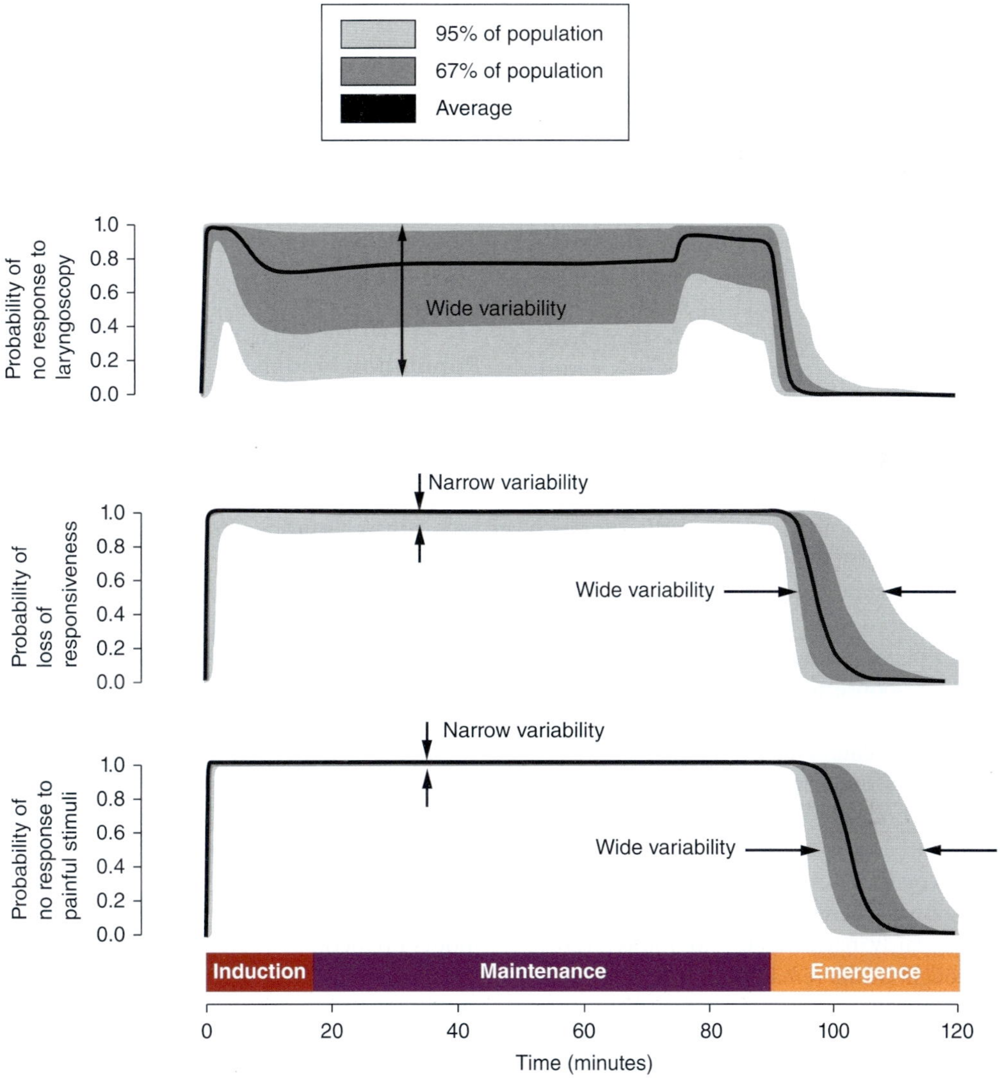

FIGURE 4–5 (Continued) Panel B: Predicted drug effects over time. Predictions include loss of response to laryngoscopy,[19] loss of responsiveness (no response to shake and shout),[17] and loss of response to a painful stimulus (30 pounds per square inch of pressure on the anterior tibia, a suggested surrogate of postoperative pain).[21] The white arrow indicates the wide variability in predictions of loss of response to laryngoscopy during the anesthetic. The blue arrows indicate the narrow range of variability for loss of responsiveness and loss of response to a painful stimulus during the anesthetic. The red arrows indicate the wide range of variability in the loss of effect once the anesthetic is terminated. Specifically, the red arrows show the variability in time required to reach a 50% probability of effect. See text for additional details. The data presented here are not real. They were created solely for the purpose of illustrating limitations to modeling drug behavior.

90-minute total intravenous anesthetic. The intravenous agents include propofol, remifentanil, and fentanyl (see figure legend for dosing scheme). The anesthetic effects include loss of response to laryngoscopy, loss of responsiveness, ventilatory depression, and loss of response to a painful stimulus (see figure legend for definitions of drug effects). To visualize the drug effect over time, the kinetic and dynamic variability presented in Figure 4–4 are combined into one plot.

During the anesthetic, although the prediction variability in drug concentrations is large (see Figure 4–5A), the corresponding prediction variability in drug effect is quite small for all effects, except for loss of response to laryngoscopy (see Figure 4–5B). This is because the anesthetic, as dosed, leads to concentrations that are near the maximal effect for each effect. Even the lowest concentration predictions for propofol, remifentanil, and fentanyl lead to a near maximal effect for loss of responsiveness and loss of response to a painful stimulus.

Loss of response to laryngoscopy is a different story. Laryngoscopy is perhaps one of the most painful stimuli encountered in the operating room and thus requires more anesthetic to blunt or block a response. Clinicians often give doses that are inadequate to block a response but use paralytics to keep patients from moving during laryngoscopy. With this dosing scheme, the probability range after induction is fairly narrow (60% to 100%, average 99%). Throughout the remainder of the anesthetic, the range quickly widens (12% to 100%, average 79%). This is because as the drug concentrations move down the slope of the response surface (Chapter 3) where a wider range of probabilities are possible.

Once the anesthetic is terminated and concentrations start to drop, variability in predictions of drug concentrations and effects becomes very large. This may explain, in part, why there is substantial variability in the time to emergence from anesthesia and time to requiring additional analgesics following surgery. For example, the range in duration of time from turning off the anesthetic and a 50% probability of loss of responsiveness (ie, emerging from anesthesia) is 4 to 17 minutes (average, 7 minutes). The time required to reach a 50% probability of loss of response to a painful stimulus (ie, loss of analgesia) is also wide, 6 to 23 minutes (average, 13 minutes).

In summary, despite the wide concentration prediction variability, model predictions suggest that this total intravenous anesthetic is effective and maintaining unresponsiveness and analgesia. Once the anesthetic is terminated, predictions become more variable, suggesting variability in the duration of various effects.

Data Collection

Population Models

Perhaps the most important limitation of models is that they do not adequately cover all medical conditions clinicians encounter. Physiologic differences between individuals in cardiac output, metabolic organ perfusion and function, age, blood pH, plasma protein concentrations, and intravascular volume status, among others, may influence anesthetic drug behavior.

Some published pharmacokinetic and pharmacodynamic models were built from studies that enrolled healthy, normal size, patients (often young), or volunteers to serve as subjects and then are extrapolated to represent an entire population. Unfortunately, frequently encountered disease states are poorly characterized in these models. For some models, but not all, drugs, age, weight, and to some extent body habitus have been integrated into model predictions. For the most part, patient conditions such as heart, liver, lung, or kidney disease, or chronic exposure to substances that influence anesthetic drugs (eg, opioids, alcohol, anxiolytics, antidepressants, nicotine) are not incorporated into models of drug behavior. For example, it is difficult to model how dehydration, blood loss, congestive heart failure, cardiomyopathy, or myocardial ischemia influence plasma drug concentrations.

A majority of models come from data where only one drug is evaluated. Anesthetics are rarely just one drug; they often involve 3 or more drugs from different classes of anesthetics such as opioids, nonopioid analgesics, sedative–hypnotics, and neuromuscular blockers. When making predictions about specific drug effects, one class of anesthetics can significantly impact the behavior of companion anesthetics (ie, influence of inhalation agents

TABLE 4–1 Selected unknown anesthetic drug interactions.

Benzodiazepines With:
Inhalation agents
Opioids
Neuromuscular blockers
Ketamine, etomidate, or sodium thiopental
Ketamine, Etomidate, or Sodium Thiopental With:
Inhalation agents
Opioids
Neuromuscular blockers
Benzodiazepines
Neuromuscular Blockers With:
Inhalation agents
Propofol
Opioids

on opioids). Recent research has characterized several common drug interactions, but many remain unknown. The previous chapter presents a summary of known and extrapolated anesthetic drug interactions. Table 4–1 presents a set of drug interactions that remain unknown, but are important to anesthesiologists.

Inadequate Data

Models of drug behavior are only as good as the data used to build them. Data collection is a difficult process with many pitfalls that may create misleading model predictions. Some examples include:

- Collecting data is expensive. Cost constraints may limit the number of data points that are measured (ie, costs associated with assays to measure drug concentrations, devices to detect drug effect).
- Collected data may not cover a clinically relevant range of drug concentrations. Limitations may include an inability to measure low concentrations (ie, below an assay detection limit) or data was not collected at high concentrations because of adverse side effects (ie, hypotension with high-dose propofol). If higher concentrations are unavailable and do not cover the dynamic range (Chapter 1), pharmacodynamic model construction is compromised.
- Data sampling may be too infrequent to capture rapid changes in concentration or effect. Rapid changes may be inadequately characterized if drug concentration or effect sampling is too slow. One challenge is that although a model can be fit to sparse data and may fit the data well, it will not make predictions of clinical value. A second challenge with sparse data is that several models may be fit to the data. Each model may fit the data well but make different predictions. Which model is best can be difficult to determine.
- It is difficult to characterize the lag time between changes in concentration and effect (known as *biophase*). Researchers have found that the lag time may be a function of how a drug is administered (ie, bolus versus infusion).
- Some effects are easily measured (ie, is the patient responsive or unresponsive?) and others are not (ie, responsive or unresponsive to skin incision?). It is unethical to explore the effect for a full range of drug concentrations on responsiveness to skin incision, so researchers use surrogates of surgical pain. Surrogate painful stimuli are reproducible and responses to them are easily measured, but their clinical correlate is not well defined. Surrogates such as loss of response to electrical tetany, hot plates, anterior tibial pressure, and shoulder squeeze are all easily measured, but they do not directly correlate with skin incision.
- Measures of sedation and loss of responsiveness are often made in the absence of a noxious stimulus. Data used from these measurements to create models that predict loss of responsiveness are inherently inaccurate. It is likely that more anesthetic will be required to achieve the same level of unresponsiveness in the presence of a noxious stimulus compared to an unstimulated state.
- Data collection may not go on long enough to adequately account for drug distribution and accumulation in peripheral tissues. This may be important once drug administration is terminated. This phenomenon is associated

with lipophilic drugs (ie, fentanyl and midazolam). After prolonged infusions, more time may be required for drug concentrations to dissipate. If a pharmacokinetic model was built from data collected during a short infusion (ie, 30 minutes) and then used to predict the concentration decline after a long infusion (ie, 10 hours), the model will predict a rapid decline in plasma concentrations when in reality, it would require a much longer period of time to dissipate.

- Data sampling from a small number of subjects may lead to undue influence from outliers and skew model predictions. For example, if plasma concentration data were collected from 6 volunteers following a 0.07 mg/kg bolus of midazolam and data from 1 volunteer had plasma concentrations much higher than the rest of the group, it will skew the model to predict higher concentrations. Reasons for this data may include a low cardiac output, plasma concentration assay error, or inadvertent dosing error among others.
- Some drugs have active metabolites (ie, morphine, ketamine), so characterizing clinically relevant concentrations in the plasma or blood may require measuring several compounds.

Model Building

Model construction empirically fits an equation to data (ie, plasma concentration over time). Terms within a mathematical expression are rearranged to create a set of model parameters (ie, volumes and clearances). To account for interindividual variability and model error, model construction involves estimating parameter variability. If data (ie, measured plasma concentrations or drug effects) have substantial scatter, model parameters may have an unreasonably wide range of variability, making predictions too vague to be clinically useful. Some published models include metrics of parameter variability, but many do not.

Model Predictions

One temptation is to use models to predict drug concentrations or effect outside the range of concentrations used to create the model. These predictions can be inaccurate. Pharmacokinetic parameters (ie, clearance) for most drugs are considered to be linear. Linear means that model parameters are the same for all plasma concentrations. If linear, the profile of drug concentration predictions over time looks similar for any dose; the time to peak concentration, half-life, rate of decline, are all identical—only the concentrations are different. For most drugs at concentrations that are clinically relevant, this is usually true. But in some instances, especially with very high doses of drugs associated with cardiovascular depression (eg, propofol 4 mg/kg), pharmacokinetic parameters may be nonlinear. Although some researchers have begun to explore this phenomenon, this element of drug behavior remains largely unknown.

In general, cardiac output significantly influences the kinetic behavior of anesthetic drugs. Reduced cardiac output from intravascular volume depletion will slow the onset of intravenous drugs but lead to higher effect-site concentrations[22,23] and accelerate the onset of inhalation agents. Unfortunately, the extent cardiac output influences drug behavior is not easily implemented in clinical settings. Cardiac output is infrequently monitored, and models that describe how cardiac output changes drug behavior have not been well validated.

REFERENCES

1. Wissing H, Kuhn I, Rietbrock S, Fuhr U. Pharmacokinetics of inhaled anaesthetics in a clinical setting: comparison of desflurane, isoflurane and sevoflurane. *Br J Anaesth*. 2000;84(4): 443-449.
2. Shafer SL, Varvel JR, Aziz N, Scott JC. Pharmacokinetics of fentanyl administered by computer-controlled infusion pump. *Anesthesiology*. 1990;73(6):1091-1102.
3. Scott JC, Stanski DR. Decreased fentanyl and alfentanil dose requirements with age. A simultaneous pharmacokinetic and pharmacodynamic evaluation. *J Pharmacol Exp Ther*. 1987;240(1):159-166.
4. Schnider TW, Minto CF, Shafer SL, et al. The influence of age on propofol pharmacodynamics. Anesthesiology, 1999. 90(6):1502-1516.
5. Schnider TW, Minto CF, Gambus PL, et al. The influence of method of administration and covariates on the pharmacokinetics of propofol in adult volunteers. *Anesthesiology*. 1998;88(5):1170-1182.

6. Roy JJ, Donati F, Boismenu D, Varin F. Concentration-effect relation of succinylcholine chloride during propofol anesthesia. *Anesthesiology*. 2002;97(5):1082-1092.
7. Plaud B, Proost JH, Wierda JM, Barre J, Debaene B, Meistelman C. Pharmacokinetics and pharmacodynamics of rocuronium at the vocal cords and the adductor pollicis in humans. *Clin Pharmacol Ther*. 1995;58(2):185-191.
8. Minto CF, Schnider TW, Shafer SL. Pharmacokinetics and pharmacodynamics of remifentanil. II. Model application. *Anesthesiology*. 1997;86(1): 24-33.
9. Minto CF, Schnider TW, Egan TW, et al. Influence of age and gender on the pharmacokinetics and pharmacodynamics of remifentanil. I. Model development. *Anesthesiology*. 1997;86(1):10-23.
10. Lerou JG, Verheijen R, Booij LH. Model-based administration of inhalation anaesthesia. 4. Applying the system model. *Br J Anaesth*. 2002;88(2):175-183.
11. Lerou JG, Dirksen R, Beneken Kolmer HH, Booij LH, Borm GF. A system model for closed-circuit inhalation anesthesia. II. Clinical validation. *Anesthesiology*. 1991; 75(2):230-237.
12. Lerou JG, Dirksen R, Beneken Kolmer HH, Booij LH., A system model for closed-circuit inhalation anesthesia. I. Computer study. *Anesthesiology*. 1991;75(2):345-355.
13. Lerou JG, Booij LH. Model-based administration of inhalation anaesthesia. 3. Validating the system model. *Br J Anaesth*. 2002;88(1):24-37.
14. Lerou JG, Booij LH. Model-based administration of inhalation anaesthesia. 1. Developing a system model. *Br J Anaesth*. 2001;86(1):12-28.
15. Lerou JG, Booij LH. Model-based administration of inhalation anaesthesia. 2. Exploring the system model. *Br J Anaesth*. 2001;86(1):29-37.
16. Cooper RA, Maddineni VR, Mirakhur RK, Wierda JM, Brady M, Fitzpatrick KT. Time course of neuromuscular effects and pharmacokinetics of rocuronium bromide (Org 9426) during isoflurane anaesthesia in patients with and without renal failure. *Br J Anaesth*. 1993;71(2):222-226.
17. Kern SE, Xie G, White JL, Egan TD. A response surface analysis of propofol-remifentanil pharmacodynamic interaction in volunteers. *Anesthesiology*. 2004;100(6): 1373-1381.
18. Johnson KB, Syroid ND, Gupta DK, et al. An evaluation of remifentanil-sevoflurane response surface models in patients emerging from anesthesia: model improvement using effect-site sevoflurane concentrations. *Anesth Analg*. 2010;111(2):387-394.
19. Bouillon TW, Bruhn J, Radulescu L, et al. Pharmacodynamic interaction between propofol and remifentanil regarding hypnosis, tolerance of laryngoscopy, bispectral index, and electroencephalographic approximate entropy. *Anesthesiology*. 2004;100(6):1353-1372.
20. Wright PM. Population based pharmacokinetic analysis: why do we need it; what is it; and what has it told us about anaesthetics? *Br J Anaesth*. 1998;80(4):488-501.
21. Johnson KB, Syroid ND, Gupta DK, et al. An evaluation of remifentanil propofol response surfaces for loss of responsiveness, loss of response to surrogates of painful stimuli and laryngoscopy in patients undergoing elective surgery. *Anesth Analg*. 2008;106(2):471-479.
22. Upton RN, Ludbrook GL, Grant C, Martinez AM. Cardiac output is a determinant of the initial concentrations of propofol after short-infusion administration. *Anesth Analg*. 1999.;89(3):545-552.
23. Upton RN, Ludbrook GL. A physiological model of induction of anaesthesia with propofol in sheep. 1. Structure and estimation of variables. *Br J Anaesth*. 1997;79(4):497-504.

CHAPTER 5

The Clinical Pharmacology of Opioids

Ken B. Johnson, MD, and Austin Healy, BS

HISTORY OF DEVELOPMENT

The first reports of opioid use date to more than 6000 years ago, when a gummy substance known as opium was extracted from poppy plants known for its mind-altering effects. In 1805, a German chemist, Friedrich Serturner, identified the active ingredient in opium. He named it morphine, after Morpheus, the Greek God of dreams. In 1853, the hypodermic needle was introduced, and morphine could be administered intravenously. Morphine was used extensively during the American Civil War, and thousands of soldiers became addicted to the drug. In 1874, morphine was modified by adding 2 acetyl groups to make heroin and in 1898 was marketed as a cough suppressant. In 1924, because of the addictive properties of opioids, nonmedical use was banned. In 1930, the synthetic opioid meperidine was introduced as an alternative to morphine to treat pain. During World War II another synthetic opioid, methadone, was developed as an alternative to morphine, and in the 1960s it was used as an adjunct to treat opioid addicts. In 1959, Janssen Pharmaceuticals developed another synthetic opioid, fentanyl, which was introduced into clinical care in 1960. Janssen went on to develop other fentanyl congeners, including sufentanil (1974) and alfentanil (1976). In 1992, Glaxo Smith Kline developed and marketed the newest of the fentanyl congeners, remifentanil.

MECHANISM OF ACTION

Opioids activate opioid receptors present throughout membranes in the brain, spinal cord, and gastrointestinal system. Opioid receptors have been most extensively studied at synaptic junctions in the spinal cord. They consist of G protein–coupled receptors that activate ion channels and allow the flux of potassium and chloride, leading to a net negative polarization of a neuron membrane. In a hyperpolarized state, neurotransmission of pain signals are reduced especially in C and Aδ fibers that detect noxious stimuli.[1] The main types of receptors are presented in Table 5–1.[2] These receptors are similar; up to 70% of their protein sequence is identical. Other types of opioid receptors exist, but their role in pain control is not well defined.[3]

DOSING REGIMENS

Opioids are administered intravenously as a bolus and/or a continuous infusion and by mouth. Sample intravenous dosing regimens for commonly used opioids are presented in Table 5–2. Dosing is often thought of as an absolute dose; for example, for postoperative pain control, 100 mcg of intravenous fentanyl is frequently used. This approach works well when most patients are about the same size (ie, 70–75 kg). As clinicians face a more diverse range in body weight, a more accurate approach is to normalize the dose to weight. Table 5–2 presents doses normalized to weight as well as common absolute doses.

Drug Preparation

With the exception of remifentanil, opioids are dispensed as liquid suspensions. Fentanyl, hydromorphone, and alfentanil are packaged so that they do

TABLE 5–1 Opioid receptor site of action and effect.

Opioid Receptor	Site of Action	Effect
μ (μ1, μ2, μ3)	Brain Spine Gastrointestinal tract	μ1: Supraspinal analgesia Physical dependence μ2: Respiratory depression Physical dependence Miosis Euphoria Reduced gastrointestinal motility μ3: Unknown
κ	Brain Spine	Spinal analgesia Sedation Miosis Inhibition of antidiuretic hormone release
δ	Brain	Analgesia Euphoria Physical dependence

Adapted, with permission, from Yaster M, Kost-Byerly S, Maxwell LG. Opioid agonists and antagonists. In: Schechter NL, Berde CB, Yaster M, eds. Pain in infants, children, and adolescents. 2nd ed. Philadelphia: Lippincott Williams & Wilkins, 2003:181-224.

TABLE 5–3 Opioid equivalencies.

Opioid	Equipotent Doses
Morphine	1 mg
Meperidine	10 mg
Methadone	1 mg
Hydromorphone	0.2 mg
Fentanyl	50 mcg
Alfentanil	500 mcg
Sufentanil	5 mcg
Remifentanil	50 mcg

not require dilution for an adult. Morphine, meperidine, and sufentanil are more concentrated and require dilution. Remifentanil comes as a lyophilized powder and requires dilution with normal saline. Because it is nearly equipotent to fentanyl, a common technique is to prepare remifentanil in concentrations of 20 to 50 mcg/mL. Opioid equivalencies are useful comparisons when considering different opioids to achieve a similar effect. Selected equivalencies are presented in Table 5–3.

TABLE 5–2 Intravenous opioid dosing regimens.

Opioid (Trade Name)	Bolus	Infusion Rate	Comments
Morphine	20–80 mcg/kg	0.01–0.05 mg/kg/h	Common bolus dose: 1–5 mg
Meperidine (Demerol)	0.2–0.7 mg/kg	None	Common bolus dose: 12.5–50 mg
Methadone	0.02–0.08 mg/kg	None	
Hydromorphone (Dilaudid)	3–14 mcg/kg	0.2–0.4 mg/kg/h	Common bolus dose: 0.2–0.4 mg
Fentanyl (Sublimaze)	1–3 mcg/kg	2.0–6.0 mcg/kg/h	Common bolus dose: 50–150 mcg
Alfentanil (Alfenta)	50–75 mcg/kg	0.5–1.5 mcg/kg/min	
Sufentanil (Sufenta)	1–2 mcg/kg	0.5–1.0 mcg/kg/h	Common bolus dose: 5-15 mcg
Remifentanil (Ultiva)	0.5–3 mcg/kg	Moderate sedation: 0.05–0.10 mcg/kg/min General anesthesia: 0.10–0.25 mcg/kg/min	Available as a lyophilized powder; dilute with 0.9% saline to 10 or 50 mcg/mL

Pharmacodynamic Models

Researchers have identified opioid concentrations that provide analgesia for a variety of noxious stimuli using pharmacodynamic models. Similar to minimum alveolar concentration levels, the C_{50}, defined as the effect-site concentration necessary to achieve an effect (ie, analgesia) in 50% of healthy adults, is used to describe opioid potency. C_{50} concentrations have been most extensively studied with remifentanil. Remifentanil C_{50} values have been identified for opioid effects to include various painful stimuli, ventilatory depression, and sedation (Table 5–4).

SIMULATIONS

Simulations provide visualization of the magnitude and time course of drug concentrations (pharmacokinetics) as well as the onset and duration of drug effects (pharmacodynamics). For purposes of illustrating opioid effects, 2 effect measures will be used: the loss of response to 30 pounds per square inch of anterior tibial pressure and a respiratory rate less than 4 breaths per minute (see Table 5–4). The loss of response to tibial pressure is used as a surrogate of moderately painful surgical stimuli. Simulations will be used to explore the behavior of commonly used opioid administered as a bolus and as a continuous infusion.

Bolus Dosing

Using published pharmacokinetic models[11-16] and sample bolus doses presented in Table 5–2, simulations of a bolus of alfentanil, fentanyl, sufentanil, remifentanil, hydromorphone, and morphine are presented in Figure 5–1. Of note is the difference in the time required to reach the peak effect-site concentration (Table 5–5). The fentanyl congeners (remifentanil, alfentanil, and sufentanil) all share a similar profile; the effect-site peaks shortly after administration. Alfentanil and remifentanil require less than 2 minutes to reach their peak, and fentanyl and sufentanil require 4 to 6 minutes. After reaching their peak, effect-site concentrations wane over the next 30 to 40 minutes. Of the fentanyl congeners, remifentanil has the most rapid drop in effect-site concentrations, whereas fentanyl has the slowest.

TABLE 5–4 Remifentanil effect-site concentrations associated with a 50% probability of selected effects (C_{50}).

Effect	Remifentanil C_{50} (ng/mL)
Analgesia	
Loss of Response to Moderate Pain	
Tibial pressure (30 PSI)	1.3[4]
Loss of Response to Severe Pain	
Electrical tetany (50 mA)	21.3[5]
Hot plate (50°C for 5 seconds)	6.1[6]
Tibial pressure (50 PSI)	7.1[6]
Laryngoscopy	6.8[6] 4.8[7]
Endotracheal intubation	4.9[7]
Esophageal instrumentation	9.8[8]
Respiratory Depression	
50% decrease in minute ventilation	3.3[9]
Respiratory rate ≤ 4 breath/min	4.2[8]
Sedation	
Sedation (OAAS < 4)[a]	12.5[5]
Loss of responsiveness (OAAS < 2)[b]	50.9[4]

mA, milliamps; OAAS, Observer's Assessment of Alertness and Sedation; PSI, pounds per square inch.[10]
[a]OAAS < 4 indicates that patients respond only after their name is called loudly and/or repeatedly (sedated).
[b]OAAS < 2 indicates that patients do not respond to moderate prodding or shaking with verbal stimulus (unresponsive).

In contrast, the profiles of hydromorphone and morphine are much different. Morphine requires up to 83 minutes to reach its peak effect-site concentration. Despite taking a long time to reach its peak, it has a quick rise to near its peak just after administration; it reaches 70% of its peak within 5 minutes. Hydromorphone requires less time (15 minutes) to reach its peak effect-site concentration, but like morphine, the time course of the effect-site concentration is much slower to dissipate compared to the fentanyl congeners.

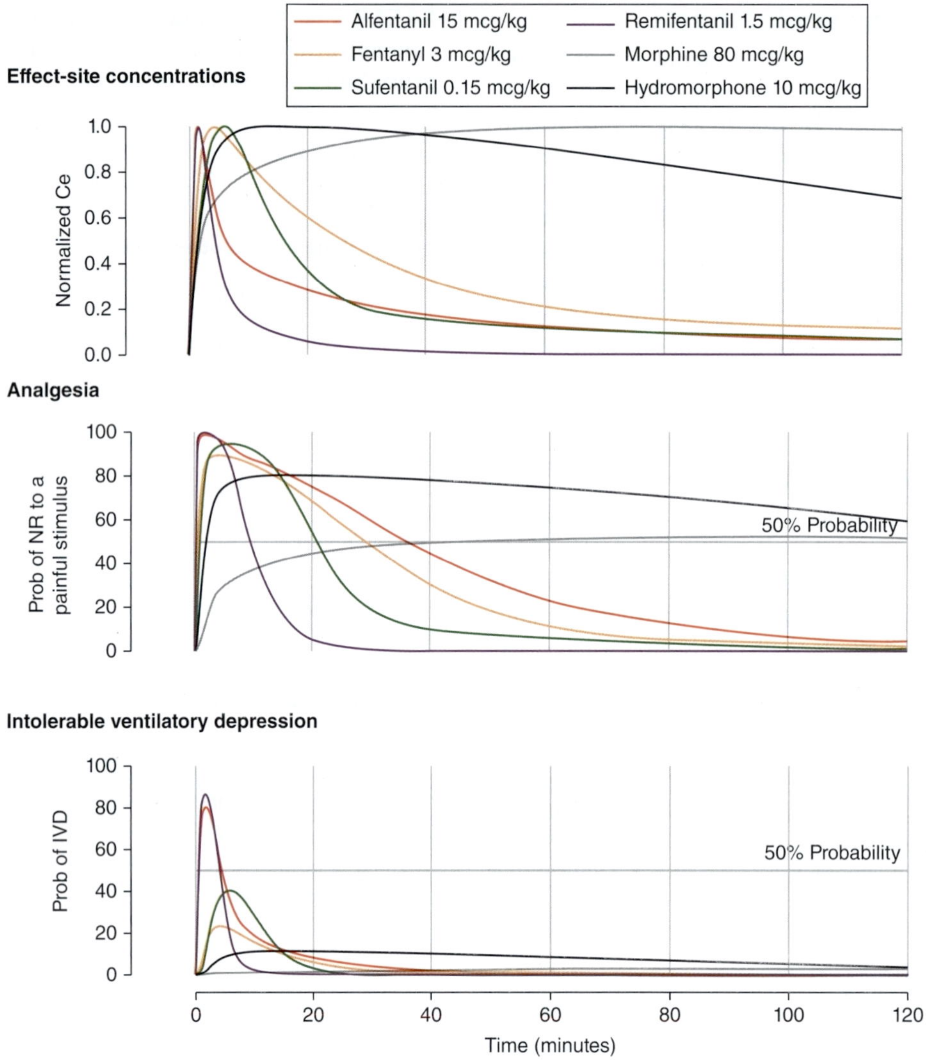

FIGURE 5–1 Simulations of selected opioid bolus doses. The top plot is the normalized effect-site concentration (Ce) over 2 hours following a bolus dose of alfentanil, fentanyl, sufentanil, remifentanil, hydromorphone, and morphine. The effect-site concentrations were normalized (the peak Ce for each bolus was set to 1) to better illustrate the kinetic differences between each drug. The middle plot is the probability (Prob) of no response (NR) to a painful stimulus. The painful stimulus is a surrogate of moderate postsurgical pain—30 pounds per square inch of pressure on the anterior tibia. The bottom plot is the probability of intolerable ventilatory depression (IVD) defined as intolerable ventilatory rate less than 4 breaths per minute. The light gray lines in the middle and bottom plot represent the 50% probability for each effect.

For discussion purposes, onset and duration of effect are characterized in terms of the time required to reach and maintain a 50% and 90% probability of effect. For a 50% probability of analgesic effect, the fentanyl congeners as dosed have a rapid onset (1 minute or less) with a duration of 9 to 36 minutes. For morphine, the onset time is slow (more than 30 minutes) with a duration of up to 2 hours. For hydromorphone, the onset time is faster than morphine (within 2 minutes) with a duration of up

TABLE 5–5 Analgesic effect following an intravenous bolus of selected opioids.

	Alfentanil 15 mcg/kg	Fentanyl 3.0 mcg/kg	Sufentanil 0.15 mcg/kg	Remifentanil 1.5 mcg/kg	Morphine 0.08 mg/kg	Hydromorphone 0.01 mg/kg
Time to Peak Ce (min):	< 2	4	5	< 2	83	15
Onset Time (min):						
Time to Probability > 50%	< 1	< 1	1	< 1	38	2
Time to Probability > 90%	< 1	–	8	< 1	–	–
Duration (min):						
Probability > 50%	36	28	20	9	122	143
Probability > 90%	6	–	3	5	–	–

to 2 hours. For a 90% probability of analgesic effect, remifentanil and alfentanil have a rapid onset (less than 1 minute) and short duration (5–6 minutes). The sufentanil dose leads to a slower onset and brief duration at this level of effect. As dosed, fentanyl, hydromorphone, and morphine never achieve this level of effect.

Clinical Implications

- Unlike slower onset opioids, with the rapid onset of effect following a bolus dose of remifentanil or alfentanil, there is little time for carbon dioxide to accumulate and offset the respiratory depressant effects of opioids. This may lead to more profound respiratory depression with alfentanil and remifentanil, although, from an analgesic standpoint, these doses are near equipotent with longer acting analgesics.
- Although alfentanil and remifentanil have a rapid onset, the duration of effect is much longer with alfentanil (see Table 5–5). In fact, alfentanil may last longer than a fentanyl bolus (see Figure 5–1).

With regard to intolerable ventilatory depression, remifentanil and alfentanil have a rapid onset (less than 2 minutes) and short duration (4–5 minutes) where the probability is greater than 50% (see Figure 5–1). The probability of ventilatory depression is less (never achieves a 50% probability) with the other opioids as dosed.

Figure 5–2 presents simulated effect-site concentrations over time following various bolus doses of fentanyl. In this set of simulations, it is assumed that the pharmacokinetics are linear; thus, the time to reaching the peak effect-site concentration and the rate of decline has the same profile regardless of the dose. As expected, the onset and duration of effects are a function of dose (Table 5–6). For the 50% probability of analgesic effect, all doses except 1 mcg/kg have a rapid onset (1 minute or less), and the duration increases as a function of dose. With the exception of the 5 mcg/kg dose, none of the fentanyl bolus doses achieve a probability greater than 90%. The 5 mcg/kg dose exceeded the 90% probability within 1 minute and lasts for 19 minutes. None of the bolus doses lead to significant ventilatory depression, except the 5 mcg/kg dose, where it exceeded the 50% probability within 2 minutes and lasted 7 minutes.

Continuous Infusion Dosing

Clinical pharmacologists have characterized the pharmacokinetic behavior of opioid infusions using context-sensitive half-time. The context-sensitive

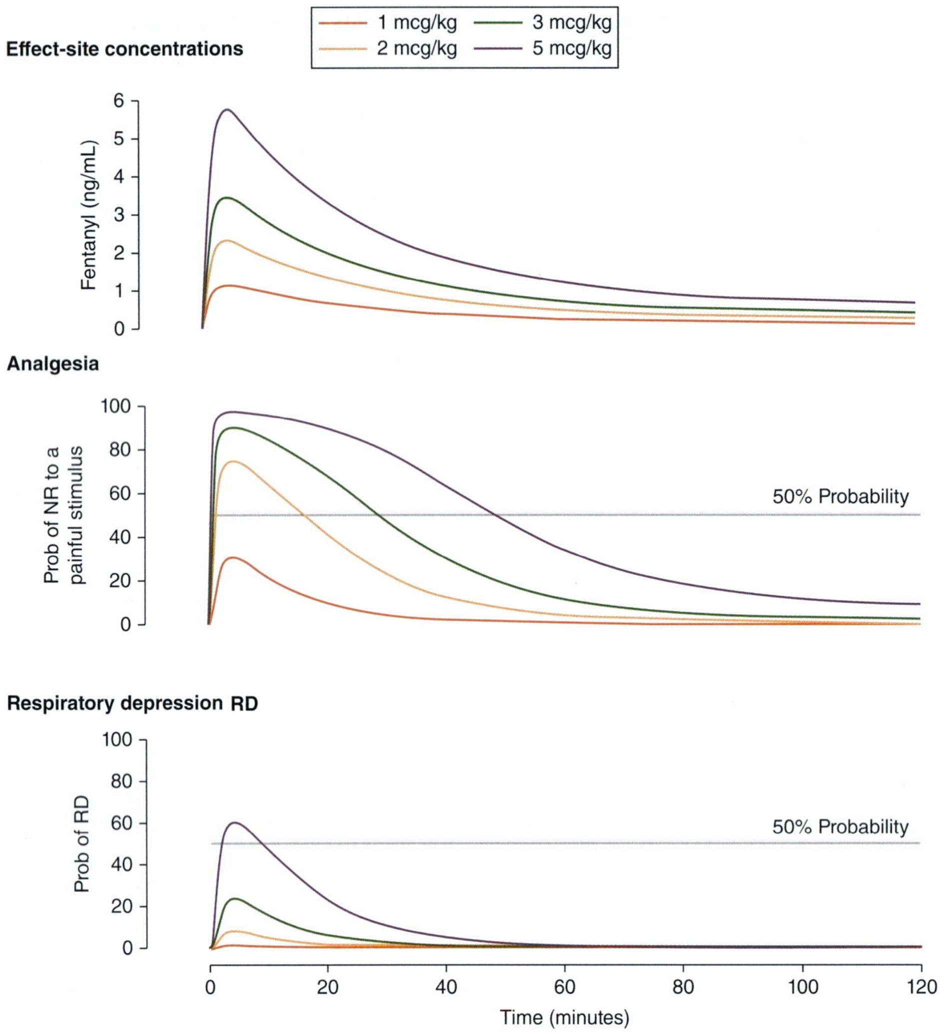

FIGURE 5–2 Simulations of selected fentanyl bolus doses. The simulations assume linear pharmacokinetics. The top plot is the effect-site concentration over a 2-hour time window following a 1-, 2-, 3-, and 5-mcg/kg bolus. The middle plot is the probability (Prob) of no response (NR) to a painful stimulus. The painful stimulus is a surrogate of moderate postsurgical pain—30 pounds per square inch of pressure on the anterior tibia. The bottom plot is the probability of intolerable ventilatory depression (IVD) defined as intolerable ventilatory rate less than 4 breaths per minute. The light gray lines in the middle and bottom plot represent the 50% probability for each effect.

TABLE 5–6 Descriptors of analgesic effect following various bolus doses of intravenous fentanyl.

50% or Greater Probability of No Response to a Moderately Painful Stimulus	1 mcg/kg	2 mcg/kg	3 mcg/kg	5 mcg/kg
Onset Time (min):	–	1	1	< 1
Duration of effect (min):	–	17	28	49

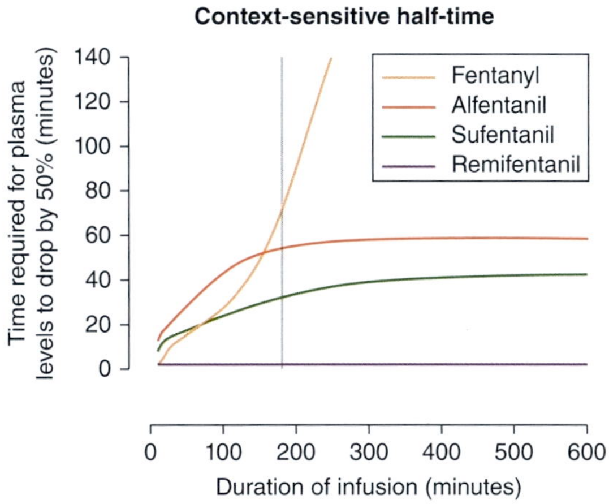

FIGURE 5–3 Context-sensitive half-time for selected opioids. The vertical axis represents the time required for the plasma concentration to decrease by 50% (the 50% decrement time) once an infusion is terminated as a function of the duration of a continuous infusion. The horizontal axis represents the duration of an infusion up to 600 minutes. The gray vertical line represents the 3-hour mark.

half-time for the fentanyl congeners is presented in Figure 5–3. This plot presents the time required for the plasma concentration to decrease by 50% once an infusion is terminated. It provides a qualitative comparison of opioid behavior as a function of infusion duration. For longer infusions, the context-sensitive half-times differ according to the unique pharmacokinetic features of each opioid. For example, remifentanil has a rapid decline independent of infusion duration. By contrast, fentanyl has the largest increase in the context-sensitive half-time as a function of infusion duration. For example, for a 4-hour infusion, the 50% decrement time is more than 2 hours. Alfentanil and sufentanil are different from fentanyl in that as the infusion duration increases, the context-sensitive half-time eventually reaches a plateau (ie, 45 minutes for sufentanil and 60 minutes for alfentanil). Fentanyl, in contrast, never reaches a plateau; the context-sensitive half-time continues to increase exponentially as the infusion duration increases.

Clinical Implications

- The context-sensitive half-time is useful when selecting an opioid for a continuous infusion of long duration.
- If a prolonged decline in opioid concentrations is an analgesic goal, then fentanyl is ideal. For example, following a procedure associated with severe postoperative pain in patients who remain intubated and mechanically ventilated, a fentanyl infusion is useful.
- If a predictable decline within 1 hour of terminating an opioid infusion is desirable, then sufentanil or alfentanil are reasonable choices. For example, following a procedure associated with moderate postoperative pain, which requires a timely emergence from anesthesia, turning off a sufentanil or alfentanil infusion 30 to 45 minutes prior to the end of surgery will provide a predictable decline in opioid concentrations when it is time to emerge from anesthesia.

Figure 5–4 presents simulations of a 3-hour infusion for the fentanyl congeners dosed according to infusion rates for general anesthesia presented in Table 5–2. Of note is the difference in the time required to reach the maximal effect-site concentration during the infusion (Table 5–7). Fentanyl, sufentanil, and alfentanil, unlike remifentanil, all require significant time to approach 90% of the maximal effect-site concentration achieved during the 3-hour infusion (ie, 22 minutes versus more than 2 hours).

Clinical Implications

- With the exception of remifentanil, effect-site concentrations do not plateau but continually rise during the infusion. This may be important when titrating an opioid infusion during a procedure associated with dynamic changes in surgical stimulus. Once the infusion is turned off, the context-sensitive half-times range from 5 minutes to 48 minutes, with fentanyl requiring the most time and almost double of what is required by sufentanil.

A significant limitation of the context-sensitive half-time is that it does not provide an estimate of analgesic effect. In Figure 5–3, the context-sensitive half-times for a 3-hour infusion (gray line) are all different but do not provide information regarding the onset and duration of effect. As with the simulations

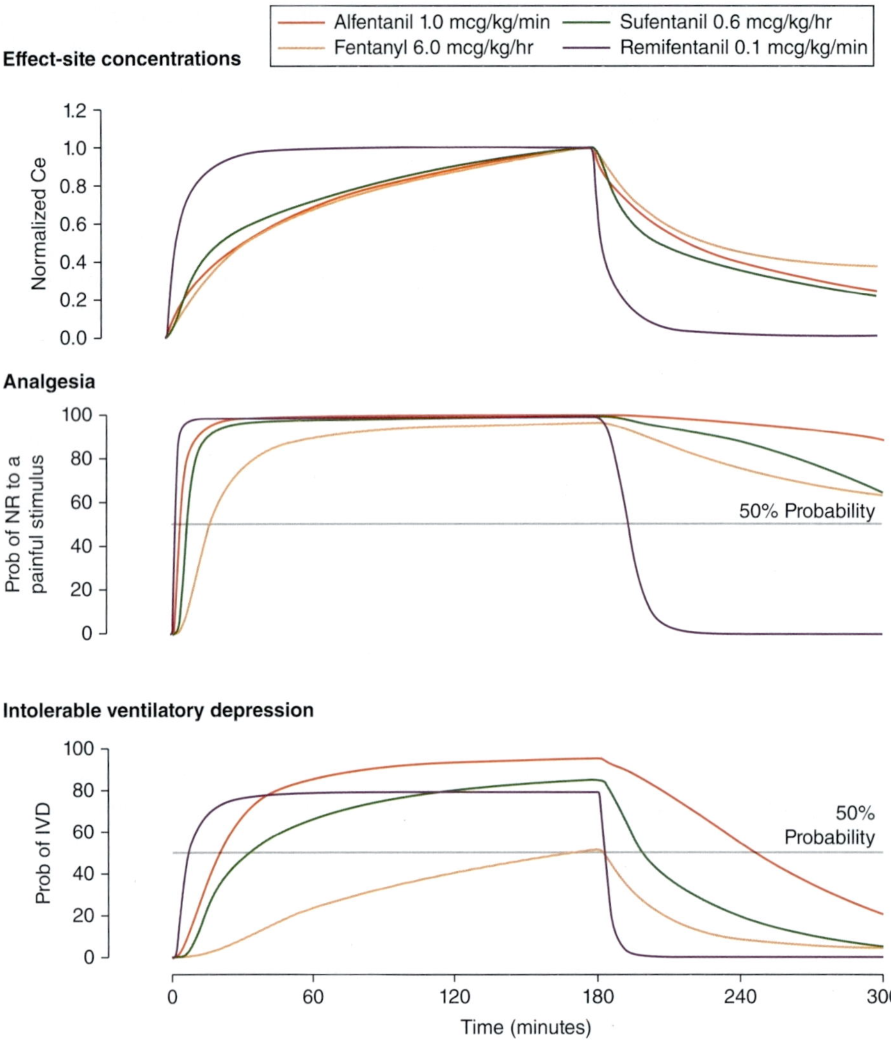

FIGURE 5–4 Simulations of selected opioid infusions. The top plot is the normalized effect-site concentration (Ce) over a 5-hour time window following a 3-hour infusion of alfentanil, fentanyl, sufentanil, and remifentanil. The effect-site concentrations were normalized (the peak Ce for each infusion was set to better illustrate the kinetic differences between each drug. The middle plot is the probability (Prob) of no response (NR) to a painful stimulus. The bottom plot is the probability of intolerable ventilatory depression (IVD) defined as an intolerable ventilatory rate less than 4 breaths per minute. The horizontal light gray lines in the middle and bottom plot represent the 50% probability for each effect.

of bolus doses, pharmacodynamic models are required to explore these features of drug behavior.

Analgesic Effect

To achieve an analgesic effect, the fentanyl congeners as dosed have a fairly rapid onset; 2 to 17 minutes to exceed a 50% probability of analgesia and all of them eventually exceed a 90% probability of effect (see Table 5–7). Fentanyl requires the most time (more than 1 hour to reach a 90% probability of effect). Once the infusion is turned off, remifentanil drops below 90% almost immediately and below 50% within 13

TABLE 5–7 Analgesic and respiratory effects following a 3-hour infusion.

	Alfentanil 1 mcg/kg/min	Fentanyl 6 mcg/kg/hr	Sufentanil 0.6 mcg/kg/hr	Remifentanil 0.2 mcg/kg/min
Effect-Site Concentrations				
Time to 90% of Peak Ce **Minutes after start of infusion**	128	136	124	21
Context–Sensitive Half-Time **Time to 50% of Peak Ce** **Minutes after infusion is turned off**	40	48	27	5
Analgesia				
Onset Time **Minutes after start of infusion**				
Time to Probability > 50%	4	17	7	2
Time to Probability > 90%	12	64	16	4
Offset Time **Minutes after infusion is turned off**				
Time to Probability < 50%	220	237	150	13
Time to Probability < 90%	111	21	50	5
Intolerable Ventilatory Depression				
Onset Time **Minutes after start of infusion**				
Time to Probability > 50%	20	170	33	7
Time to Probability > 90%	81	–	–	–
Offset Time **Minutes after infusion is turned off**				
Time to Probability < 50%	67	3	19	3
Time to Probability < 90%	11	–	–	–

minutes. For the others, after 3 hours of drug accumulation, the analgesic effects linger for several hours. Sufentanil has the shortest profile, dropping below 50% in less than 1 hour. Alfentanil behaves very similarly to fentanyl, with a slow decline in analgesic effect taking close to 4 hours to drop below a 50% probability of effect. This is interesting to consider given that alfentanil was once thought of as a rapid-acting opioid. When administered as a bolus, it is rapid acting. However, when administered as an infusion, it behaves more like fentanyl with a prolonged duration of effect.

Ventilatory Depression

As dosed, all of the fentanyl congeners achieve significant ventilatory depression, but only alfentanil exceeds a 90% probability of effect. This is a dose-dependent phenomenon; the other fentanyl congeners would exceed a 90% probability of effect with higher infusion rates. The onset is relatively quick with remifentanil and alfentanil (7 and 20 minutes, respectively) and slower with sufentanil and fentanyl. Once the infusion is turned off, the probability of ventilatory depression quickly wanes for remifentanil. By contrast, this effect slowly dissipates for the other fentanyl congeners, with alfentanil requiring the most time (more than an hour to drop below a 50% probability).

Clinical Implications

- These simulations illustrate the potential value of using a bolus followed by an infusion at the start of a procedure to quickly achieve target concentrations. By contrast to an infusion, a bolus dose can attain a target concentration (and its associated effect) in a short period of time (seconds to minutes). The infusion can then maintain concentrations without a prolonged ramp-up time, as is the case with sufentanil (16 minutes) and fentanyl (64 minutes).
- Onset of drug effect within seconds to minutes is more consistent with clinical practice, because anesthesiologists often seek to induce and maintain selected drug effects quickly to facilitate airway instrumentation and block responses to surgical stimuli. A comparison of a sufentanil bolus followed by an infusion with a simple infusion is presented in Figure 5–5. In this example, the bolus and infusion exceeds a 90% probability of analgesia within 30 seconds and then maintains that level of effect for the entire 3 hours.

The consequence of using a bolus can become evident once a surgical procedure is completed. Analgesic effects are substantially increased. The times required to drop below a 90% and 50% probability of analgesia are 76 and 190 minutes, respectively. This is considerably longer than with a simple sufentanil infusion (see Table 5–7). The ventilatory depressant effects are also prolonged; the time required to drop below a 50% probability of intolerable ventilatory depression increases from 19 to 34 minutes. This is of concern when attempting to minimize respiratory depression prior to emergence from anesthesia. To offset these prolonged effects, a common clinical practice is to turn off the infusion 45 minutes prior to the end of a procedure. This allows for the probability of ventilatory depression to drop below 50% while maintaining a high probability of analgesia.

COMMON CLINICAL USES

Intravenous opioids are a mainstay of anesthetic techniques for intraoperative and postoperative analgesia. They are primarily used in conjunction with other anesthetics but can be used as a single agent. The major challenge when titrating opioids is to achieve an adequate level of analgesia while avoiding unwanted respiratory depression, among other adverse side effects. This is especially important during emergence from general anesthesia and treating postoperative pain.

Intraoperatively, opioids are often dosed using intermittent boluses. Boluses are used in anticipation of or in response to an increase in noxious stimuli. With this dosing technique, the analgesic effect is episodic, with peaks of analgesia followed by periods of minimal analgesic effect. If continuous level of analgesia is desired, a continuous infusion may be more effective. In Figure 5–6, a bolus technique with fentanyl is compared with a continuous infusion technique with remifentanil. The simulation assumes a 2-hour period of noxious stimuli. Fentanyl is intermittently dosed at the start (1.5 mcg/kg) followed by 2 additional doses of 1 mcg/kg at 45 and 90 minutes. Remifentanil is dosed at the start (1 mcg/kg) followed by a continuous infusion dosed at 0.2 mcg/kg/min. Figure 5–6 illustrates the difference in analgesic effect over the 2-hour period. The fentanyl dosing provides brief episodes above the 50% probability of analgesic effect. By contrast, the remifentanil dosing provides a continuous 2-hour time window above the 90% probability of analgesic effect.

Some important limitations of this simulation merit discussion. First, opioids are rarely administered as a sole agent. These simulations do not account for the analgesic effect of other anesthetics or the synergistic interactions opioids have with other anesthetics. These interactions can significantly enhance the analgesic and ventilatory depressant

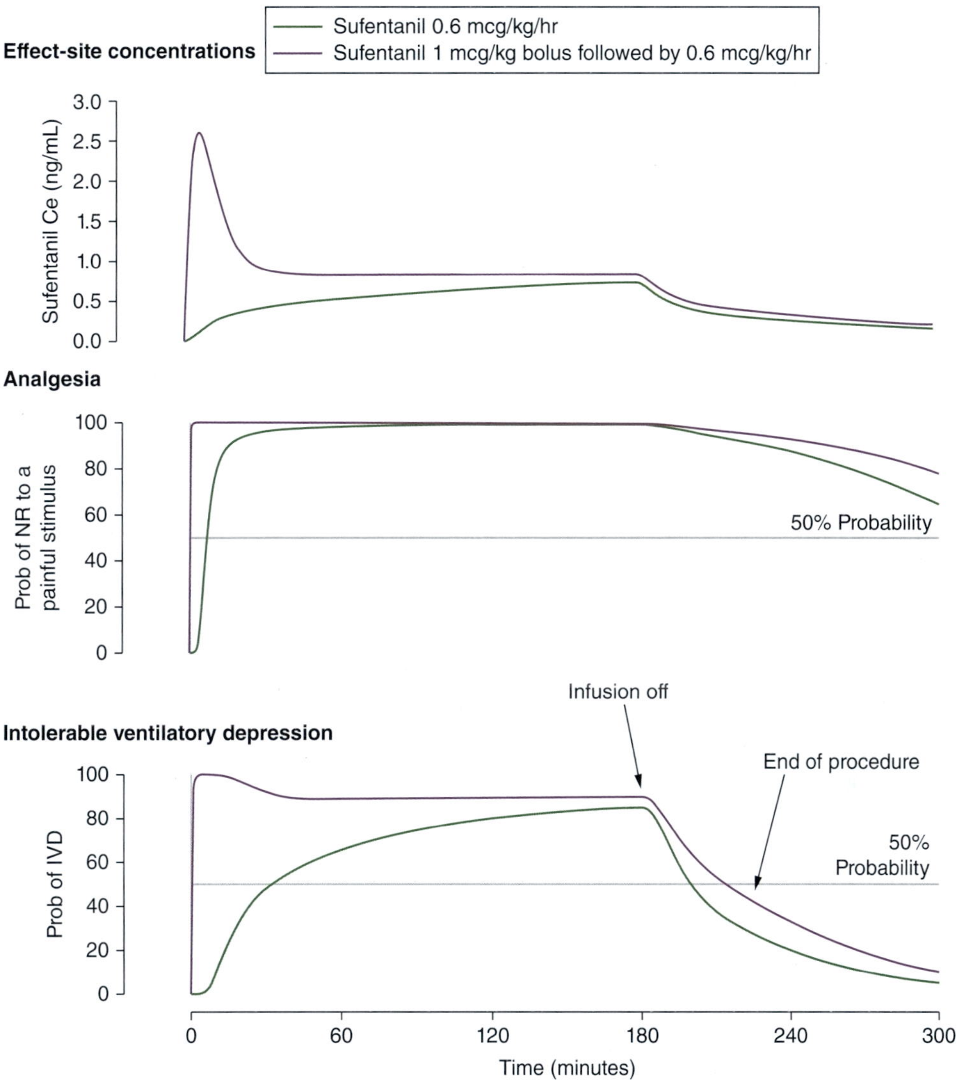

FIGURE 5–5 Simulations of a sufentanil infusion versus a bolus followed by an infusion. The top plot is effect-site concentration (Ce) over a 5-hour time window. The middle plot is the probability (Prob) of no response (NR) to a painful stimulus. The bottom plot is the probability of intolerable ventilatory depression (IVD) defined as an intolerable ventilatory rate less than 4 breaths per minute. The horizontal light gray lines in the middle and bottom plot represent the 50% probability for each effect.

effects of both the fentanyl and remifentanil. Second, if the 2-hour procedure is associated with significant postoperative pain, these dosing techniques will not provide adequate analgesic effect after 2 hours. Additional analgesics, known as "transition opioids" will be required to bridge the analgesia requirements from the end of the procedure into the recovery period.

ADVERSE EFFECTS

Acute Opioid Tolerance and Hyperalgesia: Is It real?

One concern with high-dose intraoperative opioid use is the development of acute tolerance or hyperalgesia[17] leading to increased postoperative

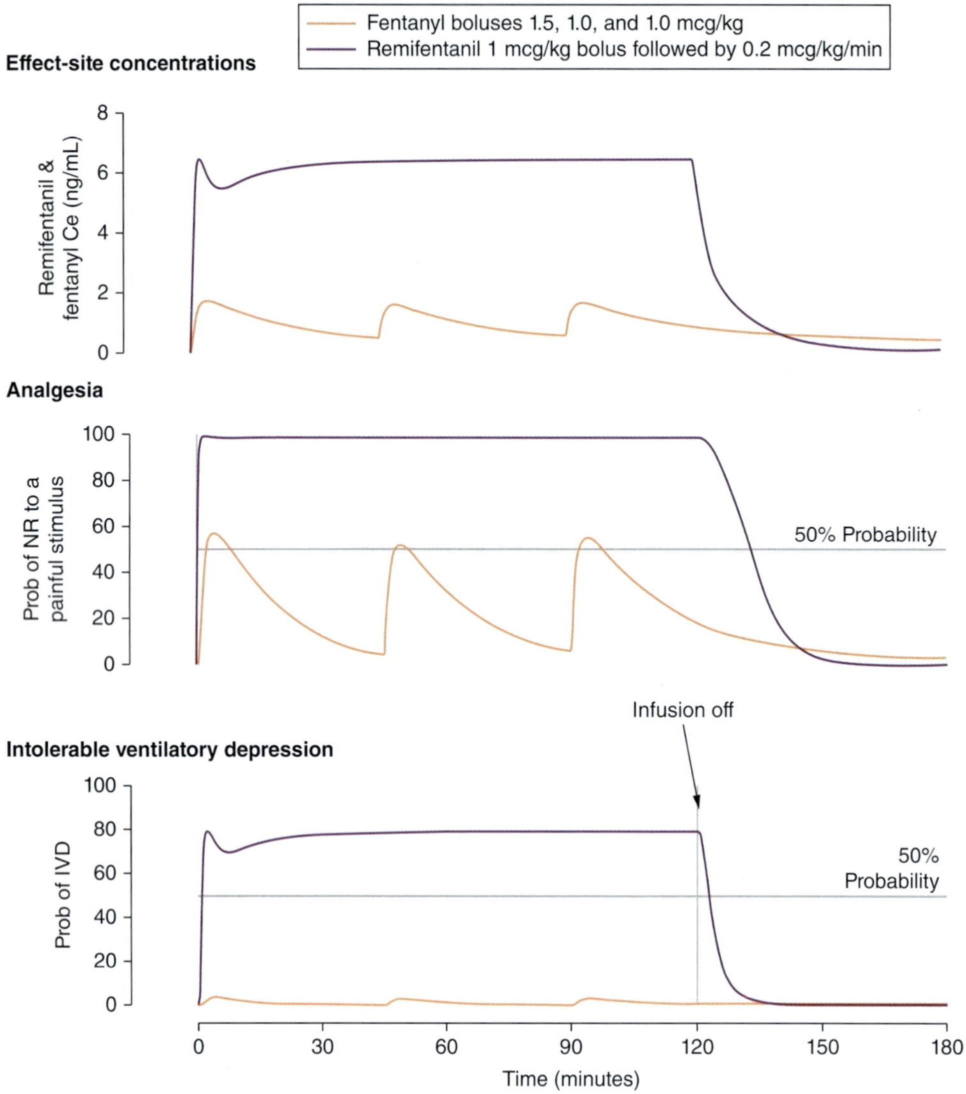

FIGURE 5–6 Simulations of a 2-hour remifentanil infusion versus a set of intermittent fentanyl boluses (1.5 mcg/kg at the beginning, 1 mcg/kg 45 minutes later, and 1 mcg/kg 90 minutes later. The top plot is effect-site concentration (Ce) over a 3-hour time window. The middle plot is the probability (Prob) of no response (NR) to a painful stimulus. The bottom plot is the probability of intolerable ventilatory depression (IVD) defined as an intolerable ventilatory rate less than 4 breaths per minute. The light gray lines in the middle and bottom plot represent the 50% probability for each effect.

opioid requirements. Numerous studies have explored this question in both animal and human studies. Remifentanil has been implicated as an analgesic that initially provides effective analgesia, but whose effect wanes, increasing postoperative opioid requirements.[18] Thought to develop within 2 to 8 hours,[19] acute opioid tolerance may be a function of exposure (continuous infusion, consistently maintaining high opioid concentrations, versus bolus dosing, resulting in short bursts of high opioid concentrations). One theory considered was that changes in opioid receptor function lead to a paradoxical increase in the sensitivity to painful stimuli. The consensus, however, is that opioid tolerance does not exist; several studies have been unable to measure the development of acute opioid tolerance.[20,21]

REFERENCES

1. Fine PG, Portenoy RK. *The Endogenous Opioid System*: New York: McGraw-Hill; 2004.
2. Corbett AD, Henderson G, McKnight AT, Paterson SJ. 75 years of opioid research: the exciting but vain quest for the Holy Grail. *Br J Pharmacol.* 2006;147(suppl 1): S153-S162.
3. Snyder SH. Opiate receptor revisited. *Anesthesiology.* 2007;107(4):659-661.
4. Johnson KB, Syroid ND, Gupta DK, et al. An evaluation of remifentanil-sevoflurane response surface models in patients emerging from anesthesia: model improvement using effect-site sevoflurane concentrations. *Anesth Analg.* 2010;111(2):387-394.
5. Kern SE, Xie G, White JL, Egan TD. A response surface analysis of propofol-remifentanil pharmacodynamic interaction in volunteers. *Anesthesiology.* 2004;100(6): 1373-1381.
6. Manyam SC, Gupta DK, Johnson KB, et al. Opioid-volatile anesthetic synergy: a response surface model with remifentanil and sevoflurane as prototypes. *Anesthesiology.* 2006;105(2):265-278.
7. Mertens MJ, Olofsen E, Engbers FH, Burm AG, Bovill JG, Vuyk J. Propofol reduces perioperative remifentanil requirements in a synergistic manner: response surface modeling of perioperative remifentanil-propofol interactions. *Anesthesiology.* 2003;99(2):345-359.
8. Lapierre CD, Johnson KB, Randall B, White JL, Egan TD. An exploration of combinations of remifentanil and propofol that lead to a loss of response to esophageal instrumentation, a loss of responsiveness, and/or onset of intolerable ventilatory depression. *Anesth Analg.* 2011;113(3):490-499.
9. Nieuwenhuijs DJ, Olofsen E, Romberg RR, et al. Response surface modeling of remifentanil-propofol interaction on cardiorespiratory control and bispectral index. *Anesthesiology.* 2003;98(2):312-322.
10. Chernick DA, Gillings D, Laine H, et al. Validity and reliability of the Observer's Assessment of Alertness/Sedation Scale: study with intravenous midazolam. *J Clin Psychopharmacol.* 1990;10(4):244-251.
11. Minto CF, Schnider TW, Egan TD, et al. Influence of age and gender on the pharmacokinetics and pharmacodynamics of remifentanil. I. Model development. *Anesthesiology.* 1997;86(1):10-23.
12. Egan TD, Minto CF, Hermann DJ, Barr J, Muir KT, Shafer SL. Remifentanil versus alfentanil: comparative pharmacokinetics and pharmacodynamics in healthy adult male volunteers. *Anesthesiology.* 1996;84(4): 821-833.
13. Shafer SL, Varvel JR, Aziz N, Scott JC. Pharmacokinetics of fentanyl administered by computer-controlled infusion pump. *Anesthesiology.* 1990;73(6):1091-1102.
14. Dershwitz M, Walsh JL, Morishige RJ, et al. Pharmacokinetics and pharmacodynamics of inhaled versus intravenous morphine in healthy volunteers. *Anesthesiology.* 2000;93(3):619-628.
15. Drover DR, Angst MS, Valle M, et al. Input characteristics and bioavailability after administration of immediate and a new extended-release formulation of hydromorphone in healthy volunteers. *Anesthesiology.* 2002;97(4):825-836.
16. Gepts E, Shafer SL, Camu F, et al. Linearity of pharmacokinetics and model estimation of sufentanil. *Anesthesiology.* 1995;83(6):1194-1204.
17. Angst MS, Clark JD. Opioid-induced hyperalgesia: a qualitative systematic review. *Anesthesiology.* 2006;104 (3):570-587.
18. Guignard B, Bossard AE, Coste C, et al. Acute opioid tolerance: intraoperative remifentanil increases postoperative pain and morphine requirement. *Anesthesiology.* 2000;93(2):409-417.
19. Simonnet G. Acute tolerance to opioids: methodological, theoretical and clinical implications. *Pain.* 2009;142(1-2):3-4.
20. Angst MS, Chu LF, Tingle MS, Shafer SL, Clark JD, Drover DR. No evidence for the development of acute tolerance to analgesic, respiratory depressant and sedative opioid effects in humans. *Pain.* 2009;142(1-2): 15-26.
21. Cortinez LI, Brandes V, Munoz HR, Guerrero ME, Mur M. No clinical evidence of acute opioid tolerance after remifentanil-based anaesthesia. *Br J Anaesth.* 2001; 87(6):866-869.

[illegible]

1. [illegible]
2. [illegible] Handb Exp Pharmacol. 2008;(182):471–487.
3. [illegible]
4. [illegible] Kern SE. Flexible interaction model for complex interactions of multiple anesthetics. Anesthesiology. 2006;105:286–296.
5. Kern SE, Xie G, White JL, Egan TD. A response surface analysis of propofol-remifentanil pharmacodynamic interaction in volunteers. Anesthesiology. 2004;100:1373–1381.
6. Manyam SC, Gupta DK, Johnson KB, et al. Opioid-volatile anesthetic synergy: a response surface model with remifentanil and sevoflurane as prototypes. Anesthesiology. 2006;105:267–278.
7. Mertens MJ, Olofsen E, Engbers FH, Burm AG, Bovill JG, Vuyk J. Propofol reduces perioperative remifentanil requirements in a synergistic manner: response surface modeling of perioperative remifentanil-propofol interactions. Anesthesiology. 2003;99:347–359.
8. LaPierre CD, Johnson KB, Randall BR, White JL, Egan TD. An exploration of remifentanil-propofol combinations that lead to a loss of response to esophageal instrumentation, a loss of responsiveness, and/or onset of intolerable ventilatory depression. Anesth Analg. 2011;113(3):490–499.
9. [illegible]
10. [illegible]
11. [illegible]
12. [illegible]
13. [illegible]
14. [illegible]
15. [illegible]
16. [illegible] Anesthesiology. [illegible]
17. Angst MS, Clark JD. Opioid-induced hyperalgesia: a qualitative systematic review. Anesthesiology. 2006;104:570–587.
18. Guignard B, Bossard AE, Coste C, et al. Acute opioid tolerance: intraoperative remifentanil increases postoperative pain and morphine requirement. Anesthesiology. 2000;93(2):409–417.
19. Simonnet G. Acute tolerance to opioids: methodological, theoretical and clinical implications. Pain. 2009;142:3–4.
20. Angst MS, Chu LF, Tingle MS, Shafer SL, Clark JD, Drover DR. No evidence for the development of acute tolerance to analgesic, respiratory depressant and sedative opioid effects in humans. Pain. 2009;142(1–2):17–26.

CHAPTER

6

Intravenous Sedative–Hypnotics

Aaron Freeman, BS, and Ken B. Johnson, MD

HISTORY OF DEVELOPMENT

Sedative–hypnotics are a relatively new class of anesthetics, beginning with the introduction of sodium thiopental in the early 1930s. Since then, several sedative–hypnotics have been introduced (Table 6–1), with more in the drug development pipeline, such as remimazolam, fospropofol, and isomers of etomidate. Goals of these modified drugs include fast metabolism and breakdown as well as creating "soft" drugs with safer profiles. A major goal in developing methoxycarbonyl-etomidate is the removal of adrenocortical suppression by modifying the pyrrole ring in etomidate. Fospropofol is water-soluble as opposed to propofol, which is administered as an oil–water emulsion. In 2008, fospropofol was approved by the US Food and Drug Administration, although many clinical trials are still underway for specific uses of the drug.[1]

MECHANISM OF ACTION AND DRUG EFFECTS

Most sedative–hypnotics work via the γ-aminobutyric acid (GABA) receptor complex by enhancing the effect of GABA (Figure 6–1), the major inhibitory neurotransmitter in the central nervous system. GABA receptors are transmembrane, made up of 5 subunits (2 α, 2 β, 1 γ), with a central pore. There are several types of each subunit, leading to a variety of slightly different GABA receptors. Overall, there are 2 types: type A, a chloride channel, and type B, a potassium channel. Type A receptors are very similar to other ligand-linked ion channels (eg, serotonin and nicotinic acetylcholine receptors) and are commonly found on the postsynaptic cleft of a neuron junction. As chloride passes through the GABA receptor channel, neuronal cell wall membranes are hyperpolarized (stabilizing the resting membrane state), producing an inhibitory effect on action potentials. Mild potentiation of GABA type A receptor function leads to anxiolysis, whereas more pronounced potentiation of receptor function leads to sedation and loss of responsiveness. Of note, GABA triggers GABA type A receptors at sites between the α and β subunits.

Other sedatives, such as dexmedetomidine and clonidine produces an analgesic effect by selective α2-adrenoreceptor agonism leading to presynaptic inhibition of norepinephrine release decreasing sympathetic tone (Figure 6–2). Sedation and anxiolysis are likely mediated through α2-adrenoreceptor agonism in an area of the brain called the locus coeruleus.

Tables 6–2 through 6–7 detail the mechanism of action and drug effects of selected sedative–hypnotics used in anesthetic practice. These data are important when formulating a complete drug regimen. For example, propofol has hypnotic but no analgesic effects, unlike ketamine. Benzodiazepines produce anxiolysis and anterograde amnesia, but they are slow to reach peak effect, have prolonged drug effect, and cause dependency and withdrawal. Thus benzodiazepines are more common as an adjunct to another anesthetic.[2,3]

PHARMACOKINETICS AND PHARMACODYNAMICS

Although sedative–hypnotics have similar effects, there are several differences in their pharmacologic behavior. In this section, simulations will be used to illustrate differences in their front end (distribution

TABLE 6–1 History of sedative–hypnotics.

Drug	Year of Discovery	Year of First Clinical Use	Details
Sodium thiopental	1930	1934	Popular for many years for the induction of anesthesia. However, the use in the United States as part of a 3-drug cocktail for lethal injection of death row inmates caused the major supplier to stop sales to the United States. This has limited availability of the drug.
Benzodiazepines	1955	1957	Well known for positive drug effects that include sedation, anticonvulsant properties, and muscle relaxation. However, dependence and withdrawal symptoms have limited their use.
Ketamine	1962	1970	After approval was a popular battlefield anesthetic. However, unpleasant awakening/dissociation has limited use. Illicit use led to classification as a Schedule III controlled substance.
Etomidate	1964	1972	Used for sedation in the intensive care unit until studies showed increased mortality rates due to adrenocortical suppression and inhibition of protein synthesis.[4]
Propofol	1973	1983 (current formulation)	Negative side effects of various formulations led to the current lipid emulsion form. Propensity for bacterial growth led to the addition of EDTA or sodium metabisulfite to prevent bacterial growth. The drug is very popular for induction of anesthesia due to quick action and elimination along with a decrease in intracranial pressure, decreased metabolism of oxygen by the brain and anticonvulsant effects.[5]
Dexmedetomidine	1970s	1999	The D-steroisomer of medetomidine was used for years as an α2-receptor agonist in veterinary medicine. The drug was approved by the FDA for use in humans in 1999.

EDTA, ethylenediaminetetraacetic acid; FDA, US Food and Drug Administration.

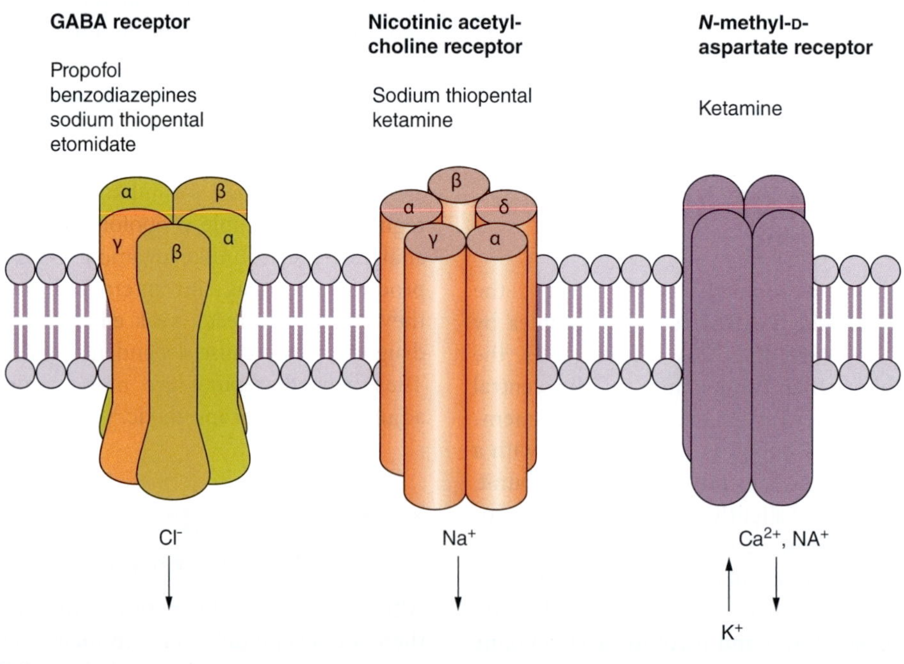

FIGURE 6–1 Schematic diagram of postsynaptic cleft transmembrane receptors, the sedative–hypnotics that act on each receptor and the ions each receptor allows to pass through.

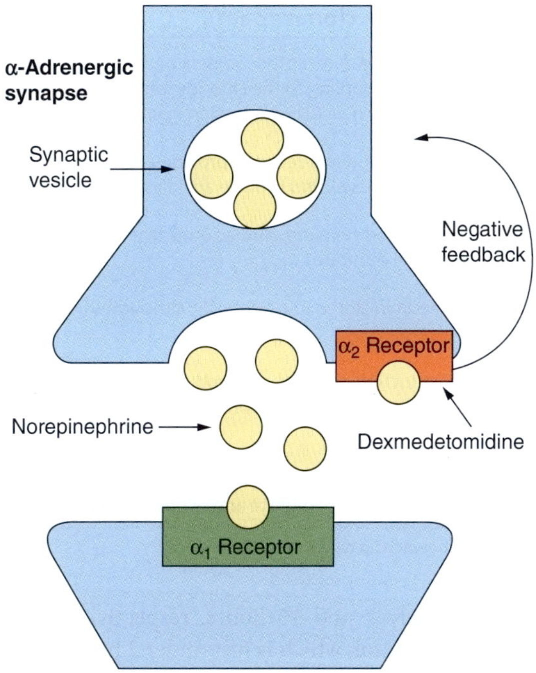

FIGURE 6–2 Schematic diagram of the α-adrenergic synapse and site of action for dexmedetomidine.

and redistribution) and back end (elimination) kinetics. Pharmacokinetic simulations assume a 30-year-old, 78-kg, and 180-cm tall male.

Bolus Dosing

When administered as a bolus, simulations of the front-end kinetics reveal that propofol, sodium thiopental, and etomidate reach peak effect-site concentrations (Ce) more quickly than other sedatives, whereas ketamine and midazolam are considerably slower to reach peak Ce (Figure 6–3, Table 6–8). Simulations of back-end kinetics reveal that after reaching their peak Ce, concentrations of propofol and etomidate diminish quickly. By comparison, sodium thiopental, ketamine, and midazolam have slower elimination and distribution, leading to slower declines in drug concentrations.

Continuous Infusion Dosing

When administered as a continuous infusion, each sedative–hypnotic has a unique profile. A key point is that without a bolus, each sedative has a sharp increase in drug concentration over approximately 15 minutes (Figure 6–4, Table 6–9). Similar to the bolus dosing, propofol and etomidate reach 90% of their maximal peak concentrations more quickly

TABLE 6–2 Sodium thiopental.

Mechanism of action	Sodium thiopental, a barbiturate, acts on the GABA-A receptor and may inhibit nicotinic acetylcholine receptors in the CNS.[6]
CNS	Sodium thiopental causes significant decreases in CBF, $CMRO_2$, and ICP. It also causes increased CPP. It has no analgesic effect and can actually lower the pain threshold.
Cardiovascular	Sodium thiopental causes moderate heart rate increase and moderate MAP decrease. Baroreceptor response is necessary for maintaining cardiac output. Absence due to hypovolemia, congestive heart failure, or β-adrenergic blockade can cause a severe drop in cardiac output and blood pressure.
Respiratory	Sodium thiopental causes profound respiratory depression with a small decrease in bronchodilation.
Clinical uses	Sodium thiopental is used as an intravenous induction agent, for treatment of elevated ICP, and for neuroprotection from focal cerebral ischemia. Thiopental is not a complete anesthetic, lacking the ability to produce amnesia, analgesia, and reflex suppression.
Adverse effects	Injection of thiopental into the intra-arterial space can cause extreme pain/tissue damage. It can also cause laryngospasm and generally depresses the respiratory system. It can cause allergic reactions in rare cases.

CBF, cerebral blood flow; $CMRO_2$, cerebral metabolic rate of oxygen; CNS, central nervous system; CPP, cerebral perfusion pressure; GABA-A, γ-aminobutyric acid type A; ICP, intracranial pressure; MAP, mean arterial pressure.

TABLE 6–3 Benzodiazepines (midazolam, diazepam, lorazepam, clonazepam).

Mechanism of action	Benzodiazepines bind to unique receptor sites on the GABA-A receptor complex between the α and γ subunits. This binding increases the efficiency of GABA coupling to the chloride ion channel. Since benzodiazepines only modulate this effect, there is a "ceiling" in CNS depression from these drugs.
CNS	Benzodiazepines reduce brain $CMRO_2$, prevent/control grand mal seizures, provide anterograde amnesia, serve as mild muscle relaxants at the spinal cord level, and provide anxiolysis.
Cardiovascular	Benzodiazepines produce slight decreases in arterial blood pressure, cardiac output, and peripheral vascular resistance. They may cause a slight increase in heart rate.
Respiratory	Benzodiazepines are respiratory depressants when administered intravenously, although this is generally insignificant via other pathways.
Clinical uses	Benzodiazepines are used for anxiolysis, sedation, induction of anesthesia, and suppression of seizure activity, and they may be used to treat insomnia and epilepsy.[7] Effects can quickly be reversed with the benzodiazepine antagonist flumazenil.
Adverse effects	Benzodiazepines cause pain during injection, particularly diazepam due to the organic solvent, propylene glycol. Benzodiazepines are also associated with dependence and withdrawal symptoms.

$CMRO_2$, cerebral metabolic rate of oxygen; CNS, central nervous system; GABA-A, γ-aminobutyric acid type A.

than the other sedatives. Once the 1-hour infusion is terminated, propofol and etomidate quickly dissipate, while the other sedatives require more time to decrease. Of note, sodium thiopental, midazolam, and dexmedetomidine require a substantial amount of time to reach 10% of the maximal Ce: approximately 7 and 15 hours, respectively, compared to propofol, which is just under 2 hours.

Pharmacodynamics

To put the bolus dosing into clinical context, an estimate of the duration of effect can be used. For

TABLE 6–4 Ketamine.

Mechanism of action	Is an antagonist of the *N*-methyl-D-aspartate (NMDA) receptor, which functions as an ion channel. Ketamine also interacts with phencyclidine binding sites that inhibit NMDA receptor function, interacts with selected opioid receptors (μ, Δ, and κ), muscarinic receptors, voltage-gated calcium channels, and monoaminergic receptors. It has S and R isomers, both of which are pharmacologically active and can produce anesthesia, dysphoria, analgesia, and dissociation. The S isomer is up to 3 times more analgesic than the R isomer. At high doses, ketamine also behaves as a local anesthetic by blocking sodium channels in a comparable fashion to lidocaine or procaine.
CNS	Increases $CMRO_2$, CBF, and ICP.
Cardiovascular	Increases arterial blood pressure, heart rate, and cardiac output due to stimulation of the sympathetic nervous system. Ketamine also blocks reuptake of epinephrine. It increases pulmonary artery pressure and myocardial work. These can be useful properties in patients with acute hypovolemic shock.
Respiratory	Causes minimal respiratory depression with significant bronchodilation.
Clinical uses	Induction and maintenance of anesthesia, but unpleasant emergence limits its use. Ketamine is a potent analgesic. Ketamine can be administered via oral, rectal, intravenous, or epidural routes, making it useful in cases of mentally challenged or uncooperative pediatric patients. A popular use is administration in subanalgesic doses in order to limit or reverse opioid tolerance.[7]
Adverse effects	Psychological effects of ketamine are the major limiting-factor of use. Common experiences include vivid dreams, hallucinations, out-of-body experiences, and a general dissociative mental state. Combination with benzodiazepines can limit these symptoms.[8]

CBF, cerebral blood flow; $CMRO_2$, cerebral metabolic rate of oxygen; CNS, central nervous system; ICP, intracranial pressure.

TABLE 6–5 Etomidate.

Mechanism of action	Etomidate binds to a subunit of the GABA-A receptor, which increases the receptor's affinity for GABA. It can produce disinhibitory effects on extrapyramidal motor activity, resulting in a 30%–60% chance of myoclonus.
CNS	Etomidate is a potent cerebral vasoconstrictor. It decreases CBF and ICP. It does not share the neuroprotective properties of propofol and thiopental.
Cardiovascular	Etomidate infusions are characterized by cardiovascular stability. There is a modest to no decrease in systemic blood pressure due to systemic vascular resistance (these can be exaggerated during hypovolemia). There are minimal changes in heart rate and cardiac output.
Respiratory	Etomidate induces mild ventilatory depression, much less than propofol. This depression can be exaggerated in combination with inhaled anesthetics or opioids.
Clinical uses	Intravenous induction of anesthesia. Etomidate is often used in patients who have compromised myocardial contractility.
Adverse effects	More frequent deaths in ICU patients led to the discovery that etomidate suppresses adrenocortical function by inhibiting synthesis of cortisol. A portion of etomidate, specifically its pyrrole ring, inhibits 11-β-hydroxylase, an enzyme known to play a key role in steroid synthesis. Following only a routine induction dose, etomidate can suppress adrenal function up to and beyond 24 hours. This can be dangerous in septic and critically ill patients who require steroids to maintain their immune function and metabolic homeostasis. Consider abandoning etomidate as an induction drug for septic patients or at a minimum, providing supplemental corticosteroid therapy following etomidate administration. Etomidate can cause myoclonic movement. This can be reduced by premedication with benzodiazepines, but at the cost of prolonged emergence. Etomidate can cause pain on injection due to the organic solvent propylene glycol. Premedication with benzodiazepines and opioids can reduce pain on injection. Etomidate is often associated with postoperative nausea and vomiting, usually requiring addition of an antiemetic.

CNS, central nervous system; CBF, cerebral blood flow; GABA-A, γ-aminobutyric acid type A; ICP, intracranial pressure.[2,3]

TABLE 6–6 Propofol.

Mechanism of action	Propofol potentiates GABA-A receptor function by slowing channel closing time, blocks sodium channels, and may influence the endogenous cannabinoid system.
CNS	Propofol is a sedative–hypnotic but not an analgesic. It decreases CBF and $CMRO_2$. It also decreases ICP and IOP, found to be protective during focal ischemia. Propofol also has anticonvulsant effects, although some twitching and movement can occur during induction.
Cardiovascular	Propofol produces a significant decrease in systemic blood pressure and profound vasodilation in both arterial and venous circulation. It inhibits the baroreflex response and can contribute to a small increase in heart rate.
Respiratory	Propofol is responsible for significant respiratory depression, with high probability of apnea with induction doses. It also causes significant reduction in upper airway reflexes.
Clinical uses	Intravenous induction and maintenance of anesthesia, sedation (popular for mechanically ventilated patients), and as an antiemetic.
Adverse effects	Preservative-free propofol use is associated with higher infection rates in ICU patients. The FDA has approved the use of propofol in the United States with addition of either EDTA or sodium metabisulfite. Propofol formulations are also stored under nitrogen atmospheres to prevent growth. Propofol can also cause some pain on injection; this effect can be lessened by preinjection or mixed injection with lidocaine. Studies have also shown that addition of remifentanil can also reduce pain on injection. Propofol infusion syndrome is a very rare but often fatal condition that can occur with propofol infusions over 48 hours in high doses (> 4 mg/kg/h).[5,9,10]

CBF, cerebral blood flow; $CMRO_2$, cerebral metabolic rate of oxygen; CNS, central nervous system; EDTA, ethylenediaminetetraacetic acid; FDA, US Food and Drug Administration; GABA-A, γ-aminobutyric acid type A; ICP, intracranial pressure; ICU, intensive care unit; IOP, intraocular pressure.[2,3]

TABLE 6–7 Dexmedetomidine.

Mechanism of action	Dexmedetomidine is a selective α2-adrenergic receptor agonist. It is the pharmacologically active R-enantiomer of medetomidine, a drug that has been used for decades in veterinary medicine as a sedative
CNS	When administered systemically, dexmedetomidine produces analgesic effects by α2-adrenoreceptor agonism and the subsequent presynaptic inhibition of norepinephrine release that decreases sympathetic tone within the spinal cord. The additional effects of sedation and anxiolysis are likely mediated through α2-adrenoreceptor agonism in an area of the brain called the locus coeruleus. Sedation resembles a sleep state more than other anesthetics. It also decreases CBF without significant change in ICP and $CMRO_2$.
Cardiovascular	Dexmedetomidine produces moderate decreases in heart rate, systemic vascular resistance, and systemic blood pressure. This may cause symptomatic bradycardia and/or hypotension.
Respiratory	Dexmedetomidine produces very little effect on ventilatory function with a small to moderate decrease in tidal volume but little effect on respiratory rate. Dexmedetomidine can produce upper airway obstruction after sedation.
Clinical uses	Dexmedetomidine may be used for short-term sedation of intubated/ventilated patients. It can be used as an adjunct in general anesthesia. It can also be used as an adjunct with benzodiazepines to treat acute alcohol withdrawal symptoms.[11]
Adverse effects	Dexmedetomidine's cardiovascular effects are highly variable. Dosing should be carefully titrated to avoid adverse cardiovascular effects.

CNS, central nervous system; CBF, cerebral blood flow; $CMRO_2$, cerebral metabolic rate of oxygen; ICP, intracranial pressure.[2,3]

example, consider the combined pharmacokinetic and pharmacodynamic simulations presented in Figures 6–5 and 6–6. They present the predicted Ce from a range of propofol bolus doses and the resultant estimated effect in terms of the probability loss of responsiveness (LOR). These plots are especially helpful in mapping the Ce that corresponds to a given effect. For example, Figures 6–5 and 6–6 show that a propofol Ce of 4 to 6 mcg/mL corresponds to LOR. Of note, lower doses (0.5 to 1 mg/kg) do

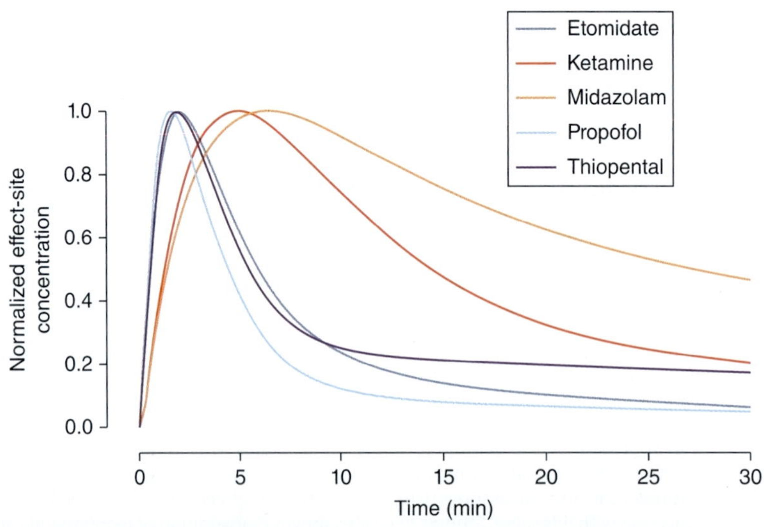

FIGURE 6–3 Simulations of predicted effect-site concentrations (Ce) following a bolus dose of etomidate, ketamine, midazolam, propofol, and thiopental. For comparison purposes, maximal Ces have been normalized to 1. Simulations were based on published pharmacokinetic models for etomidate,[12] ketamine,[13,14] midazolam,[15] propofol,[16] and thiopental.[17]

TABLE 6–8 Selected time points of interest based on pharmacokinetic simulations of common bolus doses of sedative–hypnotics.[a]

	Time to 90% of Peak Ce (minutes)	Time to Peak Ce (minutes)	Time to 20% of Peak Ce via Elimination and Distribution (minutes)	Time to 10% of Peak Ce via Elimination and Distribution (minutes)
Propofol	1	1.5	7.5	11
Sodium thiopental	1	2	18	73
Etomidate	1.5	2	11	20
Ketamine	3	5	30	64
Midazolam	4	6.5	95	232

Ce, effect-site concentration.
[a]When administered as a bolus dose, presented in Figure 6–3.

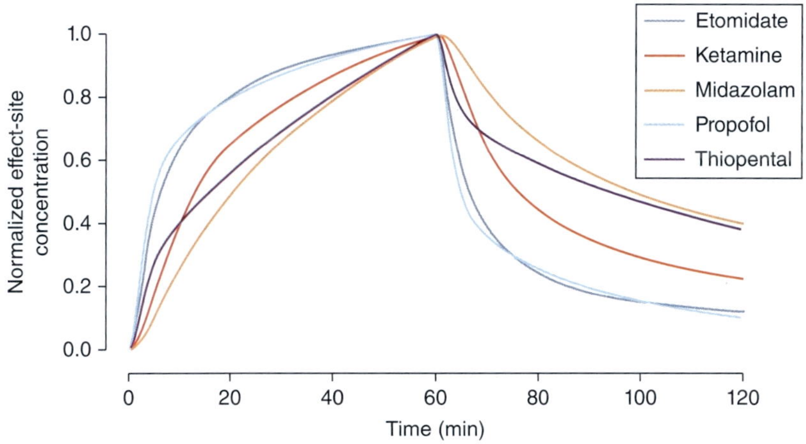

FIGURE 6–4 Simulations of predicted effect-site concentrations (Ce) for a 1-hour infusion of etomidate, ketamine, midazolam, propofol, thiopental, and dexmedetomidine. For comparison purposes, maximal Ces have been normalized to 1. Simulations were based on published pharmacokinetic models for etomidate,[12] ketamine,[13,14] midazolam,[15] propofol,[16] and thiopental.[17]

TABLE 6–9 Selected time points of interest based on pharmacokinetic simulations of common infusion rates of sedative–hypnotics.[a]

	Time to 90% of Peak Ce (minutes)	Time to 20% of Peak Ce via Elimination and Distribution (minutes)	Time to 10% of Peak Ce via Elimination and Distribution (minutes)
Propofol	35	88	119
Sodium thiopental	49	245	920
Etomidate	32.5	85	167
Ketamine	44.5	127	225
Midazolam	50	244	462
Dexmedetomidine	49	397	758

Ce, effect-site concentration.
[a]When administered as a 1-hour infusion, presented in Figure 6–4.

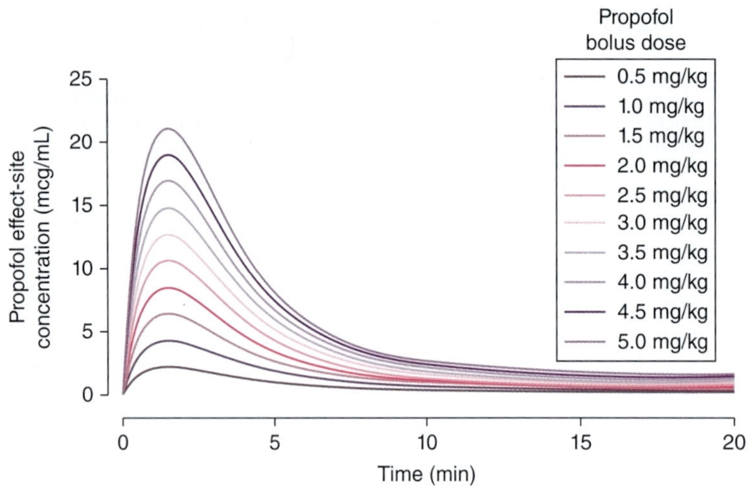

FIGURE 6–5 Simulations of predicted propofol effect-site concentrations (Ce) for a range of propofol bolus doses (0.5-5.0 mg/kg). Simulations were based on a pharmacokinetic model for propofol.[16]

not achieve a clinically suitable level of LOR for induction of anesthesia, whereas the others do with increasing duration of effect (Table 6–10). Thus, the bolus dose of propofol may be important to consider, especially when a prolonged duration of effect may have adverse effects such as unintended LOR during moderate sedation or prolonged effect when managing a difficult airway.

Figures 6–7 and 6–8 show dosage-specific Ce values and probability LOR for infusions of propofol. As seen in the figures, a Ce value greater than 4 mcg/mL leads to a probability LOR in the high 90s. This range is achieved using a 150 mcg/kg/min infusion, although it takes approximately 38 minutes to reach those values, showing a need for a bolus or higher initial infusion rate if quick LOR is needed (Table 6–11).

Increasing the dose for an infusion by 50 mcg/kg/min leads to a delay between 3 and 4.5 minutes for reaching 50% probability LOR over previous doses,

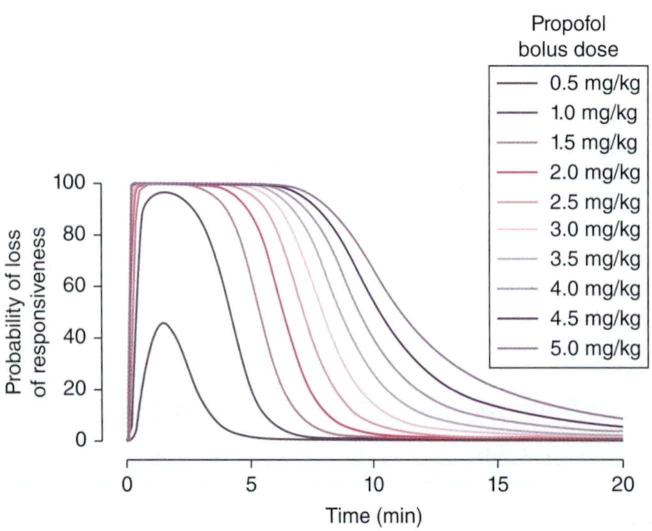

FIGURE 6–6 Simulations of the predicted probability loss of responsiveness (LOR) for a range of propofol boluses (0.5-5.0 mg/kg). Simulations were based on pharmacokinetic and pharmacodynamic models for propofol.[16-17]

TABLE 6–10 Selected pharmacokinetic and pharmacodynamic data of interest.[a]

Dose (mg/kg)	Peak Ce (mcg/mL)	Maximum Probability of LOR (%)	Time to 50% Probability of LOR (minutes)	Time to 10% Probability of LOR (minutes)
0.5	2.1	45	NA	3.5
1.0	4.2	96	4.0	5.5
1.5	6.4	100	5.5	7.0
2.0	8.5	100	6.5	8.0
2.5	10.6	100	7.0	9.0
3.0	12.7	100	8.0	10.0
3.5	14.8	100	9.0	12.0
4.0	16.9	100	9.5	14.0
4.5	19.1	100	10.0	16.0
5.0	21.2	100	11.0	18.0

Ce, effect-site concentration; LOR, loss of responsiveness.
[a]For a range of bolus propofol doses, presented in Figures 6–5 and 6–6.

showing slight exponential properties. The time required to reach the 10% of maximal concentration has a similar exponential tendency, going from a 4.5-minute delay over previous dose up to 9 minutes. However, at the highest infusion rate, there is only an 8-minute delay over the previous dose, showing a potential ceiling to the exponential behavior.

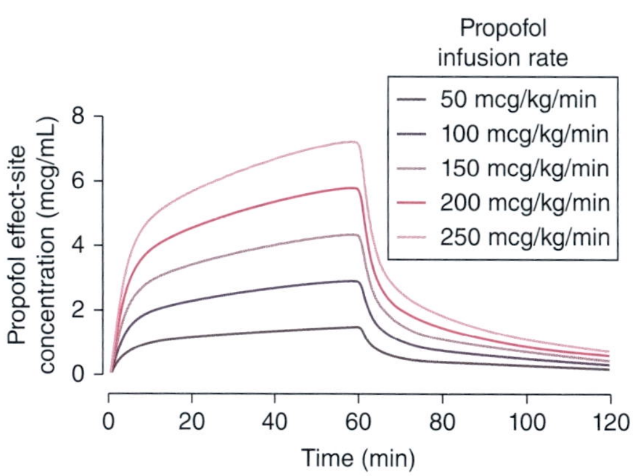

FIGURE 6–7 Simulations of predicted propofol effect-site concentration (Ce) for a range of infusion rates from 50 to 250 mg/kg/min. Simulations were based on a pharmacokinetic model for propofol.[16]

Pharmacokinetics of Prolonged Infusions

Figure 6–9 shows a 24-hour infusion of propofol compared to dexmedetomidine and midazolam. Propofol shows a clear advantage in onset of action

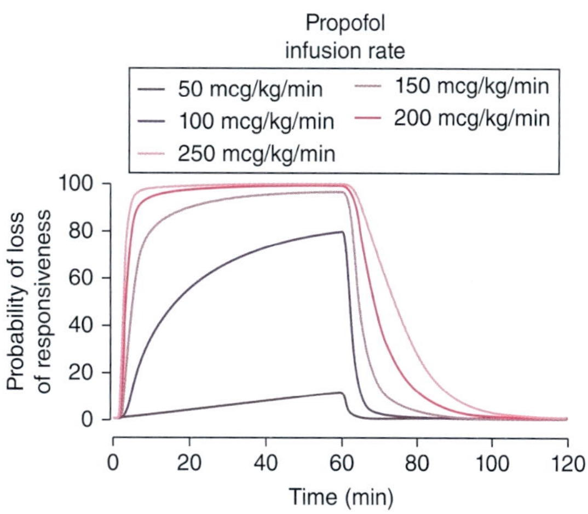

FIGURE 6–8 Simulations of the predicted probability of loss of responsiveness (LOR) for a range of propofol infusion rates (50 to 250 mg/kg/min). Simulations were based on published pharmacokinetic and pharmacodynamic models for propofol.[16-17]

TABLE 6–11 Selected pharmacokinetic and pharmacodynamic data of interest for a range of propofol infusion rates.[a]

Infusion Rate (mg/kg/min)	Peak Ce (mcg/mL)	Maximum Probability of LOR (%)	Time to 50% probability of LOR Once Infusion is Terminated (minutes)	Time to 10% Probability of LOR Once Infusion is Terminated (minutes)
50	1.5	11	NA	1
100	2.9	80	2	5
150	4.3	97	5	12
200	5.8	99	8	21
250	7.2	100	14	29

Ce, effect-site concentration; LOR, loss of responsiveness.
[a]Presented in Figures 6–7 and 6–8.

during infusions, with midazolam second and dexmedetomidine last.

After this extended infusion, propofol reaches 10% max Ce after 8 hours. Dexmedetomidine takes nearly 18 hours. Midazolam takes just under 11 hours. These properties show propofol's potential for use in a continuous infusion.

Importance of a Bolus Followed by Infusion

Figures 6–10 through 6–12 show the effect of variable length infusions of propofol on the probability LOR (loss of consciousness) using a 2-mg/kg bolus followed immediately by a 150-mg/kg/min infusion. Front-end kinetics in this case are identical, and only length of infusion differs.

During the infusion, although the Ce value only goes up slightly, the tissues retain some propofol, leading to delayed elimination and distribution from the central compartment. Figure 6–12 shows how this increases the time to reach both 50% and 5% probability LOR and acts in a linear manner for both values. This gives insight into the delay in awakening and lingering effects, depending on length of infusion for propofol.

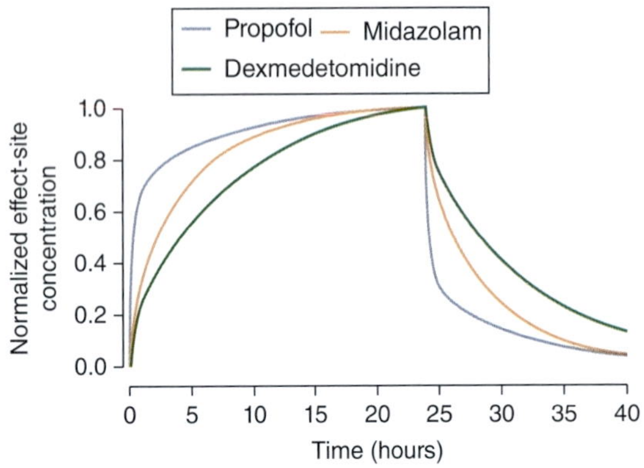

FIGURE 6–9 Simulations of predicted effect site concentrations (Ce) for a 24-hour infusion of propofol, midazolam, and dexmedetomidine. For comparison purposes, maximal Ces have been normalized to 1. Simulations were based on published pharmacokinetic models for. propofol,[16] midazolam,[15] and dexmedetomidine.[18,19]

Context-Sensitive Half-Time

Figure 6–13 shows elimination from the blood after variable infusion lengths for each drug. Propofol has the fastest elimination, followed by etomidate and ketamine. Thiopental, dexmedetomidine, and midazolam respectively have the slowest elimination rates at the longer infusion times (longer than 350 minutes).

CLINICAL USES

With the exception of dexmedetomidine, all the listed drugs can be used for intravenous induction of anesthesia. Some sedative–hypnotics have multiple uses including sedation, anxiolysis, and reduction of increased intracranial pressure (Tables 6–2 through 6–7).

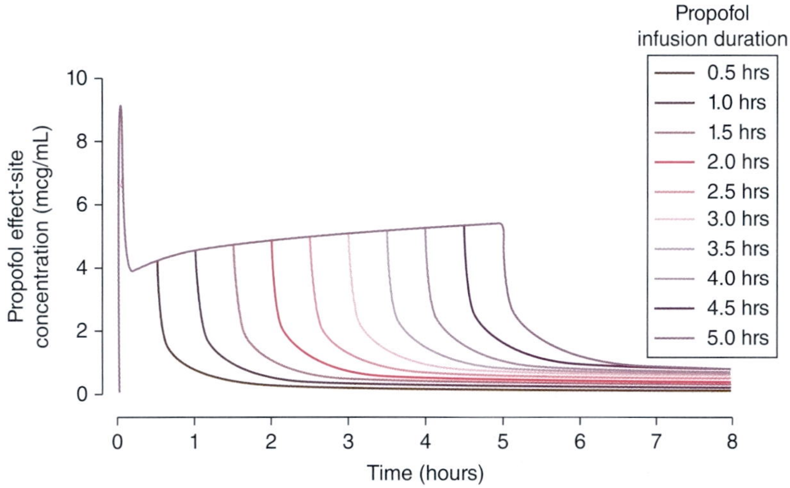

FIGURE 6–10 Simulations of propofol effect site concentrations following a 2-mg/kg bolus dose followed by an infusion of 150 mg/kg/min. The infusion was continued for variable lengths ranging from 30 minutes to 5 hours. Simulations were based on a published pharmacokinetic model for propofol.[16]

ADVERSE EFFECTS

Adverse effects of sedative–hypnotics are largely responsible for the popularity of each drug. For example, while ketamine has a good drug profile with reasonable kinetics, unpleasant awakening has made it much less popular. Patients often feel disconnected after surgery and can have vivid dreams and hallucinations. Other adverse effects are associated with mortality rather than patient experience. Etomidate must be used carefully due to adrenocortical suppression. Use of etomidate was connected with higher mortality in the intensive care unit due to inhibition of cortisol and corticosterone synthesis.[4] However, some of the listed side effects are extremely rare such as propofol infusion syndrome (PRIS). While extremely

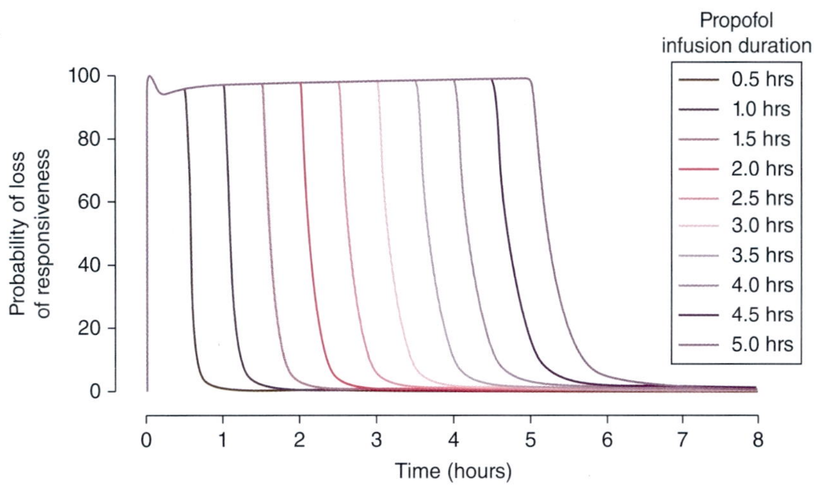

FIGURE 6–11 Simulations of the predicted probability of loss of responsiveness (LOR) for a 2-mg/kg propofol bolus dosefollowed by an infusion of 150 mg/kg/min. The infusion was continued for variable lengths ranging from 30 minutes to 5 hours. Simulations were based on a published pharmacokinetic model for propofol.[16-17]

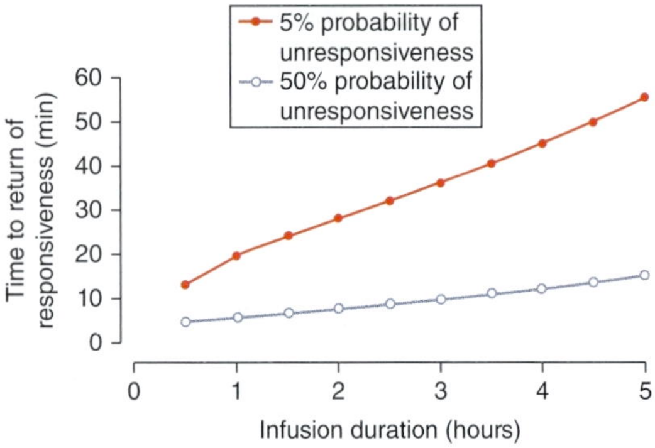

FIGURE 6–12 Simulations of the time required to reach a 50 and then 5% probability of loss of responsiveness once a propofol infusion is terminated. Propofol dosing included a 2-mg/kg bolus dose followed by an infusion rate of 150 mg/kg/min infusion ranging from 30 minutes to 5 hours. Simulations were based on a published pharmacokinetic model for propofol.[16]

uncommon, during high-dose infusions over long periods of time, it poses a higher risk. Some articles suggest that lactic acidosis is a potential warning sign. Risk factors for PRIS include young age, mitochondrial disease, fatty acid oxidation defects, critical illness of central nervous system or respiratory origin, exogenous catecholamine or glucocorticoid administration, or inadequate carbohydrate

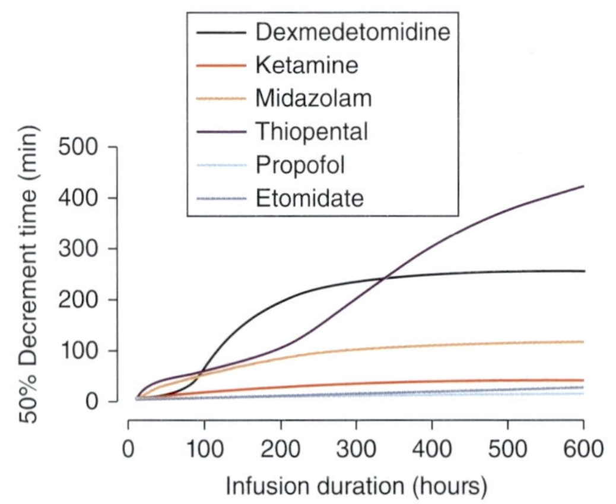

FIGURE 6–13 Context sensitive half time (also known as the 50% decrement time) for selected sedative–hypnotics. Simulations were based on a published pharmacokinetic models for dexmedetomidine,[19,20] etomidate,[12] ketamine,[13,14] midazolam,[15] propofol,[21] and thiopental.[18]

intake.[9] Monitoring of pH, lactate, and creatine kinase levels are recommended in cases where long-term high dose infusions are absolutely necessary.[10] Adverse effects are presented in Tables 6–2 through 6–7.

REFERENCES

1. Bengalorkar GM, Bhuvana K, Sarala N, Kumar TN, et al. Fospropofol: clinical pharmacology. *J Anaesthesiol Clin Pharmacol.* 2011;27(1):79-83.
2. Barash PG, Cullen BF, Stoelting RK. *Clinical Anesthesia.* 5th ed. Philadelphia: Lippincott Williams & Wilkins; 2006.
3. Stoelting RK, Miller, RD. *Basics of Anesthesia.* 5th ed. Philadelphia: Churchill Livingstone Elsevier; 2007.
4. Ball C, Westhorpe R. Intravenous induction agents: etomidate. *Anaesth Intensive Care.* 2002;30(4):405.
5. Baker MT, Naguib M. Propofol: the challenges of formulation. *Anesthesiology.* 2005;103(4):860-876.
6. Weber M, Motin L, Gaul S, et al., Intravenous anaesthetics inhibit nicotinic acetylcholine receptor-mediated currents and Ca2+ transients in rat intracardiac ganglion neurons. *Br J Pharmacol.* 2005;144(1):98-107.
7. Quibell R, Prommer EE, Mihalyo M, et al. Ketamine*. *J Pain Symptom Manage.* 2011;41(3) 640-649.
8. Jennings PA, Cameron P, Bernard S. Ketamine as an analgesic in the pre-hospital setting: a systematic review. *Acta Anaesthesiol Scand.* 2011;55(6):638-643.
9. Wong JM. Propofol infusion syndrome. *Am J Ther* 2010;17(5):487-491.
10. Fudickar A, Bein B, Tonner PH. Propofol infusion syndrome in anaesthesia and intensive care medicine. *Curr Opin Anaesthesiol.* 2006;19(4):404-410.
11. Muzyk AJ, Fowler JA, Norwood DK, Chilipko A. Role of alpha2-agonists in the treatment of acute alcohol withdrawal. Ann Pharmacother. 2011;45(5):649-657.
12. Arden JR, Holley FO, Stanski DR. Increased sensitivity to etomidate in the elderly: initial distribution versus altered brain response. *Anesthesiology.* 1986;65(1):19-27.
13. Ihmsen H, Geisslinger G, Schuttler J. Stereoselective pharmacokinetics of ketamine: R(-)-ketamine inhibits the elimination of S(+)-ketamine. *Clin Pharmacol Ther.* 2001;70(5):431-438.
14. Persson J. The ketamine enigma. *Acta Anaesthesiol Scand.* 2008;52(4):453-455.
15. Albrecht S, Ihmsen H, Hering W, et al. The effect of age on the pharmacokinetics and pharmacodynamics of midazolam. *Clin Pharmacol Ther.* 1999;65(6):630-639.

16. Schnider TW, Minto CF, Gambus PL, et al. The influence of method of administration and covariates on the pharmacokinetics of propofol in adult volunteers. *Anesthesiology*. 1998;88(5):1170-1182.
17. Kern SE, XIE G, White JL, Egan TD. A response surface analysis of propofol-remifentanil pharmacodynamic interaction in volunteers. *Anesthesiology*. 2004; 100(6):1373-81.
18. Stanski DR, Maitre PO. Population pharmacokinetics and pharmacodynamics of thiopental: the effect of age revisited. *Anesthesiology*. 1990;72(3):412-422.
19. Dyck JB, Maze M, Haack C, Azarnoff DL, Vuorilehto L, Shafer SL. Computer-controlled infusion of intravenous dexmedetomidine hydrochloride in adult human volunteers. *Anesthesiology*. 1993;78(5):821-828.
20. Potts AL, Anderson BJ, Holford NH, Vu TC, Warman GR. Dexmedetomidine hemodynamics in children after cardiac surgery. *Paediatr Anaesth*. 2010;20(5):425-433.
21. Marsh B, White M, Morton N, Kenny GN. Pharmacokinetic model driven infusion of propofol in children. *Br J Anaesth*. 1991. 67(1):41-48.

C H A P T E R

7

Opioid and Benzodiazipine Reversal Agents

Tyler Call, MD

INTRODUCTION

Opioid and benzodiazepine antagonists are an important component of an anesthesiologists' armamentarium. Anesthesiologists rely on these agents for rapid reversal of adverse effects such as respiratory depression and loss of responsiveness. This may be especially important in the context of restoring ventilation in hypoxic patients either by antagonizing the ventilatory depressant effect of opioids or antagonizing the sedating properties of benzodiazepines so that patients can be prompted to breathe. Furthermore, select antagonists may also play an important role in other pathologic conditions, including tumor progression in selected types of cancer. This chapter will provide a brief overview of commonly used opioid and benzodiazepine antagonists. A summary of each reversal agent is presented in Table 7–1.

NALOXONE

History

First synthesized in 1961, naloxone is indicated for the complete or partial reversal of opioid sedation and respiratory depression. It is also indicated for suspected opioid intoxication and has been proposed as an adjunctive agent in the management of septic shock.[1]

Mechanism of Action

Naloxone is a pure opioid antagonist. Although its mechanism of action is not fully understood, in vitro studies suggest that it competes for the μ, κ, and σ opiate receptor sites of the central nervous system (CNS). When administered in the absence of opioid activity, it has no effect.[1]

Dosing

The most rapid onset of action is achieved by intravenous (IV) injection. Intramuscular (IM) or subcutaneous (SQ) injections are also possible but may have unreliable absorption patterns. Endotracheal administration is also an option when intravascular access is unavailable. Because the duration of action for many opioids is longer than that of naloxone, patients should be closely monitored following administration.[1]

Adults

For opioid overdose, an initial IV dose of 0.4 to 2 mg may be given. This may be repeated at 2- 3-minute intervals. In the case of postoperative respiratory depression, naloxone hydrochloride can be injected in 0.04- to 0.2-mg increments at 2-minute intervals until the desired reversal is achieved. Excessive or rapid reversal can induce nausea, vomiting, sweating, or circulatory arrest.[1]

Children

In suspected opioid overdose, an initial dose of 0.01 mg/kg is given. A subsequent dose of 0.1 mg/kg may be given if the initial dose does not result in adequate clinical improvement. In children with postoperative opioid respiratory depression, IV naloxone can be administered in 0.005- to 0.01-mg increments at 2- to 3-minute intervals until adequate reversal is achieved. Children should be monitored for at least 24 hours following administration.[1]

Onset/Duration of Action

Onset of action for IV administration is approximately 2 minutes, and its half-life is approximately 1 hour in adults[2] and approximately 3 hours in neonates.[1,3,4] An adult study showed that 5 mcg/kg of IV

TABLE 7–1 Summary of reversal agent dosing.

Naloxone for reversal of respiratory depression[1]
Adults: 0.04–0.2 mg IV given every 2 minutes, titrated to effect
IV infusion: 2-mg naloxone in 500 mL 0.9% sodium chloride; rate titrated to effect
Children: 0.005–0.01 mg IV given every 2 minutes, titrated to effect
Flumazenil for reversal of benzodiazepine sedation[5]
Adults: 0.2 mg IV given every 1 min, titrated to effect (up to 1 mg)
Pediatrics: 0.01 mg/kg given every 1 min, titrated to effect (up to 0.05 mg/kg)
Subcutaneous methylnaltrexone[6]
8 mg SQ (38–62 kg)
12 mg SQ (62–114 kg)
0.15 mg/kg for patients < 38 kg or > 114 kg
Nalbuphine
For analgesia: 10 mg IV up to 30 mg total[7]
For opioid-induced side effects: 2 to 3 mg IV[8]

IV, intravenous; SQ, subcutaneous.

naloxone effectively reversed respiratory depression produced by morphine for 79 minutes.[9]

Pharmacokinetics/Pharmacodynamics:

Naloxone does cross the placenta, and protein binding is relatively weak. Hepatic metabolism primarily by glucuronide conjugation produces naloxone-3-glucuronide as the major metabolite.[1]

Clinical Applications

For the anesthesiologist, naloxone is most often used to partially reverse opioid-induced sedation and respiratory depression. This is done by careful titration to desired effect. Naloxone has been used in some instances to increase blood pressure for several hours in patients with septic shock; however, improved survival has not been demonstrated.[1]

Adverse Effects

Given the relatively short half-life of naloxone, patients should be closely monitored beyond its duration of action to ensure adequate respiratory function and consciousness. Caution should be used when administering naloxone to newborns of mothers who have been dependent on opioids as precipitation of an acute withdrawal syndrome may occur. Patients who are physically dependent on opioids are also at risk for withdrawal syndrome. Signs of acute withdrawal may include tachycardia, diarrhea, pain, fever, rhinnorhea, sweating, nausea, vomiting, trembling, abdominal pain, and hypertension. In the neonate, convulsions, irritability, and hyperactive reflexes may be noted. Complications, including pulmonary edema, hypertension, cardiac dysrhythmias, cerebral aneurysm rupture, and cardiac arrest and sudden death, have been reported.[10,11] The antihypertensive effects of clonidine can be antagonized by naloxone, producing sudden hypertension.[12] Careful, slow titration of naloxone is recommended to prevent undesired side effects.[12]

FLUMAZENIL

History

First characterized in 1981,[13] flumazenil is indicated for complete or partial reversal of the sedative effects of benzodiazepines.[5]

Mechanism of Action

Flumazenil is a competitive antagonist for the benzodiazepine recognition site on the γ-aminobutyric acid (GABA)–benzodiazepine receptor complex.[5] It effectively reverses the effects of all benzodiazepines without altering their kinetics or bioavailability.[14]

Dosing

Like naloxone, flumazenil should be carefully titrated to effect to reduce the chance of adverse effects. In adults, the recommended dose is 0.2 mg IV given over 15 seconds. If desired effects are not obtained, an additional 0.2 mg/min may be given up to a total dose of 1 mg. In studies where more than 1 mg of flumazenil was given, withdrawal-like events were 2 to 5 times more likely. No more than 3 mg should be given in 1 hour. In patients who are tolerant to benzodiazepines, slower titration rates of 0.1 mg/min and decreased total flumazenil dosing may reduce the frequency of agitation and confusion. Patients who are physically dependent on benzodiazepines are at high risk for withdrawal seizures, and thus flumazanil should be used with extreme caution in this population.[5]

In children, the recommended initial dose is 0.01 mg/kg (up to 0.2 mg) IV given over 15 seconds. If desired effects are not obtained, an additional 0.01 mg/kg (up to 0.2 mg) may be given at 1-minute intervals to a maximum total dose of 0.05 mg/kg or 1 mg (whichever is lower).[5] Flumazenil is metabolized by the liver and excreted through the kidneys.[13]

Onset/Duration of Action

Onset of benzodiazepine reversal is usually noted within 2 minutes after injection. Peak effect occurs between 6 and 10 minutes. Half-life is approximately 1 hour.[5,15] Duration of action and degree of reversal is related to dose and plasma concentrations.

Clinical Applications

Flumazenil is used to partially or completely reverse the sedating effects of benzodiazepines. In general, dose totals of 0.1 to 0.2 mg produce partial antagonism. Dose totals of 0.4 to 1 mg may produce complete reversal in patient who have received standard sedating doses of benzodiazepines.[5] Flumazenil may also be titrated to reverse benzodiazepine overdose.

Adverse Effects

Flumazanil may precipitate acute withdrawal syndrome in patients who have been chronically taking benzodiazepines.[16] Those patients who have either been taking benzodiazepines long term or who have overdosed on cyclic antidepressants are at increased risk for developing seizures with the administration of flumazenil.[5] It is possible to have recurrence of benzodiazepine effects such as sedation after flumazenil has been eliminated when longer acting benzodiazines were administered.

METHYLNALTREXONE

History

In 1978, Leon Goldberg was asked by a colleague to help with a case of a patient who was refusing morphine for his cancer pain because of severe constipation. Goldberg proposed a targeted opioid receptor antagonist for treatment of this condition. Screening of thousands of previously synthesized opioid-like molecules led to a compound called *N*-methyl-naltrexone (MNTX), which was synthesized by Boehringer Ingleheim.[17,18] Today, MNTX is indicated for the treatment of opioid-induced constipation in patients with advanced illness who have had insufficient response to laxative therapy while receiving palliative care.[6]

Mechanism of Action

MNTX is a selective peripherally acting μ-opioid receptor antagonist. Its quaternary amine inhibits its ability to cross the blood-brain barrier. This allows MNTX to antagonize the μ receptors of the gastrointestinal tract with no effect of the opioid-mediated analgesic effects of the CNS.[6,19]

Dosing

Recommended dosing for subcutaneous MNTX bromide is 8 mg SQ for patients weighing 38 to 62 kg and 12 mg SQ for patients weighing 63 to 114 kg. For patients who weigh less than 38 kg or more than 114 kg, 0.15 mg/kg is recommended. Recommended injection sites include abdomen, thighs, or upper arms, with rotation of injection sites. The recommended schedule for dosing is one injection every other day as needed, with no more than 1 injection in a 24-hour period.[6] Patients with severe renal impairment, defined as a creatinine clearance of less than 30 mL/min, should have 50% of the calculated dose, as 50% of MNTX is eliminated in the urine.[6,19]

Onset and Duration of Action

Peak concentrations are achieved at 30 minutes, and studies indicate that 30% of patients experience laxation within 30 minutes of a dose.[6] Terminal half-life is 8 hours.[6,20]

Pharmacokinetics/Pharmacodynamics

A dose ranging study showed that at a dose of less than 0.05 mg/kg produced a laxative response in 10% of patients, while doses greater than 0.25 mg/kg produced a laxative response in 70% of patients.[21] Another study showed that 48% of patients had laxation within 4 hours after the first study dose of 0.15 mg/kg of body weight.[22]

Clinical Applications

MNTX is currently indicated for the treatment of opioid-induced constipation in patients with advanced illness who have had insufficient response to laxative therapy while receiving palliative care.[6] It does not appear to have any affect on central analgesia or appear to precipitate withdrawal.[22] Recent studies suggest that MNTX may be beneficial in the treatment of cancer patients.[23-25]

Adverse Effects

MNTX may cause diarrhea and should not be administered in the setting of persistent diarrhea.[6] Abdominal pain, flatulence, nausea, dizziness, and increased body temperature occurred slightly more frequently in patients who received MNTX compared to those who received placebo.[22] Rare cases of gastrointestinal perforation have been reported in patients with advanced illness and conditions that may compromise the structural integrity of the gastrointestinal tract.[6]

NALBUPHINE

History

In an effort to produce narcotic analgesics with reduced abuse potential, several semisynthetic opioid agonist–antagonists were developed. One of these agents was nalbuphine. First approved for the United States in 1979, nalbuphine remains as the only opioid analgesic that is not presently controlled under the Controlled Substances Act.[26] Indicated for the relief of moderate to severe pain,[7] nalbuphine has also been shown to be effective in reversing or reducing opioid-induced respiratory depression,[27-33] nausea,[34] pruritus,[8,35-37] and other unwanted side effects.[27]

Mechanism of Action

Nalbuphine is both a κ-opioid receptor agonist and a μ-opioid receptor antagonist.[7,27] Both κ and μ receptors are involved in nociception. Morphine, hydromorphone, fentanyl, and methadone all act primarily on the μ-opioid receptor thus nalbuphine inhibits the effects of these opioids while producing analgesia through κ-opioid receptors.

Dosing

Recommended dosing for analgesia is 10 mg for a 70-kg patient given intravenously, subcutaneously, or intramuscularly, repeated every 3 to 6 hours as needed. Nalbuphine is approximately equipotent to morphine.[7,38] Dosing protocols for pruritus, nausea, respiratory depression, and other opioid-induced side effects are not well established; however, studies indicate that titration and careful consideration of unique patient factors are warranted.[27,32] In one study, optimal dosing for the treatment of pruritus was seen at 2 to 3 mg IV in patients who had received intrathecal morphine for cesarean section.[8] Another study showed decreased nausea (45% compared to 65%) in patients who were given 0.01-mg nalbuphine per 1 mg of morphine in patient-controlled analgesia when compared to patients who received only morphine.[34] Neither of these studies showed increased pain scores in the nalbuphine groups. Nalbuphine has been shown to have a ceiling effect at doses greater than 30 mg, where increasing doses do not increase analgesia or increase respiratory depression.[7,27]

Onset/Duration of Action

Onset of action occurs in 2 to 3 minutes with IV injection and in less than 15 minutes with SQ or IM injection. Duration of action is between 3 and 6 hours.[7]

Pharmacokinetics/Pharmacodynamics

Nalbuphine is hepatically metabolized and excreted primarily through the feces. Plasma elimination half-life of IV nalbuphine is approximately 2 to 3 hours.[38] Pharmacokinetic studies in young adults, elderly adults, children, and neonates have shown plasma elimination half-lives of 1.9, 2.3, 0.9, and 4.1 hours, respectively.[27,39,40]

Clinical Applications

Nalbuphine is indicated for the treatment of moderate to severe pain. However, studies support its use for the treatment and prevention of opioid-induced prurituis, respiratory depression, tolerance and dependence, nausea, and urinary retention. It is also an acceptable treatment for labor pain.[27]

Adverse Effects

Considerations when using nalbuphine for analgesia include the ceiling effect where doses greater than 30 mg produce no additional analgesia. This effect limits the use of nalbuphine in extremely painful procedures. Transitioning to a μ-opioid receptor agonist must be done with careful planning as the μ antagonist effects of nalbuphine may increase μ agonist dose requirements. Nalbuphine may cause respiratory depression at the dose of 10 mg, especially in patients with impaired respiration. More rarely, severe allergic reactions have been reported, and severe fetal bradycardia has been reported with the use of nalbuphine during labor.[7]

REFERENCES

1. Naloxone product information. Hospira. January, 2007.
2. Wang DS, Sternbach G, Varon J. Nalmefene: a long-acting opioid antagonist. clinical applications in emergency medicine. *J Emerg Med.* 1998;16(3):471-475.
3. Moreland TA, Brice JEH, Walker CHM, et al. Naloxone pharmocokinetics in the newborn. *Fr J Clin Pharmacol.* 1980;9:609-612.
4. Stile IL, Fort M, Wurzburger RJ, et al. The pharmacokinetic of naloxone in the premature newborn. *Dev Pharmacol Ther.* 1987;10:454-459.
5. Flumazenil product information. Hikma Farmacutica. April, 2009.
6. Relistor (methylnaltexone bromide) product information. Wyeth Pharmaceuticals. September, 2010.
7. Nalbuphine hyrochloride product information. Hospira. August, 2007.
8. Somrat C, Oranuch K, Ketchada U, et al. Optimal dose of nalbuphine for treatment of intrathecal-morphine incuced pruritus after caesarean section. *J Obstet Gynaecol Res.* 1999;25(3):209-213.
9. Johnstone RE, Jobes DR, Kennell EM, et al. Reversal of morphine anesthesia with naloxone. *Anesthhsiology.* 1974;41(4):361-367.
10. Michaelis LL, Hickey PR, Clark PR, et al. Ventricular irritability associated with the use of naloxone hydrochloride. *Ann Thorac Surg.* 1974;18;608.
11. Taff RH. Pulmonary edema following naloxone administration in a patient without heart disease. *Anesthesiology.* 1983;59:576.
12. Anderson JA. Reversal agents in sedation and anesthesia: a review. *Anesth Prog.* 1988;35:43-47.
13. Hunkeler W, Mohler H, Pieri L, et al. Selective antagonists of benzodiazepines. *Nature.* 1981;290: 514-516.
14. O'Boyle C, Lambe R, Darragh A, Taffe W, et al. Ro15-1788 antagonizes the effects of diazepam in man without affecting its bioavailability. *Br J Anaesth.* 1983;55:349-355.
15. Whitwam JG. Flumazenil: a benzodiazepine antagonist. *BMJ.* 1988; 297:999.
16. Ashton H. Benzodiazepine withdrawal: an unfinished story. *Gr Med J.* 1984;288:1135-1140.
17. Methylnaltrexone. http://en.wikipedia.org/wiki/Methylnaltrexone. April, 2011.
18. Quaternary salts of normorphine and its acylated derivatives. US patent 3101339, Karl Zeile and Kurt Freter. Issued 1963-0820. assigned to C.H. Boehringer Sohn.
19. Hendrikx J, Beijnen J, Schellens J. Methylnaltrexone. *Oncologist.* 2009;14:679-682.
20. Moss J, Rosow CE. Development of peripheral opioid antagonists' new insights into opioid effects. *Mayo Clin Proc.* 2008; 83:1116-1130.
21. Portenoy RK, Thomas J, Moehl Boatwright ML, et al. Subcutaneous methylnaltexone for the treatment of opioi-induced constipation in patients with advanced illness: a double-blind, randomized, parallel group, dose-ranging study. *J Pain Symptom Manage.* 2008;35:458-468.
22. Thomas J, Karver S, Cooney GA, et al. Methylnaltrexone for opioid-induced constipation in advanced illness. N Engl J Med. 2008; 358(22):2332-2343.
23. Wang CZ, Li XL, Sun S, et al. Methylnaltrexone, a peripherally acting opioid receptor antagonist, enhances tumoricidal effects of 5-Fu on human carcinoma cells. *Anticancer Res.* 2009;29(8);2927-2932.
24. Singleton PA, Mambetsariev N, Lennon FE, et al. Methylnaltrexone potentiates the anti-angiogenic effects of mTOR inhibitors. *J Angiogen Res.* 2010;2(1):5.
25. Mathew B, Lennon F, Siegler J, et al. The novel role of the mu receptor in lung cancer progression: a laboratory investigation. *Anesth Analg.* 2011;112:558–567.
26. Nalbuphine. http://en.wikipedia.org/wiki/Nalbuphine. April, 2011.
27. Gunion MW, Marchionne AM, Anderson CT. Use of the mixed agonist-antagonist nalbuphine in opioid analgesia. *Acute Pain.* 2004;6:29-39.
28. Cohen SE, Ratner EF, Kreitzman TR, et al. Nalbuphine is better than naloxone for treatment of side effects after epidural morphine. *Anesth Analg.* 1992;75:747-752.
29. Baxter AD, Samson B, Penning J, et al. Prevention of epidural morphine-induced respiratory depression with intravenous nalbuphine infusion in post-thoracotomy patients. *Can J Anaesth.* 1989;36:503-509.
30. Penning JP, Samson G, Baxter AD. Reversal of epidural morphine-induced respiratory depression and pruritus with nalbuphine. *Can J Anaesth.* 1988;35:599-604.
31. Jaffe RS, Moldenhauer CC, Hug CC, et al. Nalbuphine antagonism of fentanyl-induced ventilatory depression: a randomized trial. *Anesthesiology.* 1988;68:254-260.
32. Bailey PL, Clark NJ, Pace NL, et al. Antagonism of postoperative opioid-induced respiratory depression: nalbuphine versus naloxone. *Anesth Analg.* 1987;66: 1109-1114.

33. Blaise GA, McMichan JC, Nugent M, et al. Nalbupine produces side-effects while reversing narcotic-induced respiratory depression by nalbuphine. *Anesth Analg.* 1986;65;S19.
34. Yeh YC, Lin TF, Chang HC, et al. Combination of low-dose nalbuphine and morphine in patient-controlled analgesia decreases incidence of opioid-related side effects. *J Formos Med Assoc.* 2009;108(7):548-553.
35. Kjellberg F, Tramer MR. Pharmacological control of opioid-induced pruritus: a quantitative systematic review of randomized trials. *Eur J Anaesthesiol.* 2001;18(6): 346-357.
36. Charuluxananan S, Kyokong O, Lomboonviboon W, et al. Nalbuphine versus ondansetron for prevention of intrathecal morphine-induced pruritus after cesarean delivery. *Anesth Analg.* 2003;96(6):1789-1793.
37. Yeh YC, Lin TF, Lin FS, et al. Cobination of opioid agonist and agonist-antagonist: patient-controlled analgesia requirement and adverse events among different-ratio morphine and nalbuphine admixtures for postoperative pain. *Br J Anaesth.* 2008;101(4):542-548.
38. Schmidt WK, Tam SW, Shotzberger GS, et al. Nalbuphine. *Drug Alcohol Dep.* 1985;14:339-362.
39. Jaillon P, Gardin ME, Lecocq B, et al. Pharmacokinetics of nalbuphine in infants, young healthy volunteers, and elderly patients. *Clin Pharmacol Ther.* 1989;46:226-233.
40. Nicolle E, Devillier P, Delanoy B et al. Therapeutic monitoring of nalbuphine: transplacental transfer and estimated pharmacokinetics in the neonate. *Eur J Clin Pharmacol.* 1996;49:485-489.

C H A P T E R

8

Potent Inhaled Agents

Ken B. Johnson, MD, and Nathan Birgenheier, MD

HISTORY OF DEVELOPMENT

The discovery of inhalation anesthetics has a colorful history and began as early as the late 1700s with nitrous oxide. One initial use was in the treatment of dental pain and was later in combination with oxygen as an anesthetic. Chloroform was discovered in 1831 by an obstetrician, James Simpson, who used it to relieve labor pain for Queen Victoria for her eighth and ninth deliveries in the mid-1800s. Although diethyl ether was discovered in the 1600s, it was not used as an anesthetic until the mid-1800s in the United States, most notably by William Morton at Massachusetts General Hospital in Boston, to successfully anesthetize a patient for a mandibular tumor resection. In search of better anesthetics, development of additional agents continued. Ethyl chloride, an agent used as a topical anesthetic to freeze painful tissue, was later found to render patients unconscious. Additional agents developed during the late 1800s were ethylene and cyclopropane, and during the early 1900s, divinyl ether was developed.

Major drawbacks to these early inhaled agents were they were pungent, flammable, and with selected drugs, associated with substantial hepatoxicity and/or cardiotoxicity, making them less desirable to use. In the 1950s, fluorinated hydrocarbons were introduced as nonflammable alternatives and have remained the mainstay of potent inhaled agents. Since then, numerous fluorinated hydrocarbon compounds have been evaluated, with several introduced into clinical use (enflurane, methoxyflurane, and halothane). Those with the best kinetic profile and minimal toxic side effects remain in use today (isoflurane, sevoflurane, and desflurane).

MECHANISM OF ACTION AND DRUG EFFECTS

The mechanism of action for potent inhaled agents is not well understood and has been the subject of debate since the agents were discovered to be anesthetics. Unlike intravenous anesthetics, where pharmacologic action is associated with a drug binding to a receptor and triggering an effect, potent inhaled agents do not appear to have specific receptor targets. There are several theories. Researchers have suggested that potent inhaled agents deform lipid membranes such that they alter function of lipid proteins that play a role in neurotransmitter function within synaptic clefts. Inhaled anesthetics may act at multiple sites, making it difficult to pin down their exact mechanism, but it may be best described by physical chemistry (ie, swelling of nerve cell walls) and not chemical bonding between a drug and receptor.[1]

PHARMACOKINETICS AND PHARMACODYNAMICS

Pharmacokinetics

Important elements of inhaled agent pharmacokinetics are presented in Chapter 2. Inhaled agent kinetics (time course of drug concentration in response to dose) are a function of drug delivery as well as pulmonary ventilation and perfusion. A detailed description of factors that influence inhaled agent pharmacokinetics is presented in Figure 8–1.

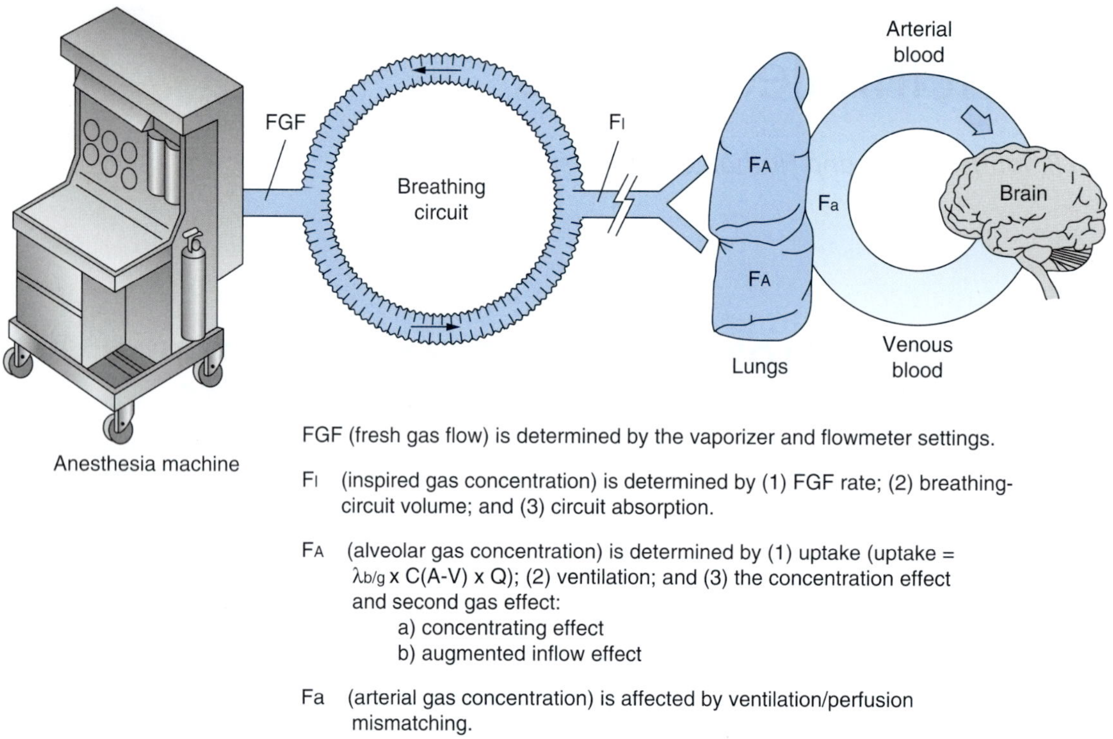

FIGURE 8–1 Schematic representation of factors that influence inhalation agent pharmacokinetics. The inspired (inhalation agent delivered is a function of vaporizer setting, fresh gas flow, and circuit volume. The alveolar drug concentration is a function of anesthetic uptake, pulmonary ventilation, and the second gas effect and concentration effect (Chapter 2). Uptake is determined by the blood–gas partition gas coefficient, the difference in drug partial pressure between the alveolar gas and venous blood, and the cardiac output (specifically the rate of blood perfusion of ventilated alveoli). Arterial drug concentration is a function of lung ventilation and perfusion. Drug delivery to the central nervous system is a function of arterial drug concentration, tissue perfusion, and blood–tissue partition coefficients. Drug uptake at tissues of interest (ie, brain and spinal cord) is dependent on the partial pressure difference between arterial blood and tissue. (Reproduced with permission from Butterworth JF, Mackey DC, Wasnick JD: Morgan, Mikhail, & Murray, Clinical Anesthesiology, 5th edition. McGraw-Hill, 2013.)

Key Points

1. Factors that influence drug uptake include alveolar ventilation, blood–gas partition coefficients (Table 8–1), and cardiac output. Alveolar ventilation is a function of the tidal volume, dead space volume, and respiratory rate. Figure 8–2 presents a set of simulations that plot the predicted effect-site concentration of isoflurane for 3 different alveolar minute volumes (3, 6, and 12 L/min). The time required to reach 90% of the maximal effect-site concentration was 36, 19, and 12 minutes, respectively, for each alveolar minute volume. As will be described below, the effect-site concentration is not to be confused with the end-tidal concentration, especially during non–steady-state conditions.
2. The blood–gas partition coefficient is a reflection of drug solubility. The coefficient represents the ratio of gas amount (drug) in air versus blood. For example, the blood–gas coefficient for desflurane is 0.42, indicating that at equilibrium at 37°C, a certain volume of blood (eg, 5 mL) will hold 42% of the

TABLE 8–1 Minimum alveolar concentration for selected inhaled agents and nitrous oxide.

Inhaled Agent	Minimum Alveolar Concentration (MAC)[a]	Blood–Gas Partition Coefficient
Isoflurane	1.15%	1.4
Desflurane	6.0%	0.42
Sevoflurane	1.71%	0.65
Nitrous oxide	104%	0.47
Xenon	71%	0.11

[a]MAC is defined as no skeletal muscle movement in response to a noxious stimulus in 50% of patients. MAC values assume an atmospheric pressure of 760 mm Hg. Anesthetics delivered at higher altitudes require higher MAC values to achieve an equivalent effect.

desflurane of an equivalent volume of air (eg, 5 mL).[1]

3. Anesthetics with a low blood–gas partition coefficient (low solubility) quickly reach maximal content in blood and have a rapid onset and offset time (ie, nitrous oxide) compared to those with a high blood–gas coefficients (ie, isoflurane).
4. Inhalation agent elimination is a function of primarily by exhalation once delivery is terminated. Other factors include biotransformation and loss from skin tissue to air directly. Both of these contribute little to the rate of partial pressure drop once drug is discontinued. Biotransformation is minimal for modern inhalation agents but was more pronounced with highly metabolized drugs previously used, such as methoxyflurane and to a lesser extent halothane.[1]
5. Like delivery, elimination from the brain via the lungs is largely dependent on central nervous system perfusion, cardiac output, tissue–blood and blood–gas partition coefficients, lung perfusion and ventilation, and the removal of drug from the anesthesia circuit. Anesthesiologists can influence this process using a few techniques to enhance drug removal. Some of these include increasing fresh gas flow to wash out exhaled drug via the drug scavenging system and ensuring adequate ventilation and lung perfusion (typically using blood pressure and heart rate as a surrogate measure of cardiovascular function).
6. Researchers have devised a tool to hasten volatile anesthetic removal involving rebreathing carbon dioxide to increase cerebral blood flow and double minute volume while avoiding hypocarbia.[2,3] Using this technique, elevating the partial pressure of carbon dioxide, via a rebreathing circuit, to 55 mm Hg and hyperventilating decreased emergence times for isoflurane; this worked to a lesser extent for sevoflurane and desflurane. For example, in 20 patients undergoing anterior cruciate ligament repair, wake-up times were 50% faster (7 minutes earlier) with hyperventilation hypercarbia. This device may be useful for rapid emergence following anesthetics with a long duration; procedures that require high-dose inhaled agents; or abrupt, perhaps unanticipated, end to surgery.
7. Given that volatile anesthetics are lipid soluble, one concern is the accumulation of drug with prolonged drug delivery. Figure 8–3 presents a simulation of sevoflurane with the vaporizer set to 2% for 1, 4, and 8 hours. Once the delivery was terminated and the vaporizer set to 0%, predictions from this simulation suggest that all of the concentrations will decrease by 50% in 5 to 6 minutes for drug delivery ranging from 1 to 8 hours (the 50% decrement time). However, it is important to point out that at the end of a 1-, 4-, and 8-hour anesthetic, the peak concentrations are progressively higher (1.6 vol%, 1.9 vol%, and 1.95 vol%).

Pharmacodynamics

Minimum alveolar concentration (MAC) is a measure of volatile anesthetic potency and is used to compare the concentration–effect relationship between volatile anesthetics (see Table 8–1). MAC is defined as the concentration necessary to render a patient immobile in the presence of a supranoxious stimulus (ie, skin incision) at sea level with normal

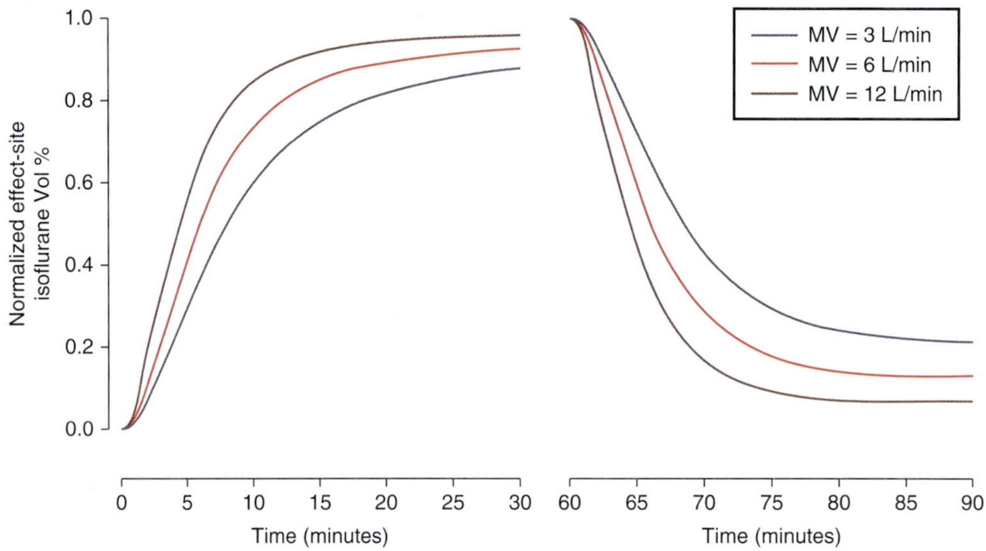

FIGURE 8–2 Simulation of the influence of alveolar ventilation on isoflurane pharmacokinetics. Isoflurane is delivered with the vaporizer set to 1.2% for 1 hour. The vertical axis is normalized to 1.0. Effect-site concentrations (vol%) are presented for an alveolar minute volume (MV) of 3, 6, and 12 L/min. The first 20 minutes after starting drug delivery and 20 minutes following termination of drug delivery are presented in the left and right columns, respectively. Simulations assume a 30-year-old, 183-cm, 100-kg male; a fresh gas flow of 2 L/min; a MV of 6 L/min; and a normal cardiac output. The vaporizer is set at 1.2% for isoflurane, 2% for sevoflurane, and 6% for desflurane. Simulations used the following published pharmacokinetic and pharmacodynamic parameters to predict end-tidal and effect-site concentrations and drug effects: Johnson KB, Syroid ND, Gupta DK, et al. Evaluation of remifentanil sevoflurane response surface models in patients emerging from anesthesia: model improvement using effect-site sevoflurane concentrations. *Anesth Analg*, 2010;111(2): 387-394; Lerou JG, Dirksen R, Beneken Kolmer HH, et al. A system model for closed-circuit inhalation anesthesia. I. Computer study. *Anesthesiology*. 1991;75(2):345-355; Lerou JG, Dirksen R, Beneken Kolmer HH, et al. A system model for closed-circuit inhalation anesthesia. II. Clinical validation. *Anesthesiology*. 1991;75(2):230-237; Lerou JG, Booij LH. Model-based administration of inhalation anaesthesia. 1. Developing a system model. *Br J Anaesth*. 2001;86(1):12-28; Lerou JG, Booij LH. Model-based administration of inhalation anaesthesia. 2. Exploring the system model. *Br J Anaesth*. 2001;86(1):29-37; Lerou JG, Booij LH. Model-based administration of inhalation anaesthesia. 3. Validating the system model. *Br J Anaesth*. 2002;88(1):24-37; Lerou JG, Verheijen R, Booij LH. Model-based administration of inhalation anaesthesia. 4. Applying the system model. *Br J Anaesth*. 2002;88(2):175-183; and Wissing H. Volatile anesthetic pharmacokinetics. *Br J Anaesth*. 2000;84:443-493.

atmospheric pressure (760 mm Hg) and normal body temperature (37°C).

Key Points

1. MAC is similar to the C_{50} presented in Chapter 1. Of note, the MAC (or C_{50}) does not describe the entire concentration–effect curve. The slope of concentration versus effect is required to fully understand this relationship; however, clinicians often use 1.3 MAC as the amount of inhalation agent necessary to prevent movement in 95% of patients and 0.3 MAC as the concentration when patients emerge from anesthesia.[1]
2. MAC and any other pharmacodynamic parameter, for that matter, that describes an effect at a given effect-site concentration is an estimate of drug concentration at the site of action (likely at the brain or spinal cord). Many monitors display MAC based on the end-tidal concentration of a volatile anesthetic. End-tidal concentrations are a

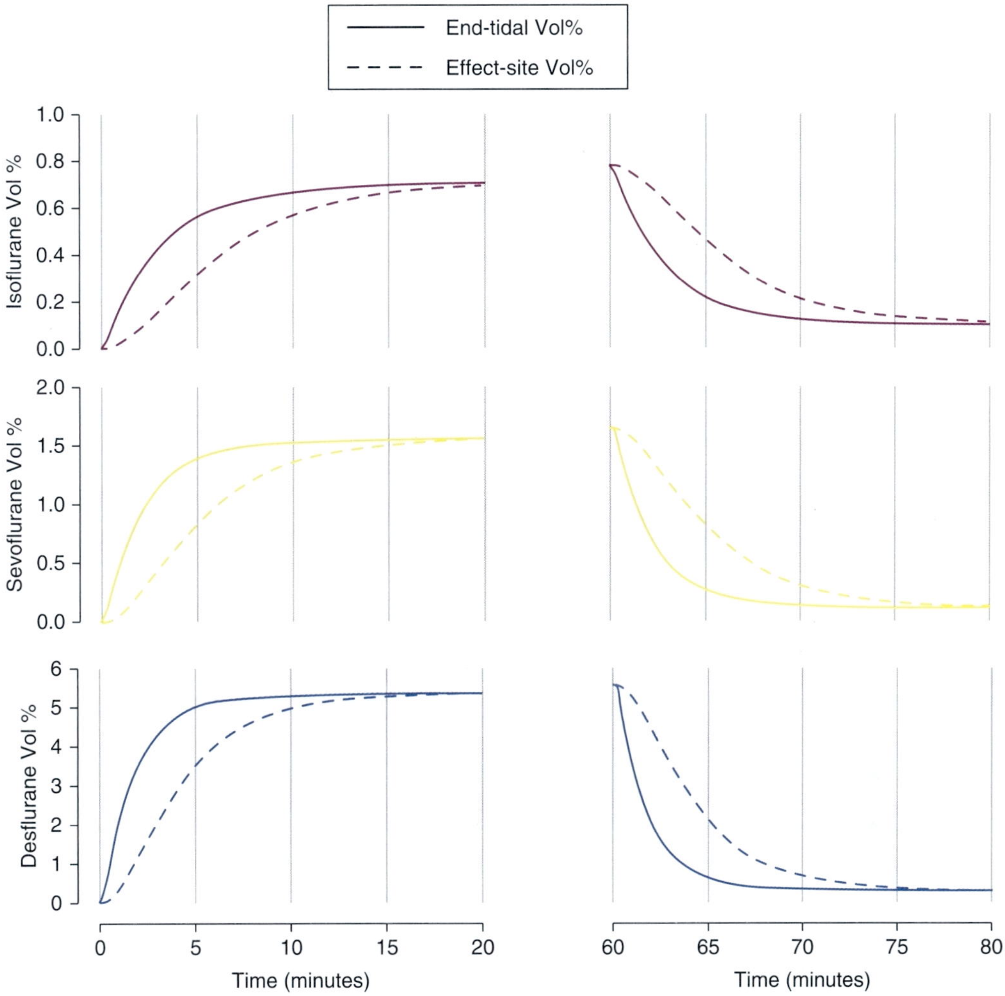

FIGURE 8–3 Simulation of non–steady-state conditions for volatile agent levels delivered over 1 hour. End-tidal and effect-site vol % are presented as solid and dashed lines, respectively. The first 20 minutes after starting drug delivery and 20 minutes following termination of drug delivery are presented in the left and right columns, respectively. Simulations assumed the same conditions and patient demographics as in Figure 8–2.

surrogate estimate of effect-site concentrations and are only reasonable at near–steady-state conditions. During induction, emergence, or large adjustments in vaporizer settings, displayed MAC values will likely misrepresent effect-site concentrations. Caution should be used when interpreting these values under non–steady-state conditions to make clinical decisions. Consider the simulations presented in Figure 8–4. This set of simulations presents the time course of end-tidal and effect-site concentrations (vol%) for isoflurane, sevoflurane, and desflurane. During non–steady-state conditions, the effect-site levels lag behind the end-tidal levels. The time required for the effect-site concentrations to achieve 90% of the end-tidal concentrations are presented in Table 8–2. Under routine conditions with fresh gas flow, minute ventilation, and cardiac output, the effect-site

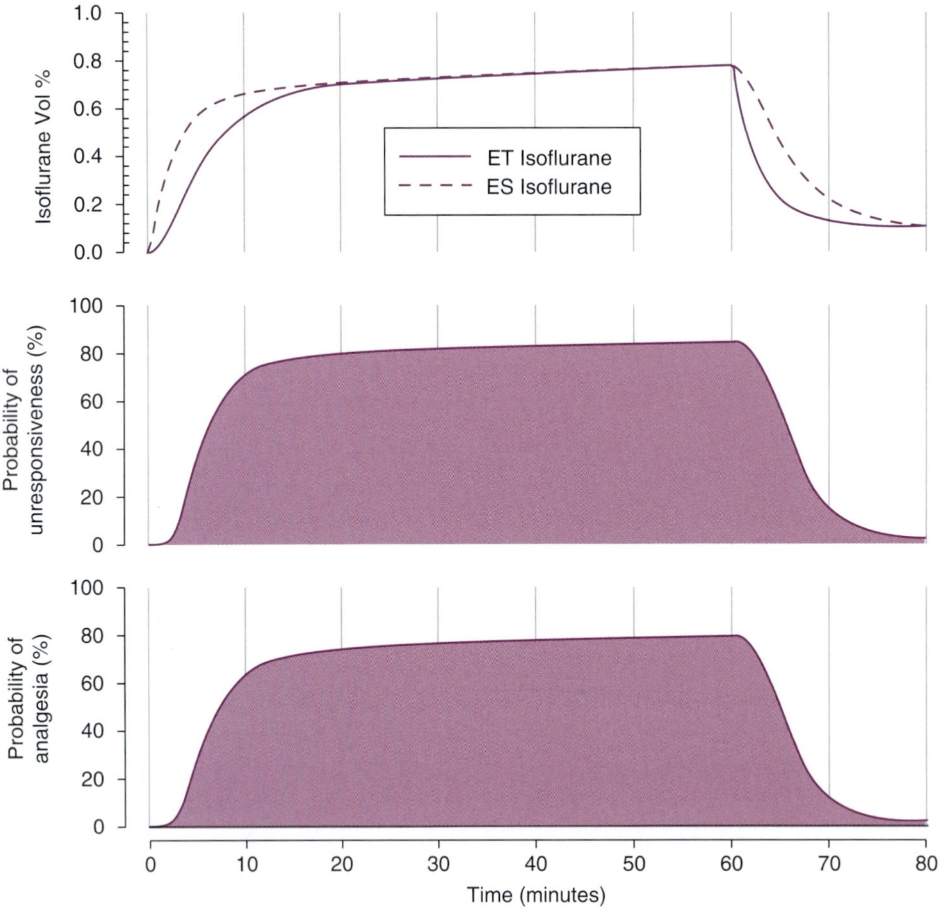

FIGURE 8–4 Simulation of isoflurane end-tidal (ET) and effect-site (ES) concentrations (vol%), loss of responsiveness, and loss of response to a painful stimulus for a 1-hour delivery with the vaporizer set at 1.2%. Simulations assumed the same conditions and patient demographics as in Figure 8–2.

concentration can take up to 10 minutes to approximate the end-tidal concentration. This may explain why patients remain unresponsive for a time during emergence from anesthesia despite the measured end-tidal concentration reading 0 vol%.

3. Not all effects follow the same concentration–effect curve. As with opioids, the concentration–effect relationship for loss of responsiveness, adverse effects (ie, severe cardiac depression), or electroencephalogram burst suppression are not identical.

4. MAC is used to describe loss of response to a supranormal noxious stimulus (skin incision). Other methods of describing drug effect include dividing up anesthetic effects into sedation/hypnosis, analgesia, and neuromuscular blockade. Volatile anesthetics produce all of these effects to varying degrees. A simulation of a 1-hour administration of isoflurane with the vaporizer set to 1.2% is presented in Figure 8–5. This figure presents predictions of drug concentrations and selected effects, namely loss of responsiveness

TABLE 8–2 Simulations of the time required for effect-site concentrations to achieve 90% of end-tidal concentrations under non–steady-state conditions.

Inhaled Agent	Time Required for Effect-Site Concentrations to Reach 90% of End-Tidal Concentrations (vol%)[a]
Isoflurane	13 minutes
Desflurane	9 minutes
Sevoflurane	11 minutes

[a]Simulations assume a fresh gas flow of 2 L/min, a minute volume of 6 L/min, and normal cardiovascular function.

and loss of response to a moderately painful stimulus (30 pounds per square inch of pressure over the anterior tibia). Of note, the loss of response to laryngoscopy and tracheal intubation is substantially more stimulating than tibial pressure. As dosed, isoflurane achieves less than 4% of a probability of blocking the response to laryngoscopy and tracheal intubation.

5. The MAC equivalents of simultaneous administration of multiple inhalation agents are additive. For example, 0.5 MAC of nitrous oxide and 0.5 MAC of isoflurane yield 1.0 MAC of combined anesthetic effect. When administering nitrous oxide at 66%, it reduces the MAC of volatile anesthetics by up to 50%.

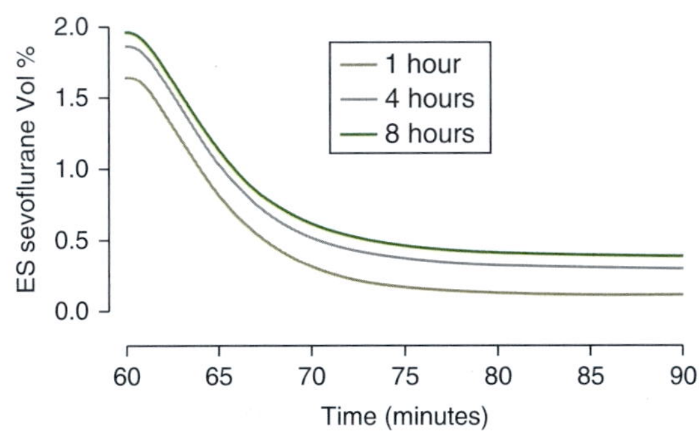

FIGURE 8–5 Simulation of sevoflurane effect-site (ES) concentrations (vol%) following a 1-, 4-, and 8-hour anesthetic with the vaporizer set to 2%. This simulation illustrates the impact of drug accumulation on decrement time. Of note, the 50% decrement time (time required to reach 50% of the ES concentration just prior to terminating the anesthetic) was within 5 to 6 minutes for the 1-, 4-, and 8-hour anesthetics. Simulations assumed the same conditions and patient demographics as in Figure 8–2.

CLINICAL PHARMACOLOGY OF SELECTED INHALATION AGENTS

Isoflurane

Isoflurane, $C_3H_2ClF_5O$, is nonflammable isomer of enflurane yet has substantially different properties. It has a pungent odor, making it difficult to use for inhalational induction.

Isoflurane increases cerebral blood flow and intracranial pressure at MAC levels greater than 1. It also decreases cerebral metabolic rate and can produce electrical silence (burst suppression) on the electroencephalogram at MAC of 2 or greater.

Isoflurane has minimal cardiovascular depression, maintains cardiac output but does decrease systemic vascular resistance and blood pressure, and mimics ischemic preconditioning when administered for a brief period prior to an ischemic insult. Thus it may play a role in preserving myocardium at risk of injury from perioperative occlusive injury.[4,5] Isoflurane is also a coronary vasodilator. A theoretical risk is that dilating disease-free coronary arteries may excessively divert blood flow from diseased coronary arteries, putting myocardium at risk for ischemia (coronary steal syndrome). However, isoflurane remains a commonly used anesthetic in patients with known or suspected cardiac disease.

Isoflurane, like other potent inhaled agents, is a bronchodilator, but because of its pungent odor may irritate airway structures. Isoflurane suppresses ventilatory function. It reduces tidal volume but increases respiratory rate. The overall net effect is a decrease in minute volume. Isoflurane blunts the response to hypoxia and hypercarbia.

Sevoflurane

Sevoflurane, $C_4H_3F_7O$, is widely used in adults and pediatric patients and is not as pungent as other potent inhaled agents, making it more suitable for mask induction of anesthesia. It has a relatively low blood–gas partition coefficient (0.65), allowing for rapid onset.

Like other potent inhaled agents, sevoflurane increases cerebral blood flow and intracranial pressure at normocarbia. It also decreases cerebral metabolic rate and can produce electrical silence (electroencephalogram burst suppression) at MAC of 2 or greater.

Sevoflurane reduces cardiac contractility, cardiac output, systemic vascular resistance, and blood pressure, but to a lesser extent than with isoflurane. It does not cause coronary artery steal syndrome.

Sevoflurane is a bronchodilator and suppresses ventilatory function similar to isoflurane. It reduces tidal volume but increases respiratory rate. The overall net effect is a decrease in minute volume. Sevoflurane blunts the response to hypoxia and hypercarbia.

Desflurane

Desflurane, $C_3H_2F_6O$, although chemically similar to isoflurane, has much different physiochemical properties. Because of its high vapor pressure and ability to boil at room temperatures at high altitudes, it requires a special vaporizer. Because of a low blood–gas partition coefficient, it has a fast onset. With a low solubility, alveolar and blood partial pressures quickly equilibrate, making it easy to titrate to desired partial pressures.

Like other potent inhaled agents, desflurane increases cerebral blood flow and intracranial pressure but also decreases cerebral metabolic rate, reducing the cerebral blood flow requirements to maintain brain–tissue metabolism.

Desflurane is similar to isoflurane in terms of its cardiovascular profile; although it maintains cardiac output, it does decrease systemic vascular resistance and blood pressure. It does not dilate coronary arteries. Caution should be used with quickly increasing desflurane, because it may lead to a catecholamine surge and a worrisome increase in heart rate and blood pressure.[6,7]

Desflurane, because of its pungent odor, may irritate airway structures, leading to laryngospasm and excessive salivation. Desflurane suppresses ventilatory function (decreased minute volume) by decreasing tidal volume but increasing respiratory rate, and it also blunts the response to hypoxia and hypercarbia.

Nitrous Oxide

Nitrous oxide (N_2O) is a nonflammable gas at room temperature. It requires a high concentration to achieve an effect (ie, MAC = 104%), making it potentially unsafe to use because increasing doses may lead to inadequate oxygen delivery. Nitrous oxide increases cerebral blood flow, cerebral oxygen consumption, cerebral blood volume, and a small increase in intracranial pressure.

Similar to desflurane, nitrous oxide stimulates the sympathetic nervous system and increases cardiovascular tone. Although it is a direct myocardial depressant, the increase in catecholamines offsets this effect resulting in minimal change in hemodynamics.

Nitrous oxide reduces tidal volume but increases respiratory rate. The overall net effect is a minimal change in minute volume. It also blunts the response to hypoxia.

SELECTED ADVERSE EFFECTS FROM INHALED ANESTHETICS

Postoperative Nausea and Vomiting

Volatile anesthetics and nitrous oxide are implicated in higher rates of postoperative nausea and vomiting when compared to intravenous techniques with propofol.[8-10]

Methionine Synthase Inhibition

Nitrous oxide inhibits vitamin B_{12}–dependent enzymes (such as thymidylate synthase, methionine synthase) by altering vitamin B_{12}. Thymidylate synthase is required for DNA synthesis, and methionine synthase is required for myelin formation. Clinicians often avoid nitrous oxide in pregnant women because of possible teratogenic effects.

Air-Containing Cavities

Nitrous oxide is 35 times more soluble than nitrogen. Nitrous oxide will diffuse into air-containing cavities faster than nitrogen will diffuse out. This may lead to volume expansion within the air-containing cavity (ie, increasing the size of a pneumothorax, air embolism, or pneumocephalus), or if the volume is fixed, it may lead to increasing pressure (ie, diffusion into the cuff of an endotracheal tube increasing pressure on tracheal mucosa).[1]

Pulmonary Hypertension

Nitrous oxide increases pulmonary vascular resistance and should be avoided in patients with preexisting pulmonary hypertension.

Fluoride Toxicity

Fluoride is a metabolite of volatile anesthetics and known to be nephrotoxic. Compared to isoflurane and desflurane, sevoflurane has a high metabolism (5%), leading to potentially high fluoride levels. Clinical use of sevoflurane, however, has not been associated with renal dysfunction.

Compound A

Compound A (flouromethyl-2,2-diflouro-1-triflouromethylvinyl ether) is a degradation product of sevoflurane in barium hydroxide and soda lime used to capture carbon dioxide. Compound A is nephrotoxic in a rodent model, but this toxicity has not been established in humans. Conditions that lead to compound A accumulation include a desiccated carbon dioxide absorber, elevated temperature, high sevoflurane concentrations, and prolonged anesthetics. Despite little evidence to support it, clinicians recommend providing fresh gas flows of 2 L/min or more to wash out accumulations of compound A and to avoid sevoflurane in patients with known renal disease.

Carbon Monoxide Poisoning

Desflurane is degraded by dried-out carbon dioxide absorbers made from barium hydroxide, and to a lesser extent, from sodium hydroxide into carbon monoxide.[11-13] This condition may occur when high fresh gas flows are left on overnight or over a weekend and dry out the carbon dioxide absorbent. Compared to other agents, carbon monoxide production is most pronounced with desflurane. While under an anesthetic, developing carbon monoxide poisoning may require an arterial blood gas analysis to detect significant carboxyhemoglobin.

Malignant Hyperthermia

Volatile anesthetics and succinylcholine are known triggers of malignant hyperthermia, a rapidly progressing hypermetabolic process within skeletal muscle due to a single-point ryanodine receptor mutation. Testing is expensive and invasive (a vastus muscle biopsy and contracture test), and it is difficult to obtain. If a patient is suspected of being susceptible to malignant hyperthermia, clinicians simply avoid triggering agents.

Postoperative Cognitive Dysfunction

Although elderly patients may emerge from anesthesia and appear neurologically intact, family members may note a subtle but persistent decline in cognitive abilities that can lead to a significantly reduced quality of life.[14] Exposure to volatile anesthetics along with nitrous oxide, ketamine, and benzodiazepines may result in increased expression of substances that are harmful to neural tissue.[15,16] Mechanisms may include abnormal neuroapoptosis (cell death) and/or faulty synaptogenesis. Specifically researchers have reported that expression of proapoptotic proteins (such as bcl-xS, bax, bix, caspase-3) that are increased in the presence of volatile anesthetics. Capsases, for example, cleave intracellular cytoskeletal structure, leading to cell death. Of the 3 commonly used volatile anesthetics, isoflurane appears to be worse than sevoflurane or desflurane in animal models of neuroapoptosis.[17,18] Transitioning these histologic findings to in vivo behavioral analysis, researchers have found that in an elderly rodent model, exposure to isoflurane results in impaired acquisition of spatial memory.[19] In addition, Alzheimer disease may also be exacerbated by various anesthetics, including volatile anesthetics,[20,21] by favoring formation of insoluble Aβ oligomers that induces caspase-3 activation, leading to increased neuroapoptosis.

REFERENCES

1. Morgan G, Mikhail M, Murray M. Inhalation anesthetics. In: *Clinical Anesthesiology*. 4th ed. New York: McGraw-Hill; 2013.
2. Sakata DJ, Gopalakrishnan NA, Orr JA, White JL, Westenskow DR. Rapid recovery from sevoflurane and

desflurane with hypercapnia and hyperventilation. *Anesth Analg*. 2007;105(1):79-82.

3. Sakata DJ, Gopalakrishnan NA, Orr JA, White JL, Westenskow DR. Hypercapnic hyperventilation shortens emergence time from isoflurane anesthesia. *Anesth Analg*. 2007;104(3):587-591.
4. Cason BA, Gamperl AK, Slocum RE, Hickey RF. Anesthetic-induced preconditioning: previous administration of isoflurane decreases myocardial infarct size in rabbits. *Anesthesiology*. 1997;87(5):1182-1190.
5. Kersten JR, Schmeling TJ, Paget PS, Gross GJ, Waltier DC. Isoflurane mimics ischemic preconditioning via activation of K(ATP) channels: reduction of myocardial infarct size with an acute memory phase. *Anesthesiology*. 1997;87(2):361-370.
6. Gormley WP, Murray JM, Trinick TR. Intravenous lidocaine does not attenuate the cardiovascular and catecholamine response to a rapid increase in desflurane concentration. *Anesth Analg*. 1996;82(2):358-361.
7. Rodig G, Keyl C, Kaluza M, Kees F, Hobbhahn J. Effects of rapid increases of desflurane and sevoflurane to concentrations of 1.5 MAC on systemic vascular resistance and catecholamine response during cardiopulmonary bypass. *Anesthesiology*. 1997;87(4):801-807.
8. Gupta A, Stierer T, Zuckerman R, Sakima N, Parker SD, Fleisher LA. Comparison of recovery profile after ambulatory anesthesia with propofol, isoflurane, sevoflurane and desflurane: a systematic review. *Anesth Analg*. 2004;98(3):632-641.
9. Mraovic B, Simurina T, Sonicki Z, Skitarelic N, Gan TJ. The dose-response of nitrous oxide in postoperative nausea in patients undergoing gynecologic laparoscopic surgery: a preliminary study. *Anesth Analg*. 2008; 107(3):818-823.
10. Visser K, Hassink EA, Bonsel GJ, Moen J, Kalkman CJ. Randomized controlled trial of total intravenous anesthesia with propofol versus inhalation anesthesia with isoflurane-nitrous oxide: postoperative nausea with vomiting and economic analysis. *Anesthesio-logy*. 2001;95(3):616-626.
11. Fan SZ, Lin YW, Chang WS, Tang CS. An evaluation of the contributions by fresh gas flow rate, carbon dioxide concentration and desflurane partial pressure to carbon monoxide concentration during low fresh gas flows to a circle anaesthetic breathing system. *Eur J Anaesthesiol*. 2008;25(8):620-626.
12. Keijzer C, Perez RS, de Lange JJ. Carbon monoxide production from desflurane and six types of carbon dioxide absorbents in a patient model. *Acta Anaesthesiol Scand*. 2005;49(6):815-818.
13. Wissing H, Kuhn I, Warnken U, Dudziak R. Carbon monoxide production from desflurane, enflurane, halothane, isoflurane, and sevoflurane with dry soda lime. *Anesthesiology*. 2001; 95(5):1205-1212.
14. Cottrell JE. We care, therefore we are: anesthesia-related morbidity and mortality: the 46th Rovenstine Lecture. *Anesthesiology*. 2008;109(3):377-388.
15. Engelhard K, Werner C, Eberspacher E, et al. The effect of the alpha 2-agonist dexmedetomidine and the N-methyl-D-aspartate antagonist S(+)-ketamine on the expression of apoptosis-regulating proteins after incomplete cerebral ischemia and reperfusion in rats. *Anesth Analg*. 2003;96(2): 524-531.
16. Creeley CE, Olney JW. The young: neuroapoptosis induced by anesthetics and what to do about it. *Anesth Analg*. 2010;110(2):442-448.
17. Yang H, Liang G, Hawkins BJ, Madesh M, Pierwola A, Wei H. Inhalational anesthetics induce cell damage by disruption of intracellular calcium homeostasis with different potencies. *Anesthesiology*. 2008;109(2):243-250.
18. Liang G, Ward C, Peng J, Zhao Y, Huang B, Wei H. Isoflurane causes greater neurodegeneration than an equivalent exposure of sevoflurane in the developing brain of neonatal mice. *Anesthesiology*. 2010;112(6):1325-1334.
19. Culley DJ, Baxter MG, Yukhananov R, Crosby G. Long-term impairment of acquisition of a spatial memory task following isoflurane-nitrous oxide anesthesia in rats. *Anesthesiology*. 2004;100(2):309-314.
20. Liang G, Wang Q, Li Y, et al. A presenilin-1 mutation renders neurons vulnerable to isoflurane toxicity. *Anesth Analg*. 2008;106(2): 492-500.
21. Whittington RA, Papon MA, Chouinard F, Planel E. Hypothermia and Alzheimer's disease neuropathogenic pathways. *Curr Alzheimer Res*. 2010;7(8):717-725.

CHAPTER

9

Neuromuscular Blocking Agents

Stephen Aniskevich, MD, Sorin J. Brull, MD, FCARCSI (Hon), and Mohamed Naguib, MB, BCh, MSc, FFARCSI, MD

HISTORY OF DEVELOPMENT

Neuromuscular blocking agents (NMBAs) were first "discovered" by the native Indian populations of South America and were used for hunting game. They called their plant-based concoction "ourari," which was later interpreted as "curare" by the early European explorers. The use of neuromuscular relaxants in medicine, however, would have to wait until the mid-1800s, when Dr Louis Sayres of New York attempted to treat the spasms associated with tetanus with a rudimentary curare preparation (Chapter 10). The first successful use of curare during surgery was described by Dr Arthur Lawen in 1912; however, it would take an additional 30 years of further refinement in anesthesia methodology, notably improved tracheal intubation techniques, before Drs Harold Griffith and Enid Johnson demonstrated successful and safe use of curare in surgery and anesthesia. After their groundbreaking work, research into NMBAs led to the development and purification of several different neuromuscular agents. Of the modern neuromuscular agents still in clinical use, succinylcholine was first synthesized in 1906, but its clinical effect was not recognized until 1949. Pancuronium was manufactured in 1964, and further research to lessen its side-effect profile led to the development of vecuronium in 1979. More recently, mivacurium and rocuronium became available for clinical use in the early 1990s.

Further research into compounds with more rapid metabolism and elimination resulted in the introduction into practice in the 1980s of vecuronium,[1] an aminosteroid, and atracurium,[2,3] a benzylisoquinolinium compound. These relaxants had little or no dependence on the kidney for elimination, and vecuronium lacked cardiovascular effects.[1] The degradation of atracurium via Hofmann elimination removed any important influence of advanced age or organ failure on the profile of the drug and greatly increased its acceptance in the clinical setting, despite its hemodynamic side-effect profile. In an attempt to decrease the histamine release associated with atracurium, one of its isomers, cisatracurium, was isolated in the mid-1990s and became widely popular in anesthesia practice.

NORMAL NEUROMUSCULAR TRANSMISSION

NMBAs act to prevent effective transmission of nerve impulses across the neuromuscular junction, the synapse interposed between the presynaptic nerve terminal and the postsynaptic muscle membrane. Under normal conditions, when a nerve impulse is transmitted along the axon and reaches the nerve terminal, it causes release of stored acetylcholine from the nerve terminal (readily releasable vesicle pool). The acetylcholine (released as quanta, each quantum containing approximately 5000 acetylcholine molecules per vesicle) then diffuses across the synaptic cleft and interacts with nicotinic acetylcholine receptors on the postsynaptic (muscle) membrane. When enough of these receptors are activated (all-or-none rule), an action potential ensues leading to muscle contraction. The adult acetylcholine receptor (Figure 9–1) consists of 2 identical α subunits, and 1 β, δ, and ε subunits each, arranged in a rosette pattern ($\alpha_2\beta\delta\varepsilon$). In fetal acetylcholine receptors, the ε subunit is replaced by a γ subunit ($\alpha_2\beta\delta\gamma$) (Figure 9–2). Acetylcholine must bind to both α subunits simultaneously in order to induce the conformational change needed to activate the receptor.

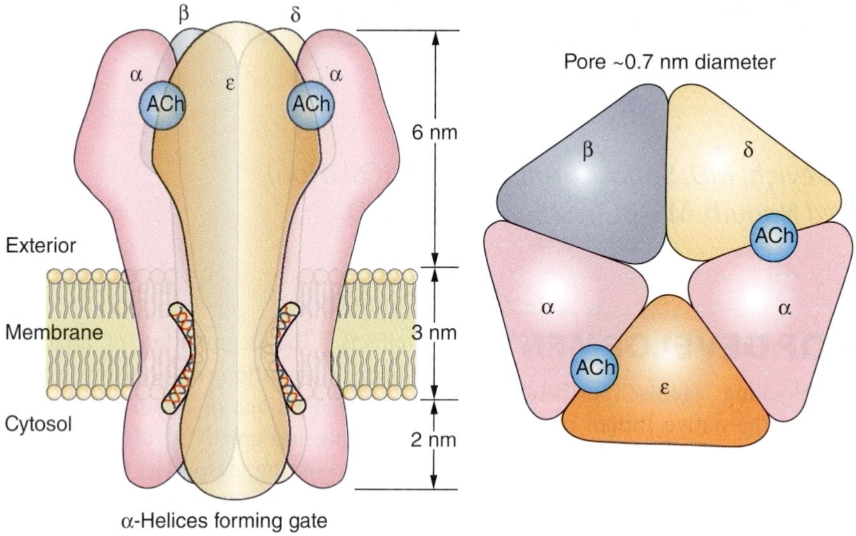

FIGURE 9–1 Adult acetylcholine receptor (AChR) consisting of 5 subunits (two identical α subunits, and one β, δ, and ε subunits each) arranged in a rosette ($\alpha_2\beta\delta\varepsilon$) pattern. The two α subunits contain the recognition sites for acetylcholine binding. (Reproduced with permission from Brull SJ, Naguib M. Review of Neuromuscular Junction Anatomy and Function. In:*The Neuroscientific Foundations of Anesthesiology*. Mashour GA, Lydic R (Editors), Oxford University Press, New York. 2011; pp:205-210.)

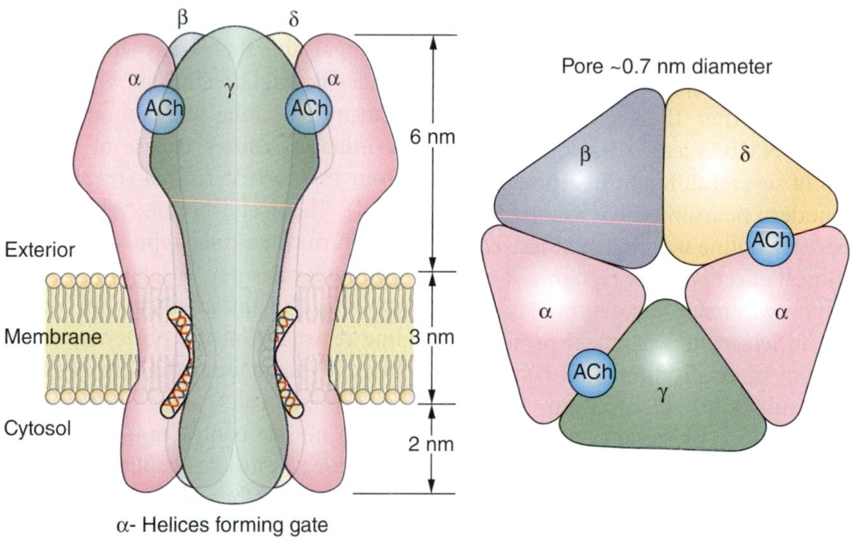

FIGURE 9–2 Fetal acetylcholine receptor (AChR) consisting of 5 subunits (two identical α subunits, and one β, δ, and γ subunits each) arranged in a rosette pattern. Note that the ε subunit is replaced by a γ subunit resulting in ($\alpha_2\beta\delta\gamma$) pattern. The two α subunits contain the recognition sites for acetylcholine binding. (Reproduced with permission from Brull SJ, Naguib M. Review of Neuromuscular Junction Anatomy and Function. In:*The Neuroscientific Foundations of Anesthesiology*. Mashour GA, Lydic R (Editors), Oxford University Press, New York. 2011; pp:205-210.)

The activated (open) receptor allows for the flow of sodium, calcium, and potassium ions across their electrochemical concentration gradients, resulting in muscle membrane depolarization and muscle fiber contraction.

Currently, there are 2 classes of NMBAs available in the clinical setting. Each prevents muscle contraction through different mechanisms.

DEPOLARIZING NEUROMUSCULAR BLOCKING AGENTS

Succinylcholine chloride (suxamethonium chloride) is the only depolarizing agent available for clinical use today. Succinylcholine acts by binding to one or both of the α subunits of the postsynaptic receptor, leading to activation of the end-plate receptor (see Figure 9–1). Since the elimination of succinylcholine from the neuromuscular junction is slower than that of acetylcholine (a few milliseconds), the effect is that of prolonged depolarization. During this period of depolarization, initial disorganized muscle contraction (evidenced clinically by muscle fasciculations) is followed by flaccid paralysis. While depolarized, the receptor is not susceptible (ie, it is desensitized) to further stimulation by acetylcholine until succinylcholine redistributes away from the neuromuscular junction. Depolarizing neuromuscular blockade is also referred to as *phase I neuromuscular block*. If large doses of succinylcholine are administered, or if the patient has an abnormal ("atypical") gene for butyrylcholinesterase, the patient may develop a neuromuscular block with the characteristics of that produced by nondepolarizing NMBAs, called *phase II neuromuscular block*. Table 9–1 describes the differences between phase I and phase II block. However, it has been shown that post-tetanic potentiation and presence of fade in response to train-of-four and tetanic stimuli (ie, phase II block) may also be characteristics of neuromuscular block after bolus administration of different doses of succinylcholine.[4] It appears that some characteristics of phase II blockade are evident following the administration of an initial dose of succinylcholine—as small as 0.3 mg/kg.[4]

TABLE 9–1 Characteristics of phase I and phase II block.

	Phase I Block	Phase II Block
Fade with tetanus	–	+
Post-tetanic potentiation	–	+
Double-burst stimulation fade	–	+
Train-of-four fade	–	+
Effect of anticholinesterases	Enhances	Reverses (may be partially effective)

Dosing Regimens

Succinylcholine is a white, odorless, crystalline powder that is readily soluble in water. In powder form, it is stable indefinitely at room temperature. Once mixed in solution, it is relatively unstable in alkaline solutions but becomes more stable in acidic solutions. For this reason, the pH of succinylcholine solution is adjusted to 3.5 to 4 by the addition of hydrochloric acid. The stability is further enhanced by refrigeration, which helps preserve its original potency. Succinylcholine is marketed premixed in solutions of 20 mg/mL for bolus administration; it is also supplied in 50-mg/mL and 100-mg/mL concentrations for preparing an infusion mixture. Additionally, succinylcholine chloride powder (chloride dihydrate) for infusion is available in 500-mg or 1000-mg vials.

Succinylcholine is an ultra–short-acting agent that is useful for inducing skeletal muscle relaxation quickly; however, a number of significant side effects need to be considered prior to its use. Succinylcholine is usually administered intravenously, but intraosseous,[5,6] intralingual,[7] and intramuscular[8] administration has been reported in special circumstances such as in patients with laryngospasm without preexisting intravenous access. The clinical utility of some of the aforementioned approaches has been debated.

Succinylcholine is a long, flexible molecule that is comprised of 2 molecules of acetylcholine joined end-to-end via their terminal acetate methyl groups.

It is positively charged and has low lipid solubility, giving it a volume of distribution roughly equivalent to the extracellular space. The potency of NMBAs is quantified by the dose required to decrease the strength of contraction in the adductor pollicis muscle (thumb adduction) by a certain percent from baseline. This is known as the effective dose (ED). Thus, the ED_{50} or ED_{95} is the dose of muscle relaxant required to decrease the strength of contraction by 50% or 95% from baseline, respectively. In some studies, the estimated ED_{95} of succinylcholine was 0.63 mg/kg.[9] Using cumulative dose-response techniques, Kopman[10] estimated that its potency to be far greater, with an ED_{95} of less than 0.3 mg/kg. The usual succinylcholine intubating dose in adults is 1 to 1.5 mg/kg intravenously (3 to 5 times the ED_{95}). When administered intramuscularly or to children, higher doses, in the range of 2 to 4 mg/kg, are often required. Administration of a defasciculating dose of a nondepolarizing neuromuscular blocking agent, such as d-tubocurarine, increases the ED_{95} requirement by roughly 50% and therefore a larger dose of succinylcholine may be needed.[9]

Figure 9–3 shows a simulation-derived example of the plasma concentration, effect-site concentration, and recovery from intravenous administration of 1.0 mg/kg or 1.5 mg/kg of succinylcholine. Following administration of an intubating dose of succinylcholine, profound paralysis occurs within 1 to 2 minutes, with spontaneous recovery occurring within 10 to 15 minutes.[11-13] The central muscles, such as the laryngeal adductor muscles, are affected faster than the peripheral muscles.[14] This may be due to rich blood flow to the central muscles.

Hydrolysis of succinylcholine by butyrylcholinesterase (also known as plasma pseudocholinesterase or plasma cholinesterase) occurs in plasma, follows first-order kinetics, and occurs rapidly in most patients. In fact, the majority of administered succinylcholine (up to 90% of the administered dose) is hydrolyzed by butyrylcholinesterase to succinylmonocholine and choline before reaching the neuromuscular junction.[15] Succinylmonocholine is known to possess a weak neuromuscular blocking ability. The elimination half-life ($t_{1/2}\beta$) of intravenous 0.5, 1.0 or 5.0 mg/kg succinylcholine is about 5 minutes in dogs, with a distribution half-life ($t_{1/2}\alpha$) of less than

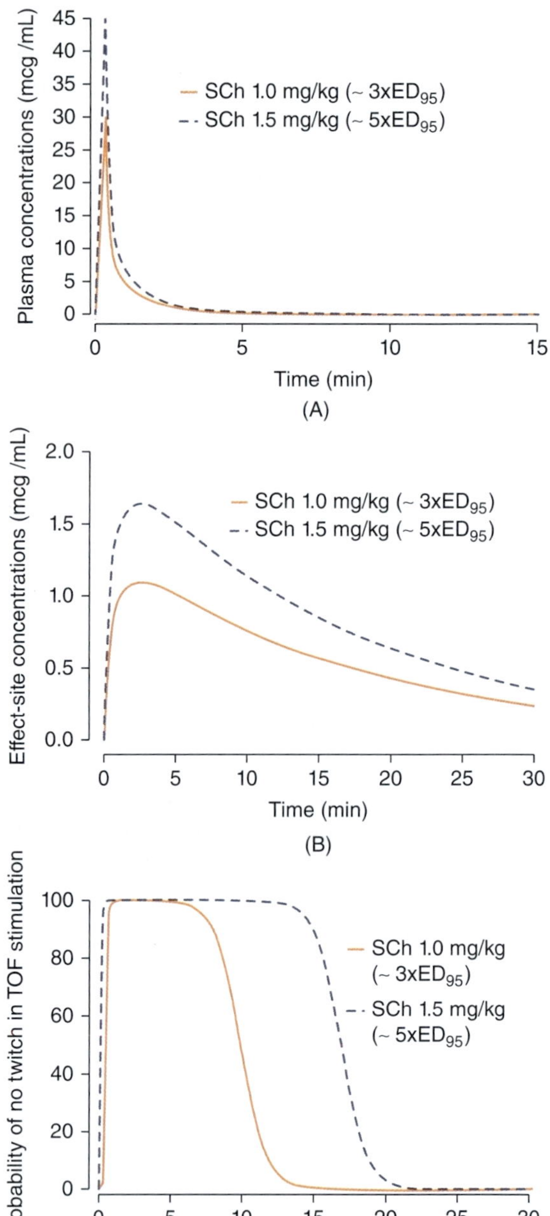

FIGURE 9–3 A, plasma concentration; B, effect-site concentration; and C, probability of no-twitch response to train-of-four (TOF) stimulation over time resulting from administration of 2 doses of succinylcholine (SCh).

1 minute.[16] In humans, the mean pharmacokinetic parameters of 1 mg/kg succinylcholine are apparent volume of distribution = 16.4 mL/kg, total body clearance = 40.5 L/min, and $t_{½}\beta$ = 16.6 s.[17] In contrast to succinylcholine, succinylmonocholine has a delayed onset of peak plasma concentration, slower distribution, and longer $t_{½}\beta$ of 1 to 3 hours.[18]

Acetylcholinesterase, which rapidly degrades acetylcholine, does not have the ability to hydrolyze succinylcholine, and the termination of the effect at the neuromuscular junction is largely due to redistribution of succinylcholine away from the neuromuscular junction along its concentration gradient into the plasma. Patients with abnormal butyrylcholinesterase activity can have significantly prolonged duration of action of succinylcholine that is correlated with butyrylcholinesterase activity.[19]

Normal individuals have 2 functional genes located on chromosome 3 that encode for pseudocholinesterase. It is estimated that 1 in 25 patients may be heterozygous "atypical," and 1 in 2500 individuals are homozygous "atypical" for the pseudocholinesterase gene.[20,21] These latter patients can have varying degrees of sensitivity to succinylcholine and may require prolonged postoperative mechanical ventilation in some cases. Quantification of the degree of abnormality (ie, enzymatic activity) can be obtained using dibucaine number testing. Dibucaine is a local anesthetic that inhibits normal butyrylcholinesterase activity to a greater degree than atypical butyrylcholinesterase. This measurement, referred to as the dibucaine number, is an approximation of the percentage of normal enzyme inhibition. In normal individuals, the dibucaine number is approximately 80, and for homozygous abnormal individuals, the dibucaine number is approximately 20. For heterozygous individuals, the dibucaine number can be anywhere between 20 and 80 but tends to cluster in the range of 40 to 60. Fluoride-resistant butyrylcholinesterase variants have also been described. The fluoride number indicates the percentage inhibition of butyrylcholinesterase in the presence of fluoride.

In addition to inherent enzyme abnormalities, a host of chronic disease states can result in decreased pseudocholinesterase synthesis and function. Liver disease, renal disease, acute burns, and sepsis have all been associated with decreased production of pseudocholinesterase. Pregnancy has also been associated with decreased butyrylcholinesterase activity and decreased absolute quantity (due to salt and water retention).[22,23] Although most genetic variants of serum butyrylcholinesterase are associated with decreased activity, some rare variants are associated with increased enzyme activity (2 to 3 times normal).[24]

Common Clinical Uses

Succinylcholine is considered by many to be the drug of choice for muscle relaxation when performing an anesthetic rapid-sequence induction and intubation. In patients who have recently consumed a meal or have certain medical conditions (eg, small bowel obstruction, severe gastroesophageal reflux disease), there is a risk of vomiting and aspiration of gastric contents into the lungs during induction of anesthesia and tracheal intubation. Because of succinylcholine's fast onset of action and high reliability in producing profound neuromuscular block (thus providing optimal intubating conditions), tracheal intubation with a cuffed tracheal tube can be achieved rapidly, thereby decreasing the likelihood of pulmonary aspiration.

Succinylcholine can also be administered via infusion in cases where profound, short-duration paralysis is needed. During such cases, succinylcholine continuous infusion should be administered via a dedicated intravenous catheter to prevent an accidental bolus and/or the development of phase II block. Continuous neuromuscular monitoring should routinely be employed along with careful titration to prevent complete loss of muscle response to stimulation. This continuous succinylcholine infusion technique, however, has lost its popularity with the introduction of the newer, intermediate-acting neuromuscular blockers.

Adverse Effects

The therapeutic benefits of succinylcholine should always be weighed against the side effects associated with its use. While still useful clinically for rapid-sequence induction and intubation, research into newer nondepolarizing NMBAs with short duration may eventually contribute to rendering succinylcholine obsolete.

Muscle fasciculations following administration of succinylcholine are very common and were first described more than 60 years ago.[25] Fasciculations are due to retrograde propagation of the action potential to the prejunctional terminal of the motor neuron (resulting in disorganized, muscle fiber contractions) and may be prevented by administering a "defasciculating" dose of nondepolarizing NMBA several minutes prior to succinylcholine. Another method of preventing or attenuating fasciculations is the "self-taming" technique, in which 5 to 10 mg of succinylcholine precedes administration of the intubating dose of succinylcholine. Administration of the defasciculating dose, however, is not devoid of potential complications; it has been associated with symptoms of muscle weakness and even respiratory paralysis, so the clinician must be ever vigilant and prepared to secure the airway emergently.

Myalgias have also been associated with succinylcholine administration, and the incidence reported in the literature varies between 2% and 89%.[26,27] Females are more likely to experience post-succinylcholine myalgias than men, while pregnancy and the extremes of age (children and adults older than 60 years of age) appear to be somewhat protective.[28,29] Interestingly, the frequency and severity of myalgias appear to be inversely proportional to the state of muscular fitness, such that athletes will experience fewer side effects.[30] Similarly, early ambulation postoperatively has been reported to increase the incidence and severity of myalgias.[31] While myalgias are thought to occur from microtrauma during fasciculations (perhaps due to the asynchronous contraction of adjacent fascicles without the opportunity for shortening of the fiber length and resulting in fiber rupture that causes pain), they are not directly related to the severity of the fasciculations themselves.[32] In many (but not all) cases, a defasciculating dose of nondepolarizing NMBA seems to be successful in ameliorating the pain associated with myalgias. Pretreatment with a prostaglandin inhibitor (lysine acetyl salicylate) has been shown to be effective in decreasing the incidence of muscle pains after succinylcholine.[33] This suggests a possible role for prostaglandins and cyclooxygenases (COX) in succinylcholine-induced myalgias. Several other classes of drugs (benzodiazepines, local anesthetics, vitamin C, dantrolene, calcium gluconate, magnesium, anticonvulsants, and nonsteroidal anti-inflammatory drugs) have been administered in an attempt to decrease postoperative myalgias with varying degrees of success.

The use of succinylcholine has been associated with increases in intraocular, intragastric, and intracranial pressures. The increase in intragastric pressure is thought to be due to the contractions of the abdominal wall musculature. Fortunately, this pressure increase is offset by a concomitant contraction of the lower esophageal sphincter, and reflux is prevented. Similarly, intracranial pressure is increased by succinylcholine, although the effect is mild and probably negligible when compared to the stimulating effects of laryngoscopy and intubation on intracranial pressures. The increase in intragastric and intracranial pressures can be attenuated by pretreatment with a nondepolarizing NMBA. Intraocular pressure (IOP) transiently increases by an average of 8 mm Hg following administration of succinylcholine, an increase that was feared detrimental to patients with open-globe injury. The exact etiology of the increase has not been fully elucidated and is not consistently prevented by administration of a defasciculating dose of nondepolarizing NMBA.[34] Extrusion of intraocular contents due to succinylcholine-induced increase in IOP, a much-feared complication, has never been reported, however. In fact, other maneuvers increase the IOP to a much greater degree: eye blinking increases IOP by 10 to 50 mm Hg,[35] coughing or vomiting increase IOP by 30 to 40 mm Hg, and pressure from the face mask during assisted ventilation may increase IOP by hundreds of mm Hg (**Figure 9–4**). Several studies of thousands of patients with open-globe injuries have failed to report any extrusion of intraocular contents from succinylcholine use.[36]

Potentially fatal increases in serum potassium levels can occur following succinylcholine administration in patients with conditions that cause an up-regulation in fetal acetylcholine receptors. Unlike adult nicotinic acetylcholine receptors, activation of the fetal subtypes ($\alpha_2\beta\delta\gamma$) may cause prolonged depolarization of the muscle cell membrane.

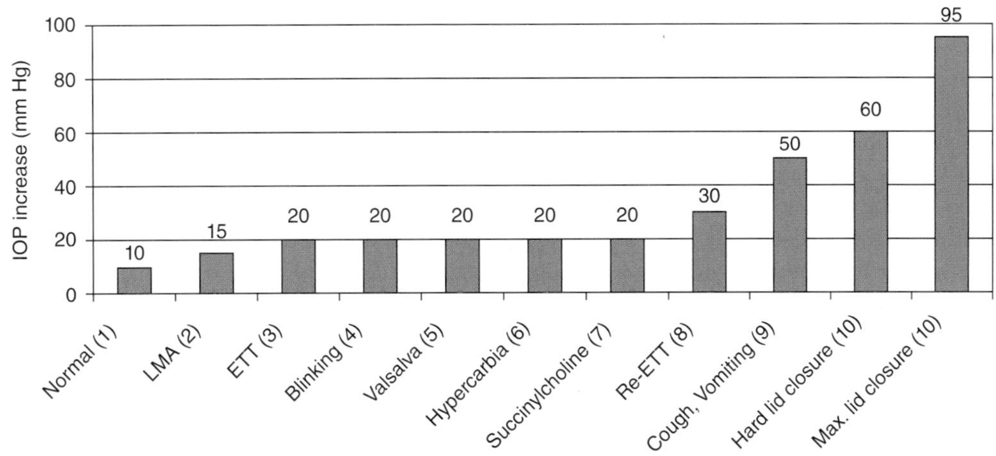

FIGURE 9–4 Mean increase in intraocular pressure (IOP) from baseline (normal = 10 mm Hg) in response to various procedures and maneuvers. The numbers in parentheses refer to the following studies:
1. Murphy DF. Anesthesia and intraocular pressure. *Anesth Analg.* 1985;64:520-530.
2. Lamb K, James MF, Janicki PK. The laryngeal mask airway for intraocular surgery: effects on intraocular pressure and stress responses. *Br J Anaesth.* 1992;69:143-147.
3. Drenger B, Pe'er J. Attenuation of ocular and systemic responses to tracheal intubation by intravenous lignocaine. *Br J Ophthalmol.* 1987;71:546-548.
4. Miller D. Pressure of the lid on the eye. *Arch Ophthalmol.* 1967;78:328-330.
5. Rafuse PE, Mills DW, Hooper PL, Chang TS, Wolf R. Effects of Valsalva's manoeuvre on intraocular pressure. *Can J Ophthalmol.* 1994;29:73-76.
6. Duncalf D, Weitzner SW. The influence of ventilation and hypercapnea on intraocular pressure during anesthesia. *Anesth Analg.* 1963;42;232-237.
7. Kelly RE, Dinner M, Turner LS, Haik B, Abramson DH, Daines P. Succinylcholine increases intraocular pressure in the human eye with the extraocular muscles detached. *Anesthesiology.* 1993;79:948-952.
8. Bithal PK, Reddy TS, Prabhakar H. Effect of repeat laryngoscopy on intraocular pressure. *Eur J Anaesthesiol.* 2004;21:496-497.
9. McGoldrick KE, Gayer SI. *Anesthesia for Ophthalmic Surgery* (Chapter 51). In: Barash PG, Cullen BF, Stoelting RK, Cahalan MK, Stock MC, eds. *Clinical Anesthesia.* 6th ed. Philadelphia: Lippincott Williams & Wilkins;, 2009:1321-1345.
10. Coleman DJ, Trokel S. Direct-recorded intraocular pressure variations in a human subject. *Arch Ophthalmol.* 1969;82:637-640.
ETT, endotracheal tube; LMA, laryngeal mask airway.

resulting in excessive potassium out-flux into the circulation.[37] Chronic denervation, prolonged bed rest, major burns, spinal cord injuries, myopathies, encephalitis, sepsis, acute renal failure, and severe trauma have all been associated with succinylcholine-induced hyperkalemia. Pretreatment with nondepolarizing NMBAs does not prevent or lessen potassium release from intracellular stores. Treatment of hyperkalemia by hyperventilation, administering calcium chloride 1.0 to 2.0 g intravenously, sodium bicarbonate 1 mmol/kg, and 10 units regular insulin in 50 mL 50% glucose for adults or, for children, 0.15 units regular insulin/kg in 1.0 mL/kg 50% glucose, should be considered any time an unexplained cardiac arrest occurs immediately following administration of succinylcholine.

Succinylcholine can mimic acetylcholine at muscarinic receptors and has been associated with a variety of cardiac dysrhythmias. Asystole and bradycardia have been well described and can usually be treated with antimuscarinic agents such as atropine and glycopyrrolate. Pediatric patients can be especially sensitive to the cardiac effects of succinylcholine, and atropine should always be administered concomitantly. Bradycardia is also common after a repeat dose of succinylcholine due to the actions of the metabolite choline, which acts to sensitize the muscarinic receptors in the myocardium.[38] Succinylcholine can also cause tachycardia and endogenous catecholamine release at higher doses.[39]

Succinylcholine is a potent trigger of malignant hyperthermia and should be avoided in anyone with a personal history of malignant hyperthermia; it should never be used in patients with a family history of the disorder. Additionally, succinylcholine can be associated with prolonged masseter muscle rigidity that can impede mouth opening, laryngoscopy, and tracheal intubation. Although there is a correlation between masseter muscle rigidity and malignant hyperthermia, and patients should be monitored closely for signs and symptoms of malignant hyperthermia should this complication occur,[40] masseter muscle spasm is not consistently associated with malignant hyperthermia.[41]

NONDEPOLARIZING NEUROMUSCULAR BLOCKING AGENTS

Nondepolarizing NMBAs cause paralysis by competitive inhibition of the postjunctional acetylcholine receptor. Only one α subunit has to be bound by a nondepolarizing NMBA to prevent the conformational change and generation of an action potential (see Figure 9–1). Because of this, there are no muscle contractions (fasciculations) prior to the onset of flaccid paralysis.

Dosing Regimens

Nondepolarizing NMBAs can be classified as benzylisoquinolinium (atracurium, doxacurium, cisatracurium, and mivacurium) or steroidal compounds (rocuronium, vecuronium, pancuronium, and pipecuronium), depending on their chemical structure. They are further subdivided, based on their duration of action, as short-, intermediate-, or long-acting. With the exception of vecuronium, nondepolarizing NMBAs are marketed in premixed liquid suspensions with concentrations that vary among individual drugs. Vecuronium is dispensed as an intravenous powder in 10-mg or 20-mg doses that must be reconstituted prior to use. Typically, vecuronium is diluted in 10 mL of sterile saline, resulting in a concentration of 1 mg/mL or 2 mg/mL, respectively.

Nondepolarizing NMBAs are almost always administered intravenously either as intermittent boluses or as continuous infusions. Intramuscular administration of nondepolarizers has been described,[42-44] but some authorities argue that this should be a route of last resort due to its slow and variable onset of action.[43-45] **Table 9–2** describes the typical intermittent and bolus doses for commonly used NMBAs.

Similar to succinylcholine, nondepolarizing NMBAs are positively charged and have low lipid solubility and therefore are distributed mostly in the extracellular fluid. Because of this, patients with significant diseases (eg, liver failure and renal failure) that result in increased total body water may require higher initial doses to achieve pharmacodynamic responses comparable to those in healthy individuals. Effects at the neuromuscular junction are terminated either by redistribution or metabolism. Onset of action generally varies depending, in general, on potency, with more potent agents having a slower onset. This delay in speed of onset occurs because there are fewer molecules per unit volume of potent NMBAs (lower molar potency) available to occupy the acetylcholine receptors.[46]

Simulations of equipotent doses of different nondepolarizing NMBAs (**Figures 9–5** through **9–8**) show the variability in onset and duration of action. Long-acting agents, such as pancuronium (see Figure 9–5), have an initial peak after intravenous administration, followed by a gradual decline in plasma and effect-site concentrations as cessation of neuromuscular block is due primarily to drug excretion. Intermediate-acting neuromuscular blocking agents such as cisatracurium (see Figure 9–6) and rocuronium (see Figure 9–7) show a more rapid decline at the effect-site, largely due to drug redistribution. Mivacurium (see Figure 9–8) has a short duration of action, and its effect is largely terminated by metabolism by butyrylcholinesterase enzyme.

Typically, NMBAs are titrated based on a measured response to nerve stimulation such as train-of-four stimulation. Adequate vigilance and intraoperative monitoring are required to decrease the incidence of residual neuromuscular block in the postoperative care unit.[47] As with succinylcholine, the central muscles (diaphragm, laryngeal, orbicularis oculi, and corrugator supercilii) are blocked first and recover faster than peripheral muscles (adductor pollicis).

TABLE 9–2 Dosing regimens of common neuromuscular blocking agents.

Drug	ED_{95}	Typical Bolus Dose for Induction	Typical Starting Infusion Dose	Studies[a]
Succinylcholine	0.30 mg/kg	1.0–1.5 mg/kg	2–15 mg/min	1, 2, 3
Mivacurium	0.08 mg/kg	0.15–0.25 mg/kg	5–8 mcg/kg/min	4, 5, 6
Atracurium	0.23 mg/kg	0.4–0.5 mg/kg	5–12 mcg/kg/min	3, 4, 5, 7
Cisatracurium	0.05 mg/kg	0.15–0.2 mg/kg	1–2 mcg/kg/min	3, 5
Rocuronium	0.30 mg/kg	0.6–1.2 mg/kg	10–12 mcg/kg/min	2
Vecuronium	0.05 mg/kg	0.08–0.1 mg/kg	1–2 mcg/kg/min	2, 3, 4
Pancuronium	0.07 mg/kg	0.06–0.1 mg/kg	20–40 mcg/kg/min	4, 8

[a]See numbered list.

1. El-Orbany MI, Joseph NJ, Salem MR, Klowden AJ. The neuromuscular effects and tracheal intubation conditions after small doses of succinylcholine. *Anesth Analg.* 2004;98:1680-1685.
2. Stoelting RK, Hillier SC, eds. Neuromuscular blocking drugs (Chapter 8). In: *Pharmacology and Physiology in Anesthetic Practice*. 4th ed. Philadelphia: Lippincott Williams & Wilkins; 2006:208-250.
3. Morgan GE, Mikhail MS, Murray MJ, eds. Neuromuscular blocking agents (Chapter 9). In: *Clinical Anesthesiology*. 4th ed. New York: McGraw-Hill; 2006.
4. Savarese JJ, Ali HH, Basta SJ, et al. The clinical neuromuscular pharmacology of mivacurium chloride (BW B1090U). A short-acting nondepolarizing ester neuromuscular blocking drug. *Anesthesiology.* 1988;68:723-732.
5. Atherton DP, Hunter JM. Clinical pharmacokinetics of the newer neuromuscular blocking drugs. *Clin Pharmacokinet.* 1999;36:169-189.
6. Caldwell JE. New skeletal muscle relaxants. *Int Anesthesiol Clin.* 1995;33:39-60.
7. McManus MC. Neuromuscular blockers in surgery and intensive care, Part 2. *Am J Health Syst Pharm.* 2001;58:2381-2395.
8. Sharpe MD. The use of muscle relaxants in the intensive care unit. *Can J Anaesth.* 1992;39:949-962.

Metabolism of nondepolarizing NMBAs (Table 9–3) is variable and will be discussed individually below. As a rule, liver and/or renal disease will increase the duration of action of the aminosteroid agents but have little effect on the metabolism of benzylisoquinolinium compounds. Mivacurium is metabolized by butyrylcholinesterase and, like succinylcholine, its effects are prolonged in patients with abnormal or decreased pseudocholinesterase activity. Atracurium and its isomer cisatracurium also undergo metabolism independent of liver or renal function. Under normal physiologic conditions, both NMBAs undergo nonenzymatic (Hofmann) degradation to yield laudanosine.[48] Hyperthermia and increase in body pH can significantly increase the rate of the Hofmann reaction, whereas hypothermia and acidosis can dramatically delay the reaction. Laudanosine is subsequently metabolized by the liver or excreted by the kidneys. It has been shown to be neuroexcitatory in animals but has little effect in humans at normal clinical doses of cisatracurium. Additionally, atracurium, but not cisatracurium, appears to undergo ester hydrolysis in the plasma by nonspecific esterases.

Pancuronium undergoes primarily renal excretion; however, some hepatic metabolism does occur. Vecuronium also undergoes hepatic metabolism but is primarily excreted in the bile, and the drug also undergoes significant (up to 25%) renal excretion. Both pancuronium and vecuronium have active metabolites that have 50% to 80% of the parent compound potency. These metabolites may play a role in residual weakness and myopathy following long-term infusions. Rocuronium elimination is primarily hepatic and biliary, with minimal renal excretion; for this reason, its pharmacokinetics is not altered significantly by renal failure. Rocuronium has no active metabolites detected in plasma or in the urine.

A number of interactions need to be considered when nondepolarizing NMBAs are administered. Hypokalemia, hypocalcemia, hypothermia, and acidosis augment neuromuscular blockade. Aminoglycoside antibiotics and magnesium also act to potentiate the actions of nondepolarizing NMBAs

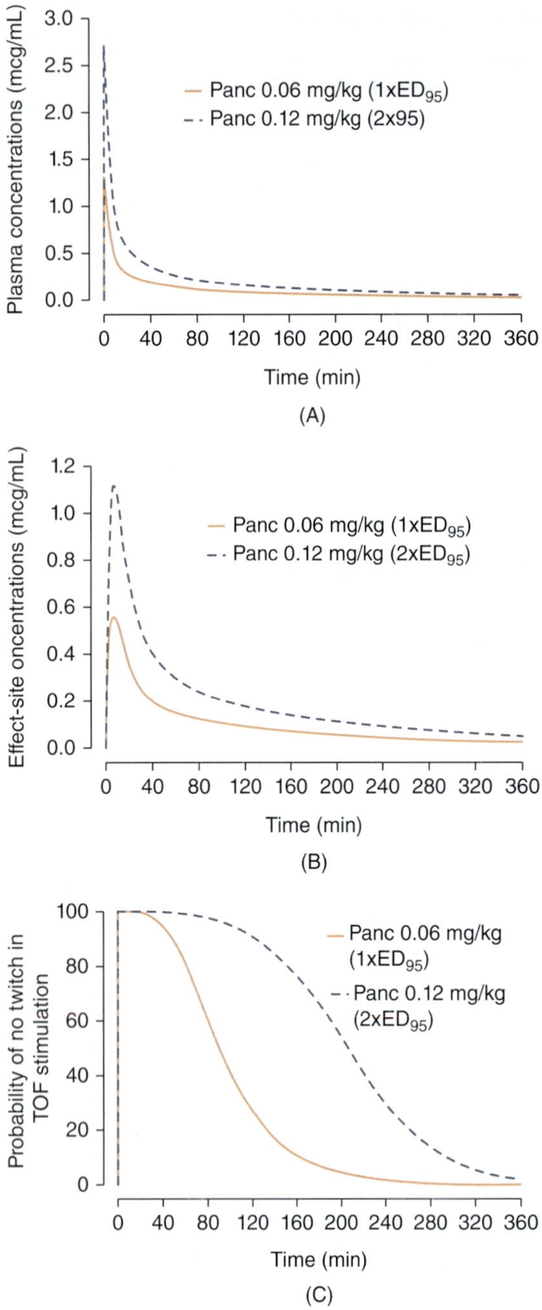

FIGURE 9–5 A, plasma concentration; B, effect-site concentration; and C, probability of no-twitch response to train-of-four (TOF) stimulation over time resulting from administration of 2 different doses of pancuronium (Panc).

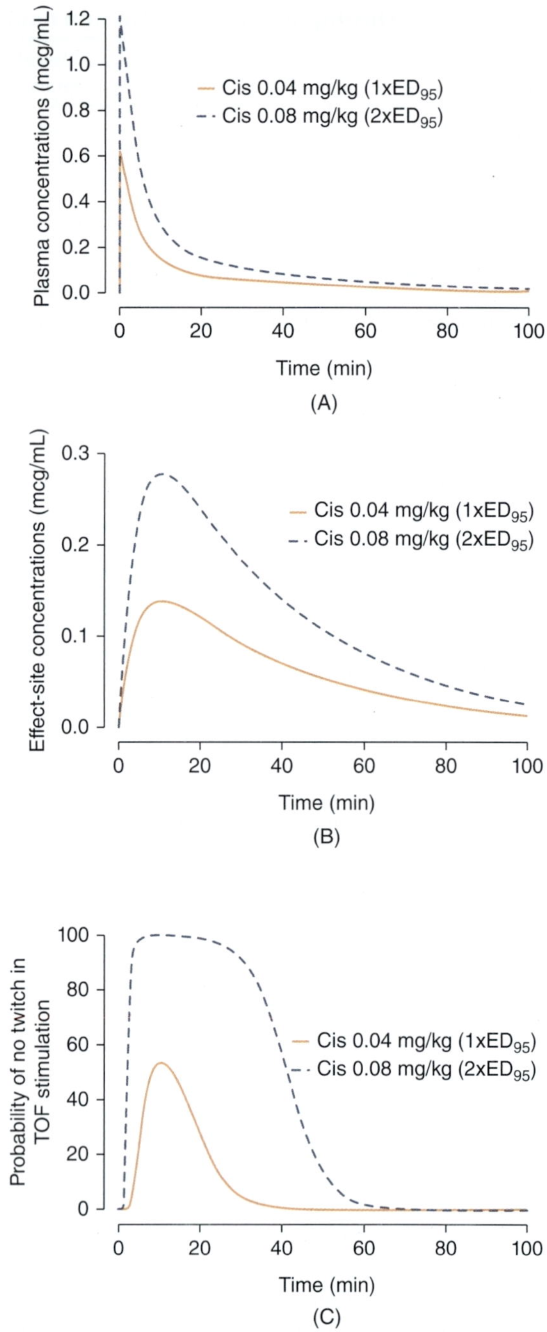

FIGURE 9–6 A, plasma concentration; B, effect-site concentration; and C, probability of no-twitch response to train-of-four (TOF) stimulation over time resulting from administration of 2 different doses of cisatracurium (Cis).

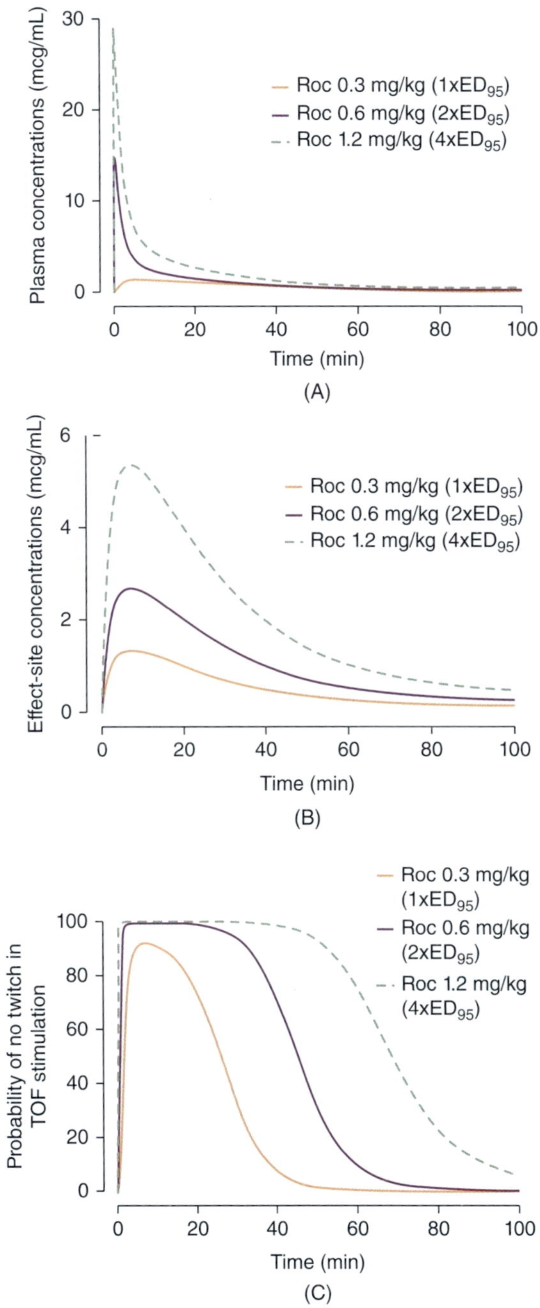

FIGURE 9–7 A, plasma concentration. B, effect-site concentration; and C, probability of no-twitch response to train-of-four (TOF) stimulation over time resulting from administration of 3 different doses of rocuronium (Roc).

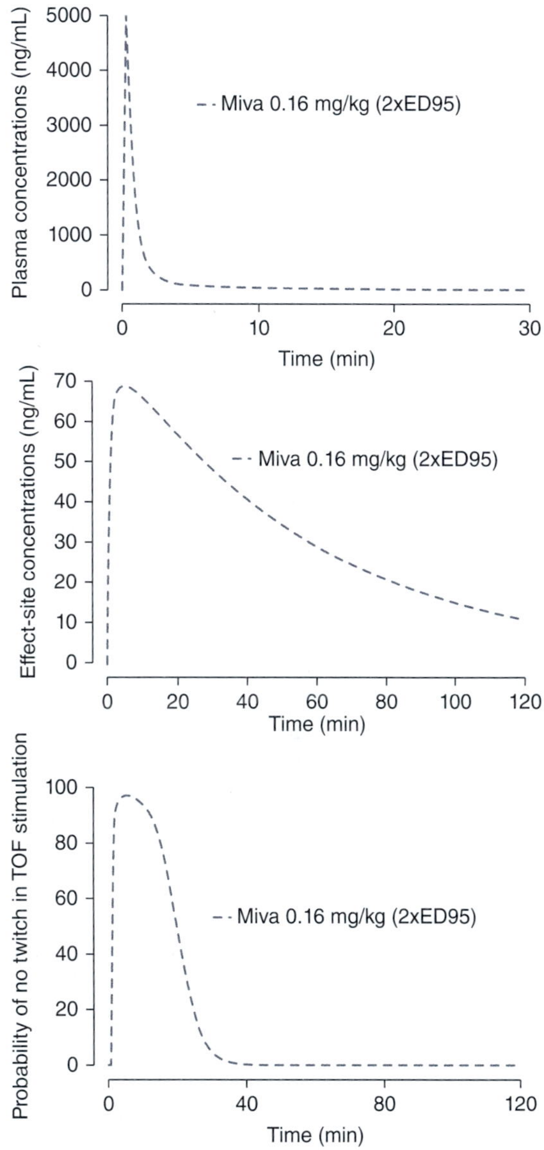

FIGURE 9–8 A, plasma concentration; B, effect-site concentration; and C, probability of no-twitch response to train-of-four (TOF) stimulation over time resulting from administration of mivacurium (Miva).

TABLE 9–3 Pharmacology of nondepolarizing neuromuscular blocking agents in healthy adults.

Drug	Onset (min)	Duration (min)	$T_{1/2}$ (min)	Primary Mechanism of Metabolism/Excretion	Noteworthy Metabolic Products	Studies[a]
Succinylcholine	1	10–15	2–4	Butyrylcholinesterase	Succinylmonocholine	1
Mivacurium	2–3	10–20	18	Butyrylcholinesterase, renal		2, 3, 4
Atracurium	3–5	20–40	12–21	Hofmann degradation, ester hydrolysis	Laudanosine, acrylate fragments	2, 4
Cisatracurium	3–5	20–35	22–35	Hofmann degradation	Laudanosine, acrylate fragments	2, 4
Rocuronium	1–2	20–35	69–100	Hepatic (bile), renal	Minimal metabolism	2, 4, 5
Vecuronium	3–5	20–35	50–110	Hepatic, some renal	3-desacetyl vecuronium	2
Pancuronium	3–5	60–90	89–161	Renal, some hepatic	3-desacetyl pancuronium	2

[a]See numbered list.

1. El-Orbany MI, Joseph NJ, Salem MR, Klowden AJ. The neuromuscular effects and tracheal intubation conditions after small doses of succinylcholine. *Anesth Analg.* 2004;98:1680-1685.
2. Stoelting RK, Hillier SC, eds. Neuromuscular blocking drugs (Chapter 8). In: *Pharmacology and Physiology in Anesthetic Practice*. 4th ed. Philadelphia: Lippincott Williams & Wilkins; 2006:208-250.
3. Savarese JJ, Ali HH, Basta SJ, et al. The clinical neuromuscular pharmacology of mivacurium chloride (BW B1090U). A short-acting nondepolarizing ester neuromuscular blocking drug. *Anesthesiology.* 1988;68:723-732.
4. Atherton DP, Hunter JM. Clinical pharmacokinetics of the newer neuromuscular blocking drugs. *Clin Pharmacokinet.* 1999;36:169-189.
5. Caldwell JE. New skeletal muscle relaxants. *Int Anesthesiol Clin.* 1995;33:39-60.

at the neuromuscular junction. Volatile inhalational agents also produce dose-dependent potentiation of neuromuscular blockade[49,50] (**Figure 9–9**). Chronic use of anticonvulsants, on the other hand, may necessitate a higher dose of nondepolarizing agents due to increased plasma protein binding of the NMBA, hepatic enzyme induction by the anticonvulsant, or proliferation of acetylcholine receptors on the muscle membrane.[51] Conversely, if administered acutely, phenytoin may act to potentiate neuromuscular blockade.[52] Propofol and opioids do not affect NMBA potency.

A number of disease states alter a patient's response to nondepolarizing NMBAs. Patients with myasthenia gravis tend to be resistant to succinylcholine but sensitive to nondepolarizing NMBAs due to the numerical decrease in acetylcholine receptors. Patients with severe burns and denervation injuries may develop resistance to nondepolarizing NMBAs. It is hypothesized that the proliferation of extrajunctional fetal receptors may play a role in the resistance.

Common Clinical Uses

Nondepolarizing NMBAs are used primarily (1) to facilitate tracheal intubation and for maintenance of muscle relaxation during surgery or (2) to facilitate mechanical ventilation in the critical care setting. Since their onset of action tends to require several minutes, with the exception of rocuronium, they are not ideal for use in rapid-sequence induction of anesthesia and tracheal intubation. The literature is replete with reports seeking to design methods to hasten the onset on nondepolarizing NMBAs. One such method to speed up onset time is to employ a "priming" dose. This entails administering a small dose (10%) of the NMBA several minutes prior to administering the intubating NMBA dose. The theory behind this technique is that the initial "priming" dose will occupy up to 70% of the

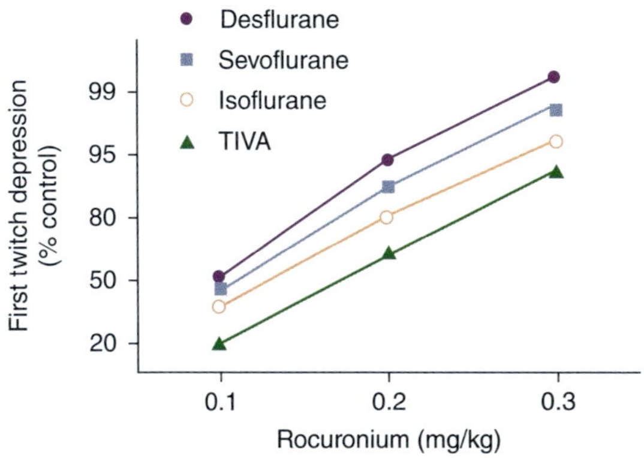

FIGURE 9–9 Cumulative dose-response curves for rocuronium-induced neuromuscular blockade during 1.5 minimum alveolar concentration anesthesia with desflurane, sevoflurane, isoflurane, and total intravenous anesthesia (TIVA). (Reproduced with permission from Wulf H, Ledowski T, Linstedt U, Proppe D, Sitzlack D. Neuromuscular blocking effects of rocuronium during desflurane, isoflurane and sevoflurane anaesthesia. *Can J Anaesth* 1998;Jun;45(6):526-32.)

available acetylcholine receptors, which will result in no appreciable decrease in the strength of striated muscle function (safety margin). This "priming" of the receptors is then followed by the rest of the intubating dose of NMBA, which will need to block only 30% of the remaining acetylcholine receptors, thus effecting a more rapid onset of neuromuscular block. However, due to the wide variability in the response of patients to the effects of most drugs, some patients may develop signs of muscle weakness even after the priming dose, placing them at risk of loss of airway protection and pulmonary aspiration of gastric contents. Alternatively, increasing the dose of rocuronium from 0.6 mg/kg (2 times the ED_{95}) to 1.2 mg/kg (4 times the ED_{95}) shortened the onset time of complete neuromuscular blockade but significantly prolonged the clinical duration (see Figure 9–7). This approach (high-dose rocuronium) has gained popularity when the use of succinylcholine is contraindicated or undesirable in patients requiring rapid-sequence induction of anesthesia and tracheal intubation.

Nondepolarizing NMBAs can also be used to mitigate some of the side effects of succinylcholine. When administered just prior to succinylcholine, they can diminish the severity of fasciculations, prevent increases in intragastric and intracranial pressure, and may lessen the pain associated with postoperative myalgia (see above).

Adverse Effects

Nondepolarizing NMBAs are associated with several side effects that should be considered prior to their use. Most commonly, incomplete reversal or failure to ensure full recovery of neuromuscular function may result in residual muscle weakness in the postoperative care unit. Clinicians cannot rely on time alone to ensure that nondepolarizing agents have been eliminated, as there is wide interindividual variability among patients.[47,53] Typically, a combination of clinical tests, such as head lift for 5 seconds, masseter muscle test, or grip strength, are used in conjunction with subjective (visual or tactile) assessment of responses to nerve stimulation (eg, train-of-four stimulation). The literature is replete with reports of patients who exhibit residual neuromuscular weakness upon arrival to the postoperative care unit, despite having received pharmacologic antagonism and having been deemed "adequately reversed."[54,55] Additionally, recent articles have reviewed the incidence and etiology, and they have offered methods to reduce the risk of postoperative residual weakness.[56,57] Until recently, it was believed that a train-of-four ratio (ie, the ratio of the fourth to the first twitches of train-of-four) of 0.7 or greater indicated adequate return of muscle strength following the use of nondepolarizing NMBAs. More recent data, however, have demonstrated that a train-of-four ratio greater than 0.9 may in fact be a more reliable measure of adequate neuromuscular recovery and patient safety. Persistent residual weakness in the recovery room associated with the use of NMBAs is often unrecognized and may be associated with an increased risk of silent aspiration, hypoxemia, need for reintubation, and prolonged stay in the recovery room.[56,57]

Atracurium is associated with histamine release, especially if doses larger than 3 times the ED_{95} are administered rapidly, and may result in hypotension and tachycardia. Bronchospasm has also been described. Like atracurium, rapid intravenous administration of mivacurium may also result in clinically significant histamine release. Cisatracurium has not been reported to release histamine and therefore is probably a better choice in patients with preexisting asthma. Significant histamine release is not associated with aminosteroid NMBA administration.

Pancuronium is associated with an increase in heart rate, thought to be due to direct vagolytic action on the heart.[58] This side effect is often useful to counteract the bradycardia associated with high-dose narcotics when performing a nitrous–narcotic anesthesia induction but should be used with caution in patients with coronary artery disease undergoing surgery. Pancuronium use has decreased substantially in clinical practice in the last decade due mostly to its long duration of action and the significant accumulation following large or repeated-dose administration.

NEWER AGENTS

Research into newer NMBAs continues even today as researchers try to discover drugs with improved safety profiles. Ideally, an NMBA should have a very rapid onset and be easily and quickly reversible while having few, if any, side effects. Based on these criteria, researchers are currently developing a new class of ultra–short-acting nondepolarizers known as the chlorofumarates. Gantacurium and CW002 are asymmetric, mixed-onium chlorofumarates with short and intermediate durations of action, respectively.[59] Interestingly, these compounds undergo rapid reversal (degradation) with the addition of the nonessential amino acid cysteine, but their effects are also antagonized by the administration of anticholinesterases. Unfortunately, it is uncertain whether these (or other related) compounds will ultimately reach the market, despite their current investigation in preclinical studies, because of the potential for histamine release in humans.

REFERENCES

1. Savage DS, Sleigh T, Carlyle I. The emergence of ORG NC 45, 1- [2 beta, 3 alpha, 5 alpha,16 beta, 17 beta)-3, 17-bis(acetyloxy)-2-(1-piperidinyl)-androstan-16-yl]-1-methylpiperidinium bromide, from the pancuronium series. *Br J Anaesth.* 1980; 52(suppl 1): 3S-9S.
2. Coker GG, Dewar GH, Hughes R, et al. A preliminary assessment of atracurium, a new competitive neuromuscular blocking agent. *Acta Anaesthesiol Scand.* 1981;25:67-69.
3. Stenlake JB, Waigh RD, Urwin J, Dewar GH, Coker GG. Atracurium: conception and inception. *Br J Anaesth.* 1983;55(suppl 1):3S-10S.
4. Naguib M, Lien CA, Aker J, Eliazo R. Posttetanic potentiation and fade in the response to tetanic and train-of-four stimulation during succinylcholine-induced block. *Anesth Analg.* 2004;98:1686-1691.
5. Moore GP, Pace SA, Busby W. Comparison of intraosseous, intramuscular, and intravenous administration of succinylcholine. *Pediatr Emerg Care.* 1989; 5:209-210.
6. Katan BS, Olshaker JS, Dickerson SE. Intraosseous infusion of muscle relaxants. *Am J Emerg Med.* 1988; 6:353-354.
7. Wisely NA, Mayall R. Intralingual succinylcholine injection provides a rapid onset of muscle relaxation in an emergency. *Anaesthesia.* 2001;56:1213.
8. Vanderveen JL, Sneddon EA, Schmidt SJ. Intramuscular succinylcholine in adults. A controlled study. *Anesthesiology.* 1963;24:765-769.
9. Szalados JE, Donati F, Bevan DR. Effect of d-tubocurarine pretreatment on succinylcholine twitch augmentation and neuromuscular blockade. *Anesth Analg.* 1990;71:55-59.
10. Kopman AF, Klewicka MM, Neuman GG. An alternate method for estimating the dose-response relationships of neuromuscular blocking drugs. *Anesth Analg.* 2000; 90:1191-1197.
11. Curran MJ, Donati F, Bevan DR. Onset and recovery of atracurium and suxamethonium-induced neuromuscular blockade with simultaneous train-of-four and single twitch stimulation. *Br J Anaesth.* 1987;59:989-994.
12. Walts LF, Dillon JB. Clinical studies on succinylcholine chloride. *Anesthesiology.* 1967;28:372-376.
13. Katz RL, Ryan JF. The neuromuscular effects of suxamethonium in man. *Br J Anaesth.* 1969;41:381-390.
14. Meistelman C, Plaud B, Donati F. Neuromuscular effects of succinylcholine on the vocal cords and adductor pollicis muscles. *Anesth Analg.* 1991;73:278-282.
15. Gissen AJ, Katz RL, Karis JH, Papper EM. Neuromuscular block in man during prolonged arterial infusion with succinylcholine. *Anesthesiology.* 1966;27: 242-249.
16. Baldwin KA, Forney R Jr. Correlation of plasma concentration and effects of succinylcholine in dogs. *J Forensic Sci* 1988;33:470-479.
17. Hoshi K, Hashimoto Y, Matsukawa S. Pharmacokinetics of succinylcholine in man. *Tohoku J Exp Med* 1993;170: 245-250.

18. Kuepper U, Musshoff F, Hilger RA, Herbstreit F, Madea B. Pharmacokinetic properties of succinylmonocholine in surgical patients. *J Anal Toxicol* 2011;35:302-311.
19. Viby-Mogensen J. Correlation of succinylcholine duration of action with plasma cholinesterase activity in subjects with the genotypically normal enzyme. *Anesthesiology.* 1980;53:517-520.
20. Lehmann H, Lidell J. Human cholinesterase: genetic variants and their recognition. *Br J Anaesth.* 1969;41:235-244.
21. Whittaker M. Plasma cholinesterase variants and the anaesthetist. *Anaesthesia.* 1980;35:174-197.
22. Robson N, Robertson I, Whittaker M. Plasma cholinesterase changes during the puerperium. *Anaesthesia.* 1986;41:243-249.
23. Leighton BL, Cheeks TG, Gross JB, et al. Succinylcholine pharmacodynamics in peripartum patients. *Anesthesiology.* 1986;64:202-205.
24. Naguib M, Gomaa M, Samarkandi AH, et al. Increased plasma cholinesterase activity and mivacurium resistance: report of a family. *Anesth Analg.* 1999; 89: 1579-1582.
25. Bourne JG, Collier HOJ, Somers GF. Succinylcholine (succinoylcholine): muscle-relaxant of short action. *Lancet.* 1952;55:1225–1229.
26. Crawford JS. Suxamethonium muscle pains and pregnancy. *Br J Anaesth.* 1971;55:677–680.
27. Ali AH. Neuromuscular block and its antagonism: clinical aspects. In: Nunn JF, Utting JE, Brown BRJ, eds. *General Anaesthesia.* 5th ed. London: Butterworths, 1989;164–184.
28. Bush GH, Roth F. Muscle pains after suxamethonium in children. *Br J Anaesth.* 1961;55:151-155.
29. Foster CA. Muscle pain that follows the administration of suxamethonium. *Br Med J.* 1960;55: 24-25.
30. Newnam PTF, Loudon JM. Muscle pain following administration of suxamethonium: the aetiological role of muscular fitness. *Br J Anaesth.* 1966;55:533-540.
31. Oxorn DC, Whatley GS, Knox JWD, Hooper J. The importance of activity and pretreatment in the prevention of suxamethonium myalgias. *Br J Anaesth.* 1992;55:200-201.
32. Wong SF, Chung F. Succinylcholine-associated postoperative myalgia. *Anaesthesia.* 2000;55:144-152.
33. Naguib M, Farag H, Magbagbeola JA. Effect of pre-treatment with lysine acetyl salicylate on suxamethonium-induced myalgia. *Br J Anaesth.* 1987;59:606-610.
34. Kelly RE, Dinner M, Turner LS, Haik B, Abramson DH, Daines P. Succinylcholine increases intraocular pressure in the human eye with the extraocular muscles detached. *Anesthesiology.* 1993;79:948-952.
35. Miller D. Pressure of the lid on the eye. *Arch Ophthalmol* 1967;78:328-330.
36. Libonati MM, Leahy JJ, Ellison N. The use of succinylcholine in open eye surgery. *Anesthesiology.* 1985;62:637-640.
37. Naguib M, Flood P, McArdle JJ, Brenner HR. Advances in neurobiology of the neuromuscular junction: implications for the anesthesiologist. *Anesthesiology.* 2002;96:202-231.
38. Shoenstadt DA, Witcher CE. Observations on the mechanism of succinyldicholine induced cardiac arrhythmias. *Anesthesiology.* 1963;24:358-362.
39. Galindo AH, Davis TB. Succinylcholine and cardiac excitability. *Anesthesiology.* 1962;23:32-40.
40. O'Flynn RP, Shutack JG, Rosenberg H, Fletcher JE. Masseter muscle rigidity and malignant hyperthermia susceptibility in pediatric patients. An update on management and diagnosis. *Anesthesiology.* 1994;80: 1228-1233.
41. Van der Spek AF, Fang WB, Ashton-Miller JA, Stohler CS, Carlson DS, Schork MA. The effects of succinylcholine on mouth opening. *Anesthesiology.* 1987;67:459-465.
42. Kaplan RF, Uejima T, Lobel G, et al. Intramuscular rocuronium in infants and children: a multicenter study to evaluate tracheal intubating conditions, onset, and duration of action. *Anesthesiology.* 1999;91: 633-638.
43. Reynolds LM, Lau M, Brown R, Luks A, Fisher DM. Intramuscular rocuronium in infants and children. Dose-ranging and tracheal intubating conditions. *Anesthesiology.* 1996;85:231-239.
44. Cauldwell CB, Lau M, Fisher DM. Is intramuscular mivacurium and alternative to intramuscular succinylcholine? *Anesthesiology.* 1994;80:320-325.
45. Donati F, Guay J. No substitute for the intravenous route. *Anesthesiology.* 2001;94:1-2.
46. Kopman AF, Klewicka MM, Kopman DJ, Neuman GG. Molar potency is predictive of the speed of onset of neuromuscular block for agents of intermediate, short, and ultrashort duration. *Anesthesiology.* 1999;90:425-431.
47. Yip PC, Hannam JA, Cameron AJ, Campbell D. Incidence of residual neuromuscular blockade in a post-anaesthetic care unit. *Anaesth Intensive Care.* 2010;38:91-95.
48. Fodale V, Santamaria LB. Laudanosine, an atracurium and cisatracurium metabolite. *Eur J Anaesthesiol.* 2002;19:466-473.
49. Miller RD, Way WL, Dolan WM, Stevens WC, Eger EI II. Comparative neuromuscular effects of pancuronium, gallamine, and succinylcholine

during forane and halothane anesthesia in man. *Anesthesiology.* 1971;35:509-514.
50. Caldwell JE, Laster MJ, Magorian T, et al. The neuromuscular effects of desflurane, alone and combined with pancuronium and succinylcholine in humans. *Anesthesiology.* 1991;74:412-418.
51. Loan PB, Connolly FM, Mirakhur RK, Kumar N, Farling P. Neuromuscular effects of rocuronium in patients receiving beta-adrenoreceptor blocking, calcium entry blocking and anticonvulsant drugs. *Br J Anaesth.* 1997;78:90-91.
52. Spacek A, Nickl S, Neiger FX, et al. Augmentation of the rocuronium induced neuromuscular block by the acutely administered phenytoin. *Anesthesiology.* 1999;90:1551-1555.
53. Claudius C, Karacan H, Viby-Mogensen J. Prolonged residual paralysis after a single intubating dose of rocuronium. *Br J Anaesth.* 2007;99: 514-517.
54. Debaene B, Plaud B, Dilly MP, Donati F. Residual paralysis in the PACU after a single intubating dose of nondepolarizing muscle relaxant with an intermediate duration of action. *Anesthesiology.* 2003;98:1042–1048.
55. Cammu G, De Witte J, De Veylder J, et al. Postoperative residual paralysis in outpatients versus inpatients. *Anesth Analg.* 2006;102:426-429.
56. Murphy GS, Brull SJ. Residual neuromuscular block: lessons unlearned. Part I: Definitions, incidence, and adverse physiologic effects of residual neuromuscular block. *Anesth Analg.* 2010;111:120-128.
57. Brull SJ, Murphy GS. Residual neuromuscular block: lessons unlearned. Part II: Methods to reduce the risk of residual weakness. *Anesth Analg.* 2010;111:129-140.
58. Miller RD, Eger EL, Stevens WC, Gibbons R. Pancuronium-induced tachycardia in relation to alveolar halothane, dose of pancuronium, and prior atropine. *Anesthesiology.* 1975;42:352-355.
59. Lien CA, Savard P, Belmont M, Sunaga H, Savarese JJ. Fumarates: unique nondepolarizing neuromuscular blocking agents that are antagonized by cysteine. *J Crit Care.* 2009;24:50-57.

CHAPTER

10

Reversal of Neuromuscular Blockade

Mohamed Naguib, MB, BCh, MSc, FFARCSI, MD, Stephen Aniskevich, MD, and Sorin J. Brull, MD, FCARCSI (Hon)

INTRODUCTION

In 1516, Peter Martyr D'Anghera (1457–1526) described in his book, *De Orbo Novo* (The New World) the effects of poisoned arrows (proven later to contain crude curare) used by South American Indians for hunting and for fighting their enemies.[1] His description clearly demonstrates the use of curare. He stated "Despite their nakedness, it must be admitted that in some places, the natives have exterminated entire groups of Spaniards, for they are ferocious and are armed with poisoned arrows." D'Anghera then goes to give more details such as, "It was discovered that their poisoned arrows contained a kind of liquid which oozed out when the point broke." Referring to the time course of the effect of curare, he reported, "Hojeda, under the influence of the poison, saw his strength ebbing ... away" and stated that, "... the strength of the poison is such, that the mere odor of it, while compounding almost kills its makers. Whoever is wounded by one of these poisoned arrows dies, but not instantly, and no Spaniard has yet found a remedy for such wounds."[1] In 1596, Sir Walter Raleigh in his book, *The Discoverie* [sic] *of the Large, Rich and Bewtiful Empyre* [sic] *of Guiana*[2] reported on this strong native arrow poison and referred to it as "Tupara, curare or ourari." This poison was later found to be derived from the rubber plant *Chondodendron tomentosum*. During the 19th century, the paralyzing effect of curare on skeletal muscles[3,4] and the antagonistic effects of physostigmine[5] were studied in several animal experiments.

The clinical utility of curare was first explored in 1912 by Arthur Läwen, a German surgeon from Leipzig, who administered 0.8 mg of curarine intramuscularly to provide relaxation for intraperitoneal surgery.[6] However, due to the lack of supplies of curarine, Läwen could not develop its clinical applications further. In 1935, King successfully extracted tubocurarine from crude curare and determined its chemical structure.[7] In 1942, Harold Griffith and Enid Johnson were the first clinicians to use curare (Intocostrin), on some 25 patients.[8]

A few years later, Dr R.E. Pleasance, in his Presidential Address to the Society of Sheffield Anaesthetists on January 15, 1948, described his clinical experience using curare.[9] Pleasance never mentioned the need for antagonizing the residual effects of curare in his patients. In fact, he stated that, during recovery, "there is no evidence that curare has any latent toxicity. It is completely and fairly rapidly eliminated." It should be noted, however, that when curarization was initially introduced, tracheal intubation was the exception in routine surgical practice, and most patients undergoing anesthesia were breathing spontaneously.

It is interesting to note that the Intocostrin package insert in 1943 stated, "When dangerous respiratory embarrassment occurs, resuscitation by. . . artificial respiration may be expected to carry the patient through the paralysis. Particularly one should be certain that an airway exists. Prostigmin [neostigmine] is also a physiologic antidote; the respiratory paralysis if not too profound is removed by this drug." Nevertheless, no dosage for neostigmine was suggested at that time. It was not until 1948 that intravenous administration of neostigmine 1 mL of a 1:2000 dilution (0.5 mg) to treat moderate curare overdosage was suggested by E.R. Squibb and Sons. At that time, the use of neostigmine to antagonize the effects of curare on neuromuscular function was gaining momentum. In the same year, Burke and colleagues stated, in one of the early papers on the use of neostigmine for antagonism of d-tubocurarine, that "the use of neostigmine will shorten the period for the necessity of artificial respiration, but its administration should be considered as an adjuvant to treatment rather than as a substitute."[10] The recommendation for neostigmine dosages came from Prescott and colleagues in 1946.[11] They stated "[I]f [P]rostigmin is to be effective, doses of the order of 5 mg or more must be used. Atropine 1.3 mg should also be given, to balance the parasympathomimetic action of [P]rostigmin."

Inadequate recovery of neuromuscular function at the end of surgery was therefore common in the mid-1950s. It was termed *neostigmine-resistant curarization*[12] and was attributed to mechanisms (such as depression of the acetylcholine cholinesterase system) other than the presence of a profound block induced by d-tubocurarine that could not be antagonized with neostigmine.[13] Therefore, it was not surprising that the use of neuromuscular blockers in 1950s was associated with a mortality rate 6 times greater (1:370 anesthetics) than the mortality rate when neuromuscular blockers were avoided (1:2100 anesthetics).[14] Furthermore, 63% of deaths that involved the use of a neuromuscular blocker were caused by respiratory failure. To date, perioperative management of neuromuscular blocking drugs remains suboptimal, and significant patient weakness in the recovery room associated with the residual effects of neuromuscular blocking drugs still occurs.[15]

CRITERIA FOR ADEQUATE RECOVERY FROM A NEUROMUSCULAR BLOCKADE

The current consensus is that a train-of-four (TOF) ratio of at least 0.9 should be attained prior to tracheal extubation. At this level of recovery, esophageal tone, pharyngeal coordination,[16] hypoxic ventilatory drive,[17] and muscle strength[18] appear to return toward baseline. A TOF ratio of less than 0.9 in unanesthetized volunteers has been associated with difficulty in speaking and swallowing as well as with visual disturbances.[18]

PROBLEMS OF RESIDUAL NEUROMUSCULAR BLOCKADE

Postanesthetic morbidity in the form of incomplete reversal and residual postoperative weakness (also known as "residual paralysis" or "residual curarization") is a frequent occurrence. A recent survey indicated that anesthesia providers have very different opinions about the best way to clinically demonstrate adequate recovery from neuromuscular block, and more than 75% of the respondents from both the United States and Europe believed that postoperative residual weakness was a significant anesthetic complication.[15] A 45% incidence of postoperative residual neuromuscular blockade in patients arriving in the postanesthesia care unit was reported in 2003.[19] This incidence is significantly higher following the use of long-acting (~70%–74%) compared to intermediate-acting (~35%–54%) neuromuscular blocking drugs.[20] In addition, the incidence of critical respiratory events in the postoperative care unit remained a significant 0.8%.[21] Thus, it is possible that as many as 112,000 patients annually in the United States are at risk for adverse events associated with undetected residual neuromuscular blockade.[22] Monitoring the effects of neuromuscular blockers ensures their appropriate intraoperative use, effective antagonism, and prevention of residual neuromuscular weakness.

SYNAPTIC PLASTICITY OF THE NEUROMUSCULAR JUNCTION

Synaptic plasticity is the "ability of individual synaptic junctions to respond [to change in strength in response] to either use or disuse."[23] The plasticity of neuromuscular junction is dependent on a highly orchestrated mechanism involving the (1) synthesis, storage, and release of acetylcholine from motor nerve endings (presynaptic region) at the neuromuscular junction; (2) binding of acetylcholine to nicotinic receptors on the muscle membrane (postsynaptic region) and generation of action potentials; and (3) rapid hydrolysis of acetylcholine by the enzyme acetylcholinesterase, which is present in the synaptic cleft.[24]

ACETYLCHOLINESTERASE AT THE NEUROMUSCULAR JUNCTION

At the neuromuscular junction, the acetylcholinesterase enzyme is responsible for the rapid hydrolysis of released acetylcholine, thereby controlling the duration of receptor activation.[25] Approximately 50% of the released acetylcholine is hydrolyzed during its diffusion across the synaptic cleft, before reaching nicotinic acetylcholine receptors located on the postsynaptic muscle membrane. The efficiency of acetylcholinesterase depends on its unusually high catalytic activity, which is one of the highest known.[25] The active site of acetylcholinesterase lies near the bottom of a deep and narrow gorge that reaches halfway into the protein (**Figure 10–1**).[26] A second anionic (peripheral) site is located at the top of the active site gorge and is probably involved in electrostatic interactions with acetylcholine.[26,27] Acetylcholine must enter this cleft in the enzyme to the active site.[28]

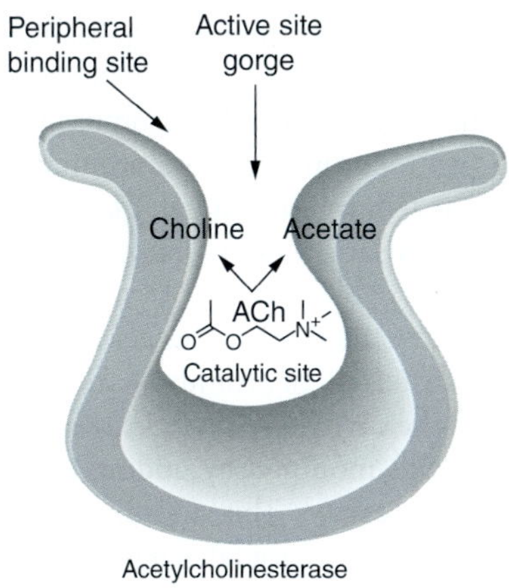

FIGURE 10–1 The enzyme acetylcholinesterase (AChE). The active catalytic site (lined with hydrophobic amino acid side chains) lies near the bottom of a deep and narrow cleft (gorge). Acetylcholine (ACh) must enter this cleft in the enzyme, which is blocked by a mobile ring of molecules more than 97% of the time. Molecular dynamics simulations showed that the entrance to the cleft opens and shuts so frequently that any ACh molecules lingering nearby may have ample chances to diffuse in.[28] AChE promotes hydrolysis of ACh by forming an acetyl-AChE intermediate with the release of choline and then hydrolysis of the intermediate to release acetate. This reaction is antagonized by AChE inhibitors such as neostigmine, edrophonium, and pyridostigmine, thereby increasing the concentration of ACh.

Acetylcholinesterase is highly concentrated at the neuromuscular junction but is also present in a lower concentration throughout the length of muscle fiber membrane.[29] The distribution of acetylcholinesterase molecules at the neuromuscular junction closely matches the distribution of nicotinic acetylcholine receptors.[30]

In addition to acetylcholinesterase, butyrylcholinesterase is also present at the neuromuscular junction at low concentrations.[31] Butyrylcholinesterase is synthesized by the liver and is found in the plasma and is responsible for metabolism of succinylcholine, mivacurium, procaine, chloroprocaine, tetracaine, cocaine, and heroin. The exact function of butyrylcholinesterase at the neuromuscular junction is not known, but there is evidence that butyrylcholinesterase may act as a poison scavenger (eg, cocaine poisoning), protecting the integrity of acetylcholinesterase.[32]

MECHANISMS OF REVERSAL

Inhibition of Acetylcholinesterase

Enzymatic inhibition is an indirect mechanism for antagonizing the residual effects of neuromuscular blockers; it affects neither the rate of elimination of the neuromuscular blocker from the body, nor the plasma or tissue (biophase) concentration of the neuromuscular blocking agent. Acetylcholinesterase inhibitors (eg, neostigmine and, less commonly, edrophonium and pyridostigmine) are used clinically to antagonize the residual effects of neuromuscular blockers and to accelerate recovery from nondepolarizing neuromuscular blockade. This antagonism results in a decrease in the rate of acetylcholine hydrolysis and in increase in acetylcholine concentrations. The increased amount of acetylcholine competes with the residual unbound (free) molecules of the neuromuscular blocking drug for the available unoccupied nicotinic acetylcholine receptors at the neuromuscular junction. This mechanism of antagonism has a ceiling effect.[33,34] Once the inhibition of acetylcholinesterase is maximal, administering additional doses of an acetylcholinesterase inhibitor (eg, neostigmine) will serve no useful purpose. If neostigmine is administered at a deep level of neuromuscular blockade (ie, no response to TOF stimulation), the concentration of neuromuscular agent will be high at the neuromuscular junction; even with full cholinesterase antagonism, the amount of free acetylcholine at the junction will be insufficient to effectively compete with the neuromuscular agent. Indeed, administering additional neostigmine at this point may in fact worsen neuromuscular recovery.[35] This underscores the limitations of neostigmine (or any other acetylcholinesterase inhibitor) in clinical practice and explains, in part, the high incidence of postoperative residual neuromuscular blockade.[20]

Pharmacokinetics of Acetylcholinesterase Inhibitors

The pharmacokinetic parameters of the acetylcholinesterase inhibitors are listed in Table 10–1.[36-39] The elimination half-life of edrophonium is similar to that of neostigmine and pyridostigmine,[38] although the duration of action of pyridostigmine is somewhat longer.[36,37] Renal excretion accounts for about 50% of the elimination of neostigmine and about 75% of that of pyridostigmine and edrophonium. Renal failure decreases the plasma clearance of neostigmine, pyridostigmine, and edrophonium as much as, if not more than, that of the long-acting neuromuscular blockers.

Selective Relaxant-Binding Agent (Sugammadex)

Encapsulation of free molecules of rocuronium and vecuronium (steroidal-type muscle relaxant agents) represents an innovative approach for antagonizing the effects of neuromuscular blockers. Sugammadex is a modified γ-cyclodextrin (Figure 10–2).[40-43] Cyclodextrins are cyclic dextrose units joined through 1 to 4 glycosyl bonds that are produced from starch or starch derivatives using cyclodextrin glycosyltransferase. The 3 natural unmodified cyclodextrins consist of 6-, 7-, and 8-cyclic oligosaccharides and are called α-, β-, and γ-cyclodextrin, respectively. Their 3-dimensional structures, which resemble a hollow, truncated cone or a doughnut, have a hydrophobic cavity and a hydrophilic exterior because of the presence of polar hydroxyl groups. Hydrophobic interactions trap the drug into the cyclodextrin cavity (the doughnut hole), resulting in formation of a water-soluble guest–host complex.

Compared with α- and β-cyclodextrins, γ-cyclodextrin exhibits more favorable properties with regard to steroidal relaxant interaction in terms of the size of its internal cavity, water solubility, and bioavailability. This is because the α- and β-cyclodextrins have smaller lipophilic cavities (diameter < 0.65 nm) and form less stable complexes with the bulky aminosteroid neuromuscular blocker molecule (eg, rocuronium or vecuronium; molecular width, ~ 0.75 nm). In contrast, the γ-cyclodextrin molecule has a larger lipophilic cavity (0.75–0.83 nm in diameter).[40]

To improve the fit of the larger, rigid structure of the aminosteroid neuromuscular blocker molecule within the cavity of γ-cyclodextrin, the sugammadex ring was modified by adding 8 side chains to extend the cavity. This modification allowed the 4 hydrophobic steroidal rings of rocuronium to be better accommodated within the hydrophobic cavity. Addition of negatively charged carboxyl groups at the end of each of the 8 side chains serves

TABLE 10–1 Pharmacokinetic parameters for neostigmine, pyridostigmine, and edrophonium in anesthetized patients.

Cholinesterase Inhibitor	Clearance (mL/kg/min)	Volume of Distribution (mL/kg)	Elimination Half-Time (min)
Neostigmine[39]	9.2 ± 2.6	740 ± 200	77.8 ± 47
Edrophonium[39]	9.2 ± 2.6	1100 ± 200	110 ± 34
Pyridostigmine[37]	8.6 ± 1.7	1100 ± 300	112 ± 12

Data are presented as mean ± SD.

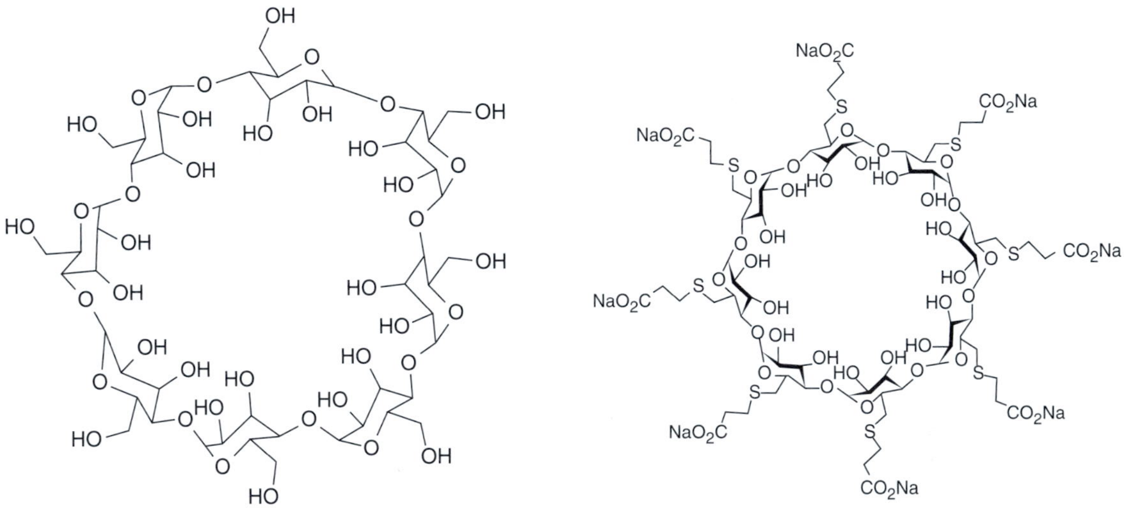

A B

FIGURE 10–2 A, γ-cyclodextrin and B, sugammadex [6^{A},6^{B},6^{C},6^{D},6^{E},6^{F},6^{G},6^{H}-octakis-S-(2-carboxyethyl)-6^{A},6^{B},6^{C},6^{D},6^{E},6^{F},6^{G},6^{H}-octathio-γ-cyclodextrin octasodium salt], a modified γ-cyclodextrin.

2 purposes. First, the repellent forces of the negative charges keep propionic acid side chains from being disordered, thereby allowing the cavity to remain open until encapsulation. Second, these negatively charged carboxyl groups enhance the electrostatic binding to the positively charged quaternary nitrogen of rocuronium, rendering the complexation irreversible (see Figure 10–2).[40,41]

These modifications resulted in sugammadex, a compound that is highly water soluble and that contains a hydrophobic cavity large enough to encapsulate steroidal neuromuscular blocking drugs, especially rocuronium.[40-43] The aqueous solution of sugammadex has a pH of approximately 7.5 and osmolality of 300 to 500 mOsm/kg. Sugammadex exerts its effect by forming very tight complexes in a 1:1 ratio with steroidal neuromuscular blocking agents (rocuronium > vecuronium >> pancuronium).[40-43] The intermolecular (van der Waals) forces, thermodynamic (hydrogen) bonds, and hydrophobic interactions of the sugammadex–rocuronium complex make it very tight.[40] The sugammadex–rocuronium complex has a very high association rate and a very low dissociation rate. Estimates are that for every 30 million sugammadex–rocuronium complexes, only one complex dissociates.

Pharmacokinetics of Sugammadex

Sugammadex is biologically inactive.[44-46] When administered by itself to volunteers who had not received a neuromuscular blocking agent, doses of 0.1 to 8.0 mg/kg of sugammadex had a clearance rate of 120 mL/min, an elimination half-life of 100 minutes, and a volume of distribution of 18 L.[45] Approximately 75% of the sugammadex dose was eliminated through the urine. The clearance of sugammadex/rocuronium complex is 109 mL/min.[47] Between 59% and 80% of total dose of sugammadex is excreted in the urine in the first 24 hours after administration.[45] The kinetics of sugammadex appear to be dose dependent, in that clearance increased and elimination half-life decreased, when the sugammadex dose was increased from 0.15 to 1.0 mg/kg.[45] The clearance of sugammadex decreases with advancing age, and this reduction is correlated with reduced creatinine clearance seen in the elderly.[47] In elderly patients (age > 75 year), sugammadex clearance is decreased by 50% compared with adult (18–64 year) patients

(52 versus 103 mL/min) and by approximately 30% compared with older (65–74 year) patients (52 versus 76 mL/min).[47]

In the absence of sugammadex, rocuronium is eliminated mainly by biliary excretion (> 75%) and to a lesser degree by renal excretion (10%–25%). The plasma clearance of sugammadex alone is approximately three times lower than that of rocuronium alone.[48] In volunteers, the plasma clearance of rocuronium was decreased by a factor of greater than 2 after administration of a dose of sugammadex of equal or greater than 2.0 mg/kg.[45] This prolongation is due to the biliary route of excretion, which becomes unavailable for the rocuronium–sugammadex complex, and rocuronium clearance decreases to a value approaching the glomerular filtration rate (120 mL/min). As noted earlier, after administration of sugammadex, the plasma concentration of free rocuronium decreases rapidly, but the total plasma concentration of rocuronium (both free and bound to sugammadex) increases due to redistribution of free rocuronium from the peripheral compartments to the plasma (Figure 10–3).[47,49]

The soluble nature of the sugammadex–rocuronium complex results in urinary excretion of the complex as the major route of elimination of rocuronium (65%–97% of the administered dose).[45,48] Excretion is rapid, with approximately 70% of the dose being excreted within 6 hours and more than 90% within 24 hours. Renal excretion of rocuronium is increased by more than 100% after administration of 4 to 8 mg/kg of sugammadex.[48]

Sugammadex does not bind to human plasma proteins and erythrocytes to a significant extent. Metabolism of sugammadex is at most very limited, and the drug is predominantly eliminated unchanged by the kidneys. In patients with substantial renal impairment, clearance of sugammadex and rocuronium decreased by factors of 16 and 3.7, respectively, relative to clearance in healthy subjects, and the elimination half-lives were increased by factors of 15 and 2.5, respectively. The effectiveness of dialysis in removing sugammadex and rocuronium from plasma has not been demonstrated consistently. Therefore, sugammadex administration should be avoided in patients with a creatinine clearance less than 30 mL/min.

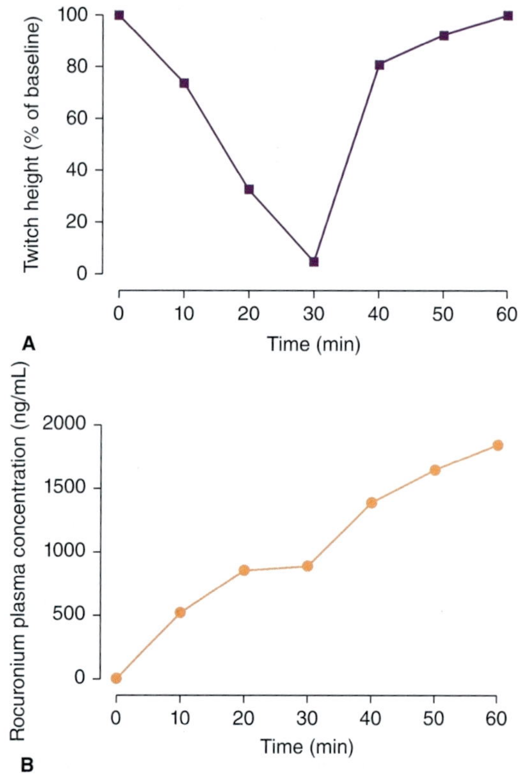

FIGURE 10–3 Relationship between rocuronium plasma concentration and twitch height. Rocuronium-induced block was reversed while the rocuronium infusion was ongoing. Note the increase in the total plasma concentration of rocuronium (free and complexed) and recovery of twitch height, even though the infusion rate of rocuronium was maintained. (Reproduced with permission from Epemolu O, Bom A, Hope F, Mason R: Reversal of neuromuscular blockade and simultaneous increase in plasma rocuronium concentration after the intravenous infusion of the novel reversal agent Org 25969. *Anesthesiology* 2003;Sep;99(3):632-637.)

CLINICAL PHARMACOLOGY

Acetylcholinesterase Inhibitors

Recovery from nondepolarizing neuromuscular blockade depends primarily on several factors: (1) the depth of blockade when reversal is attempted, (2) the anticholinesterase used, (3) the dose of anticholinesterase administered, (4) the rate of clearance of the neuromuscular blocker from plasma, and (5) the choice of anesthetic agents administered and depth of anesthesia.

Rate of Spontaneous Clearance of the Neuromuscular Blocker

The plasma concentrations of neuromuscular blocking drugs with a short duration of action (mivacurium) decrease more rapidly than those with an intermediate (cisatracurium and rocuronium) or long duration of action (pancuronium and d-tubocurarine), and consequently, the recovery of neuromuscular function is more rapid (Figure 10–4). Spontaneous recovery from mivacurium-induced neuromuscular block is very rapid, because the drug is hydrolyzed by plasma cholinesterase at a rate approximately 80% of that of succinylcholine.[50] Simulations in Figure 10–5 depict the time from administration of equipotent doses (twice the effective dose to produce 95% effect, $2 \times ED_{95}$) of mivacurium, cisatracurium, rocuronium, and pancuronium to a 95% probability of spontaneous recovery to TOF of 0.9. As expected, this recovery time is a function of the type of neuromuscular blocker. In the aforementioned simulations, the average times for spontaneous TOF 95% recovery were 30, 55, 65, and 320 minutes for mivacurium, cisatracurium, rocuronium, and pancuronium, respectively.

Figure 10–6 presents simulated effect-site and plasma concentrations over time following 2 different bolus doses of neostigmine. Following administration of an anticholinesterase, two processes contribute to recovery of neuromuscular function. The first is the antagonism induced by the effect of the anticholinesterase at the neuromuscular junction; and the second is the decrease in plasma concentration of the neuromuscular blocker due to redistribution and elimination.[34,51] Therefore, the more rapid the elimination of the neuromuscular blocker (see Figure 10–4), the faster will be the recovery of adequate neuromuscular function after

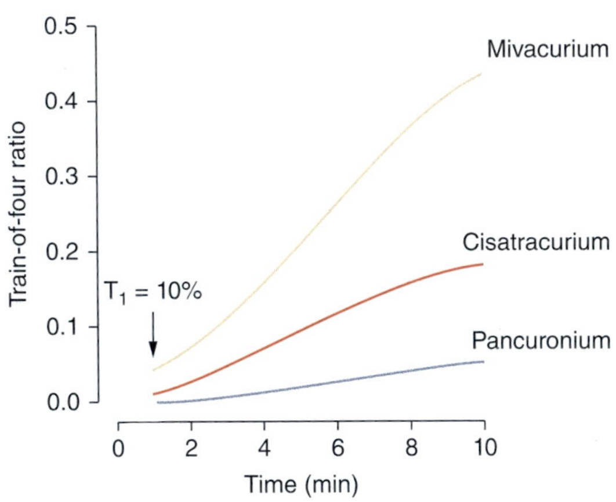

FIGURE 10–4 Comparative mean spontaneous recovery following bolus administration of equipotent doses ($2 \times ED_{95}$) of pancuronium, cisatracurium, and mivacurium following the return of the first twitch height (T_1) to 10% of baseline.

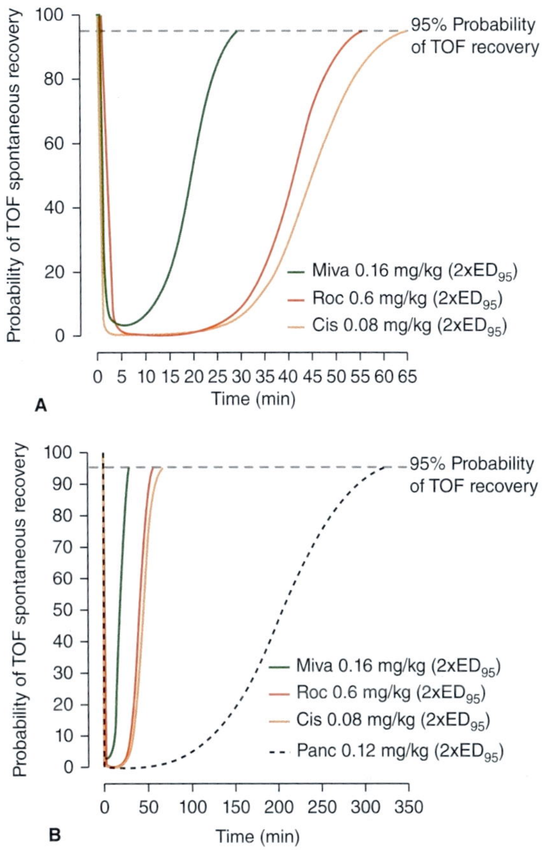

FIGURE 10–5 A, simulations depicting the probability of spontaneous recovery of equipotent doses of mivacurium (Miva is a short-acting neuromuscular blocker), rocuronium (Roc), and cisatracurium (Cis) (Roc and Cis are intermediate-acting neuromuscular blockers) to a train-of-four (TOF) ratio of 0.9. B, the simulated spontaneous recovery of equipotent doses pancuronium (Panc; a long-acting neuromuscular blocker) is included for comparison.

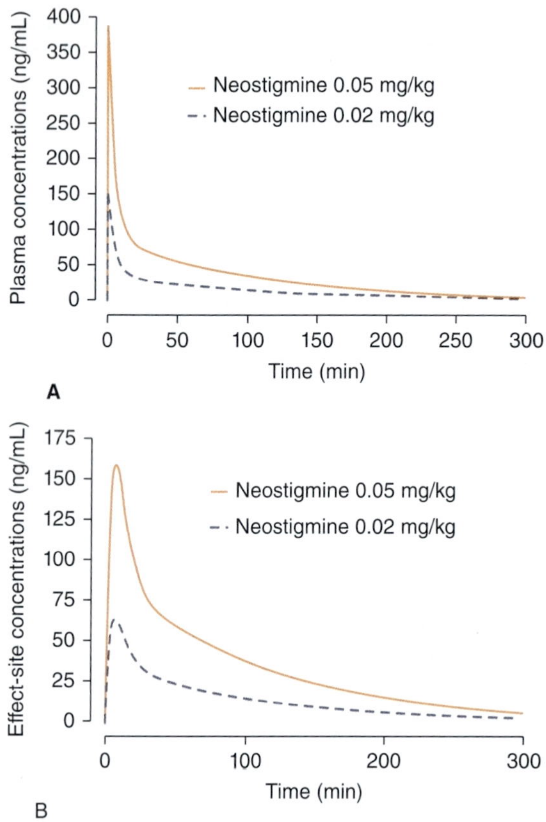

FIGURE 10–6 A and B, simulations of two different bolus doses of neostigmine.

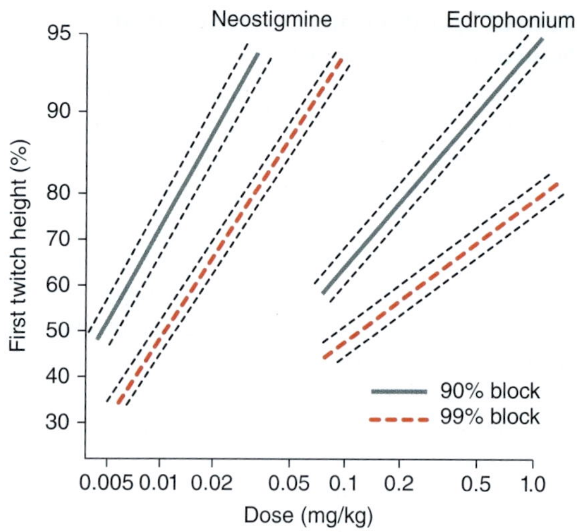

FIGURE 10–7 Reversal of atracurium-induced blockade. First-twitch height (T_1) versus dose was measured 10 minutes after administration of neostigmine and edrophonium given at either 1% (99% block) or 10% (90% block) T_1 recovery from atracurium. Thin dashed lines represent the standard error of estimate for the mean. (Reproduced with permission from Donati F, Smith CE, Bevan DR: Dose-response relationships for edrophonium and neostigmine as antagonists of moderate and profound atracurium blockade. *Anesth Analg* 1989;Jan;68(1):13-19.)

administration of an antagonist. The ease and rapidity of antagonism of short- and intermediate-acting neuromuscular blockers (mivacurium, atracurium, vecuronium) explain the lower incidence of inadequate neuromuscular function in the postoperative period as compared with long-acting neuromuscular blockers (pancuronium).[20,52,53]

Depth of Neuromuscular Blockade

As a general rule, it is recommended that antagonism of residual neuromuscular blockade be attempted when there is evidence of spontaneous recovery (preferably a TOF of 4, corresponding to a recovery of the first TOF twitch, T_1 to 25% of baseline)[54] as detected by a conventional nerve stimulator (which requires the clinician to evaluate the evoked response visually or tactilely).

Antagonism of a shallow degree of blockade requires less doses of neostigmine (Figure 10–7) and is associated with faster recovery of neuromuscular function than is antagonism of deep blockade.[55] During recovery from vecuronium-induced blockade, administration of 0.04-mg/kg neostigmine at the reappearance of the fourth response of TOF (ie, a TOF count of 4), as opposed to a TOF count of 2, resulted in a faster recovery in healthy patients.[56,57]

Anticholinesterase drugs

Edrophonium has a more rapid onset than neostigmine or pyridostigmine when used to reverse residual neuromuscular blockade.[58,59] Edrophonium (0.5–1 mg/kg) was as effective as neostigmine (40 µg/kg) in reversing moderate neuromuscular blockade (< 90% twitch depression, corresponding to a TOF count of 1) from pancuronium, atracurium and vecuronium.[60] Edrophonium (1 mg/kg, but not 0.5 mg/kg) was as effective as neostigmine in antagonizing deep blockade (> 90% twitch depression) from pancuronium, atracurium and vecuronium, but was not as effective in reversing profound (99% twitch depression) atracurium blockade (see

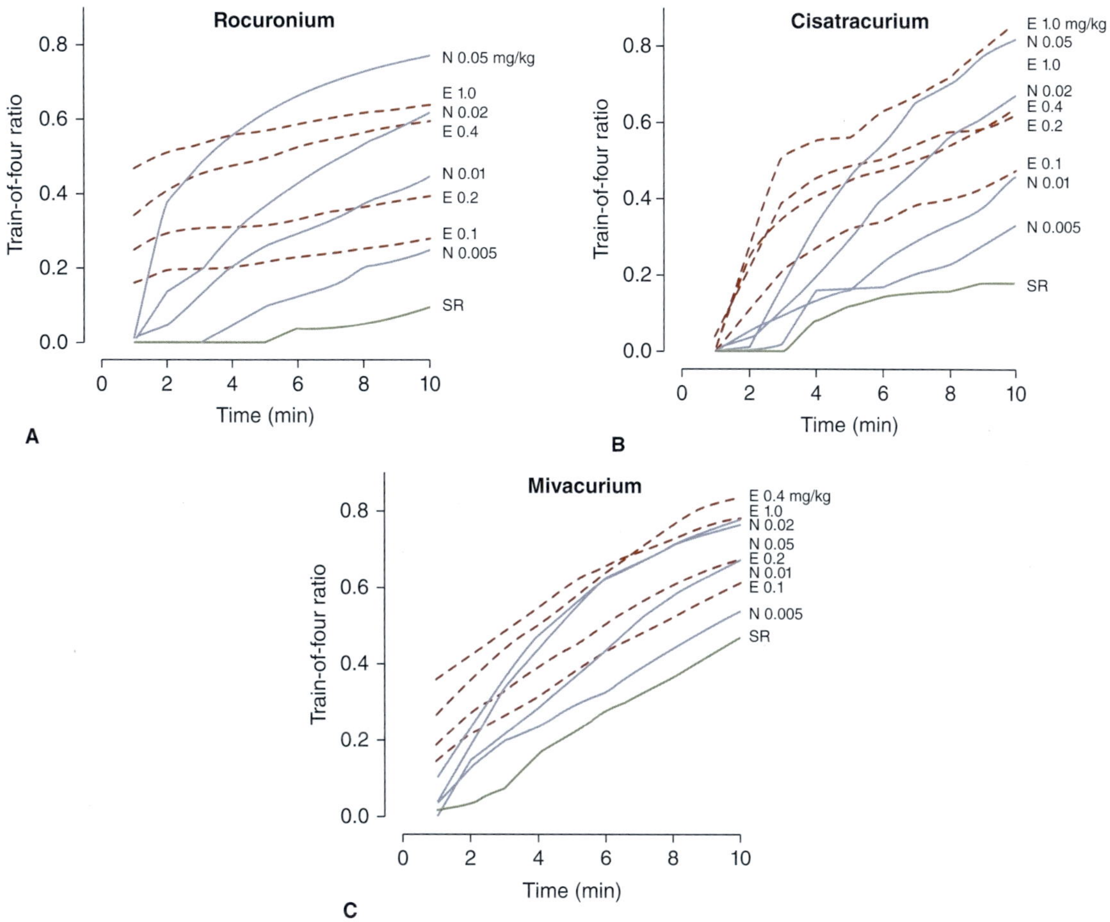

FIGURE 10–8 A–C, mean train-of-four (TOF) ratio versus time after administration of various doses of neostigmine (N) or edrophonium (E). Antagonism of neuromuscular blockade was attempted when first twitch height (T_1) had reached 10% of its control value. The neuromuscular blockers used were rocuronium,[61] cisatracurium,[62] or mivacurium.[63] From Naguib et al.[61-63] SR, spontaneous recovery. (Data from Naguib M, Abdulatif M, al-Ghamdi A: Dose-response relationships for edrophonium and neostigmine antagonism of rocuronium bromide (ORG 9426)-induced neuromuscular blockade. *Anesthesiology* 1993;79:739-745. Naguib M, Riad W: Dose-response relationships for edrophonium and neostigmine antagonism of atracurium and cisatracurium-induced neuromuscular block. *Can J Anaesth* 2000;47:1074-1081. Naguib M, Abdulatif M, al-Ghamdi A, Hamo I, Nouheid R: Dose-response relationships for edrophonium and neostigmine antagonism of mivacurium-induced neuromuscular block. *Br J Anaesth* 1993;71:709-714.)

Figure 10–7).[55,60] Edrophonium (1 mg/kg) was less effective than 50 mcg/kg of neostigmine at reversing rocuronium-induced TOF fade (**Figure 10–8A**).[61] However, this difference was not evident with cisatracurium (see Figure 10–8B), atracurium,[62] or mivacurium (see Figure 10–8C).[63] Dose-response curves for edrophonium and neostigmine are not parallel, meaning that potency ratios may differ; they may differ for single-twitch versus TOF responses, may change over time (ie, 5 minutes versus 10 minutes after administration), and may depend on the relaxant being antagonized.[61] For example, 10 minutes after reversal from a rocuronium-induced blockade (at T_1 = 10%), neostigmine was 27.7 times as potent as edrophonium in achieving the ED_{50} of the TOF.[61] Corresponding potency ratios for atracurium, cisatracurium, and mivacurium were 13, 11.8, and 10.4, respectively.[62,63]

Mixing antagonists is not advisable. Neostigmine and edrophonium do not potentiate each other; in fact, their effects in combination may not even be additive.[64] Therefore, when inadequate reversal occurs, one should not administer a different anticholinesterase but should ensure that ventilation is supported until adequate neuromuscular function is achieved.

Anticholinesterase Dose

Within limits, increasing the dose of an anticholinesterase will result in faster complete recovery from a nondepolarizing-induced neuromuscular block (see Figure 10–8). Studies have demonstrated that a dose of 40 mcg/kg of neostigmine (administered at T_1 of 5%–10% recovery) sufficiently antagonizes residual neuromuscular blockade, and there is no further advantage in using higher doses (eg, 80 mcg/kg) of neostigmine [65,66] or administering a second dose of neostigmine.[67] In fact, administration of a second dose of neostigmine could result in a depolarizing block.[35] It is recommended that the maximal dose of neostigmine be 70 mcg/kg. The maximum effective dose for edrophonium appears to be 1.0 mg/kg.[60,68] Antagonism of residual neuromuscular blockade induced by the various nondepolarizing neuromuscular blockers is similar in children and adults.[69] When neostigmine is administered to antagonize a stable level of blockade maintained by continuous infusion of vecuronium, cisatracurium, rocuronium, or mivacurium, the rate and degree of recovery are not different from those following bolus administration of each neuromuscular blocker alone.[70-72]

Choice of Anesthetic Agents Administered and Depth of Anesthesia

Volatile inhalational anesthetics potentiate the neuromuscular blocking effect of nondepolarizing neuromuscular blockers.[73] The magnitude of this potentiation depends on (1) the duration of anesthesia,[74-76] (2) the specific volatile anesthetic used,[77] and (3) the concentration of volatile anesthetic.[78] The rank order of potentiation of neuromuscular block by volatile inhalational anesthetics is desflurane > sevoflurane > isoflurane > halothane > nitrous oxide–opioid or propofol. Therefore, the efficacy of acetylcholinesterase inhibitors is decreased in the presence of anesthetizing concentrations of inhaled anesthetics.[79,80] For example, rocuronium reversal by neostigmine is faster during anesthesia with propofol than with sevoflurane.[80] Reversal during anesthesia with isoflurane is faster than with desflurane or sevoflurane.[81] Withdrawal of the volatile anesthetic at the end of surgery will speed pharmacologic reversal of the neuromuscular blocking agent.[82]

Sugammadex

Sugammadex is the first selective relaxant-binding agent. It exerts no effect on acetylcholinesterases or on any receptor system in the body, thus eliminating the need for anticholinergic drugs and their adverse side effects. Sugammadex, when administered in appropriate doses, reverses neuromuscular block to a TOF ratio greater than or equal to 0.9 within 3 minutes from any depth of neuromuscular blockade induced by rocuronium or vecuronium.[83] During rocuronium- or vecuronium-induced neuromuscular blockade, intravenous administration of sugammadex results in rapid removal of free (unbound) rocuronium or vecuronium molecules from the plasma. This creates a concentration gradient favoring movement of the remaining rocuronium or vecuronium molecules from the extravascular space (including neuromuscular junction) back into the plasma, where they are encapsulated by free sugammadex molecules. Unbound sugammadex molecules also enter the tissues and form a complex with the rocuronium or vecuronium molecules. This results in an increased total plasma concentration of rocuronium or vecuronium (both free and bound to sugammadex)[47,49] or vecuronium.

The efficacy of sugammadex in antagonizing different levels of rocuronium- or vecuronium-induced neuromuscular blockade has been demonstrated in several clinical studies.[48,84-90] At appropriate doses, no reappearance of neuromuscular weakness ("recurarization") has been reported in human studies. Figure 10–9A depicts the simulated plasma concentrations following administration of 2-mg/kg sugammadex or 0.05-mg/kg neostigmine. Following administration of rocuronium, simulations in Figure 10–9B demonstrate that when 2-mg/kg sugammadex is administered at reappearance of the second twitch of the TOF ratio (which corresponds to T_1 of ~ 10%–15% of the control height), complete TOF recovery occurred in 45 seconds, whereas administration of 0.05-mg/kg neostigmine requires

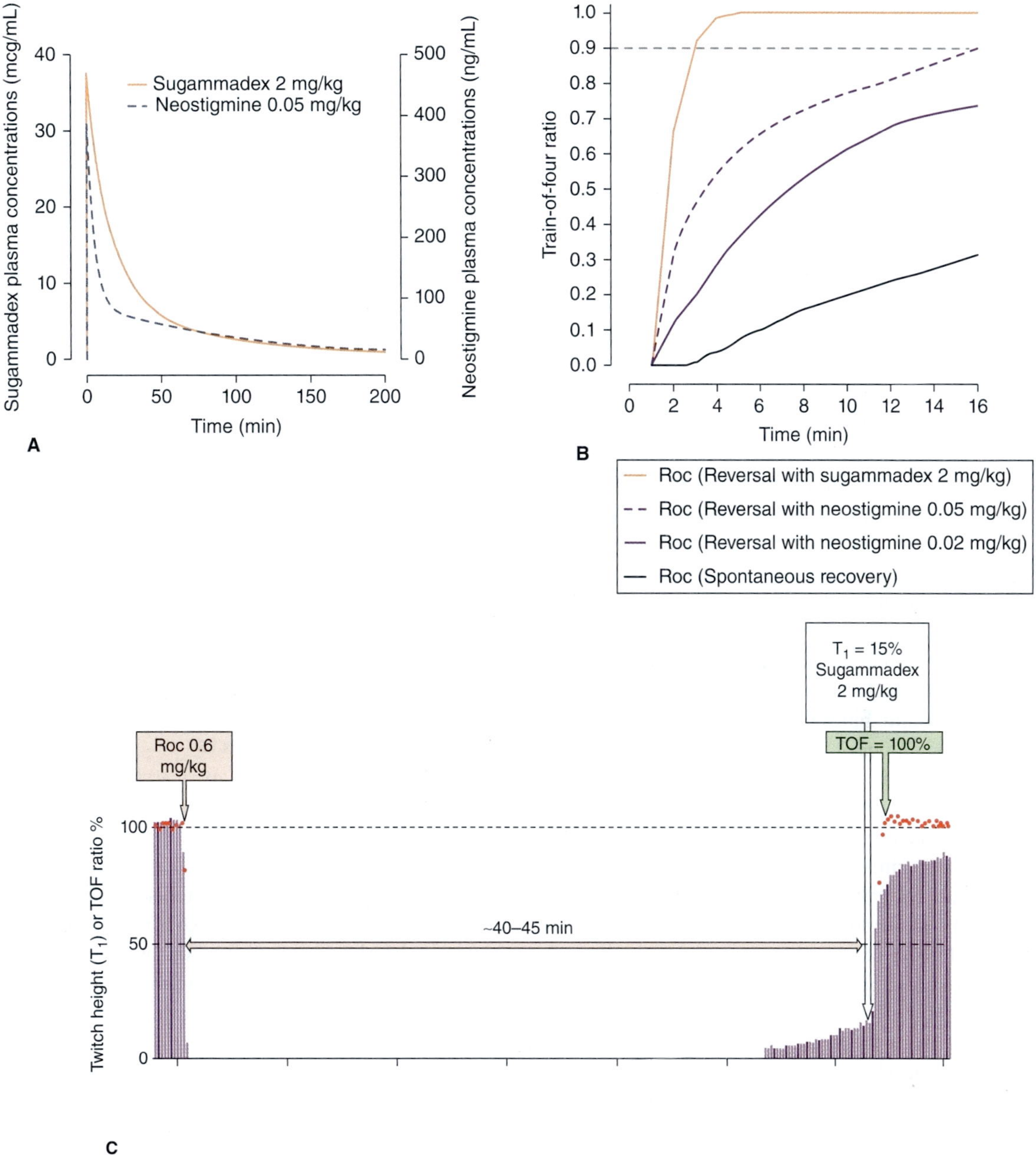

FIGURE 10–9 A, simulated plasma concentrations following 2-mg/kg sugammadex or 0.05-mg/kg neostigmine. B, when 2-mg/kg sugammadex is administered at reappearance of the second twitch (T_2) of the train-of-four (TOF) ratio (which corresponds to T_1 of ~ 10%–15% of the control height), complete TOF recovery occurred in 45 seconds, whereas administration of 0.05-mg/kg neostigmine required 16 minutes on average to reach a TOF ratio of 0.9. C, acceleromyographic recording of the recovery of the twitch height and TOF ratio after administration of 2 mg/kg of sugammadex at 15% twitch recovery from a rocuronium (Roc)-induced neuromuscular blockade. Complete neuromuscular recovery (TOF ratio of 100%) occurred 45 seconds later. Red dots indicate the TOF ratio. The failure of first twitch (T_1) to return to baseline height is probably a drift artifact.

16 minutes on average to reach a TOF ratio of 0.9. Stimulations also show that using a smaller dose of neostigmine will not be sufficient to attain adequate recovery (see Figure 10–9B).

With profound blockade induced by rocuronium or vecuronium, larger doses of sugammadex (8–16 mg/kg) are required for adequate and rapid recovery. In **Figure 10–10**, the speed of recovery from 1.2 mg/kg of rocuronium followed 3 minutes later by 16 mg/kg of sugammadex is compared with the speed of spontaneous recovery from 1.0 mg/kg of succinylcholine in surgical patients.[83] The total time from administration of rocuronium until recovery of the TOF ratio to ≥ 0.9 was shorter than that needed for a similar degree of spontaneous recovery from succinylcholine-induced blockade (see Figure 10–10).

Published data indicate that if the TOF count is 2 during recovery from rocuronium-induced neuromuscular blockade, administering 2 mg/kg of sugammadex would be sufficient to produce adequate neuromuscular recovery (TOF ratio ≥ 0.9). Similarly, 4 mg/kg of sugammadex is sufficient to produce adequate neuromuscular recovery from a deeper blockade (1–2 post-tetanic count). A still more profound blockade would require a greater dose of sugammadex, in the range of 8 to 16 mg/kg.

Sugammadex is ineffective in reversing succinylcholine as well as benzylisoquinolinium neuromuscular blockers such as mivacurium, atracurium, and cisatracurium because it cannot form inclusion complexes with these drugs.[91] Therefore, if neuromuscular blockade must be reestablished after the administration of sugammadex, one of the benzylisoquinolinium neuromuscular blockers or succinylcholine should be considered. As discussed earlier, after full recovery from neuromuscular blockade, significant numbers (~80%) of nicotinic acetylcholine receptors at the neuromuscular junction are still occupied by the neuromuscular blocker.[92] Therefore, it is expected that if the neuromuscular blockade needs to be reestablished after the use of sugammadex, a situation similar to "pretreatment or priming" will be present, which would result in a delayed onset of succinylcholine effects (ie, antagonism of depolarizing blockers) and potentiation of the effects (ie, faster onset and prolonged duration) of benzylisoquinolinium neuromuscular blockers.[93-95]

DRUG INTERACTIONS WITH ACETYLCHOLINESTERASE INHIBITORS

The effect of succinylcholine (1 mg/kg) was prolonged from 11 to 35 minutes when it was given 5 minutes after administration of neostigmine (5 mg).[96] This can be explained partly by the inhibition of butyrylcholinesterase by neostigmine. Butyrylcholinesterase is also inhibited, but to a lesser extent, by pyridostigmine. Ninety minutes after neostigmine administration, butyrylcholinesterase activity returns to less than 50% of its baseline value.

SIDE EFFECTS

Acetylcholinesterase Inhibitors

Inhibition of acetylcholinesterase not only increases the concentration of acetylcholine at the neuromuscular junction (nicotinic site) but also at all other synapses at which acetylcholine is a transmitter. Despite its adverse side effects, however, neostigmine is still the anticholinesterase agent most widely used by anesthesiologists worldwide.[97]

Cardiovascular Side Effects

Only the nicotinic effects of acetylcholinesterase inhibitors are desired. Therefore, the muscarinic effects must be attenuated by atropine or glycopyrrolate.[98] To minimize the muscarinic cardiovascular side effects of acetylcholinesterase inhibitors, an anticholinergic agent should be coadministered with the acetylcholinesterase inhibitor. Atropine (7–10 mcg/kg) matches the onset of action and pharmacodynamic profile of the rapid-acting edrophonium (0.5–1.0 mg/kg),[98] and glycopyrrolate (7–15 mcg/kg) matches the slower-acting neostigmine (40–70 mcg/kg) and pyridostigmine.[58,99] In patients with preexisting cardiac disease, glycopyrrolate may be preferable to atropine,[100] and the acetylcholinesterase inhibitor and anticholinergic should be administered slowly (eg, over 2–5 minutes). In all cases, administration of acetylcholinesterase inhibitors and anticholinergic agents should be slow (over 2–3 minutes) in order to decrease the peak plasma concentrations of these agents, thereby limiting their side effects.

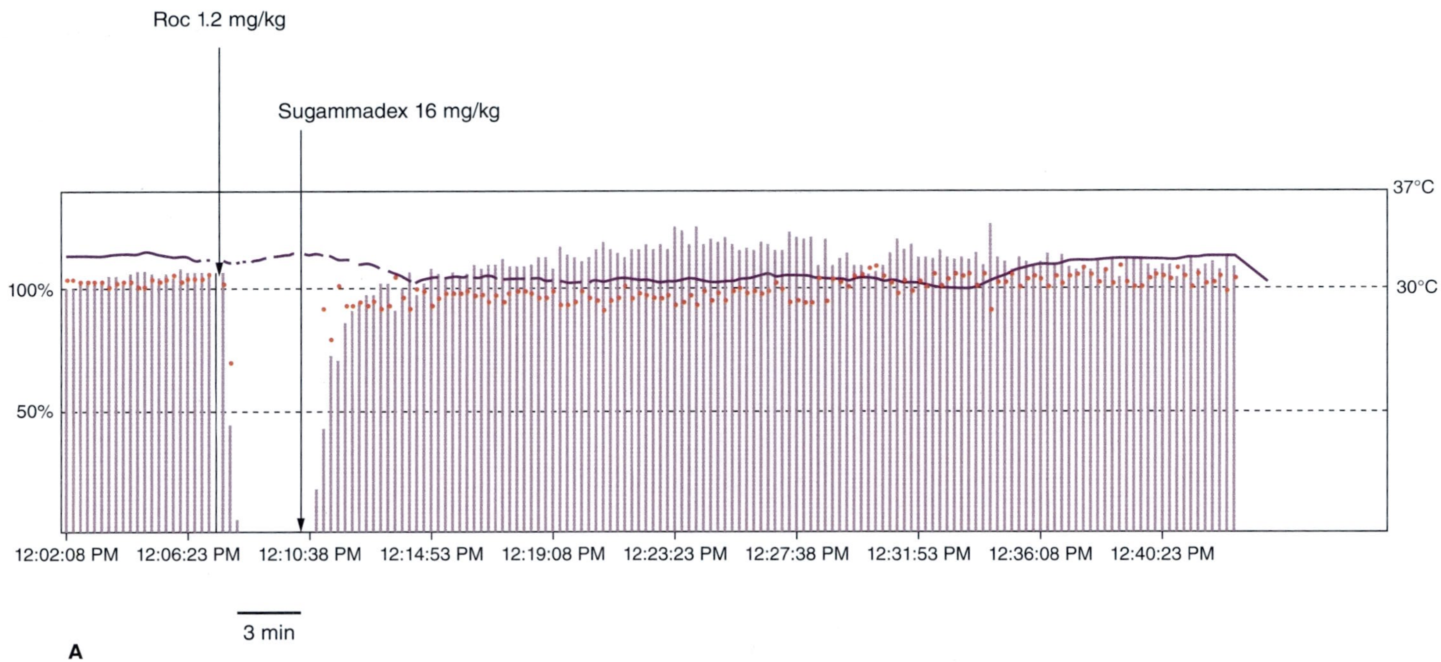

FIGURE 10–10 A, recovery of the twitch height and train-of-four (TOF) ratio after intravenous administration of 1.2 mg/kg of rocuronium (Roc), followed 3 minutes later by 16 mg/kg of sugammadex. Recovery to a first twitch height (T_1) of 90% and a TOF ratio of 0.94 occurred 110 seconds later. The onset–offset time with this sequence (ie, the time from the end of the injection of rocuronium to a T_1 recovery to 90%) was 4 minutes and 47 seconds.

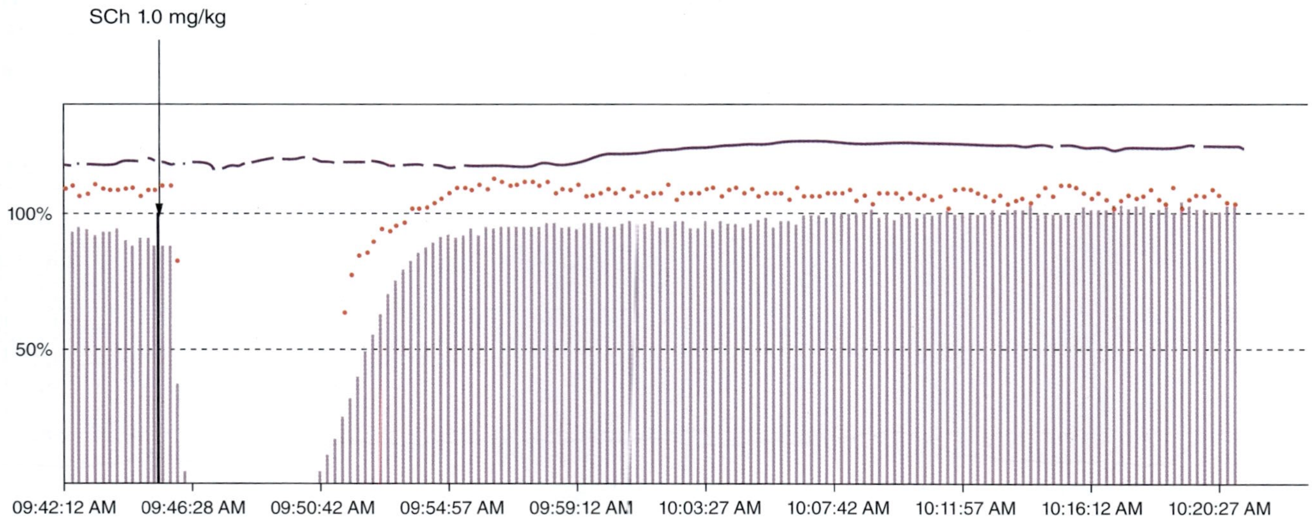

B

FIGURE 10–10 (*Continued*) B, the effects of administering 1.0 mg/kg of succinylcholine (SCh), with spontaneous recovery to a T_1 of 90% occurring after 9 minutes and 23 seconds. (Reproduced with permission from Naguib M: Sugammadex: another milestone in clinical neuromuscular pharmacology. *Anesth Analg* 2007;Mar;104(3):575-581.)

Pulmonary and Alimentary Side Effects

Administration of acetylcholinesterase inhibitors is associated with bronchoconstriction, increased airway resistance, increased salivation, and increased bowel motility (muscarinic effects). Anticholinergic agents tend to reduce these effects. Findings on whether neostigmine increases the incidence of postoperative nausea and vomiting differ;[101] neostigmine has been described both as having antiemetic properties[102] and as having no effect on the incidence of postoperative nausea and vomiting.[103]

Sugammadex

Reccurrence of Neuromuscular Weakness ("Recurarization")

It is important to distinguish between "postoperative residual weakness" due to inadequate antagonism of neuromuscular blockade[104] and the term "recurarization," which means the reccurrence of muscle paralysis (to some degree) after adequate recovery. It should be noted that even after a documented recovery to TOF of 0.9, a significant number of nicotinic acetylcholine receptors are still occupied with the neuromuscular blocker until complete elimination from the body occurs.[92] When recovery is suboptimal, administering drugs that potentiate the effects of neuromuscular blockers (eg, aminoglycoside and tetracycline antibiotics, magnesium and calcium, local anesthetics, and antidysrhythmics) can exacerbate undetected residual block.[105] Likewise, hypoxia, hypercarbia, and hypothermia potentiate residual neuromuscular block and may result in significant morbidity.

It should be noted, however, that all drugs behave in a dose-response manner.[106] A temporary decrease in TOF response (reccurrence of neuromuscular weakness) was also observed after reversal of muscle relaxation with an inadequate dose of sugammadex.[107,108] Figure 10–11 displays the simulations of the effect of different doses of sugammadex in antagonizing a profound neuromuscular block. In this simulation, it was assumed that 1.2-mg/kg rocuronium was administered, and 5 minutes later, different doses of sugammadex were administered. These simulations show that recurarization can only occur with sugammadex in situations in which inadequate does (< 1 mg/kg) were administered.

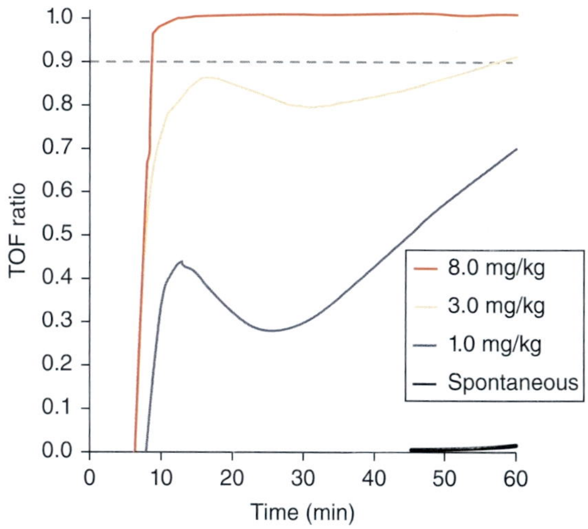

FIGURE 10–11 Simulations of the effect of different doses of sugammadex during a rocuronium-induced profound neuromuscular block. In this simulation, it was assumed that 1.2-mg/kg rocuronium was administered at time 0 and 5 minutes later, different doses of sugammadex were administered. These simulations show that reoccurrence of neuromuscular weakness can only occur after inadequate doses of sugammadex were administered. Note the time required to reach a train-of-four (TOF) ratio of 0.9 with different simulations. It took less than 3 minutes following 8-mg/kg sugammadex, but nearly an hour after 3-mg/kg sugammadex.

Safety and Tolerability

Common adverse effects associated with sugammadex administration include dysgeusia (metal or bitter taste), hypotension, diarrhea, headache, and polyuria. Sugammadex has been approved for clinical use in several European countries since 2009. As of 2014, sugammadex is used clinically in over 70 countries. However, the US Food and Drug Administration issued a "not approvable" letter (August, 2008) in response to the sugammadex new drug application, citing concerns about hypersensitivity and allergic reactions. Although the incidence of such reactions reported in all studies was less than 1%, one healthy volunteer experienced a hypersensitivity reaction after the first exposure to sugammadex that resulted in discontinuation of the sugammadex infusion. Allergic reactions have been reported in a patient who had never been exposed to sugammadex.[109] Ingestion of cyclodextrins molecules that are present in many foods might predispose to these hypersensitivity reactions.[110]

REFERENCES

1. MacNutt FA. *De Orbe Novo, the eight decades of Peter Martyr D'Anghera*. New York and London: G.P. Putnam's Sons/The Knickerbocker Press; 1912:365-393.
2. Raleigh W. *The Discoverie of the Large, Rich and Bewtiful Empyre of Guiana*. Manchester, UK: Manchester University Press; 1997:59-60 [transcribed, annotated, and introduced by Neil L. Whitehead].
3. Brodie BC. Experiments and observations on the different modes in which death is produced by certain vegetable poisons. Philosophical Transactions of the Royal Society of London. 1811;101:178-208.
4. Bernard C. Action du curare et de la nicotine sur le systeme nerveux et sur le systeme musculaire. *C R Soc Biol*. 1850;2:195.
5. Pal J. Physostigmin ein Gegengift des Curare. *Zentralbl Physiol*. 1900;14:255-258.
6. Läwen A. Über die Verbindung der Lokalanästhesie mit der Narkose, über hohe Extraduralanästhesie und epidurale Injektionen anästhesierender Lösungen bei tabischen Magenkrisen. *Beitr Klin Chir*. 1912;80: 168-180.
7. King H. Curare alkaloids. I. Tubocurarine. *J Chem Soc*. 1935;57:1381-1389.
8. Griffith H, Johnson GE. The use of curare in general anesthesia. *Anesthesiology*. 1942;3:418-420.
9. Pleasance RE. Curare. *Br J Anaesth*. 1948;21:2-23
10. Burke JC, Linegar CR, Frank MN, McIntyre AR. Eserine and neostigmine antagonism of d-tubocurarine. *Anesthesiology*. 1948;9:251-257.
11. Prescott F, Organe G, Rothbotham S. Tubocurarine chloride as an adjunct to anaesthesia. *Lancet*. 1946;2: 80-84.
12. Hunter AR. Neostigmine-resistant curarization. *Br Med J*. 1956;2:919-921.
13. Burchell GB, Lamont S. The application of a regime for the treatment of neostigmine resistant curarization. *Br J Anaesth*. 1959;31:182-185.
14. Beecher HK, Todd DP. A study of deaths with anesthesia and surgery based on a study of 599,548 anesthesias in ten institutions 1948-1952, inclusive. *Ann Surg*. 1954;140:2-33.
15. Naguib M, Kopman AF, Lien CA, Hunter JM, Lopez A, Brull SJ. A survey of current management of neuromuscular block in the United States and Europe. *Anesth Analg*. 2010;111:110-119.
16. Sundman E, Witt H, Olsson R, Ekberg O, Kuylenstierna R, Eriksson LI. The incidence and mechanisms of pharyngeal and upper esophageal dysfunction in partially paralyzed humans: pharyngeal videoradiography and simultaneous manometry after atracurium. *Anesthesiology*. 2000;92:977-984.
17. Eriksson LI. The effects of residual neuromuscular blockade and volatile anesthetics on the control of ventilation. *Anesth Analg*. 1999;89:243-251.
18. Kopman AF, Yee PS, Neuman GG. Relationship of the train-of-four fade ratio to clinical signs and symptoms of residual paralysis in awake volunteers. *Anesthesiology*. 1997;86:765-771.
19. Debaene B, Plaud B, Dilly MP, Donati F. Residual paralysis in the PACU after a single intubating dose of nondepolarizing muscle relaxant with an intermediate duration of action. *Anesthesiology*. 2003;98:1042-1048.
20. Naguib M, Kopman AF, Ensor JE. Neuromuscular monitoring and postoperative residual curarisation: a meta-analysis. *Br J Anaesth*. 2007;98:302-316.
21. Murphy GS, Szokol JW, Marymont JH, Greenberg SB, Avram MJ, Vender JS. Residual neuromuscular blockade and critical respiratory events in the postanesthesia care unit. *Anesth Analg*. 2008;107:130-137.
22. Brull SJ, Naguib M, Miller RD. Residual neuromuscular block: rediscovering the obvious. *Anesth Analg*. 2008;107:11-14.
23. Hughes JR. Post-tetanic potentiation. *Physiol Rev*. 1958;38:91-113.
24. Naguib M, Flood P, McArdle JJ, Brenner HR. Advances in neurobiology of the neuromuscular junction: implications for the anesthesiologist. *Anesthesiology*. 2002;96:202-231.
25. Rosenberry TL. Acetylcholinesterase. *Adv Enzymol Relat Areas Mol Biol*. 1975;43:103-218.
26. Sussman JL, Harel M, Frolow F, et al. Atomic structure of acetylcholinesterase from Torpedo californica: a prototypic acetylcholine-binding protein. *Science*. 1991;253:872-879.
27. Nolte HJ, Rosenberry TL, Neumann E. Effective charge on acetylcholinesterase active sites determined from the ionic strength dependence of association rate constants with cationic ligands. *Biochemistry*. 1980;19:3705-3711.
28. Zhou HX, Wlodek ST, McCammon JA. Conformation gating as a mechanism for enzyme specificity. *Proc Natl Acad Sci U S A*. 1998;95:9280-9283.
29. Cresnar B, Crne-Finderle N, Breskvar K, Sketelj J. Neural regulation of muscle acetylcholinesterase is exerted on the level of its mRNA. *J Neurosci Res*. 1994;38:294-299.
30. Hall ZW, Sanes JR. Synaptic structure and development: the neuromuscular junction. *Cell*. 1993; 72(suppl):99-121.
31. Blondet B, Carpentier G, Ferry A, Chatonnet A, José C. Localization of butyrylcholinesterase at the neuromuscular junction of normal and acetylcholinesterase knockout mice. *J Histochem Cytochem*. 2010;58:1075-1082.

32. Duysen EG, Stribley JA, Fry DL, Hinrichs SH, Lockridge O. Rescue of the acetylcholinesterase knockout mouse by feeding a liquid diet; phenotype of the adult acetylcholinesterase deficient mouse. *Brain Res Dev Brain Res*. 2002;137:43-54.
33. Bartkowski RR. Incomplete reversal of pancuronium neuromuscular blockade by neostigmine, pyridostigmine, and edrophonium. *Anesth Analg*. 1987;66:594-598.
34. Beemer GH, Goonetilleke PH, Bjorksten AR. The maximum depth of an atracurium neuromuscular block antagonized by edrophonium to effect adequate recovery. *Anesthesiology*. 1995;82:852-858.
35. Payne JP, Hughes R, Al Azawi S. Neuromuscular blockade by neostigmine in anaesthetized man. *Br J Anaesth*. 1980;52:69-76.
36. Cronnelly R, Stanski DR, Miller RD, Sheiner LB, Sohn YJ. Renal function and the pharmacokinetics of neostigmine in anesthetized man. *Anesthesiology*. 1979;51:222-226.
37. Cronnelly R, Stanski DR, Miller RD, Sheiner LB. Pyridostigmine kinetics with and without renal function. *Clin Pharmacol Ther*. 1980;28:78-81.
38. Morris RB, Cronnelly R, Miller RD, Stanski DR, Fahey MR. Pharmacokinetics of edrophonium in anephric and renal transplant patients. *Br J Anaesth*. 1981;53:1311-1314.
39. Morris RB, Cronnelly R, Miller RD, Stanski DR, Fahey MR. Pharmacokinetics of edrophonium and neostigmine when antagonizing d-tubocurarine neuromuscular blockade in man. *Anesthesiology*. 1981;54:399-401.
40. Bom A, Bradley M, Cameron K, et al. A novel concept of reversing neuromuscular block: chemical encapsulation of rocuronium bromide by a cyclodextrin-based synthetic host. *Angew Chem*. 2002;41:266-270.
41. Adam JM, Bennett DJ, Bom A, et al. Cyclodextrin-derived host molecules as reversal agents for the neuromuscular blocker rocuronium bromide: synthesis and structure-activity relationships. *J Med Chem*. 2002;45:1806-1816.
42. Tarver GJ, Grove SJ, Buchanan K, et al. 2-O-substituted cyclodextrins as reversal agents for the neuromuscular blocker rocuronium bromide. *Bioorg Med Chem*. 2002;10:1819-1827.
43. Cameron KS, Clark JK, Cooper A, et al. Modified gamma-cyclodextrins and their rocuronium complexes. *Org Lett*. 2002;4:3403-3406.
44. Zhang MQ. Drug-specific cyclodextrins: the future of rapid neuromuscular block reversal? *Drugs Future*. 2003;28:347-354.
45. Gijsenbergh F, Ramael S, Houwing N, van Iersel T. First human exposure of Org 25969, a novel agent to reverse the action of rocuronium bromide. *Anesthesiology*. 2005;103:695-703.
46. Sorgenfrei IF, Norrild K, Larsen PB, et al. Reversal of rocuronium-induced neuromuscular block by the selective relaxant binding agent sugammadex: a dose-finding and safety study. *Anesthesiology*. 2006; 104:667-674.
47. McDonagh DL, Benedict PE, Kovac AL, et al. Efficacy, safety, and pharmacokinetics of sugammadex for the reversal of rocuronium-induced neuromuscular blockade in elderly patients. *Anesthesiology*. 2011; 114:318-329.
48. Sparr HJ, Vermeyen KM, Beaufort AM, et al. Early reversal of profound rocuronium-induced neuromuscular blockade by sugammadex in a randomized multicenter study: efficacy, safety, and pharmacokinetics. *Anesthesiology*. 2007;106:935-943.
49. Epemolu O, Bom A, Hope F, Mason R. Reversal of neuromuscular blockade and simultaneous increase in plasma rocuronium concentration after the intravenous infusion of the novel reversal agent Org 25969. *Anesthesiology*. 2003;99:632-637.
50. Savarese JJ, Ali HH, Basta SJ, et al. The clinical neuromuscular pharmacology of mivacurium chloride (BW B1090U). A short-acting nondepolarizing ester neuromuscular blocking drug. *Anesthesiology*. 1988; 68:723-732.
51. Caldwell JE, Robertson EN, Baird WL. Antagonism of vecuronium and atracurium: comparison of neostigmine and edrophonium administered at 5% twitch height recovery. *Br J Anaesth*. 1987;59:478-481.
52. Berg H, Roed J, Viby-Mogensen J, et al. Residual neuromuscular block is a risk factor for postoperative pulmonary complications. A prospective, randomised, and blinded study of postoperative pulmonary complications after atracurium, vecuronium and pancuronium. *Acta Anaesthesiol Scand*. 1997;41:1095-1103.
53. Bevan DR, Smith CE, Donati F. Postoperative neuromuscular blockade: a comparison between atracurium, vecuronium, and pancuronium. *Anesthesiology*. 1988;69:272-276.
54. O'Hara DA, Fragen RJ, Shanks CA. Reappearance of the train-of-four after neuromuscular blockade induced with tubocurarine, vecuronium or atracurium. *Br J Anaesth*. 1986;58:1296-1299.
55. Donati F, Smith CE, Bevan DR. Dose-response relationships for edrophonium and neostigmine as antagonists of moderate and profound atracurium blockade. *Anesth Analg*. 1989;68:13-19.

56. Dhonneur G, Rebaine C, Slavov V, Ruggier R, De Chaubry V, Duvaldestin P. Neostigmine reversal of vecuronium neuromuscular block and the influence of renal failure. *Anesth Analg*. 1996;82:134-138.
57. Brull SJ, Murphy GS. Residual neuromuscular block: lessons unlearned. Part II: Methods to reduce the risk of residual weakness. *Anesth Analg*. 2010;111:129-140.
58. Cronnelly R, Morris RB, Miller RD. Edrophonium: duration of action and atropine requirement in humans during halothane anesthesia. *Anesthesiology*. 1982;57:261-266.
59. Miller RD, Van Nyhuis LS, Eger EI II, Vitez TS, Way WL. Comparative times to peak effect and durations of action of neostigmine and pyridostigmine. *Anesthesiology*. 1974;41:27-33.
60. Rupp SM, McChristian JW, Miller RD, Taboada JA, Cronnelly R. Neostigmine and edrophonium antagonism of varying intensity neuromuscular blockade induced by atracurium, pancuronium, or vecuronium. *Anesthesiology*. 1986;64:711-717.
61. Naguib M, Abdulatif M, al-Ghamdi A. Dose-response relationships for edrophonium and neostigmine antagonism of rocuronium bromide (ORG 9426)-induced neuromuscular blockade. *Anesthesiology*. 1993;9:739-745.
62. Naguib M, Riad W. Dose-response relationships for edrophonium and neostigmine antagonism of atracurium and cisatracurium-induced neuromuscular block. *Can J Anaesth*. 2000;47:1074-1081.
63. Naguib M, Abdulatif M, al-Ghamdi A, Hamo I, Nouheid R. Dose-response relationships for edrophonium and neostigmine antagonism of mivacurium-induced neuromuscular block. *Br J Anaesth*. 1993;71:709-714.
64. Naguib M, Abdulatif M. Priming with anti-cholinesterases–the effect of different combinations of anti-cholinesterases and different priming intervals. *Can J Anaesth*. 1988;35:47-52.
65. Jones JE, Hunter JM, Utting JE. Use of neostigmine in the antagonism of residual neuromuscular blockade produced by vecuronium. *Br J Anaesth*. 1987;59:1454-1458.
66. Harper NJ, Wallace M, Hall IA. Optimum dose of neostigmine at two levels of atracurium-induced neuromuscular block. *Br J Anaesth*. 1994;72:82-85.
67. Magorian TT, Lynam DP, Caldwell JE, Miller RD. Can early administration of neostigmine, in single or repeated doses, alter the course of neuromuscular recovery from a vecuronium-induced neuromuscular blockade? *Anesthesiology*. 1990;73:410-414.
68. Engbaek J, Ording H, Ostergaard D, Viby-Mogensen J. Edrophonium and neostigmine for reversal of the neuromuscular blocking effect of vecuronium. *Acta Anaesthesiol Scand*. 1985;29:544-546.
69. Fisher DM, Cronnelly R, Sharma M, Miller RD. Clinical pharmacology of edrophonium in infants and children. *Anesthesiology*. 1984;61:428-433.
70. Gencarelli PJ, Miller RD. Antagonism of org NC 45 (vecuronium) and pancuronium neuromuscular blockade by neostigmine. *Br J Anaesth*. 1982;54:53-56.
71. Kopman AF, Kopman DJ, Ng J, Zank LM. Antagonism of profound cisatracurium and rocuronium block: the role of objective assessment of neuromuscular function. *J Clin Anesth*. 2005;17:30-35.
72. Lessard MR, Trepanier CA, Rouillard JF. Neostigmine requirements for reversal of neuromuscular blockade following an infusion of mivacurium. *Can J Anaesth*. 1997;44:836-842.
73. Saitoh Y, Toyooka H, Amaha K. Recoveries of post-tetanic twitch and train-of-four responses after administration of vecuronium with different inhalation anaesthetics and neuroleptanaesthesia. *Br J Anaesth*. 1993;70:402-404.
74. Miller RD, Way WL, Dolan WM, Stevens WC, Eger EI II. The dependence of pancuronium- and d-tubocurarine-induced neuromuscular blockades on alveolar concentrations of halothane and forane. *Anesthesiology*. 1972;37:573-581.
75. Miller RD, Crique M, Eger EI II. Duration of halothane anesthesia and neuromuscular blockade with d-tubocurarine. *Anesthesiology*. 1976;44:206-210.
76. Kelly RE, Lien CA, Savarese JJ, et al. Depression of neuromuscular function in a patient during desflurane anesthesia. *Anesth Analg*. 1993;76:868-871.
77. Rupp SM, Miller RD, Gencarelli PJ. Vecuronium-induced neuromuscular blockade during enflurane, isoflurane, and halothane anesthesia in humans. *Anesthesiology*. 1984;60:102-105.
78. Gencarelli PJ, Miller RD, Eger EI II, Newfield P. Decreasing enflurane concentrations and d-tubocurarine neuromuscular blockade. *Anesthesiology*. 1982;56:192-194.
79. Morita T, Tsukagoshi H, Sugaya T, Saito S, Sato H, Fujita T. Inadequate antagonism of vecuronium-induced neuromuscular block by neostigmine during sevoflurane or isoflurane anesthesia. *Anesth Analg*. 1995;80:1175-1180.
80. Reid JE, Breslin DS, Mirakhur RK, Hayes AH. Neostigmine antagonism of rocuronium block during anesthesia with sevoflurane, isoflurane or propofol. *Can J Anaesth*. 2001;48:351-355.
81. Lowry DW, Mirakhur RK, McCarthy GJ, Carroll MT, McCourt KC. Neuromuscular effects of rocuronium

during sevoflurane, isoflurane, and intravenous anesthesia. *Anesth Analg*. 1998;87:936-940.
82. Baurain MJ, d'Hollander AA, Melot C, Dernovoi BS, Barvais L. Effects of residual concentrations of isoflurane on the reversal of vecuronium-induced neuromuscular blockade. *Anesthesiology*. 1991;74:474-478.
83. Naguib M. Sugammadex: another milestone in clinical neuromuscular pharmacology. Anesth Analg. 2007;104:575-581.
84. Shields M, Giovannelli M, Mirakhur RK, Moppett I, Adams J, Hermens Y. Org 25969 (sugammadex), a selective relaxant binding agent for antagonism of prolonged rocuronium-induced neuromuscular block. *Br J Anaesth*. 2006;96:36-43.
85. Suy K, Morias K, Cammu G, et al. Effective reversal of moderate rocuronium- or vecuronium-induced neuromuscular block with sugammadex, a selective relaxant binding agent. *Anesthesiology*. 2007;106:283-288.
86. Groudine SB, Soto R, Lien C, Drover D, Roberts K. A randomized, dose-finding, phase II study of the selective relaxant binding drug, sugammadex, capable of safely reversing profound rocuronium-induced neuromuscular block. *Anesth Analg*. 2007;104:555-562.
87. de Boer HD, Driessen JJ, Marcus MA, Kerkkamp H, Heeringa M, Klimek M. Reversal of rocuronium-induced (1.2 mg/kg) profound neuromuscular block by sugammadex: a multicenter, dose-finding and safety study. *Anesthesiology*. 2007;107:239-244.
88. Puhringer FK, Rex C, Sielenkamper AW, et al. Reversal of profound, high-dose rocuronium-induced neuromuscular blockade by sugammadex at two different time points: an international, multicenter, randomized, dose-finding, safety assessor-blinded, phase II trial. *Anesthesiology*. 2008;109:188-197.
89. Flockton EA, Mastronardi P, Hunter JM, et al. Reversal of rocuronium-induced neuromuscular block with sugammadex is faster than reversal of cisatracurium-induced block with neostigmine. *Br J Anaesth*. 2008;100:622-630.
90. Lee C, Jahr JS, Candiotti KA, Warriner B, Zornow MH, Naguib M. Reversal of profound neuromuscular block by sugammadex administered three minutes after rocuronium: a comparison with spontaneous recovery from succinylcholine. *Anesthesiology*. 2009;110:1020-1025.
91. de Boer HD, van Egmond J, van de Pol F, Bom A, Booij LH. Sugammadex, a new reversal agent for neuromuscular block induced by rocuronium in the anaesthetized Rhesus monkey. *Br J Anaesth*. 2006;96:473-479.
92. Waud BE, Waud DR. The relation between tetanic fade and receptor occlusion in the presence of competitive neuromuscular block. *Anesthesiology*. 1971;35:456-464.
93. Naguib M. Different priming techniques, including mivacurium, accelerate the onset of rocuronium. *Can J Anaesth*. 1994;41:902-907.
94. Naguib M, Abdulatif M, Selim M, al-Ghamdi A. Dose-response studies of the interaction between mivacurium and suxamethonium. *Br J Anaesth*. 1995;74 26-30.
95. Bom AH, Hope F. A higher than required dose of sugammadex prevents the creation of a situation similar to "priming." *Anesthesiology*. 2007:A989.
96. Sunew KY, Hicks RG. Effects of neostigmine and pyridostigmine on duration of succinylcholine action and pseudocholinesterase activity. *Anesthesiology*. 1978;49:188-191.
97. Suresh D, Carter JA, Whitehead JP, Goldhill DR, Flynn PJ. Cardiovascular changes at antagonism of atracurium. Effects of different doses of premixed neostigmine and glycopyrronium in a ratio of 5:1. Anaesthesia. 1991;46:877-880.
98. Bowman WC. *Pharmacology of Neuromuscular Function*. 2nd ed. London: Butterworth-Heinemann; 1990.
99. Salem MG, Richardson JC, Meadows GA, Lamplugh G, Lai KM. Comparison between glycopyrrolate and atropine in a mixture with neostigmine for reversal of neuromuscular blockade. Studies in patients following open heart surgery. *Br J Anaesth*. 1985;57:184-187.
100. van Vlymen JM, Parlow JL. The effects of reversal of neuromuscular blockade on autonomic control in the perioperative period. *Anesth Analg*. 1997;84:148-154.
101. Ding Y, Fredman B, White PF. Use of mivacurium during laparoscopic surgery: effect of reversal drugs on postoperative recovery. *Anesth Analg*. 1994;78:450-454.
102. Boeke AJ, de Lange JJ, van Druenen B, Langemeijer JJ. Effect of antagonizing residual neuromuscular block by neostigmine and atropine on postoperative vomiting. *Br J Anaesth*. 1994;72:654-656.
103. Hovorka J, Korttila K, Nelskyla K, et al. Reversal of neuromuscular blockade with neostigmine has no effect on the incidence or severity of postoperative nausea and vomiting. *Anesth Analg*. 1997;85: 1359-1361.
104. Viby-Mogensen J, Jorgensen BC, Ording H. Residual curarization in the recovery room. *Anesthesiology*. 1979;50:539-541.

105. Fuchs-Buder T, Tassonyi E. Magnesium sulphate enhances residual neuromuscular block induced by vecuronium. *Br J Anaesth*. 1996;76:565-566.
106. Naguib M. Sugammadex may replace best clinical practice: a misconception. *Anesth Analg*. 2007;105:1506-1507.
107. Eleveld DJ, Kuizenga K, Proost JH, Wierda JM. A temporary decrease in twitch response during reversal of rocuronium-induced muscle relaxation with a small dose of sugammadex. *Anesth Analg*. 2007;104:582-584.
108. Duvaldestin P, Kuizenga K, Saldien V, et al. A randomized, dose-response study of sugammadex given for the reversal of deep rocuronium- or vecuronium-induced neuromuscular blockade under sevoflurane anesthesia. *Anesth Analg*. 2010;110:74-82.
109. Menendez-Ozcoidi L, Ortiz-Gomez JR, Olaguibel-Ribero JM, Salvador-Bravo MJ. Allergy to low dose sugammadex. *Anaesthesia*. 2011;66:217-219.
110. Munro IC, Newberne PM, Young VR, Bar A. Safety assessment of [gamma]-cyclodextrin. *Regul Toxicol Pharmaco*l. 2004;39:3-13.

CHAPTER 11

Perioperative Pain Adjuncts

Daniel Gammon, MD, and Byron Bankhead, MD

INTRODUCTION

Perioperative pain control remains one of the primary concerns for surgical patients, surgeons, and anesthesiologists. Traditionally, opiates have been the medications used for the treatment of perioperative pain. However, as our knowledge of molecular nociception has expanded, it has become apparent that multiple receptor subtypes are involved in the neurochemical basis for pain (Figure 11–1). As perioperative physicians, anesthesiologists exploit this knowledge by using pharmacologic agents in addition to opiates to control surgical pain.

This multimodal approach to perioperative pain control has gained popularity. Common perioperative pain adjuncts include ketamine, gabapentin, pregabalin, clonidine, and dexmedetomidine, neuraxial blocks, peripheral nerve blocks, systemic nonsteroidal anti-inflammatory drugs, tricyclic antidepressants, and local anesthetics.

In addition to opiate-sparing effects, adjuncts may be useful in 2 clinical scenarios: (1) achieving safe and effective analgesia for the opiate tolerant surgical patient, and (2) reducing patients' risk of having chronic postsurgical pain syndromes after undergoing procedures that place them at risk for chronic pain.

Opiate-Tolerant Surgical Patients

The recent increased interest in multimodal pain control is in part a consequence of the steady rise in opiate use since the late 1990s. A review examining the trends of opiate use in the United States from 1997 to 2007 revealed some alarming trends.[1] While constituting only 4.6% of the world's total population in 2007, Americans were consuming 80% of the global prescription opioid supply. The average sale of opioids per person in the United States increased 402% from 1997 to 2007. Opiate use, both prescribed and illicit, may be more prevalent in surgical patients than these numbers suggest.

In tolerant patients, opiates used to treat surgical pain are less effective and potentially more dangerous, because patients often require excessive doses to achieve analgesia that are associated with adverse effects in opioid-naive patients. Thus, the benefits of pain control adjuncts are of particular interest to perioperative physicians. The evidence regarding the use of these agents in opiate-tolerant surgical patients will be discussed below.

Prevention of Chronic Pain

There is evidence that perioperative pain adjuncts may aid in the prevention of chronic postsurgical pain. Certain surgeries, such as thoracotomies and limb amputations, can produce chronic pain syndromes in as many as 30% to 50% of patients who undergo these procedures.[2] The limited data pertaining to the use of pain control adjuncts for the prevention of chronic pain syndromes after surgery will be reviewed for selected agents.

KETAMINE

History of Development

Ketamine was invented in the early 1960s as part of an effort to find a safer alternative to phencyclidine for the induction of anesthesia. It was first given to humans in 1963.[3] As an anesthetic agent, it was unique in many ways. In doses of 1 to 2 mg/kg, it produced general anesthesia with minimal respiratory depression and often caused tachycardia and hypertension. Ketamine was commonly used

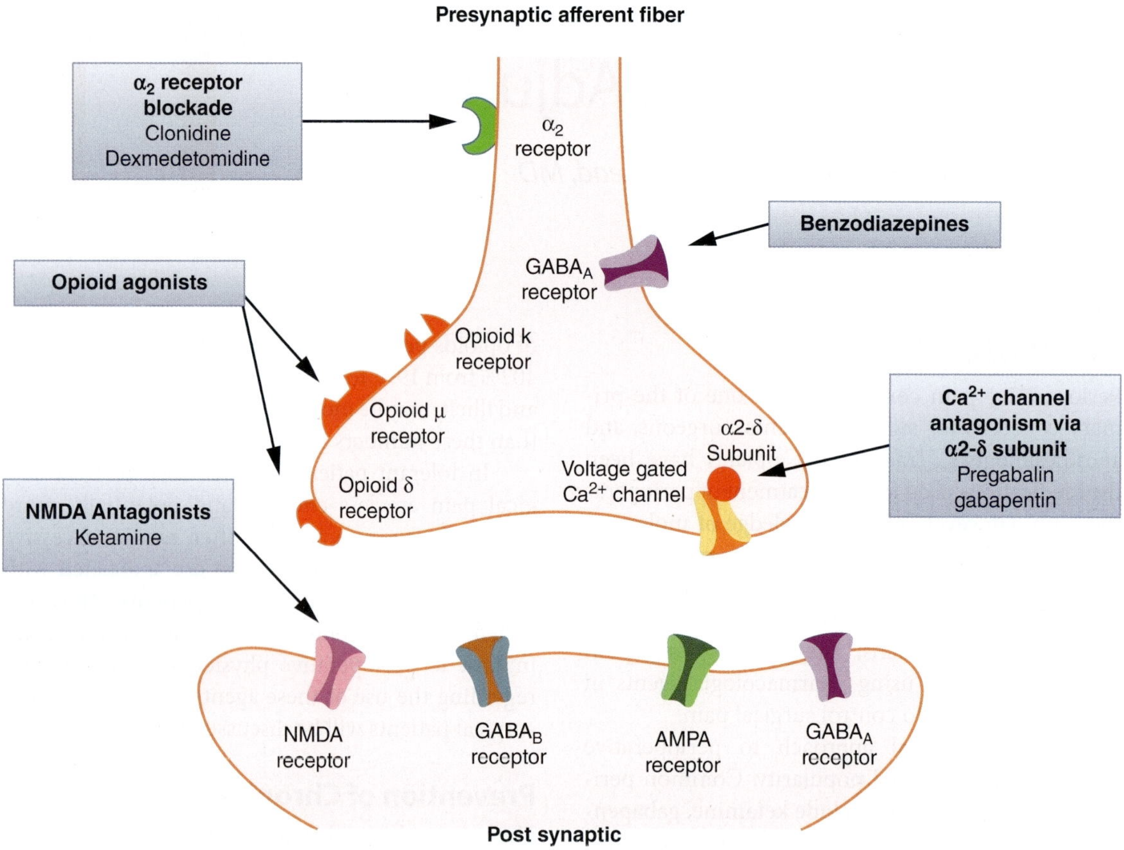

FIGURE 11–1 Schematic representation of the various receptor subtypes present on nociceptive neurons. AMPA, -amino-3-hydroxyl-5-methyl-4-isoxazole-propionate; GABA, γ-aminobutyric acid; NMDA, *N*-methyl-D-aspartate.

as an induction agent, but its tendency to cause dysphoria and hallucinations in large doses made it unpopular. Ketamine was supplanted first by thiopental and then by propofol as a routine induction agent for humans. In addition to ketamine's current use as a perioperative pain adjunct, ketamine is also used today for sedation of pediatric and burn patients, as a secondary treatment for bronchospasm, and as an agent for the induction of anesthesia in patients with decompensated hemorrhagic or septic shock.

Mechanism of Action

Ketamine is primarily a *N*-methyl D-aspartate (NMDA) receptor antagonist. NMDA receptors are ion channels that have excitatory properties. Specifically, it is a noncompetitive NMDA receptor calcium channel pore antagonist and also interacts with phencyclidine (PCP) binding sites that inhibit NMDA receptor function.[4] It also interacts with selected opioid receptors (μ, δ, and κ), muscarinic receptors, voltage-gated calcium channels, and monoaminergic receptors.[4] As a pain adjunct, ketamine reduces both nociceptive and opioid-based hyperalgesia, likely at the spinal cord level.[5] It has S and R enantiomers, both of which are pharmacologically active and can produce anesthesia, dysphoria, analgesia, and dissociation.[3] The S enantiomer is up to 3 times as analgesic as the R enantiomer. At high doses, ketamine also behaves as a local anesthetic by blocking sodium channels in a comparable fashion to lidocaine or procaine.[6]

In addition to its acute effects, perioperative ketamine may reduce pain over prolonged periods of time.[7] Preliminary work indicates that when administered to chronic pain patients, some feel relief with ketamine for up to 24 hours after receiving ketamine while others do not. The mechanism is not well defined.

Kinetics and Metabolism

Onset of Action

In general, ketamine has a rapid onset of effect, reaching peak effect-site concentrations within 5 minutes of a bolus dose. Because ketamine is often prepared as a racemic mixture and has active metabolites, it is difficult to truly characterize its pharmacokinetics and even more so its pharmacodynamics. Pharmacokinetic models exist but are only able to predict plasma concentrations of ketamine and its metabolites. Effect-site concentrations and predictions of drug effect are difficult to estimate given that drug effect can be from either the parent drug, its metabolites, or both.

Intravenous ketamine has a short α and β half-life, approximately 7 minutes and 2 to 4 hours, respectively, when given as a bolus. Consider the simulation of a low-dose intravenous bolus, 0.2 mg/kg, typical of ketamine use as an adjunct. It reaches peak effect-site concentrations (near 0.4 mcg/mL) within 5 minutes and then has a relatively slow decline in concentration (Figure 11–2). With bolus dosing, ketamine rapidly distributes to peripheral tissues (the initial rapid drop in concentration) followed by a redistribution from peripheral tissues back into the plasma and secondarily by hepatic biotransformation.[8] As a continuous infusion, ketamine's kinetic profile is described as an initial rapid rise in effect-site concentrations followed by a long, slow rise to reach near steady-state conditions. A typical continuous infusion–dosing scheme for ketamine used as an adjunct (0.2 mg/kg/h) is presented in Figure 11–3. In this simulation, the effect-site concentrations from a 2- and 8-hour infusion illustrate the slow rise to near steady-state concentrations (ie, not much change in concentration over time). Peak plasma concentrations for the 2- and 8-hour infusion are 0.15 and 0.2 mcg/mL respectively. Also of note with ketamine is its notable back-end kinetics.

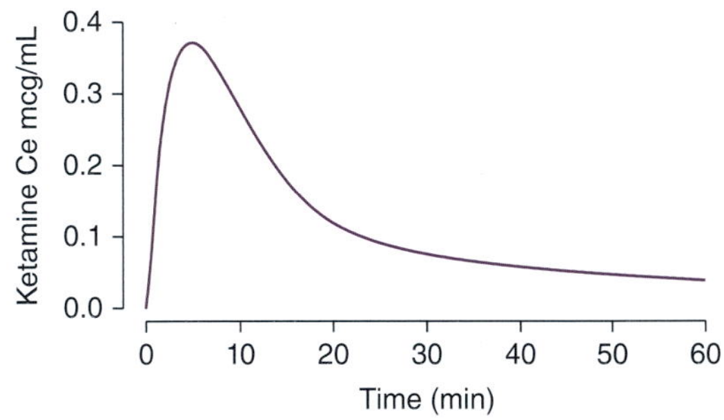

FIGURE 11–2 Simulation of an induction bolus dose of ketamine (1 mg/kg) to a 100-kg, 183-cm male. Concentrations were predicted using previously published pharmacokinetic parameters. Ce, effect-site concentration. (Ihmsen H, Geisslinger G, Schuttler J. Stereoselective pharmacokinetics of ketamine: R(–)-ketamine inhibits the elimination of S(+)-ketamine. *Clin Pharmacol Ther.* 2001;70(5):431-438; Persson J. The ketamine enigma. *Acta Anaesthesiol Scand.* 2008;52(4):453-455; Persson J, Hasselstrom J, Maurset A, et al. Pharmacokinetics and non-analgesic effects of S- and R-ketamines in healthy volunteers with normal and reduced metabolic capacity. *Eur J Clin Pharmacol.* 2002;57(12):869-875; and Voss, LJ, Baas CH, Hansson L, Steyn-Ross DA, Steyn-Ross M, Sleigh JW. Investigation into the effect of the general anaesthetics etomidate and ketamine on long-range coupling of population activity in the mouse neocortical slice. *Eur J Pharmacol.* 2012;689(1-3):111-117). Simulation limitations: ketamine is an enantiomer and has active metabolites. This simulation does not account for differences between R and S isomers, which are known to have different pharmacologic properties (White PF, Schuttler J, Shafer A, et al. Comparative pharmacology of the ketamine isomers. Studies in volunteers. *Br J Anaesth.* 1985;57(2):197-203) nor does it account for the active ketamine metabolite, norketamine.

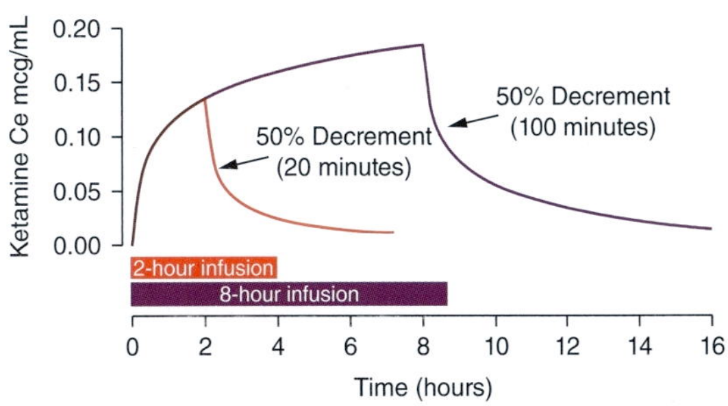

FIGURE 11–3 Simulation of a continuous ketamine infusion (0.2 mg/kg/h) to a 100-kg, 183-cm male. The 50% decrement time was calculated as the time required for the effect-site concentration (Ce) to decrease by 50% once the infusion was terminated.

Following 2- and 8-hour infusions, its context sensitive half-time ranges from 20 to 100 minutes. Thus, for long infusions, patients may have persistent effect-site concentrations well into their recovery period.

Metabolism

Ketamine is metabolized by hepatic microsomal enzymes cytochrome P CYP3A4, and to a lesser extent by CYP2B6 and CYP2C9, into pharmacologically active metabolites, primarily norketamine and to a lesser extent dehydronorketamine. The S enantiomer of ketamine is more rapidly metabolized than the R enantiomer.[9] The kidney excretes 90% of ketamine metabolites. Ketamine and its metabolites are 50% to 70% protein bound.[10]

Dosing Regimens

Ketamine is commercially available under multiple names (Ketalar, Ketaject, Ketaset, Vetalar) and comes prepared as a hydrochloride salt in doses of 10 or 100 mg/mL. As a pain adjunct, ketamine can be administered via intravenous and intramuscular routes.

A wide range of dosing strategies has been studied. Common dosing regimens include a preincision 0.1- to 0.5-mg/kg bolus followed by repeated hourly intraoperative 0.1- to 0.3-mg/kg boluses or a 0.1- to 0.5-mg/kg/h infusion. Postoperative ketamine administered as a continuous infusion or via patient-controlled analgesia has also been studied.[11] Interestingly, a Cochrane meta-analysis review of ketamine as a perioperative pain adjunct reported a ceiling to the morphine-sparing effect for ketamine; doses of ketamine greater than 0.5 mg/kg over the first 24 hours did not result in additional opiate sparing.

Indications

The US Food and Drug Administration (FDA) has approved ketamine for induction and maintenance of general anesthesia but not as a perioperative pain adjunct. Perioperative subanesthetic doses of intravenous ketamine, administered as boluses or as continuous infusions, represent an off-label application. Epidural ketamine has been studied as a pain adjunct but does not have FDA approval. Spinal administration is not recommended given potential concerns for neurotoxicity.

Low-dose ketamine has little to no hemodynamic effect. The effect of low-dose ketamine on the minimum alveolar concentration (MAC) of volatile anesthetics is unknown. From the author's personal experience, intravenous ketamine given in doses exceeding 0.5 mg/kg intraoperatively or given as a bolus near the end of a general anesthetic may delay emergence from anesthesia, particularly in the opiate-naive patient.

While the intraoperative effects of low-dose ketamine may be subtle, the postoperative effects of subanesthetic ketamine are more pronounced. A Cochrane meta-analysis showed that perioperative ketamine administration decreased rescue analgesic requirements over the first 24 hours by an average of 30% to 50%.[11] Ketamine may also suppress hyperalgesia after high-dose intraoperative opiate infusions.[4]

Despite these apparent advantages, the Cochran review did not demonstrate a reduction in postoperative acute pain scores with low-dose ketamine.[11-13] This may be attributed to the subjectivity of pain scoring systems used and the heterogeneity of studies included in the meta-analyses. Anecdotal experience suggests that perioperative ketamine may improve a patient's satisfaction with pain management, even if the reported pain scores (Visual Analog Score [VAS]) remain unchanged.

Although ketamine as a pain adjunct has been extensively studied, only a few studies have explored its effectiveness in managing perioperative pain in opiate-dependent patients. Most notably, Loftus et al found that a preincision of 0.5 mg/kg bolus followed by an intraoperative continuous infusion of 10 mcg/kg/min in opiate-tolerant surgical patients undergoing spine surgery reduced morphine use by 30% over the first 48 hours following surgery. This study also reported that this regimen reduced pain scores by 25% in the postanesthesia care unit.[14]

Some investigators have explored the use of ketamine to minimize the risk of developing chronic pain after surgery. Whether ketamine directly or indirectly, via its opiate-sparing and hyperalgesia-reducing effects, lowers the risk of developing chronic postsurgical pain is unknown.

For example, in a randomized study of patients undergoing total hip arthroplasty, one group received a 0.5-mg/kg bolus prior to incision followed by a 24-hour ketamine infusion of 2 mcg/kg/min. A second group received a saline bolus and infusion. The ketamine group used fewer opiates over the first 24 hours and reported less pain in the operative hip at both 30 days and 180 days postoperatively.[15] Subanesthetic doses of intravenous ketamine used in patients undergoing surgery for rectal adenocarcinoma produced similar reductions in pain scores even at 12 months postoperatively but only in the patients who received intraoperative total intravenous ketamine doses that exceeded 0.5 mg/kg.[13] Lastly, the Loftus study of perioperative ketamine for opiate-tolerant patients undergoing complex spine surgery not only demonstrated the acute pain benefits mentioned above but also showed patients in the ketamine arm had reduced pain scores at the 6-week postoperative visit.[14]

Limited data regarding perioperative ketamine for the prevention of chronic pain in other high-risk surgical patients has not shown benefit. Perioperative ketamine has been specifically studied for the prevention of chronic pain after thoracotomy and limb amputation, and it failed to reduce the incidence of chronic postoperative pain following these procedures.[16,17]

Adverse Effects

Ketamine is well known for its psychomimetic adverse effects. For example, large bolus doses of 1 to 2 mg/kg of intravenous ketamine produce dysphoria, emergence delirium, or hallucinations in 30% of patients.[3] However, with low-dose ketamine (< 0.5 mg/kg), adverse psychomimetic effects are uncommon, although sedation on emergence and diplopia may occur.[11] The incidence of postoperative nausea and vomiting was reduced with ketamine in studies that specifically measured that end point.

Contraindications

No known contraindications exist for low-dose ketamine. However, possible risks of increased sympathetic tone, increased intracranial pressure from cerebral vasodilation, and increased emergence delirium must be weighed against the potential benefits of using low-dose ketamine to improve perioperative pain control.

GABAPENTIN AND PREGABALIN

History of Development

Gabapentin and pregabalin are lipophilic γ-aminobutyric acid (GABA) analogs and were initially developed as anticonvulsant drugs. Through various case reports in the 1990s and early 2000s, both drugs were found to have analgesic properties. Further studies proved that these drugs were particularly useful for the treatment of neuropathic pain. Consequently, gabapentin received FDA approval in 2002 for the treatment of postherpetic neuralgia, and pregabalin received FDA approval in 2004 for the treatment of pain associated with diabetic peripheral neuropathy as well as for postherpetic neuralgia. In 2007, pregabalin became the first drug specifically approved by the FDA for the treatment of fibromyalgia.[18]

Mechanism of Action

Although gabapentin and pregabalin are structurally derived from the inhibitory neurotransmitter GABA, they do not directly bind to GABA receptors in the central nervous system. Instead, they bind to the α-2-δ subunit of voltage-dependent calcium channels in the periphery, spinal cord, and brain. The resultant decrease in calcium influx reduces the release of several neurotransmitters, including glutamate, norepinephrine, dopamine, and serotonin.[19] It is through this α-2-δ calcium channel mechanism that gabapentin and pregabalin are thought to exert their anticonvulsant, anxiolytic, and analgesic effects.

Kinetics and Metabolism

Onset of Action

Gabapentin is maximally absorbed through the gastrointestinal tract 3 hours after ingestion. Its oral bioavailability after a single dose of 300 to 600 mg is approximately 50%. This absorption is limited by a saturable, dose-dependent active transport mechanism, such that the percentage of the drug that is bioavailable decreases with increasing doses. Onset of action following consumption by mouth is within 1 to 3 hours. It is less than 3% protein bound with a volume of distribution of 0.6 L/kg.

Pregabalin is rapidly absorbed through the gastrointestinal tract, resulting in peak blood concentrations within 1 hour of ingestion. Bioavailability exceeds 90% and is independent of dose. Onset of action following consumption by mouth is also within 1 to 3 hours. It is not protein bound and has a volume of distribution of 0.5 L/kg. Pregabalin's elimination half-life ranges from 4 to 7 hours. It is important to note that pregabalin's binding affinity for the α-2-δ receptor is 6 times greater than that of gabapentin.[19]

Metabolism

Gabapentin is not metabolized, and instead is removed almost completely by renal excretion, with an elimination half-life of 5 to 9 hours.[20]

Pregabalin, like gabapentin, is not metabolized and is eliminated almost exclusively by renal excretion.

Dosing Regimens

Gabapentin exists as its brand name formulation, Neurontin, or as a generic equivalent. It is formulated in oral capsules and tablets, with strengths ranging from 100 to 800 mg per pill. An oral solution of 250 mg/5 mL is also available. As a perioperative pain adjunct, the appropriate dose for gabapentin is largely unknown. Investigational strategies using a single preoperative dose range from 300 to 1200 mg. Multidose studies have most commonly used 600 mg 3 times a day, beginning on the day of surgery and continuing until postoperative day 2 or 3.

Pregabalin can be found only as its brand name formulation, Lyrica. It is available in oral capsules, with strengths ranging from 25 to 300 mg per capsule. The appropriate dose for pregabalin as a perioperative pain adjunct is unknown. Investigational preoperative doses range from 75 to 600 mg, but single preoperative doses of 150 to 300 mg are most common.[20]

As described above, both gabapentin and pregabalin are eliminated almost exclusively by renal excretion. Consequently, both drugs should be given in decreased doses in patients with impaired creatinine clearance.

Indications

Gabapentin and pregabalin have been approved for the treatment of partial seizures and for a variety of chronic pain conditions. The administration of gabapentin or pregabalin as a perioperative adjunct for the treatment of acute pain constitutes an unlabeled use.

The intraoperative effects of preoperative gabapentin and pregabalin administration are largely unknown. These drugs appear to have little to no effect on intraoperative hemodynamics. No data on alterations of MAC with gabapentin or pregabalin exist. Limited data suggest that the addition of preoperative gabapentin at doses greater than 400 mg can partially blunt the sympathetic response to laryngoscopy.[20] No data on gabapentin's or pregabalin's effect on the timing of emergence from anesthesia exist.

The preoperative administration of gabapentin and pregabalin has a measurable opiate-sparing and analgesic effect postoperatively. Meta-analyses of perioperative gabapentin and pregabalin suggest their use results in a 20% to 60% reduction in opiate requirements over the first 24 hours postoperatively and a significant reduction of pain scores (Visual Analog Score; VAS).[21,22] There are also data to suggest that perioperative use of gabapentin and pregabalin reduces movement-evoked pain in the postoperative period, which may lead to accelerated postoperative functional recovery.

At present, there are no studies that specifically examine the effectiveness of using gabapentin or pregabalin to control perioperative pain in opiate-tolerant patients. Nevertheless, the analgesic and opiate-sparing effects of gabapentin and pregabalin make these drugs theoretically appealing for the management of opiate-tolerant surgical patients, especially because of the decreased analgesic benefit and narrowed therapeutic index of opiates in this patient population.

Several studies have shown gabapentin or pregabalin to be effective in reducing the risk of chronic pain after particular types of surgery. This has been demonstrated with gabapentin in patients undergoing hysterectomy, and with pregabalin in patients undergoing total knee arthroplasty, mastectomy, and lumbar discectomy.[23-25] However, a study in which a 30-day perioperative course of gabapentin was administered to patients having surgical limb amputations failed to show a reduction of stump pain and/or phantom limb pain at 3-month and 6-month follow-up appointments.[26] No other data that specifically pertains to the use of perioperative gabapentin or pregabalin for the prevention of chronic pain in high-risk surgery patients currently exist.

Adverse Effects

The long-term use of gabapentin and pregabalin is associated with somnolence and dizziness, with reported incidences as high as 25%.[20] These adverse effects are less common when gabapentin and pregabalin are used over a brief duration in the perioperative setting. The majority of the randomized control trials examining perioperative gabapentin or pregabalin show no difference in their side-effect profiles when compared to placebo.[20] A few perioperative trials did report more frequent sedation with gabapentin, and a single trial reported more frequent headache and dizziness with pregabalin.[20]

Contraindications

In their capacity as perioperative pain adjuncts, the contraindications for the use of gabapentin and pregabalin are not well defined. When deciding whether to use these medications, the small increased risk of sedation or other adverse effects must be weighed against the possible benefit of improved pain control for the individual patient.

CLONIDINE AND DEXMEDETOMIDINE

History of Development

Clonidine was first synthesized in 1965. It was used initially as a nasal decongestant and subsequently as an antihypertensive.[27] Over the past 4 decades, clonidine has been used for a wide variety of clinical applications, including the treatment of opiate withdrawal, prevention of myocardial ischemia, and as a pain adjunct. As an analgesic, clonidine has been administered intrathecally, epidurally, orally, topically, intramuscularly, and intravenously. It is also used as an additive to local anesthetics to enhance the duration and efficacy of peripheral nerve blocks.[27]

Dexmedetomidine is the pharmacologically active R enantiomer of medetomidine, a drug that has been used for decades in veterinary medicine as a sedative.[28] Dexmedetomidine differs from clonidine in its high-binding specificity for the α-2-adrenoreceptor. In 1999, the FDA approved the use of dexmedetomidine infusion for sedation in intubated patients in the intensive care unit.[28] Dexmedetomidine received FDA approval in 2008 for use in nonintubated patients as a sedative prior to and/or during surgery or other procedures.

Mechanism of Action

Clonidine and dexmedetomidine are α-2-adrenoreceptor agonist drugs that have sympatholytic, anxiolytic, and analgesic properties. Clonidine is a partial agonist, with an α-2–to–α-1 selectivity ratio of 39:1, while dexmedetomidine is a highly specific full agonist, with an α-2–to–α-1 selectivity ratio of 1600:1.[28] α-2-Adrenoreceptors are ubiquitous throughout the body, and can be found in the brain, the spinal cord, and the peripheral nerves. When clonidine and dexmedetomidine are given systemically, analgesic effects are due to α-2-adrenoreceptor agonism and the subsequent presynaptic inhibition of norepinephrine release that decreases sympathetic tone within the spinal cord.[28] The additional effects of sedation and anxiolysis are likely mediated through α-2-adrenoreceptor agonism in an area of the brain called the locus coeruleus.[27]

Kinetics and Metabolism

Onset of Action

Clonidine can be administered via a variety of routes to achieve analgesia; this section will focus on intravenous administration. Onset of action with intravenous dosing is rapid, within 5 minutes. Intravenous clonidine has an α half-life of 10 minutes from redistribution and a β half-life of 8 to 10 hours from elimination. It is between 20% and 40% protein bound and has a volume of distribution of 2 to 3 L/kg.

The onset of action of dexmedetomidine following a slow intravenous bolus (1 mcg/kg over 20 minutes) is within 5 minutes. Following an intravenous bolus, dexmedetomidine levels quickly rise but then fall slowly, with an α half-life of 6 minutes and a terminal β half-life of 2 hours from redistribution and elimination, respectively. It is 94% protein bound and has a volume of distribution of 1.6 L/kg.

When dosed as an infusion, dexmedetomidine exhibits linear kinetics in doses ranging from 0.2 to 0.7 mcg/kg/h and has a particularly long context sensitive half-life. Consider the simulation of a 2- and 8-hour infusion at 0.4 mcg/kg/h presented in Figure 11–4. Just after the infusion is started, there is a steep climb in plasma concentrations for the first 30 minutes, followed by a decrease in the rate of rise reaching a peak concentration of approximately 0.5 ng/mL. Even with the 8-hour infusion, however, plasma concentrations continue to rise, reaching a peak concentration of near 0.9 ng/mL. The context sensitive half-times (50% decrement times) for the 2 infusions are 20 and 200 minutes, respectively; this suggests that with long infusions, there is substantial tissue drug accumulation, which may lead to prolonged effect long after the infusion is terminated.

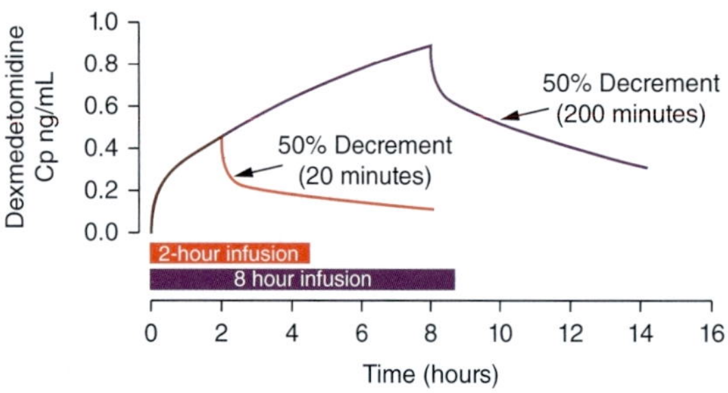

FIGURE 11–4 Simulation of a continuous dexmedetomidine infusion (0.4 mcg/kg/h) to a 100-kg, 183-cm male. Concentrations were predicted using previously published pharmacokinetic parameters (Dyck JB, Maze M, Haack C, Vuorilehto L, Shafer SL. The pharmacokinetics and hemodynamic effects of intravenous and intramuscular dexmedetomidine hydrochloride in adult human volunteers. *Anesthesiology*. 1993;78(5):813-820). The 50% decrement time was calculated as the time required for the plasma concentration (Cp) to decrease by 50% once the infusion was terminated.

Metabolism

Approximately 60% of clonidine is excreted in the urine unchanged, while the remaining 40% undergoes hepatic biotransformation (hepatic microsomal enzyme CYP2D6).

Dexmedetomidine undergoes almost complete hepatic biotransformation (hepatic microsomal enzyme CYP2D6) before urinary excretion.

Dosing Regimens

Clonidine can be given as oral tablets, transdermal patches, or injection (via the intramuscular, intravenous, epidural, and intrathecal routes). Intravenous clonidine is manufactured in 100 or 500 mcg/mL stock solutions, under the brand name Duraclon. Most studies of intravenous perioperative clonidine used preoperative bolus doses of 0.5 to 2 mcg/kg. However, the primary goal of using perioperative clonidine in these studies was to achieve anxiolysis or sedation, not analgesia.[29] Intravenous clonidine has also been given as a perioperative infusion for analgesia, with an intraoperative loading dose of 5 mcg/kg, followed by an infusion of 0.3 mcg/kg/h.[29]

Dexmedetomidine is administered only intravenously. It is produced in 2-mL vials with a concentration of 100 mcg/mL under the brand name Precedex. The standard dilution for clinical use is 4 mcg/mL, which requires adding 48 mL of normal saline to the 2-mL stock solution for a total volume of 50 mL. Common dosing strategies for dexmedetomidine include intravenous infusions of 0.2 to 0.7 mcg/kg/h, with or without a preinfusion loading dose of 1 mcg/kg given over 10 minutes. Some authors have recommended against a loading dose, given the potential risks of initial hypertension and subsequent hypotension and bradycardia that seem to be associated with rapid intravenous administration of dexmedetomidine.[28]

Indications

Clonidine, as an intravenous (and epidural) drug, has been approved for the treatment of severe cancer pain for patients who have inadequate analgesia with conventional opiate therapies. Clonidine's use as an intravenous perioperative pain adjunct constitutes an unlabeled use.

Dexmedetomidine is approved for the sedation of intubated critically ill patients and for nonintubated patients requiring sedation prior to and/or during surgery or other procedures. Administering dexmedetomidine for the purposes of perioperative pain management represents an unlabeled use.

Perioperative clonidine use is associated with decreased heart rate and blood pressure in the intraoperative period. Clonidine can blunt the sympathetic response to both laryngoscopy and surgical stimulation.[29] Intravenous clonidine for preoperative anxiolysis has been well studied, and some authors believe it to be superior for sedation, postoperative pain control, and postoperative nausea and vomiting prevention when compared with preoperative benzodiazepine administration.[30] Animal and human data suggest that intravenous clonidine in 1- mcg/kg doses or greater may result in 15%- to 40%-reductions in the MAC of volatile anesthetics.[29]

The available clinical data regarding perioperative clonidine used specifically to reduce the consumption of opiates and to improve pain scores are quite limited. The authors of a study on intravenous clonidine's analgesic effects after major spine surgery demonstrated that an intraoperative bolus of 5 mcg/kg followed by an infusion of 0.3 mcg/kg/h of clonidine resulted in a significant decrease in postoperative morphine consumption and decreased postoperative pain scores when compared to placebo.[29]

As with clonidine, the addition of dexmedetomidine to a general anesthetic may result in intraoperative hypotension and bradycardia. Intraoperative dexmedetomidine infusions may increase the risk of mild to moderate hypotension in the postoperative period. The precise interaction between dexmedetomidine and MAC for inhalational anesthetics is not known, but the limited available data suggest that dexmedetomidine doses of 0.2 to 0.8 mcg/kg/h may result in an approximate 20% reduction of MAC.[31] Despite its profound sedative properties, dexmedetomidine is associated with only limited respiratory depression.[28] Specific information on timing the emergence from anesthesia when dexmedetomidine is used as an adjunct is lacking.

Multiple clinical studies have shown perioperative dexmedetomidine infusions to result in decreased opiate use and decreased pain scores in the postanesthesia care unit.[27,31,32] However, data regarding the analgesic mechanism of dexmedetomidine following systemic administration are conflicting. Some data suggest that these postoperative benefits may be related to an opiate synergy effect and/or the anxiolytic properties of dexmedetomidine rather than an intrinsic analgesic effect of dexmedetomidine itself.[28]

At present, there are no studies that specifically address the use of intravenous clonidine or dexmedetomidine as perioperative pain adjuncts for opiate tolerant surgical patients. As with the other systemic pain adjuncts discussed in this chapter, the opiate-sparing and non-opiate analgesic effects of these α-2-adrenoreceptor agonists may be particularly beneficial for the management of perioperative pain in the opiate-tolerant surgical patient.

No data on the use of clonidine or dexmedetomidine for the prevention of chronic pain after surgery currently exists. There are, however, multiple investigations underway to evaluate the utility of these agents for the prevention and treatment of chronic postoperative pain syndromes. These studies include an investigation of epidural clonidine and its effect on postoperative hyperalgesia as well as a separate trial examining the use of dexmedetomidine for the control of postoperative pain in thoracotomy patients.[26]

Adverse Effects

There are a very limited number of studies that have examined intravenous clonidine specifically as a perioperative pain adjunct. Consequently, the adverse effects of intravenous clonidine as a perioperative pain adjunct are not well known. When used for other clinical applications, clonidine is known to have the adverse effects of sedation, dry mouth, hypotension, and bradycardia, as well as rebound hypertension if long-term clonidine treatment is abruptly discontinued.

Dexmedetomidine's potent α-2-adrenoreceptor agonism results in a centrally mediated inhibition of the sympathetic nervous system. Because of this sympatholysis, the use of dexmedetomidine in critical care patients doubles the risk of hypotension (28% versus 13%) and bradycardia (7% versus 3%) when compared to placebo. In the intraoperative setting, there have been case reports of severe hypotension, bradycardia, and cardiac arrest in patients receiving general anesthesia with dexmedetomidine used as an adjunct.[33,34]

Contraindications

When considering the use of clonidine or dexmedetomidine as perioperative pain adjuncts, the potential benefits for pain management must be weighed carefully against the potential risks of excessive sedation, hypotension, and bradycardia. Careful patient selection is critical to the appropriate perioperative use of these medications.

NONSTEROIDAL ANTI-INFLAMMATORY DRUGS AND ACETAMINOPHEN

Several nonsteroidal anti-inflammatory drugs (NSAIDs) and acetaminophen have been developed that are of potential use as an adjunct in managing postoperative pain. This section will briefly review ketorolac, celecoxib, and acetaminophen.

History of Development

The first NSAID, sodium salicylate, was discovered in 1763 and led to the development of acetylsalicylic acid (ASA; aspirin). Given the gastric toxicity associated with ASA, nonsalicylate NSAIDs such as phenylbutazone were developed in the 1950s but were associated with bone marrow toxicity. Indomethacin was developed in the 1960s. Subsequently, numerous NSAIDs have been developed to optimize drug kinetics (ie, longer lasting), fewer adverse side effects, and more pronounced anti-inflammatory effect. Today, numerous NSAIDs are available, some of which are useful in the perioperative period.

Ketorolac was first approved for use in 1990. It was the first parenteral NSAID indicated for postoperative pain. Ketorolac is typically used to provide postoperative analgesia and reduction of postoperative emesis through inhibition of prostaglandin-mediated amplification of irritants on sensory pathways. Ketorolac is often given as one component of a multimodal approach to pain management, but it has particular importance when an opioid-sparing approach to pain management is indicated.

Celecoxib has a colorful history. The FDA first approved celecoxib in the United States in 1998. It was licensed for use in acute pain, various types of arthritis, painful menstruation, and ankylosing spondylitis, among other indications. In 2009, Scott Rueben, a pain researcher working with cyclooxygenase-1 (COX-2) inhibitors, revealed that he had fabricated many of the results in several studies that exaggerated the analgesic effects of this class of drugs. Despite this setback, the drug has been found to be an effective analgesic and is the only COX-2 inhibitor approved for use in the United States.

Precursors to acetaminophen, also known as paracetamol, had been developed as early as 1886 (acetanilide) but found to be toxic because of cyanosis from methemoglobinemia. In 1947, researchers found that paracetamol was an active metabolite of acetanilide yet had minimal adverse side effects. Since the discovery of acetaminophen, it has been widely used to treat mild pain and fever. The intravenous formulation of acetaminophen was approved in the United States in 2011.

Mechanism of Action

NSAIDs block the synthesis of prostaglandins from arachidonic acid. Arachidonic acid is converted to various prostaglandins and leukotrienes throughout the body (Figure 11–5). Arachidonic acid is converted to prostaglandins along 2 pathways, the constitutive and the inducible. The constitutive pathway provides prostaglandins and thromboxane A_2 that play a role in various physiologic functions such as protection of gastric mucosa, platelet function, renal function, and bronchomotor tone. Conversion along this pathway is via COX-1. The inducible pathway

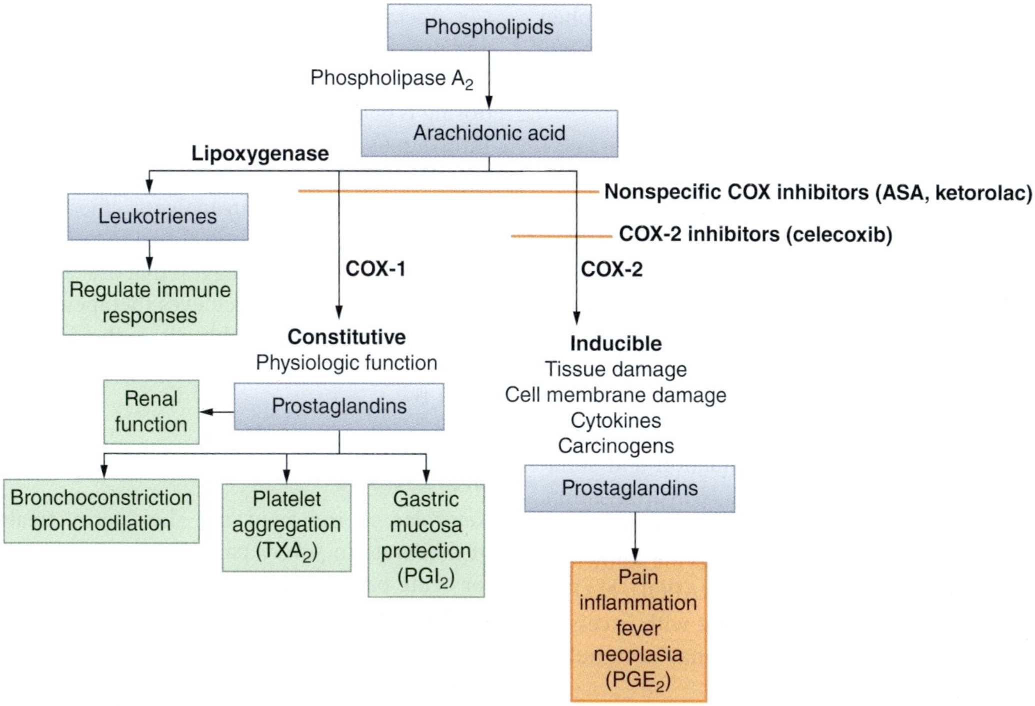

FIGURE 11–5 Schematic representation of the phospholipid/arachidonic/prostaglandin pathway. ASA, acetylsalicylic acid; COX,= cyclooxygenase (also known as prostaglandin-endoperoxide synthase); PGE_2, prostaglandin E_2; PGI_2, prostacyclin I_2; TXA_2, thromboxane A_2.

is triggered by trauma, cell wall damage, cytokines, and carcinogens, among other stimuli, that create prostaglandins associated with pain, fever, inflammation, and possible neoplasia. Conversion along this pathway is via COX-2.

Ketorolac is a nonsteroidal anti-inflammatory nonselective COX inhibitor that inhibits both COX-1 and COX-2. Celecoxib is a nonsteroidal anti-inflammatory selective COX inhibitor that inhibits COX-2 but not COX-1. The therapeutic effect of ketorolac and celecoxib are mediated by the inhibition of COX enzymes that convert arachidonic acid to prostaglandins.

Acetaminophen, although not considered a NSAID, also works via similar mechanisms. Although these mechanisms are not well defined, they have been linked to COX inhibition, specifically COX-2 inhibition,[35] central modulation of the serotonin system,[36] and endogenous cannabinoid receptors.[37,38]

Kinetics and Metabolism

Onset of Action

Ketorolac has a rapid onset time with the time to peak concentration between 1 and 3 minutes with a 6-hour half-life. It is a racemic mixture, with the S form having analgesic properties. It is highly protein bound (99%) and has a small volume of distribution—13 L in healthy adults.

Celecoxib reaches peak plasma concentrations within 3 hours of oral administration and has an effective half-life of 11.5 hours. It is highly protein bound (97%) and has an apparent volume of distribution at steady state of 400 L, suggestive of extensive distribution to peripheral tissues.

With acetaminophen, the onset of analgesia with oral administration is approximately 11 minutes[39] but can be inconsistent. In contrast, the onset of analgesia with intravenous administration is 3 minutes with a bolus and 5 minutes with a dose administered over 15 minutes.[39,40] Acetaminophen has low protein binding (10%–25%) and an apparent 0.7 to 1.0 L/kg volume of distribution.[41-45]

Metabolism

Ketorolac undergoes hepatic metabolism (hydroxylation and conjugation) and is primarily excreted in the urine.

Celecoxib is primarily metabolized in the liver by CYP2C9; it is conjugated to celecoxib glucuronide and then excreted in the bile. Drugs known to inhibit CYP2C9 (such as fluconazole) may result in elevated celecoxib plasma concentrations.

Acetaminophen undergoes hepatic metabolism primarily through glucuronidation and sulfation and to a lesser extent through *N*-hydroxylation. *N*-hydroxylation creates a toxic intermediate metabolite via CYP2D6 hepatic microenzyme known as *N*-acetyl-*p*-benzo-quinone imine (NAPQI). NAPQI is typically rapidly metabolized, but with excessive doses (ie, > 4000 mg in 1 day), it may accumulate and cause liver damage.[46]

Dosing Regimens

Ketorolac is available both in intravenous and oral forms. For the intravenous route, initial dosing is 30 mg, followed by 15 to 30 mg every 6 to 8 hours, not to exceed 120 mg per day. For the oral route, initial dosing is 20 mg followed by 10 mg every 4 to 6 hours, not to exceed 40 mg per day. Since ketorolac is a nonspecific COX inhibitor and has several adverse side effects that may occur with prolonged use, maximal duration of intravenous and oral dosing should not exceed 2 and 5 days, respectively. Doses should be decreased in patients older than 65 years and in patients with renal failure. Ketorolac is commonly used in with pediatric patients[47] and administered either intramuscularly (0.75 mg/kg) or intravenously (1 mg/kg load followed by 0.5 mg/kg every 6 hours).

Celecoxib is dosed as 400 mg by mouth initially and then 200 mg twice a day as needed for acute pain in adults. Dosing guidelines recommend that lowest effective dose be used for the shortest duration of time because of the risk of thrombotic cardiovascular events and/or severe gastrointestinal effects (eg, ulceration, bleeding, perforation).

Acetaminophen is available both in intravenous and oral forms. For the intravenous route, dosing is 1000 mg every 6 hours as needed. For the oral route, dosing is 650 to 1000 mg every 4 to 6 hours as need. Intravenous acetaminophen should be considered for patients who cannot tolerate oral medications. There is little difference in analgesic efficacy between oral and intravenous routes if therapeutic levels are achieved. Some studies suggest that oral administration of acetaminophen achieves therapeutic plasma concentrations less reliably than the intravenous route[39] while other studies demonstrate equivalent effect.[48]

Indications

Ketorolac is indicated for short-term treatment of moderate to severe pain. Celecoxib is indicated for acute pain in adults, osteoarthritis, rheumatoid arthritis, dysmenorrhea, and familial adenomatous polyposis. Acetaminophen is indicated for temporary relief of fever and minor aches and pains. Acetaminophen in combination with the 2 NSAIDs is an effective way to minimize toxic doses of either and has been found to provide better postoperative pain control than either drug administered by itself.[49]

Adverse Effects

Nonsteroidal Anti-inflammatory Drugs

There are numerous side effects with anti-inflammatory agents that anesthesiologists should consider when administering them in the perioperative arena. The primary source of adverse effects is the disruption of important balances between selected prostaglandins that mediate vasomotor and bronchomotor tone as well as platelet function, among other important physiologic functions.

Cardiovascular Effects Both COX-1 and COX-2 inhibitors are associated with cardiovascular injury. The mechanisms are not well defined, but thought to be a function of vasomotor tone dysregulation and abnormal platelet function via changes in thromboxane A_2 and prostacyclin PGI2. Specifically, COX-2 inhibitors are associated with an increased risk of arterial thrombotic events leading to myocardial injury or stroke. Caution should be used in their administration to patients with known cardiovascular disease. In addition, NSAIDs can exacerbate preexisting hypertension or lead to new-onset hypertension, cause fluid retention, or exacerbate congestive heart failure; each of these effects may increase the incidence of adverse cardiovascular events. Furthermore, celecoxib increases the risk of myocardial infarct and stroke in patients who have had recent (ie, within the past 10–14 days) coronary artery bypass graph procedures.

Gastrointestinal Effects COX inhibitors, especially nonspecific ones, are associated with gastrointestinal side effects that include gastric ulceration, bleeding, and perforation, primarily because of COX-1 mediated gastric protection. Caution should be used in their administration to patients with known gastric disease and in the elderly.

Renal Dysfunction Renal toxicity from NSAIDs primarily involves reduced renal blood flow resulting in medullary ischemia. Prostaglandins sensitive to NSAIDs (via COX-1) regulate renal blood flow.[50] Although less likely, NSAIDs use can also lead to allergic nephritis and tubulointerstitial nephritis. Caution should be used with administering NSAIDs to patients with advanced age, renal hypoperfusion, hypovolemia, sepsis, or major surgery, given that they are more likely to develop acute renal failure.

Bone Healing COX inhibitors may influence bone and soft tissue healing. Ketorolac may also have important adverse effects on bone healing. Inhibition of COX by daily administration of celecoxib or ketorolac for 5 weeks reduced new bone ingrowth by about 60% in one recent study.[51] However, other recent studies have shown no difference in nonunions following spinal fusion surgeries in groups treated with ketorolac compared to controls.[52] Thus, use of NSAIDs should be reduced or avoided in patients undergoing procedures associated with a high incidence of nonunion.

Platelet and Hematologic Function Arguably the most relevant clinical side effect of ketorolac is prolonged bleeding. Because ketorolac acts on prostaglandin synthesis in platelets, prolonged bleeding is possible. This effect is usually reversible within 1 to 2 days after discontinuation of therapy, although the platelet effects do last for the life of the platelet. Because of this effect, ketorolac should be avoided in patients who are at high risk for postoperative bleeding or in patients whose outcome would be compromised by even small amounts of bleeding in specific anatomic locations. By contrast, celecoxib does not alter platelet counts or inhibit platelet aggregation.

Allergic Reactions One concern with celecoxib is its potential for an allergic reaction in patients with a known allergy to sulfonamide antibiotics. Although celecoxib has a sulfonamide moiety, a meta-analysis of 11,000 patients suggested that patients with a sulfonamide allergy are more likely to have an allergic reaction in general (eg, equally sensitive to placebo, a non–sulfonamide-containing NSAID, or celecoxib) than patients without a sulfonamide sensitivity, but did not have a specific heightened sensitivity to celecoxib.[53] This finding warrants further investigation given that current recommendations are to avoid administering celecoxib to patients with this allergy.

Acetaminophen

The primary adverse effect associated with acetaminophen is hepatic toxicity. Hepatic injury can occur when the dose exceeds 4000 mg in a 24-hour period, if combined with other acetaminophen-containing drugs, or if administered to patients who consume more than 3 alcoholic drinks per day. Overdoses can be treated with (1) oral administration of charcoal just after ingestion and (2) acetylcysteine if measured plasma acetaminophen concentrations are elevated (ie, > 20 mg/mL, 16 hours after injection) or alanine aminotransferase or aspartate aminotransferase levels are elevated (ie, greater than> 50 IU/L).

Contraindications

For ketorolac, contraindications are:

- Complete or partial syndrome of nasal polyps or angioedema

- Bronchospastic or other allergic reactions to aspirin or other NSAIDs
- Renal dysfunction

For celecoxib, contraindications are:

- Known sulfonamide sensitivity
- History of asthma or other allergic-type reaction to aspirin or other NSAIDs
- Coronary artery bypass graft surgery (perioperative use)

For acetaminophen, contraindications are:

- Liver failure or liver problems
- Consumption of alcohol (> 3 drinks per day)

MULTIMODAL ANALGESICS

History of Development

Tramadol was developed by a German pharmaceutical company, Grünenthal, in 1962. After 15 years of research and development, tramadol was marketed as an analgesic different from conventional opioids because of its multimodal action. Some 25 years later, Grünenthal, in conjunction with Johnson & Johnson, released tapentadol in 2008. Like tramadol, it is also marketed as an analgesic different from conventional opioids because of its multimodal action.

Mechanism of Action

Tramadol is a weak μ-opioid agonist but has an active metabolite, O-desmethyltramadol, which is a more potent μ-receptor agonist. Hence, tramadol is a prodrug, much like codeine. In addition to its opioid receptor agonism, tramadol has several other mechanisms of action that may affect analgesia. Based on animal model studies, some of these include a serotonin-releasing agent,[54] norepinephrine reuptake inhibitor,[55] NMDA receptor antagonist,[56] and nicotinic and muscarinic acetylcholine receptor antagonist.[57-59] In addition, tramadol is a 5-HT_{2C} receptor antagonist.[60] This serotonin receptor inhibits the release of dopamine and norepinephrine. Tramadol also is a transient receptor potential V1 (TRPV1) receptor agonist.[61] TRPV1 also known as the capsaicin receptor or vanilloid-1 receptor, helps modulate pain.

Tapentadol is a centrally acting analgesic that also acts as a weak μ opioid receptor agonist and an inhibitor of norepinephrine reuptake. Binding at the μ opioid receptor results in inhibition of the ascending pain pathway, while an increased level of norepinephrine is thought to modify the descending pain pathway.[62]

Of note, drugs that inhibit the reuptake of serotonin and norepinephrine in the absence of any μ receptor agonism, provide an analgesic effect. For example, the antidepressant–antianxiety medication duloxetine, a selective serotonin and norepinephrine reuptake inhibitor, reduces opioid requirements in patients undergoing total knee arthoplasty.[63]

Kinetics and Metabolism

Onset of Action

Tramadol has an onset time with the time to peak concentration in 2 to 2.5 hours and a half-life of 6 hours. It is a racemic mixture with 4 isomers, with 1 isomer 4 times as potent than the others at the μ receptor.[64] It is 20% protein bound and has a small volume of distribution, 2.7 L/kg in healthy adults.

Tapentadol has an onset time with the time to peak concentration in 75 minutes with a half-life of 4 hours. It has a 540 L volume of distribution and is 20% protein bound.[65] Unlike tramadol, its metabolites have no analgesic effect.

Metabolism

Tramadol undergoes hepatic metabolism that involves both conjugation and the isoenzymes CYP2D6 and CYP3A4. CYP2D6 inhibitors, such as amitriptyline, paroxetine, and fluoxetine, as well as CYP3A4 inhibitors, such as erythromycin, encountered in the perioperative environment may reduce tramadol clearance and increase the risk of adverse events such as serotonin syndrome or seizures. It should be noted that up to 6% of the population has increased activity of CYP2D6. This may lead to increased analgesic effect because of rapid metabolism of tramadol to its active metabolite O-desmethyltramadol.

Tapentadol also undergoes hepatic metabolism that involves both conjugation and the CYP450 isoenzyme system. The majority of metabolism involves conjugation with glucuronic acid, but some drug is metabolized by the CYP2C9, CYP2C19, and CYP2D6 isoenzymes.

Dosing Regimens

Tramadol is dosed as 50 to 100 mg by mouth as needed for pain relief every 4 to 6 hours, not to exceed 400 mg per day. Tramadol 50 to 100 mg by mouth just prior to surgery is a useful adjunct for perioperative pain control.

Tapentadol is dosed as 75 to 100 mg by mouth as needed for pain relief every 4 to 6 hours, not to exceed 600 mg per day. Tapentadol 100 mg by mouth just prior to surgery is also a useful adjunct for perioperative pain control.

Indications

Tramadol and tapentadol are indicated moderate to severe acute and chronic pain. Other uses, among several, include treatment for fibromyalgia, diabetic neuropathy, and osteoarthritis.

Adverse Effects

Serotonin Syndrome

A worrisome adverse side effect with tramadol is its interaction with other serotonergic drugs such as selective serotonin reuptake inhibitors, serotonin norepinephrine reuptake inhibitors, monoamine oxidase inhibitors, and strong opioids, as well as the herbal remedy St. John's wort. Excessive serotonin can be life threatening. Caution should be used when administering tramadol and tapentadol in patients that use these medications.[66]

Seizures

Tramadol is associated with lowered seizure thresholds when administered in large doses (ie, > 600 mg).

Respiratory Depression

As multimodal agents, both tramadol and tapentadol do not rely entirely on opioid agonism to achieve analgesia. As such, there may be less respiratory depression than with other opioids at recommended doses. Higher doses of these agents, however, can cause worrisome respiratory depression. Use of tramadol and tapentadol may be an attractive alternative when managing postoperative pain in patients with known or suspected respiratory compromise such as severe sleep apnea or impaired lung function.[66]

Gastrointestinal Effects

Among the most common side effects from tramadol and tapentadol are nausea, vomiting, and constipation. Although it was once thought that this class of drugs may be advantageous in patients suffering from nausea, vomiting, and constipation, recent work suggests that tapentadol has a similar incidence of gastrointestinal side effects when compared to other opioids.[67]

Contraindications

Contraindications include:

- Hypersensitivity to central acting opioids or psychotropic drugs.
- Known or suspected elevated intracranial pressure. As a mild respiratory depressant, elevated arterial carbon dioxide levels can lead to increased intracranial pressure.

SUMMARY

The body of evidence supporting the use of ketamine, gabapentin, pregabalin, clonidine, dexmedetomidine, ketorolac, celecoxib, acetaminophen, tramadol, and tapentadol for the management of acute perioperative pain is limited but expanding. One drug that was not included in this chapter is lidocaine. It also has analgesic properties when administered as a continuous infusion perioperatively.[68,69] Lidocaine is discussed in more detail in the local anesthetic chapter.

The available data regarding the use of these agents as perioperative pain adjuncts is summarized in Table 11–1. Despite the limited amount of available data, all of these drugs show some degree of promise as analgesic adjuncts, and additional studies evaluating their specific benefits and limitations continue to emerge.

TABLE 11–1 Summary of selected perioperative pain adjuncts.

Adjunct	Suggested Perioperative Dosing	Precautions
Ketamine	**Intraoperative/postoperative** **Route: IV** **Bolus:** 0.1–0.5 mg/kg **Infusion:** 0.1–0.2 mg/kg/h	
Gabapentin	**Preoperative** **Route: PO** **Dose:** 300–900 mg; consider continuing postoperatively 300–600 mg 3 times a day for 2–3 days	
Pregabalin	**Preoperative** **Route: PO** **Dose:** 75–150 mg; consider continuing postoperatively 50–100 mg 2 times a day for 2–3 days	
Clonidine	**Intraoperative**	
	Route: IV	Consider infusion only (no bolus); may cause hypotension
	Slow bolus: 0.5–2 mcg/kg	Administer bolus dose over 10 minutes
	Infusion: 0.3 mcg/kg/h	
Dexmedetomidine	**Intraoperatively/postoperative in ICU**	
	Route: IV	Consider infusion only (no bolus); may cause hypotension
	Slow bolus: 1 mcg/kg	Administer bolus dose over 10 minutes
	Infusion: 0.2–0.7 mcg/kg/h	Consider infusion only (no bolus)
Ketorolac	**Intraoperative/postoperative**	Numerous precautions (see text)
	Route: IV **Dose:** 15–30 mg every 6–8 hours	Not to exceed 120 mg/day. Maximal duration: 2 days
	Route: PO **Initial dose:** 20 mg followed by 10 mg every 4–6 hours	Not to exceed 40 mg/day. Maximal duration: 5 days
Celecoxib	**Preoperative**	
	Route: PO **Dose:** 200–400 mg; consider continuing postoperatively 200 mg twice a day	Use the lowest effective dose for the shortest length of time (minimize thrombotic cardiovascular risk); avoid in patients with sulfa sensitivity
Acetaminophen	**Intraoperative/postoperative**	
	Route: IV: **Dose:** 1000 mg every 6 hours	Maximal daily dose not to exceed 4000 mg/day
	Route: PO **Dose:** 650–1000 mg every 4–6 hours	

(Continued)

TABLE 11–1 Summary of selected perioperative pain adjuncts. (*Continued*)

Adjunct	Suggested Perioperative Dosing	Precautions
Tramadol	**Preoperative** **Route:** PO **Dose:** 50–100 mg; consider continuing postoperatively 50–100 mg every 4–6 hours	Maximal daily dose not to exceed 400 mg/day
Tapentadol	**Preoperative** **Route:** PO **Dose:** 75–100 mg; consider continuing postoperatively 75–100 mg every 4–6 hours	Maximal daily dose not to exceed 600 mg/day
Lidocaine	**Intraoperative** **Route:** IV **Bolus:** 1.5 mg/kg **Infusion:** 2 mg/kg/h	

ICU, intensive care unit; IV, intravenous; PO, per os.

CASE SCENARIO

A 56-year-old, 178-cm, 114-kg male is scheduled for a revision of his posterior spinal fusion from T12 to L4. Past medical history includes obesity, obstructive sleep apnea, hypertension, osteoarthritis, depression, and chronic low back pain with radicular symptoms causing neuropathic pain in both legs. He has had 2 prior spine surgeries with no anesthetic complications. Medications include oxycodone/acetaminophen (Percocet; 10/325 mg 1–2 tabs q4h PRN), lisinopril (Zestril; 10 mg per day), sertraline (Zoloft; 150 mg qhs), alprazolam (Xanax; 0.5 mg q8h PRN, and a recently added time contingent preparation of oxycodone (OxyContin; 20 mg bid). His baseline VAS for pain is 7/10. Despite his self-reported high tolerance for pain, he states he had poor pain control after his 2 prior back surgeries. He is very anxious about inadequate postoperative pain management.

While perioperative pain adjuncts may produce *statistically* significant reductions in perioperative opiate requirements and pain scores in most patients, it is patients like this one who will likely derive the largest *clinically* significant benefit.

Clinicians are often more compelled to add pain adjuncts to standard anesthetics when risk factors for poor perioperative pain control are present. Risk factors include (1) opioid tolerance, (2) procedures that cause moderate to severe acute postoperative pain, (3) procedures that are high risk for creating chronic postsurgical pain syndromes, and (4) preexisting chronic pain syndromes.

In the presence of one or more risk factors, the following treatment algorithm may be warranted.

Preoperatively

1. Establish realistic pain management goals in the preoperative setting (eg, postoperative pain scores will be worse than home pain scores).
2. Administer outpatient analgesic and anxiolytic medications on the day of surgery.
3. Consider preoperative placement of regional anesthesia for perioperative pain control if possible (peripheral nerve catheter or epidural).
4. Consider pregabalin 150 mg by mouth for the typical adult and 75 mg for the elderly or those with impaired creatinine clearance.
5. Consider COX-2 inhibitors celecoxib 200-400 mg by mouth if not contraindicated by patient or type of surgery. Patients with sensitivity

to sulfonamides (compounds that contain SO_2NH_2 moiety attached to a benzene ring) should not receive celecoxib. Celecoxib along with several antibiotics and other agents contain a sulfonamide group.

6. Tramadol or tapentadol are not appropriate here, given the patient's use of a selective serotonin reuptake inhibitor. The concern is for increased serotonin levels and an increased risk of serotonin syndrome. In addition to selective serotonin reuptake inhibitors, monoamine oxidase inhibitors, serotonin norepinephrine reuptake inhibitors, and tricyclic antidepressants may all increase the risk of serotonin toxicity. Had the patient not been taking sertraline, tramadol 50 to 100 mg by mouth or tapentadol 50 to 100 mg by mouth would be appropriate.

Intraoperatively

1. Consider intravenous ketamine—a loading bolus preincision and an additional infusion for any case longer than 60 minutes. Total perioperative dose for the opioid-naive patient is 0.25 to 0.5 mg/kg. Total perioperative dose for the opioid-tolerant patient is 0.5 to 2 mg/kg.
2. Consider clonidine or dexmedetomidine; this requires careful patient selection given risks for intraoperative hypotension and bradycardia. Clonidine dosing is 0.3 mcg/kg/h infusion with or without a slow loading dose of 5 mcg/kg. Dexmedetomidine dosing is 0.2 to 0.7 mcg/kg/h infusion with or without a slow loading dose of 1 mcg/kg over 10 minutes.
3. If an epidural catheter or peripheral nerve catheter is available, employ its use prior to emergence.
4. Consider intraoperative NSAIDs (acetaminophen or ketorolac) if not contraindicated.
5. Administer an intraoperative opiate regimen of choice.

Postoperatively

1. Restart the outpatient medications for pain and anxiety as soon as possible.
2. Maximize use of regional anesthesia techniques (ie, perineural local anesthetic infusions, epidural infusions, and so on).
3. Use NSAIDs/COX-2 inhibitors and acetaminophen if not contraindicated
4. For neuropathic or poorly controlled pain, continue (or add) pregabalin 75 to 150 mg by mouth bid.
5. If an opioid-tolerant patient is doing poorly, continue the ketamine infusion postoperatively at 0.1 to 0.15 mg/kg/h on an inpatient basis. Consider transitioning to memantine, an oral NMDA antagonist.
6. Administer a postoperative opiate regimen of choice.

REFERENCES

1. Lazmaiah M, Fellows B, Ailinani H, Pampati V. Therapeutic use, abuse, and nonmedical use of opioids: a ten-year perspective. *PainPhysician*. 2010;13: 401-435.
2. Kehlet H, Jensen TS, Woolf CJ. Persistent postsurgical pain: risk factors and prevention. *Lancet*. 2006;367 (9522):1618-1625.
3. Domino EF. Taming the ketamine tiger, 1965. *Anesthesiology*. 2010;113(3):678-684.
4. Hirota K, Lambert DG. Ketamine: its mechanism(s) of action and unusual clinical uses. *Br J Anaesth*. 1996; 77(4):441-444.
5. Wilder-Smith OH, Arendt-Nielsen L. Postoperative hyperalgesia: its clinical importance and relevance. *Anesthesiology*. 2006;104(3):601-607.
6. Hirota K, Sato T, Rabito SF, Zsigmond EK, Matsuki A. Relaxant effect of ketamine and its isomers on histamine-induced contraction of tracheal smooth muscle. *Br J Anaesth*. 1996;76(2):266-270.
7. Rabben T. Skjelbred P, Oye I. Prolonged analgesic effect of ketamine, an N-methyl-D-aspartate receptor inhibitor, in patients with chronic pain. *J Pharmacol Exp Ther*. 1999;289(2):1060-1066.
8. Ihmsen H, Geisslinger G, Schuttler J. Stereoselective pharmacokinetics of ketamine: R(−)-ketamine inhibits the elimination of S(+)-ketamine. *Clin Pharmacol Ther*. 2001;70(5):431-438.
9. Kharasch ED, Labroo R. Metabolism of ketamine stereoisomers by human liver microsomes. *Anesthesiology*. 1992;77(6):1201-1207.
10. Hijazi Y, Boulieu R. Protein binding of ketamine and its active metabolites to human serum. *Eur J Clin Pharmacol*. 2002;58(1):37-40.

11. Bell RF, Dahl JB, Moore RA, Kalso EA. Perioperative ketamine for acute postoperative pain. *Cochrane Database of Systematic Reviews*. 2006, issue 1. Article no: CD004603.
12. Himmelseher S, Durieux ME. Ketamine for perioperative pain management. *Anesthesiology*. 2005; 102(1):211-220.
13. Subramaniam K., Subramaniam B, Steinbrook RA. Ketamine as adjuvant analgesic to opioids: a quantitative and qualitative systematic review. *Anesth Analg*. 2004;99(2):482-495.
14. Loftus RW, Yeager MP, Clark JA, et al. Intraoperative ketamine reduces perioperative opiate consumption in opiate-dependent patients with chronic back pain undergoing back surgery. Anesthesiology. 2010; 113(3):639-646.
15. Remerand F, Le Tendre C, Baud A, et al. The early and delayed analgesic effects of ketamine after total hip arthroplasty: a prospective, randomized, controlled, double-blind study. *Anesth Analg*. 2009;109(6): 1963-1971.
16. Duale C, Sibaud F, Guastella V, et al. Perioperative ketamine does not prevent chronic pain after thoracotomy. *Eur J Pain*. 2009;13(5):497-505.
17. Hayes C, Armstrong-Brown A, Burstal R. Perioperative intravenous ketamine infusion for the prevention of persistent post-amputation pain: a randomized, controlled trial. *Anaesth Intensive Care*. 2004; 32(3): 330-338.
18. http://www.fda.gov/NewsEvents/Newsroom/PressAnnouncements/2007/ucm108936.htm. Last accessed June 2014.
19. Gajraj NM. Pregabalin: its pharmacology and use in pain management. *Anesth Analg*. 2007;105(6):1805-1815.
20. Gilron I. Gabapentin and pregabalin for chronic neuropathic and early postsurgical pain: current evidence and future directions. *Curr Opin Anaesthesiol*. 2007;20(5):456-472.
21. Ho KY, Gan TJ, Habib AS. Gabapentin and postoperative pain—a systematic review of randomized controlled trials. *Pain*. 2006;126(1-3):91-101.
22. Tiippana EM, Hamunen K, Kontinen VK, Kalso E. Do surgical patients benefit from perioperative gabapentin/pregabalin? A systematic review of efficacy and safety. *Anesth Analg*. 2007;104(6): 1545-1556 .
23. Burke SM, Shorten GD. Perioperative pregabalin improves pain and functional outcomes 3 months after lumbar discectomy. *Anesth Analg*. 2010;110(4): 1180-1185.
24. Buvanendran A, Kroin JS, Della Valle CJ, Kari M, Moric M, Tuman KJ. Perioperative oral pregabalin reduces chronic pain after total knee arthroplasty: a prospective, randomized, controlled trial. *Anesth Analg*. 2010;110(1):199-207.
25. Kim SY, Jeong JJ, Chung WY, Kim HJ, Nam KH, Shim YH. Perioperative administration of pregabalin for pain after robot-assisted endoscopic thyroidectomy: a randomized clinical trial. *Surg Endosc*. 2010; 24(11):2776-2781.
26. Nikolajsen L, Finnerup NB, Kramp S, Vimtrup A., Keller J, Jensen TS. A randomized study of the effects of gabapentin on postamputation pain. *Anesthesiology*. 2006;105(5):1008-1015.
27. Giovannoni MP, Ghelardini C, Vergelli C, Dal Piaz V. Alpha2-agonists as analgesic agents. *Med Res Rev*. 2009;29(2):339-368.
28. Paris A Tonner PH. Dexmedetomidine in anaesthesia. *Curr Opin Anaesthesiol*. 2005;18(4):412-418.
29. Khan ZP, Ferguson CN, Jones RM. Alpha-2 and imidazoline receptor agonists. Their pharmacology and therapeutic role. *Anaesthesia*. 1999;54(2):146-165.
30. Dahmani S, Brasher C, Stany I, et al. Premedication with clonidine is superior to benzodiazepines. A meta analysis of published studies. *Acta Anaesthesiol Scand*. 2010;54(4):397-402.
31. Tufanogullari B, White PF, Peixoto MP, et al. Dexmedetomidine infusion during laparoscopic bariatric surgery: the effect on recovery outcome variables. *Anesth Analg*. 2008;106(6):1741-1748.
32. Arain SR, Ruehlow RM, Uhrich TD, Ebert TJ. The efficacy of dexmedetomidine versus morphine for postoperative analgesia after major inpatient surgery. *Anesth Analg*. 2004;98(1):153-158.
33. Ingersoll-Weng E, Manecke GR Jr, Thistlethwaite PA. Dexmedetomidine and cardiac arrest. *Anesthesiology*. 2004;100(3):738-739.
34. Sichrovsky TC, Mittal S, Steinberg JS. Dexmedetomidine sedation leading to refractory cardiogenic shock. *Anesth Analg*. 2008;106(6): 1784-1786.
35. Hinz B,Cheremina O, Brune K. Acetaminophen (paracetamol) is a selective cyclooxygenase-2 inhibitor in man. *FASEB J*. 2008;22(2):383-390.
36. Dogrul A, Seyrek M, Akgul EO, Cayci T, Kahraman S, Bolay H. Systemic paracetamol-induced analgesic and antihyperalgesic effects through activation of descending serotonergic pathways involving spinal 5-HT(7) receptors. *Eur J Pharmacol*. 2012;677(1-3): 93-101.
37. Anderson BJ. Paracetamol (Acetaminophen): mechanisms of action. *Paediatr Anaesth*. 2008;18(10): 915-921.
38. Hogestatt ED, Jonsson BA, Ermund A, et al. Conversion of acetaminophen to the bioactive N-acylphenolamine

AM404 via fatty acid amide hydrolase-dependent arachidonic acid conjugation in the nervous system. *J Biol Chem*. 2005;280(36):31405-12.
39. Moller PL, Sindet-Pedersen S, Petersen CT, Juhl GI, Dillenschneider A, Skoglund LA. Onset of acetaminophen analgesia: comparison of oral and intravenous routes after third molar surgery. *Br J Anaesth*. 2005;94(5):642-648.
40. Molle, PL, Juhl GI, Payen-Champenois C, Skoglund LA. Intravenous acetaminophen (paracetamol): comparable analgesic efficacy, but better local safety than its prodrug, propacetamol, for postoperative pain after third molar surgery. *Anesth Analg*. 2005;101(1):90-96.
41. Birmingham PK, Tobin MJ, Fisher DM, Henthorn TK, Hall SC, Cote CJ. Initial and subsequent dosing of rectal acetaminophen in children: a 24-hour pharmacokinetic study of new dose recommendations. *Anesthesiology*. 2001;94(3):385-389.
42. Birmingham PK, Tobin MJ, Henthorn TK, et al. Twenty-four-hour pharmacokinetics of rectal acetaminophen in children: an old drug with new recommendations. *Anesthesiology*. 1997;87(2):244-252.
43. Forrest JA, Clements JA, Prescott LF. Clinical pharmacokinetics of paracetamol. *Clin Pharmacokinet*. 1982;7(2):93-107.
44. Levy G. Comparative pharmacokinetics of aspirin and acetaminophen. *Arch Intern Med*. 1981;141(3 spec no): 279-281.
45. Milligan TP, Morris HC, Hammond PM, Price CP. Studies on paracetamol binding to serum proteins. *Ann Clin Biochem*. 1994;31(Pt 5):492-496.
46. Lee WM. Acetaminophen and the U.S. Acute Liver Failure Study Group: lowering the risks of hepatic failure. *Hepatology*. 2004;40(1):6-9.
47. Berde CB, Sethna NF. Analgesics for the treatment of pain in children. *N Engl J Med*. 2002;347(14):1094-1103.
48. Fenlon S, Collyer J, Giles J, et al. Oral vs intravenous paracetamol for lower third molar extractions under general anaesthesia: is oral administration inferior? *Br J Anaesth*. 2013;110(3):432-437.
49. Ong CK, Seymour RA, Lirk P, Merry AF. Combining paracetamol (acetaminophen) with nonsteroidal antiinflammatory drugs: a qualitative systematic review of analgesic efficacy for acute postoperative pain. *Anesth Analg*. 2010;110(4):1170-1179.
50. Katz, J.A. *NSAIDs and COX-2 Selective Inhibitors, Essentials of Pain Medicine and Regional Anesthesia*. 2nd ed. Philadelphia: Elsevier/Churchill Livingston3; 2005..
51. O'Keefe RJ, Tiyapatanaputi P, Xie C, et al. COX-2 has a critical role during incorporation of structural bone allografts. *Ann N Y Acad Sci*. 2006;1068:532-542.
52. Pradhan BB, Tatsumi RL, Gallina J, Kuhns CA, Wang JC, Dawson EG. Ketorolac and spinal fusion: does the perioperative use of ketorolac really inhibit spinal fusion? *Spine (Phila)*. 2008;33(19):2079-2082.
53. Patterson R, Bello AE, Lefkowith J. Immunologic tolerability profile of celecoxib. *Clin Ther*. 1999; 21(12):2065-2079.
54. Driessen B, Reimann W. Interaction of the central analgesic, tramadol, with the uptake and release of 5-hydroxytryptamine in the rat brain in vitro. *Br J Pharmacol*. 1992;105(1):147-151.
55. Sagata K, Minami K, Yanagihara N, et al. Tramadol inhibits norepinephrine transporter function at desipramine-binding sites in cultured bovine adrenal medullary cells. *Anesth Analg*. 2002;94(4):901-906.
56. Hara K, Minami K, Sata T. The effects of tramadol and its metabolite on glycine, gamma-aminobutyric acidA, and N-methyl-D-aspartate receptors expressed in Xenopus oocytes. *Anesth Analg*. 2005;100(5):1400-1405.
57. Shiga Y, Minami K, Shiraishi M, et al. The inhibitory effects of tramadol on muscarinic receptor-induced responses in Xenopus oocytes expressing cloned M(3) receptors. *Anesth Analg*. 2002;95(5):1269-1273.
58. Shiraishi M, Minami K, Uezono Y, Yanagihara N, Shigematsu A. Inhibition by tramadol of muscarinic receptor-induced responses in cultured adrenal medullary cells and in Xenopus laevis oocytes expressing cloned M1 receptors. *J Pharmacol Exp Ther*. 2001;299(1):255-260.
59. Shiraishi M, Minami K, Uezono Y, Yanagihara N, Shigematsu A, Shibuya I. Inhibitory effects of tramadol on nicotinic acetylcholine receptors in adrenal chromaffin cells and in Xenopus oocytes expressing alpha 7 receptors. *Br J Pharmacol*. 2002;136(2):207-216.
60. Ogata J, Minami K, Uezono Y, et al. The inhibitory effects of tramadol on 5-hydroxytryptamine type 2C receptors expressed in Xenopus oocytes. *Anesth Analg*. 2004;98(5):1401-1406.
61. Marincsak R., Toth BI, Czifra G, Szabo T, Kovacs L, Biro T. The analgesic drug, tramadol, acts as an agonist of the transient receptor potential vanilloid-1. *Anesth Analg*. 2008;106(6):1890-1896.
62. Tzschentke TM, Christoph T, Kogel B, et al. (–)-(1R,2R)-3-(3-dimethylamino-1-ethyl-2-methyl-propyl)-phenol hydrochloride (tapentadol HCl): a novel mu-opioid receptor agonist/norepinephrine reuptake inhibitor with broad-spectrum analgesic properties. *J Pharmacol Exp Ther*. 2007; 323(1): 265-276.
63. Ho KY, Tay W, Yeo MC, et al. Duloxetine reduces morphine requirements after knee replacement surgery. *Br J Anaesth*. 2010;105(3):371-376.

64. Goeringer KE, Logan BK, Christian GD. Identification of tramadol and its metabolites in blood from drug-related deaths and drug-impaired drivers. *J Anal Toxicol.* 1997;21(7):529-537.
65. Xu XS, Smit JW, Lin R, Stuyckens K, Terlinden R, Nandy P. Population pharmacokinetics of tapentadol immediate release (IR) in healthy subjects and patients with moderate or severe pain. *Clin Pharmacokinet.* 2010;49(10):671-682.
66. Nossaman VE, Ramadhyani U, Kadowitz PJ, Nossaman BD. Advances in perioperative pain management: use of medications with dual analgesic mechanisms, tramadol & tapentadol. *Anesthesiol Clin.* 2010;28(4):647-666.
67. Jeong ID, Camilleri M, Shin A. et al. A randomised, placebo-controlled trial comparing the effects of tapentadol and oxycodone on gastrointestinal and colonic transit in healthy humans. *Aliment Pharmacol Ther.* 2012.
68. De Oliveira GS Jr, Fitzgerald P, Streicher LF, Marcus RJ, McCarthy RJ. Systemic lidocaine to improve postoperative quality of recovery after ambulatory laparoscopic surgery. *Anesth Analg.* 2012;115(2): 262-267.
69. McCarthy GC, Megalla SA, Habib AS. Impact of intravenous lidocaine infusion on postoperative analgesia and recovery from surgery: a systematic review of randomized controlled trials. Drugs. 2010; 70(9):1149-1163.

CHAPTER

12

Local Anesthetics

Austin Wallace, MD

HISTORY

Local anesthetics have been used for centuries and represent some of the oldest drugs in the armamentarium of anesthesiologists. The story of the coca leaf and its alkaloid derivative, cocaine, is the best-known example of this. Members of the pre-Columbian Inca civilization would chew coca leaves to reduce pain and for its stimulant effects. Coca leaves are still chewed and brewed in teas in present day South American cultures. Research has found traces of coca in mummies from over 3000 years ago.[1] It is believed that shamans in the Incan culture would chew coca leaves and that the mixture of juice and saliva would be spit into the surgical site during trepanning operations. Eventually, coca was farmed for exportation to Europe starting in the 16th century. Coca wines, a blend of wine and cocaine, were popularized in the mid-1800s in Europe and eventually made an appearance in America. However, with the onset of prohibition in America, the wine in coca wine was replaced with a syrup, which became the basis for the first recipe of Coca-Cola. During the period of coca wine production in Europe, a German chemist named Albert Niemann in 1859 became the first person to isolate the primary alkaloid of coca, which he termed cocaine.[2] The first clinical use of cocaine was as an ophthalmic anesthetic by Karl Koller in 1884. Sigmund Freud, Koller's colleague, had done extensive testing of cocaine and had noted its anesthetic qualities prior to Koller's clinical use. Ultimately, the addictive properties of cocaine were recognized, and an effort was made to synthesize other local anesthetics. Einhorn developed procaine for clinical use in 1905, which became the local anesthetic of choice. Cocaine is still used even today (mostly for head, neck, and ophthalmic procedures), but its popularity is waning in the medical field. Unfortunately, most cocaine use today is as an illegal drug via snorting, smoking, or injection.

Numerous ester and amide formulations have been produced, starting in the 1890s. There was a push in the early to mid-1900s to improve the pharmacokinetics and toxicity profile of local anesthetics. Lidocaine is often considered to be the prototypical local anesthetic, and it was first used clinically in 1944 by Swedish chemist Nils Lofgren and patented in 1948.[3] Bupivacaine, another popular local anesthetic in common use today, was first synthesized in 1957 and introduced clinically in 1965. Clinicians have appreciated bupivacaine for its long duration of action but also recognized its troublesome cardiovascular toxicity profile and difficult resuscitation following inadvertent intravenous injection. In response to this, ropivacaine was developed and introduced clinically in 1996.[4] Bupivacaine consists of a racemic mixture of both S and R stereoisomers. However, ropivacaine consists of a single S stereoisomer, which shows lower potency at cardiac sodium channels and only slightly decreased anesthetic potency.

There will continue to be further research and development into the production of an ideal local anesthetic. However, one should consider that the central nervous system (CNS) and cardiovascular toxicities seen with use of a local anesthetic are in fact an extension of the drug's normal mechanism of action to undesired sites. For this reason, a perfect local anesthetic without toxicity might not be possible. Also, as local anesthetics are now being used more often via continuous infusions, and for chronic pain and cancer, development is underway to find ways to increase the duration of action via liposomal encapsulation and microspheres for sustained release.[5-8] Transcutaneous lidocaine delivery systems are already in routine use in many chronic pain clinics.

NERVE PHYSIOLOGY

Normal resting nerve membrane potential is –70 to –60 mV. This negative potential of the nerve interior is maintained by an energy-dependent Na^+/K^+ pump, primarily via potassium disequilibria (Figure 12–1). With the arrival of an appropriate nerve stimulus, the membrane becomes less negative, ultimately reaching an activation threshold of approximately –55 mV. At this point, sodium channels are converted from their resting to an opened configuration, followed by a fast inward sodium flow down its concentration gradient to depolarize the membrane to approximately +40 mV (Figure 12–2). This depolarization creates a positive feedback loop of increased sodium permeability and inward sodium current that encourages further depolarization and downstream propagation of the stimulus. The sodium channels will eventually close spontaneously to an inactivated state and potassium channels will open with an outward flow of potassium down its concentration gradient. These 2 events will shift the process toward local repolarization of the membrane. To accomplish repolarization, there is first a hyperpolarization of the membrane immediately

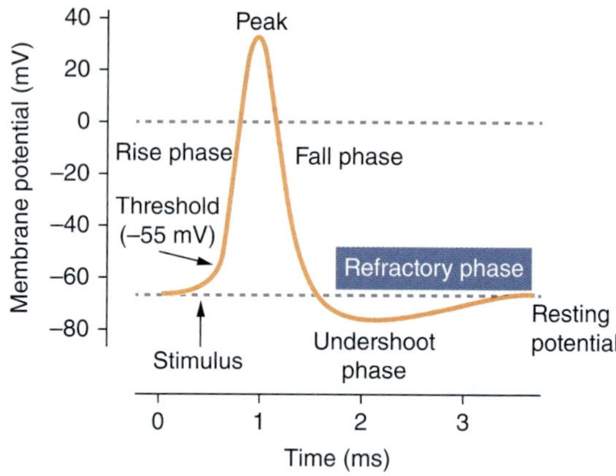

FIGURE 12–2 Schematic idealized plot of membrane voltage change during an action potential in response to a stimulus. Text labels represent the 4 phases (rising, peak, falling, and undershoot) and refractory period of the action potential. The refractory period may cross over more than one of the phases. ms, milliseconds; mV, millivolts.

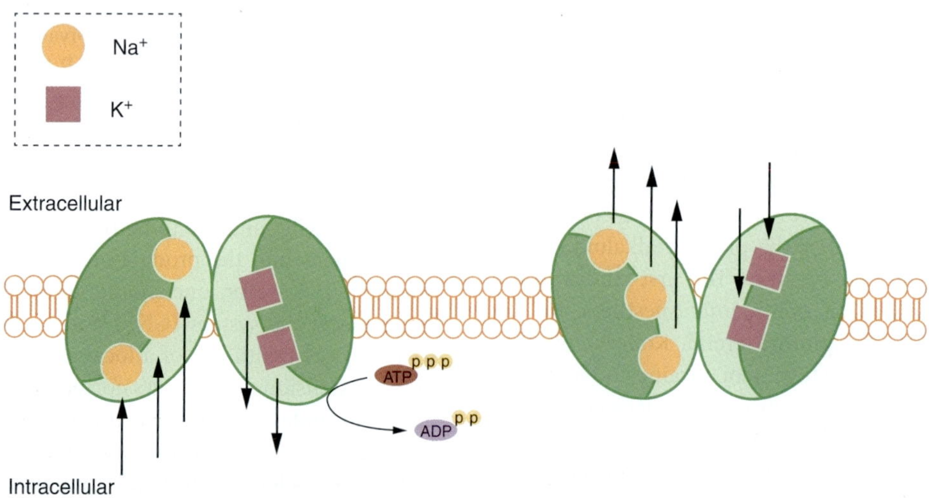

FIGURE 12–1 Schematic drawing of sodium (Na^+)/potassium (K^+) pump. The energy-dependent process transports sodium ion from intracellular cytoplasm to extracellular fluid, while at the same time transporting potassium ion from the extracellular fluid to the intracellular cytoplasm. ADP, adenosine diphosphate; ATP, adenosine triphosphate.

following an impulse that causes a refractory period during which sodium channels remain inactivated, potassium channels are still activated, and a nerve impulse cannot be conducted (see Figure 12–1). This concept explains the unidirectional aspect of nerve impulse propagation along the axon; an impulse cannot reverse direction and spread retrograde because the region behind the impulse is refractory to further stimulation. Eventually, sodium channels switch from inactivated to their resting configuration and potassium channels close, repolarizing the cell to its resting membrane potential. The Na+/K+ ATP-ase maintains this repolarized, resting state.

MECHANISM OF ACTION

The goal of local anesthesia is to induce a reversible loss of nociception within a specific region of the body. Local anesthetics accomplish this by reversibly blocking nerve impulse conduction by binding to sodium channels and inhibiting sodium influx. Local anesthetics do not affect the resting membrane potential. Instead, the local anesthetic molecule binds various receptor sites on the sodium channel, preventing sodium influx. As discussed above, there are 3 distinct channel configurations during the cycle of depolarization and repolarization: resting, open, and inactivated. The open and inactivated channel conformations bind local anesthetics better than the resting state. A weak interaction can occur between a local anesthetic molecule and the resting channel that will prevent a change to the open state—this is referred to as a tonic or resting inhibition. Nerves that are actively and repeatedly being depolarized have more of their channels in an open or inactivated state, and these nerves are therefore more susceptible to blockade by local anesthetics—this is referred to as frequency-dependent (phasic) inhibition.

Several mechanisms of local anesthetic mechanism have been proposed. It is thought that the local anesthetic molecule interacts with a binding site on the intracellular side of the sodium channel. This means that the drug must traverse the bilipid membrane to gain entry to the cell interior, and a neutral form of the drug is required to easily cross the membrane. It is also thought that local anesthetic molecules might interfere with neuronal membrane fluidity. The drug is able to expand the membrane surface and effectively close the sodium channel, thereby preventing ion passage.

Structure/Activity

The 2 available structural classes of local anesthetics include aminoesters and aminoamides (Figure 12–3). A lipophilic aromatic ring is connected to an ionizable, hydrophilic tertiary amine via either the ester or amide link. Various substitutions on these 3 portions create the wide variety of local anesthetics available today.

All local anesthetics currently used in clinical practice are weak bases, and the tertiary amine portion of the molecule can be in varying states of protonation depending on the surrounding environment's pH. Understanding the relationship between the charged and uncharged form is key to understanding the clinical effect of local anesthetics.

Looking at Table 12–1, the pKa for most clinically available local anesthetics is in the range of 7.7 to 8.9, meaning that when exposed to normal body pH of 7.4, more local anesthetic molecules will exist in the charged, ionized form. The degree of local anesthetic ionization is important, as the ionized form is active at the sodium channel receptor site and does not readily dissociate from the channel, but is also poorly lipid soluble. In contrast, the neutral form is more lipid soluble and can easily traverse nerve membranes to the site of action.

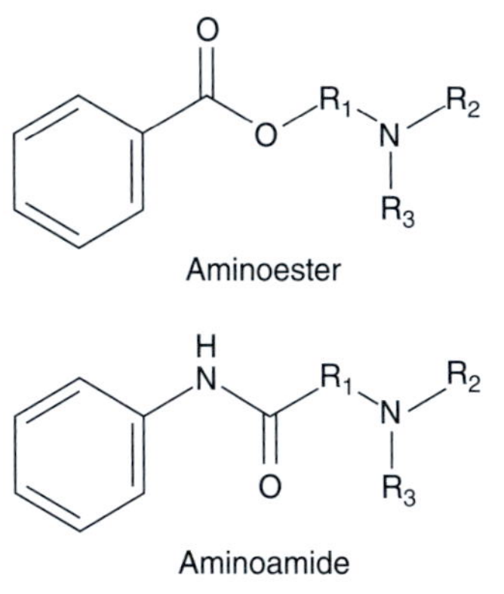

FIGURE 12–3 Schematic illustration of ester and amide local anesthetics.

TABLE 12–1 Properties of common local anesthetics.

	pKa	% Protein Binding	Speed of Onset	Duration of Action (hours)
Amides				
Lidocaine (Xylocaine)	7.8	70	Rapid	1–2
Bupivacaine (Marcaine, Sensorcaine)	8.1	96	Slow	4–8
Levobupivacaine	8.1	96	Sow	4–8
Ropivacaine (Naropin)	8.1	94	Slow	4–8
Mepivacaine (Carbocaine)	7.6	78	Slow	1.5–3
Prilocaine (Novocaine)	7.8	55	Slow	1–2
Esters				
Procaine (Citanest)	8.9	6	Slow	1
Chloroprocaine (Nesacaine)	9.0	7	Rapid	0.5
Tetracaine, Amethocaine (Pontocaine)	8.2	75	Slow	3
Benzocaine (Cetacaine)	2.5			
Cocaine	8.7			

Early studies of local anesthetics proved that a local anesthetic could more effectively block nerve transmission if the surrounding pH was more alkaline, as more molecules would be in a neutral state and able to penetrate the membrane to successfully bind the sodium channel.[9] This concept is also seen clinically as local anesthetics injected into an area of inflamed or infected tissue (with a lower pH) will not be as effective. This also explains why clinicians may choose to add bicarbonate to their local anesthetic solutions prior to injection, in an attempt to increase the pH of the local anesthetic solution, thereby increasing the proportion of uncharged molecules available. There are a lack of good data to support alkalinization of local anesthetic solutions, although it is commonly done. Some believe that along with speeding the onset time, this practice also decreases the pain patients may experience upon injection of the local anesthetic.

Lipid solubility tends to affect both duration of action and potency. As the lipid solubility of a drug increases, so does the chance that the drug will likely be taken up into other tissues. As the drug is now temporarily stored in myelin and surrounding fat/fascial compartments, the drug will be able to exit these tissues once the concentration gradient favors its movement out. Thus, the surrounding tissues act as a temporary depot of drug. Once released, the now free drug will be able to interact with nerve targets. There is a direct correlation between increasing lipid solubility and increasing affinity at the sodium channel receptor that explains the effect on potency.

Protein binding also parallels lipid solubility and, as such, the drugs with higher protein binding tend to have a longer duration of action. This increased protein binding dictates that the drug will bind not only to the sodium channel protein but also to a variety of other proteins that also act as a depot for sustained release of the drug. For example, bupivacaine binds extensively to α_1-acid glycoprotein. Looking at Table 12–1, bupivacaine has approximately 95% protein binding, whereas lidocaine has approximately 70% protein binding. This correlates with bupivacaine's longer duration of action. Protein levels can vary widely with certain disease states (eg, heart failure, liver failure, pregnancy), and all the available local anesthetics have differing levels of protein binding.

Commercial Preparations

Local anesthetics are prepared as water-soluble hydrochloride salts. The pH is decreased to approximately 4.0 to 6.4 to promote development of the cationic form, thereby increasing stability. However, as discussed above, this cationic form decreases potency and onset. Attempts at packaging local anesthetics in a higher pH solution to solve this problem have led to precipitation of the local anesthetic out of solution. Some local anesthetics come prepared with epinephrine, often at a concentration of 1:200,000 (or 5-mcg epinephrine/mL). These preparations must also be acidified because packaging them in an alkaline solution can cause oxidation of the epinephrine. Attempts have been made at adding antioxidants, such as metabisulfite (some controversy about whether it causes neurotoxicity[10]) and ethylenediaminetetraacetic acid (EDTA, associated with allergic reactions). Manufacturers have also added antimicrobials, such as paraben derivatives, which are generally avoided in neuraxial and intravenous use out of concern for cytotoxic effects and allergic reactions.

KINETICS AND METABOLISM

Local anesthetics are almost exclusively used by injecting into the tissues immediately surrounding the desired site of action. This means that systemic factors are less important to overall drug kinetics than the local factors in the area of injection. One must realize that the entirety of local anesthetic injected does not act on the nerve, as a portion of it is taken up by the bloodstream and bound by other tissue types (fat, muscle, connective tissue). The effect on the nerve is governed by uptake by these other tissues, how close the nerve is to the site of injection, intrinsic vasoactive properties of the local anesthetic drug, addition of vasoconstrictors, how easily the local anesthetic solution can flow around the nerve, and diffusion across the nerve membrane.

For example, when performing a subarachnoid block, the spinal roots are surrounded by cerebrospinal fluid, and application of a relatively small amount of local anesthetic will create the desired effect. Contrast this with performing a sciatic nerve or brachial plexus block, where the nerves are surrounded by fascial layers that must be penetrated by the drug. Because of these factors and site-to-site variability, dose-response relationships can be difficult to predict. When thinking about clinical effect of a local anesthetic, one should consider the total volume given, as well as the concentration of drug used; both will create diffusion gradients and will contribute to a successful block. Diffusion into a nerve membrane is also determined by molecular weight, pKa (discussed earlier), and lipid solubility. Molecular weights vary little between most local anesthetics. Increased lipid solubility will mean faster diffusion through nerve membranes, but it could also mean more vigorous uptake by non-neural tissue, attenuating a fast onset.

Systemic absorption of local anesthetics is linearly related to the total dose administered. The addition of vasoconstrictors (such as epinephrine) has been shown to decrease peak plasma levels of local anesthetics. Because the vasoconstrictor prevents systemic absorption, the local anesthetic demonstrates a longer duration of action. Vasoconstrictors are commonly known to be more effective at reducing blood levels when used with the shorter acting local anesthetics (lidocaine), rather than the longer acting local anesthetics (bupivacaine), which are more likely influenced by tissue and nerve binding. For example, adding 5-mcg/mL epinephrine to epidural lidocaine will increase its duration of action by 50% and decrease the peak blood level by 20% to 30%, whereas adding epinephrine to epidural bupivacaine will increase the duration by 0% to 30% and decrease the peak blood level by 10% to 20%.[11] The site of injection has also been shown to influence systemic absorption and the plasma level of local anesthetics. The highest rate of absorption is found with intercostal blocks, followed by caudal epidural, lumbar epidural, brachial plexus, and sciatic and femoral blocks. Various physicochemical properties will also affect systemic absorption, as drugs with more lipid solubility and protein binding will have lower rates of systemic absorption. Also, most local anesthetic molecules have inherent vasodilating properties that can lead to increased rates of systemic absorption. The addition of epinephrine, as described above, can attenuate this effect. Once in the venous circulation, local anesthetics are transported to lung tissue where a large portion is taken up, reducing the amount that reaches systemic circulation. Once in the systemic circulation, local anesthetics are first delivered to the vessel rich group (eg, brain, kidneys), followed by muscle and adipose tissue, based on blood flow and blood concentration gradients.

Distribution is affected by several factors. The distribution of local anesthetics follows that of a 2-compartment model, as described above, and most of the data on local anesthetic distribution comes from studies of the amides, as esters are very rapidly metabolized in the plasma. However, because of the way these local anesthetic drugs are used, one cannot assume direct correlation to classic 2-compartment modeling. We inject local anesthetics into various sites, with varying degrees of blood flow and uptake. Overall, local tissue characteristics, the physicochemical properties of the drugs being used, protein binding, lipid solubility, and local blood flow will largely determine drug distribution. Protein levels can vary widely with certain disease states (ie, heart failure, liver failure, pregnancy), and all the available local anesthetics have differing levels of protein binding. These factors should all be considered when deciding on a dose to administer each patient.

Metabolism

The clearance of amide local anesthetics is accomplished primarily by liver cytochrome P450 metabolism, and the rate of clearance is largely dictated by liver blood flow. Lidocaine has been shown to have a pharmacologically active metabolite, monoethylglycinexylidide, which is approximately one fifth as potent as the parent lidocaine but can be clinically relevant in certain disease states (eg, congestive heart failure). Ester local anesthetics are cleared by plasma and liver cholinesterases and generally have a shorter duration of action than amides. Those patients with abnormal or deficient plasma cholinesterase could likely have prolonged action of ester local anesthetics. Various disease states can also affect distribution and elimination, including such conditions as congestive heart failure, renal failure, liver failure, extremes of age, and sepsis.

DOSING REGIMENS

Dosing regimens and maximal dosing ranges for selected local anesthetics are presented in Table 12–2.

TABLE 12–2 Common dosing regimens of local anesthetics.[a]

	Maximal Dosing
Amides	
Lidocaine (Xylocaine)	4.5 mg/kg not to exceed 300 mg total dose 7 mg/kg, not to exceed 500 mg total dose with epinephrine
Bupivacaine (Marcaine, Sensorcaine)	2.5 mg/kg
Levobupivacaine (Chirocaine)	2.5 mg/kg
Ropivacaine (Naropin)	3 mg/kg 3.5 mg/kg with epinephrine
Mepivacaine (Carbocaine)	4 mg/kg 7 mg/kg with epinephrine
Prilocaine (Citanest)	7 mg/kg 8.5 mg/kg with epinephrine
Esters	
Procaine (Novocaine)	12 mg/kg, not to exceed 500–1000 mg total dose
Chloroprocaine (Nesacaine)	11 mg/kg, not to exceed 600 mg total dose 14 mg/kg, not to exceed 1000 mg total dose with epinephrine
Tetracaine, Amethocaine (Pontocaine)	1.2–1.5 mg/kg 3 mg/kg with epinephrine
Cocaine	3 mg/kg

[a]Doses are for adults only.

INDICATIONS

Local anesthetics are widely used in modern anesthetic practice. Central neuraxial delivery of local anesthetic drugs is commonly used for spinal anesthesia for abdominal, pelvic, and lower extremity surgery. Epidural local anesthetics are used for surgical anesthesia and postoperative analgesia for thoracic, abdominal, pelvic, and lower extremity surgery. Epidurals are also commonly used for obstetric analgesia.

Wound infiltration with local anesthetics is commonly used by surgeons for peri-incisional pain. New liposomal delivery formulations have been developed that increase the duration of action of infiltration analgesia. Several studies on liposomal bupivacaine have shown superior postoperative pain control following various types of surgeries.[5-8]

Peripheral nerve blocks using local anesthetics have become increasingly popular in modern anesthesiology practice and research. As part of a multimodal approach to postoperative pain control, the use of peripheral nerve blocks is increasing for upper and lower extremity orthopedic surgeries, as well as abdominal and thoracic surgeries. Advances in ultrasound technology have increased the popularity and safety profile of peripheral nerve blockade. The use of perineural catheters for several days of continued delivery of local anesthetic drugs has been widely accepted by physicians and patients.

Recently, the use of intravenous lidocaine infusions intraoperatively and postoperatively for improved postoperative pain control has gained popularity. Numerous studies have shown improved postoperative pain scores, decreased opioid consumption, improved patient satisfaction, and often a faster return of bowel function following major abdominal surgery.[12] Most authors would recommend starting with a 1.5-mg/kg lidocaine bolus at the time of anesthetic induction and then follow with an infusion of 2 mg/kg for the intraoperative course. The optimal duration of lidocaine infusion has not been determined, with some studies only running an infusion intraoperatively, while others continue an infusion for up to 4 days postoperatively. In addition to the known mechanism of action at the sodium channel, it is thought that the use of lidocaine as part of an infusion likely involves an anti-inflammatory effect that is not yet completely understood.[13]

Intravenous local anesthetics have also been used for many years in what is known as a Bier block, named for a German surgeon (August Bier) who developed the technique in the early 1900s. This technique is most commonly used for brief orthopedic procedures of the hand and forearm, such as carpal tunnel release.

Local anesthetics are also used in the management of chronic pain. Topical delivery systems have allowed lidocaine to be used in the treatment of various chronic neuropathic pain states, such as post-thoracotomy pain, amputation stump pain, intercostal neuralgia, diabetic neuropathic pain, complex regional pain syndrome, and postherpetic neuralgia.[14]

ADVERSE EFFECTS

Allergic reactions to local anesthetics are rare but can occur and can be life threatening. Between the 2 classes of local anesthetics, reactions are more common with the esters because of their p-aminobenzoic acid metabolites. A true allergic reaction to an amide is exceedingly rare. Allergic reactions to preservatives have also been described.

Direct neurotoxicity has been described with large-volume injections, injections of highly concentrated local anesthetics, and injections that produce localized pressure on the nerve and compromise its blood supply. Direct needle trauma to the nerve and intraneural injections have also led to nerve damage and should be avoided. The increasing popularity of ultrasound-guided regional anesthesia techniques will hopefully decrease the occurrence of direct nerve trauma, as well as intraneural and intravascular injections. Exposure to chloroprocaine or lidocaine used in a subarachnoid block has led to transient neurologic syndrome, a clinical diagnosis thought to involve pooling of high concentration of local anesthetics in the cauda equina space. While initial reports of this involved the use of microcatheters for continuous spinal anesthesia, it has also been described with single-shot spinal techniques. Features of this syndrome include localized back pain, as well as radiculopathies, paresthesias, and/or hypoesthesia. Intraoperative lithotomy positioning also seems to be a risk factor for transient neurologic symptoms, both when combined with spinal anesthesia and as an independent risk factor. A meta-analysis published in 2002 found that the risk for transient neurologic syndrome after spinal anesthesia with lidocaine was 6.7 times higher than if bupivacaine was used.[15]

Methemoglobinemia is a rare side effect of the use of prilocaine, usually in large doses (> 10 mg/kg). O-toluidine, a metabolite of prilocaine, can cause oxidation of hemoglobin to methemoglobin. Prilocaine is commonly used in dentistry and is found in the topical anesthetic cream, EMLA, mixed with lidocaine. Signs of methemoglobinemia include cyanosis, chocolate-colored urine, and a pulse oximetry value that approaches 85% regardless of the true value. Treatment for methemoglobinemia involves the administration of methylene blue, a reducing agent, to convert methemoglobin to hemoglobin. There have also been reports of methemoglobinemia associated with the use of several other local anesthetics, including tetracaine and benzocaine.

Finally, local anesthetic systemic toxicity (LAST) can manifest as CNS and/or cardiovascular dysfunction, ranging from mild symptoms to complete failure. Both of these can generally be prevented by avoiding intravascular injection, injecting incrementally, and using the smallest dose needed to achieve the desired clinical effect.

Signs and symptoms of CNS toxicity depend on blood levels of the local anesthetic. Early effects include circumoral numbness, metallic taste, dizziness, and tinnitus, progressing to nystagmus, twitching, convulsions, coma, cardiopulmonary arrest, and death. The convulsant activity likely stems from selective depression of inhibitory pathways, leaving unopposed excitatory activation progressing to grand mal seizures. CNS toxicity is increased by decreasing pH and increasing $PaCO_2$. It can be prevented by using appropriate doses and avoiding intravascular injection, as mentioned above. Also, premedicating with a benzodiazepine, such as midazolam, should be considered.

If signs of CNS toxicity appear, apply supplemental oxygen and instruct the patient to hyperventilate to decrease carbon dioxide levels, which will decrease blood flow to the brain. This will also raise the pH of the blood, avoiding a respiratory acidosis. Hyperventilation will also lower the extracellular potassium and hyperpolarize the neural membrane. If the patient loses consciousness or is otherwise unable to protect the airway and participate in hyperventilation, the provider should quickly call for help, assume control of the airway, and initiate hyperventilation. Benzodiazepines, barbiturates, and/or propofol should be considered for the prevention and treatment of seizures.

The cardiovascular system is significantly more resistant to local anesthetic toxicity than the central nervous system. The ratio between the dose required for cardiovascular collapse (CC) versus CNS toxicity, or the CC-to-CNS dose ratio, is approximately 7.1 for lidocaine and 2.0 for bupivacaine. This shows the lower margin of safety when using bupivacaine compared with lidocaine. It is worth mentioning that the margin of safety is even lower in pregnancy, as alterations in protein binding can lead to more unbound, pharmacologically active drug available.[16]

Cardiovascular toxicity can be very severe and quite difficult, if not impossible, to reverse. Local anesthetics produce dose-dependent decreases in contractility and cardiac electrical conduction. Also, local anesthetics can act as vasodilators. Sodium channel blockade in the cardiac conduction system leads to depressed pacemaker activity and impaired conduction of impulses throughout the myocardium. This can result in severe dysrhythmias, heart block, and hypotension.

Bupivacaine deserves special mention here as it has been recognized to produce cardiovascular toxicity that is very dangerous and difficult to reverse. Bupivacaine toxicity often presents clinically in a much more severe fashion than lidocaine, with common malignant dysrhythmias, CC, and severe hypotension. Bupivacaine displays a high degree of potency and binding affinity at the cardiac sodium channels. This increased cardiac toxicity profile of bupivacaine led to the development of ropivacaine in the 1990s. Bupivacaine contains a racemic mixture of both the R and S stereoisomers. However, ropivacaine contains only the S stereoisomer in commercial preparations. Ropivacaine is, therefore, less cardiotoxic in animal models[17,18] while maintaining a similar anesthetic potency compared to bupivacaine.

Treatment of local anesthetic-induced cardiovascular toxicity can be challenging. Special attention to the temporal relationship that occurs with these cases is crucial, as knowing that the patient has recently received a bolus of local anesthetic can eliminate wasted time in determining the cause of the CC and focus the treatment algorithm to the most effective methods for resuscitation. Initiation of Advanced Cardiac Life Support (ACLS) care with high-quality chest compressions and airway control with fraction of inspired oxygen (FiO_2) of 1.0 and hyperventilation are the first steps.

Lipid emulsion therapy has recently emerged as an effective, although incompletely understood, treatment for resuscitating a patient in CC following LAST. It is theorized that this works by delivering a bolus of lipid to bind the local anesthetic molecules, thereby sequestering them and reducing the amount available to bind cardiac sodium channels. Animal studies have shown that lipid therapy likely also accelerates the release of local anesthetic molecules already bound to myocardium, thus suggesting that it does not work only by binding free drug.[19] Other competing theories of lipid emulsion mechanism of action focus on the improved metabolic milieu created within cardiac myocytes. It has been proposed that lipid emulsion therapy might impede the local anesthetic's inhibition of acyl carnitine, which would improve mitochondrial metabolism, and a theory that lipid therapy increases calcium concentrations in cardiac myocytes and improves contractility.

Current guidelines by the American Society of Regional Anesthesia and Pain Medicine (ASRA) on the treatment of LAST conclude that standard measures of airway and seizure control be initiated first, followed by lipid therapy. The exact timing of lipid emulsion therapy remains debatable but should likely occur at the first signs of hemodynamic instability. Dosing of lipid therapy would start with a bolus of 1.5 mL/kg over 60 seconds, followed by an infusion of 0.25 to 0.5 mL/kg/min. It is necessary to continue the infusion for 10 minutes after the patient regains hemodynamic stability. The maximum dose in 30 minutes is recommended to not exceed 10 mL/kg. Propofol can be used to control seizure activity only but should not be used as a substitute for lipid therapy, as massive doses would be required which would not be prudent in a patient with hemodynamic collapse.[20,21] It should be noted on these guidelines that ACLS dosing of epinephrine in the setting of LAST is not at the standard 1-mg dose. It is believed that such large doses of epinephrine are unacceptably arrhythmogenic in these patients and that dosing should be much more conservative (approximately 1 mcg/kg). Additionally, vasopressin is not recommended.

REFERENCES

1. Rivera MA, Aufderheide AC, Cartmell LW, Torres CM, Langsjoen O. Antiquity of coca-leaf chewing in the south central Andes: a 3,000 year archaeological record of coca-leaf chewing from northern Chile., *J Psychoactive Drugs*. 2005 Dec;37(4):455-458.
2. Gootenberg P.. *Cocaine: Global Histories*. New York: Routledge; 1999;84.
3. Gordh T. Lidocaine: The Origin of a Modern Local Anesthetic. 1949. *Anesthesiology*. 2010;113(6);1433-1437.
4. Ruetsch YA, Boni T. Borgeat A. From cocaine to ropivicaine: the history of local anesthetic drugs. *Curr Top Med Chem*. 2001;1(3):175-182.
5. Bergese S, Candiotti K, Gorfine S. The efficacy of EXPAREL, a multivesicular liposomal extended-release bupivacaine. Presented at the 2011 International Anesthesia Research Society (IARS) Annual Meeting. Vancouver, British Columbia. May 21-24, 2011. Abstract S-311.
6. Onel E, Miller H, Patou G, White P. EXPAREL, a liposomal bupivacaine local analgesic, extends pain relief and decreases opioid use. Presented at the 2010 Annual Meeting of the American Society of Anesthesiologists (ASA). San Diego, CA. October 16-20, 2010.
7. Golf M, Daniels S, Onel E. A phase 3, randomized, placebo-controlled trial of DepoFoam bupivacaine (extended-release bupivacaine local analgesic) in bunionectomy. *Adv Ther.* 2011;28(9):776-788.
8. Gorfine S, Onel E, Patou G, Krivokapic Z. Bupivacaine Extended-release liposome injection for prolonged post-surgical analgesia in patients undergoing hemorrhoidectomy: a multicenter randomized, double-blind, placebo-controlled trial. *Dis Colon Rectum.* 2011;54(12):1552-1559.
9. Trevan J, Boock E. The relation of hydrogen ion concentration to the action of local anesthetics. *Br J Exp Pathol.* 8;307:1927.

10. Taniguchi M, Bollen A, Drasner K. Sodium bisulfite: scapegoat for chloroprocaine neurotoxicity? *Anesthesiology*. 2004;100(1):85-91.
11. Tucker, GT, Mather, LE. Absorption and disposition of local anesthetics. In: Cousins MJ, Bridenbaugh PO (eds). *Neural Blockade in Clinical Anesthesia and Management of Pain*. Philadelphia: JB Lippincott, 1980:45.
12. McCarthy G, Megalla S, Habib A. Impact of intravenous lidocaine infusion on postoperative analgesia and recovery from surgery: a systematic review of randomized controlled trials. *Drugs*. 2010;70(9): 1149-1163.
13. Hollmann M, Durieux M. Local anesthetics and the inflammatory response: a new therapeutic indication? *Anesthesiology*. 2000;93:858-875.
14. Devers A, Galer B. Topical lidocaine patch relieves a variety of neuropathic pain conditions: an open-label study. *Clin J Pain*. 000;16(3):205-208.
15. Eberhart LH, Morin AM, Kranke P, et al. Transient neurologic symptoms after spinal anesthesia. A quantitative systematic overview (meta-analysis) of randomized controlled studies (in German). *Anaesthetist*. 2002;51:539-546.
16. Morishima HO, Pedersen H, Finster M, et al. Bupivacaine toxicity in pregnant and nonpregnant ewes. *Anesthesiology*. 1985;63:134-139.
17. Ohmura S, Kawada M, Ohta T, Yamamoto K, Kobayashi T. Systemic toxicity and resuscitation in bupivacaine-, levobupivacaine-, or ropivacaine-infused rats. *Anesth Analg*. 2001;93(3):743-748.
18. Dony P, Dewinde V, Vanderick B, et al. The comparative toxicity of ropivacaine and bupivacaine at equipotent doses in rats. *Anesth Analgesia*. 2000;91(6):1489-1492.
19. Weinberg GL, Ripper R, Murphy P, et al. Lipid Infusion accelerates removal of bupivacaine and recover from bupivacaine toxicity in the isolated rat heart. *Reg Anesth Pain Med*. 2006;31(4): 296-303.
20. Toledo P. The role of lipid emulsion during advanced cardiac life support for local anesthetic toxicity. *Int J Obstet Anesth*. 2011;20(1):60-63.
21. Neal JM, Bernards CM, Butterworth JF, et al. ASRA practice advisory on local anesthetic systemic toxicity. *Reg Anesth Pain Med*. 2010;35(2): 152-161.

CHAPTER 13

Anesthetic Drug Interactions with Herbal Remedies

L. Lazarre Ogden, MD, Elise Heath, MD, and Gregory Wallace, MD

INTRODUCTION

As the use of herbal supplements becomes more widespread, it is vitally important that the anesthetist has a detailed understanding of potential interactions with anesthetic medications and full knowledge of the perturbations these herbal remedies can have on patient physiology in a perioperative setting. The first question to ask after reviewing conventional medications is: "Do you take any herbal supplements/medications that are not documented in your chart? It may have an impact on your surgery and/or anesthetic." The caveat is that patients do not always know *to* report supplements as medications. They may not understand the scope of properties these supplements have when not discontinued before surgery, especially when they will be exposed to a number of different medications during the perioperative and postsurgical course. A common recommendation is to refrain from taking herbal remedies for at least 2 weeks prior to surgery. This recommendation is not standard or widespread, and it is impossible to enforce due to noncompliance or emergency surgical situations. A pertinent, concise description is valuable to enhance understanding of these herbal remedies and avoid catastrophic outcomes due to inadequate consideration of these drugs effects. What follows is a review of few of the more commonly prescribed supplements that influence anesthetic drug action. A summary of these herbal remedies is presented in Table 13–1.

GARLIC (*ALLIUM SATIVUM*)

Garlic is a popular herbal supplement that is thought to aid in control of atherosclerotic disease. It is available in many different pill and capsule formulations. Its use in prevention of atherosclerotic disease is based on findings published in 1986 that it decreases thrombosis by dose-dependent inhibition of platelet aggregation inhibition, reduces blood pressure, and lowers cholesterol.[1]

Allicin and alliin (organosulfur-containing compounds) are thought to be responsible for garlic's mechanism of action. Animal studies have demonstrated a reduction of atherosclerosis, intra-arterial fat deposition, normalized lipoprotein balance, and inhibition of platelet aggregation.[2-4] Ajoene, another constituent, may cause irreversible platelet inhibition. Human studies have yielded the same results with regard to lowering cholesterol.[5,6]

Anesthetic Implications

Since garlic may potentiate effects of other anticoagulants and antiplatelet and anti-inflammatory drugs, clinicians may consider having patients stop garlic consumption 7 to 14 days prior to surgery, especially with surgical procedures associated with significant blood loss or worrisome complications from persistent unanticipated anticoagulation.

ECHINACEA (*ECHINACEA PURPUREA*)

Echinacea, purported to have immune system–stimulating properties, is derived from the daisy plant family (purple coneflower of the family Asteraceae). Common uses include prophylaxis and treatment of viral, bacterial, and fungal infections, particularly upper respiratory infections.[7-13] The mechanism is unknown, although antidepressant properties have been shown to increases in L-dopa in a rodent model.

TABLE 13–1 Summary of clinical effects, mechanisms of action, and anesthetic implication of selected herbal remedies.

Herbal Remedy	Clinical Effects	Mechanism of Action	Anesthetic Implications
Garlic (*Allium sativum*) Source: Bulb from onion-like garlic plant	Known effects: Decreased blood pressure Decreased cholesterol Decreased lipids Decreased thrombus formation	Dose-dependent platelet aggregation inhibition	Increased risk of bleeding Possible potentiation of other platelet aggregation inhibitors
Echinacea (*Echinacea purpurea*) Source: Coneflower, a flower from the daisy plant family	Purported effects: Immune system stimulant Prophylaxis/treatment of viral, bacterial and fungal infections, particularly upper respiratory infections Antidepressant	Unknown, may increase L-dopa levels	Consider avoiding in patients who require immunosuppression CYP3A4 inhibitor[a] Consider avoiding when coadministered with other potential hepatotoxic drugs
Valerian (*Valeriana officinalis*) Source: Valerian root	Purported effects: Sedation Anxiolysis Sleep aid	Potentiates GABA-ergic system	May potentiate benzodiazepines, opioids, and sedative hypnotics May cause withdrawal postoperatively with abrupt cessation
Ephedra (ma huang) Source: Ephedra plant	Known effects: Stimulant	α-1-, β-1-, and β-2-receptor agonism	Fatal cardiovascular events (myocardial infarct, stroke, death) Perioperative hemodynamic instability Catecholamine depletion Adverse cardiovascular effects when mixed with MAOIs
Ginkgo (*Ginkgo biloba*) Source: Leaf of ginkgo plant	Known effects: Improved cognitive function Antioxidant Inhibitor of platelet activation Altered vascular tone	Partially understood; flavonoids, terpenoids, and organic acids protect from oxidative damage.	Rare postoperative bleeding
St. John's wort: (*Hypericum perforatum*) Source: Shrub plant of the same name containing hypericin and hyperforin	Purported effects: Antidepressant	Inhibition of serotonin, norepinephrine and dopamine reuptake	Induction of hepatic cytochromes CYP3A4 and CYP2C9; this may decrease effect from: Warfarin Alfentanil Midazolam Lidocaine Calcium channel blockers Serotonin antagonists NSAIDS
Ginseng: (*Panax ginseng*) Source: Perennial plant of the same name containing ginsenosides a steroidal saponins	Purported effects: Protection from stress and restore homeostasis Decrease glucose levels Anticoagulation	Poorly understood, but considered similar to steroid hormones	Hypoglycemia in fasting patients Perioperative bleeding

(*Continued*)

TABLE 13–1 Summary of clinical effects, mechanisms of action, and anesthetic implication of selected herbal remedies. (*Continued*)

Herbal Remedy	Clinical Effects	Mechanism of Action	Anesthetic Implications
Kava (*Piper methysticum*) *Source:* Roots of the Kava plant	Purported effects: Sedative Anxiolytic	May influence GABA-ergic system	May potentiate sedative–hypnotics
Ginger: (*Zingiber officinale*) *Source:* Rhizome (roots) of ginger plant	Purported effects: Anti-Inflammatory Antiemetic	Potent inhibitor of thromboxane synthetase	Potential for increased risk of prolonged bleeding, especially when coadministered with NSAIDs and/or warfarin

[a]CYP3A4 inhibition decreases metabolism of many anesthetic drugs.
GABA, γ-aminobutyric acid; MAOI, monoamine oxidase inhibitor; NSAIDs, nonsteroidal anti-inflammatory drugs.

Anesthetic Implications

Since echinacea may have immune-stimulating properties, consider avoiding it in patients taking immunosuppressive drugs or in patients with autoimmune disease. Studies suggest that echinacea may be hepatotoxic and should not be used in patients with known preexisting liver disease or coadministered with other hepatotoxic medications such as methotrexate, amiodarone, ketoconazole, or anabolic steroids. Due to the risk of hepatotoxicity, it is recommended that patients do not take echinacea for longer than 8 weeks.

Echinacea is an inhibitor of the hepatic cytochrome P450 CYP3A4, an important enzyme in the metabolism of many drugs. Consumption of echinacea may lead to elevated blood levels of drugs metabolized by this cytochrome (ie, lovastatin, itraconazole, and fexofenadine).

In addition, anaphylaxis has been reported in patients with allergies to plants in the daisy family (marigold, ragweed, chrysanthemum).

VALERIAN (*VALERIANA OFFICINALIS*)

This supplement has been used as a sedative, anxiolytic, as well as a sleeping aid. It is thought to have a mechanism of action related to the neurotransmitter γ-aminobutyric acid (GABA).

Anesthetic Implications

Knowledge about patient use of this supplement is important because it can potentiate effects of benzodiazepines, sedative–hypnotics, and opioids. Via the proposed GABA mechanism, it appears to be similar to benzodiazepine in effect, and patients may experience withdrawal similar to that with benzodiazepines. Preoperatively, it is prudent to consider a drug taper prior to surgery to avoid withdrawal, which can cloud the picture if there is postoperative delirium.

EPHEDRA (MA HUANG)

Ephedra is popular for its properties as a performance-enhancing drug, to help with weight loss, and to stimulate an increase in energy. It is also used as a treatment for asthma and bronchitis. Ephedra contains alkaloids such as ephedrine, pseudoephedrine, and norephedrine; ephedrine is often the main active ingredient.[14]

Anesthetic Implications

Ephedra increases heart rate and blood pressure in dose-dependent fashion by stimulating α-1-, β-1-, and β-2-receptor activity. A major caveat is the associated reported complications (numbering in the thousands), including fatal cardiovascular events (myocardial infarct, stroke, death).[15] Perioperative hemodynamic instability associated with long-term use and consequent catecholamine depletion may also warrant attention in the perioperative period. Life-threatening episodes of hyperpyrexia, hypertension, and coma have resulted from concomitant use of ephedra and monoamine oxidase inhibitors.

There are reports of nephrolithiasis and potential kidney damage from its use as well.[16]

Ephedra use should be stopped at least 24 hours prior to surgery. Its short half-life of about 5 hours will yield up to 80% of compound excreted in the urine. Moreover, it is best to avoid use altogether in patients with cardiac disease, thyroid disease, or diabetes, or in patients who take theophylline, caffeine, or monoamine oxidase inhibitors.

GINKGO (*GINKGO BILOBA*)

This supplement is derived from the leaf of *Ginkgo biloba*. Extract from the leaves contain flavonoids, terpenoids, and organic acids. Ginkgo is used to treat cognitive disorders such as Alzheimer disease and vertigo, age-related vascular disease, macular degeneration, tinnitus, erectile dysfunction, and altitude sickness.

The mechanism of action is not well understood, but theories suggest that a combination of flavonoids and terpenoids may act synergistically to produce an antioxidant and free radical scavenging effect minimizing damage to cells from free radicals.

Cognitive improvement evidence is highlighted in a study by Le Bars et al,[17] using a randomized controlled trial comparing an extract of Ginkgo to placebo. 309 patients were evaluated in the study and findings show that the ginkgo group had statistically significant improvement on cognitive functioning tests (Alzheimer Disease Assessment Scale–cognitive subscale and Geriatric Evaluation by Relative Rating Instrument) over a 1-year study period.

In addition, ginkgo appears to alter vasoregulation, act as an antioxidant, modulate neurotransmitter and receptor activity, and inhibit platelet-activating factor.

Anesthetic Implications

Complications secondary to bleeding appear to be rare by case reports. However, evidence has surfaced with patients having had perioperative bleeding problems, including spontaneous intracranial bleeding (4 cases), spontaneous hyphema (1 case), and after laparoscopic cholecystectomy (1 case)

Anesthesiologists may consider perioperative discontinuation. The terpenoids in ginkgo have elimination half-lives after oral administration of 3 to 10 hours. The recommended cessation of ginkgo consumption is a minimum of 36 hours prior to surgery.

ST. JOHN'S WORT (*HYPERICUM PERFORATUM*)

St. John's wort is a shrub plant with a yellow 5-pedaled flower and paired oval leaves. It is commonly used to provide short-term treatment of mild to moderate depression. The active ingredients include hypericin and hyperforin. Its mechanism of action is inhibition of serotonin, norepinephrine, and dopamine reuptake by neurons.

However, in a study published by Shelton et al,[18] St. John's wort was shown to be no better than placebo in the 200 patients evaluated with various depression scoring systems. These measures included the Beck Depression Inventory, Hamilton Rating Scale for Depression, Global Assessment of Function scale, and Clinical Global Impression-Severity.

Anesthetic Implications

St. John's wort can significantly increase the metabolism of other medications used perioperatively by induction of several hepatic cytochrome P450 enzymes. CYP3A4 is induced, which metabolizes several antirejection drugs used following organ transplants. For example, metabolism of indinavir (protease inhibitor antiretroviral), ethinyl estradiol, and cyclosporine may be excessive, diminishing blood cyclosporine levels by up to 50% evidenced by 2 case reports of acute heart transplant rejection.

It may also increase the metabolism of other commonly used drugs such as alfentanil, midazolam, lidocaine, calcium channel blockers, and serotonin antagonists. Furthermore, induction of CYP2C9 may reduce the effects of warfarin, leading to a decreased anticoagulant effect and decreased efficacy of nonsteroidal anti-inflammatory drugs.

After oral administration, peak levels of hypericin were seen after 6 hours and 3.5 hours for hyperforin. Median elimination half-lives were 43.1 hours (hypericin) and 9 hours (hyperforin). It is therefore recommended to stop St. John's wort at least 5 days prior to surgery, and serious consideration should be given to longer periods of time for transplant patients.

GINSENG (*PANAX GINSENG*)

Ginseng is utilized for its purported ability to protect the body against stress and restore homeostasis. Active ingredients include ginsenosides, a group belonging to compounds called steroidal saponins. Its mechanism of action is incompletely understood, but the underlying effect is thought to be similar to that described for steroid hormones.

Perioperative considerations include bleeding and lower blood sugar levels. Because ginseng is sometimes used to lower postprandial blood glucose in patients with and without diabetes, it can be problematic in fasting patients. Ginseng has been shown to prolong coagulation time of thrombin and activated partial thromboplastin in animal models. One study (Teng et al)[19] suggested that the antiplatelet activity of ginseng was irreversible.

Considering discontinuation, studies on different ginsenosides have shown variable half-lives, between 0.8 and 7.4 hours. This suggests that ginseng should be discontinued for at least 24 hours. However, considering potential irreversible platelet inhibition, stopping 7 days before surgery may be more prudent.

KAVA (*PIPER METHYSTICUM*)

Kava (also known as kava kava) is derived from the pepper plant *Piper methysticum* and is used for its anxiolytic and sedative properties. Kava may act as a sedative–hypnotic by potentiation of the GABA system.

Anesthetic Implications

Jamieson et al,[20] found that in the laboratory animal studies, kava increased barbiturate-induced sleep. The active ingredient, kavalactone, has a dose-dependent effect on the central nervous system that includes antiepileptic, neuroprotective, and local anesthetic effects. It can potentiate the sedative effects of perioperatively administered anesthetic medications.

Kavalactones reach peak plasma levels in approximately 1.8 hours after an oral dose, and their elimination half-life is 9 hours. The common recommendation is that patients discontinue kava no less than 24 hours prior to surgery.

GINGER (*ZINGIBER OFFICINALE*)

Ginger is commonly touted as an anti-inflammatory and an antiemetic. It is thought to act directly on the gastrointestinal tract as well as inhibit peripheral and central serotonergic pathways. No significant differences, however, have been reported in a systematic review of randomized controlled trials between ginger and placebo groups on the incidence of postoperative nausea and vomiting.

Anesthetic Implications

Since ginger is a potent inhibitor of thromboxane synthetase, there is risk of prolonged bleeding time. Patients should be evaluated based on the potential for risk of bleeding, especially when nonsteroidal anti-inflammatory drugs and warfarin are used in combination with this supplement.

REFERENCES

1. Srivastava KC. Isolation and effects of some ginger components of platelet aggregation and eicosanoid biosynthesis. *Prostaglandins Leukot Med.* 1986;25(2-3):187-198.
2. Messina BA. Herbal supplements: facts and myths—talking to your patients about herbal supplements. *J Perianesth Nurs.* 2006;21:279-281.
3. Eilat S, Oestraicher Y, Rabinkov A, et al. Alteration of lipid profile in hyperlipidemic rabbits by allicin, an active constituent of garlic. *Coron Artery Dis.* 1995;6(12):985-990.
4. Abramovitz D, Gavri S, Harats D, et al. Allicin-induced decrease in formation of fatty streaks (atherosclerosis) in mice fed a cholesterol-rich diet. *Coron Artery Dis.* 1999;10(7):515-519.
5. Silagy CA, Neil HA. A meta-analysis of the effect of garlic on blood pressure. *J Hypertens.* 1994;12 (4: 463-468.
6. Elkayam A, Mirelman D, Peleg E, et al. The effects of allicin on weight in fructose-induced hyperinsulinemic, hyperlipidemic, hypertensive rats. *Am J Hypertens.* 2003;16(12):1053-1056.

7. Barrett BP, Brown RL, Locken K, et al. Treatment of the common cold with unrefined echinacea: a randomized, double blind, placebo-controlled trial. *Ann Intern Med.* 2002;137(12):939–946.
8. Echinacea (*E. angustifolia DC, E. pallida, E. purpurea*). Natural Standard Database web site: www.naturalstandard.com. Accessed June 1, 2009.
9. Fugh-Berman A. Echinacea for the prevention and treatment of upper respiratory infections. *Sem Integrative Med.* 2003;1(2):106–111.
10. O'Neil J, Hughes S, Lourie A, et al. Effects of echinacea on the frequency of upper respiratory tract symptoms: a randomized, double blind, placebo-controlled trial. *Ann Allergy Asthma Immunol.* 2008;100(4):384–388.
11. Shah SA, Sander S, White CM, et al. Evaluation of echinacea for the prevention and treatment of the common cold: a meta-analysis. *Lancet Infectious Diseases.* 2007;7(7):473–480.
12. Taylor JA, Weber W, Standish L, et al. Efficacy and safety of echinacea in treating upper respiratory tract infections in children: a randomized controlled trial. *JAMA.* 2003;290(21):2824–2830.
13. Turner RB, Bauer R, Woelkart K, et al. An evaluation of Echinacea angustifolia in experimental rhinovirus infections. *N Engl J Med.* 2005;353(4):341–348.
14. Gurley B, Wang P, Gardner S. Ephedrine-type alkaloid content of nutritional supplements containing Ephedra sinica (Ma-huang) as determined by high performance liquid chromatography. *J Pharm Sci.* 1998; 87(12):1547-1553.
15. Haller C, Benowitz N. Adverse cardiovascular and central nervous system events associated with dietary supplements containing ephedra alkaloids. *N Engl J Med.* 2000;343;1833-1838.
16. Powell T, Hsu FF, Turk J, Hruska K. Ma-huang strikes again: ephedrine nephrolithiasis. *Am J Kidney Dis* 1998;32:153-159.
17. Le Bars PL, Velasco FM, Ferguson JM, Dessain EC, Kieser M, Hoerr R. Influence of the severity of cognitive impairment on the effect of the Gnkgo biloba extract EGb 761 in Alzheimer's disease. *Neuropsychobiology.* 2002;45(1):19-26.
18. Shelton RC, Keller MB, Gelenberg A, et al. Effectiveness of St John's wort in major depression: a randomized controlled trial. *JAMA.* 2001 Apr 18; 285(15):1978-1986.
19. Teng CM, Kuo SC, Ko FN, et al. Antiplatelet actions of panaxynol and ginsenosides isolated from ginseng. *Biochim Biophys Acta.* 1989 Mar 24;990(3):315-320.
20. Jamieson DD, Duffield PH, Cheng D, Duffield AM. Comparison of the central nervous system activity of the aqueous and lipid extract of kava (Piper methysticum). *Arch Int Pharmacodyn Ther.* 1989 Sep-Oct;301:66-80.

CHAPTER 14

Vasoactive Agents

Michael Behrens, MD

INTRODUCTION

Vasoactive agents were recognized in 1895 by H.D. Rollerston, when he described a suprarenal extract as a "powerful vascular tonic."[1] Today, these drugs have an important role in anesthetics and critical care.

ADRENERGIC AGONISTS

Adrenergic receptors are classified into two commonly recognized subtypes, α and β. Many subtypes of these receptors have been described, but the most clinically important subtypes are α_1, α_2, β_1, and β_2. α_1 receptors are found primarily on smooth muscle in the vasculature where activation leads to vasoconstriction. They are also found in the genitourinary tract, intestine, as well as cardiac and liver tissue. α receptors are found in pancreatic beta cells, nerves, and platelets. They are also present on vascular smooth muscle, although to a lesser extent than α_1 receptors. β_1 receptors are found primarily in the heart and kidney. In the heart their stimulation leads to an increase in chronotropy, inotropy and atrial-ventricular node conduction velocity. Their activation in the kidney causes renin release. β_2 Receptors are prominent in smooth muscle. Activation of β_2 receptors in the vasculature results in vasodilation, while activation of the same receptors in the airways leads to bronchodilation.

Dopamine, norepinephrine, and epinephrine are endogenous adrenergic agonists synthesized from the enzymatic alteration of phenylalanine. They are most frequently used for the acute management of hypotension, although epinephrine is also indicated for use in acute bronchoconstriction and anaphylaxis. By causing vasoconstriction, these agents will alter perfusion and oxygen delivery to different organs. The clinical significance of this altered blood flow varies dramatically between patients but sometimes results in organ ischemia or ischemia of the distal extremities necessitating amputation. Tachycardia and increased myocardial oxygen consumption can lead to dysrhythmias if cardiac oxygen delivery is inadequate. Cerebral hemorrhage can occur if vasoconstriction leads to severe systemic hypertension.

Epinephrine

Epinephrine is the prototypical sympathomimetic drug and is active at both α and β receptors. At very low doses the vasodilatory effects of β_2 activation can be most prevalent, but as the dose increases the β_2 and α_1 effects dominate. Its vasoconstriction and bronchodilation properties make it an excellent drug for the treatment of anaphylaxis and it may be administered intramuscularly (IM) for the treatment of bronchoconstriction or anaphylaxis. Typical IM dosing is 300 mcg for adults and 150 mcg in children. When given IM, peak effects are seen within 15 minutes.[2] Intravenous (IV) bolus dosing effects are seen within seconds after reaching the circulation, and these effects typically last less than 5 minutes. Inhaled epinephrine can cause bronchodilation within 1 minute, but tachycardia and other systemic effects may be seen at high doses. Epinephrine is primarily eliminated by hepatic metabolism. Epinephrine causes a rise in blood glucose levels by increasing hepatic gluconeogenesis and decreasing pancreatic insulin secretion.

Norepinephrine

Norepinephrine activates both α and β receptors. It is active at α_1 receptors, although it is less potent than epinephrine and has no clinically significant β_2 effects. Its β_1 stimulation effects are equipotent to those of epinephrine. IV doses of norepinephrine have a rapid onset and offset time similar to epinephrine. It is eliminated via the same pathways as epinephrine. It is indicated for use in patients with severe hypotension due to vasodilation. In septic shock, norepinephrine causes less tachycardia and may case less splanchnic vasoconstriction than epinephrine. Although epinephrine has not been associated with worse outcomes, norepinephrine is preferred over epinephrine in the treatment of septic shock.[3]

Dopamine

Dopamine is the precursor to norepinephrine and epinephrine in catecholamine synthesis. Though it is an important neurotransmitter, it does not cross the blood-brain barrier after IV administration and is therefore not associated with clinically important central nervous system effects. It acts on α, β, and dopaminergic (D_1 and D_2) receptors. In addition to the CNS, D_1 receptors are found in the renal tubules as well as renal and mesenteric blood vessels. At low doses (< 3 mcg/kg/min), the predominant effect is vasodilation resulting from D_1 receptor activation. The increased renal blood flow is apparently offset by peripheral vasodilation via D_2 receptor attenuation of norepinephrine release shunting blood away from the kidneys. At higher doses the β_1 activity becomes more prominent, with increased myocardial contractility and a rise in systolic blood pressure. At high doses (> 10 mcg/kg/min), vasoconstriction caused by activation of α_1 receptors becomes the predominant clinical effect.

Dopamine has a rapid onset and elimination similar to epinephrine. Dopamine is metabolized by monoamine oxidase (MAO) in the liver and kidney. Its duration of action is prolonged up to 1 hour in patients taking MAO inhibitors. Dopamine is indicated in the treatment of shock states, including cardiogenic shock where its β_1 agonism could increase a low cardiac output.

Dopamine can increase urine output, and low-dose dopamine (1–3 mcg/kg/min) has been widely studied for its possible ability to prevent renal damage in low perfusion states by improving renal perfusion. However, most recent clinical data do not support the use of low-dose dopamine to preserve renal function.[3]

SYMPATHOMIMETICS

Fenoldopam

Fenoldopam is a dopamine analog that is only active on the D_1 receptor. It does not have any α or β activity, and it does not cross the blood-brain barrier. It has poor oral bioavailablity and is currently only available for parenteral administration. Its primary clinical effects are vasodilation and diuresis. It can rapidly and predictably lower blood pressure, which makes it a useful agent to treat acute and severe hypertension. It is recommended that it be administered only by continuous infusion. It has a rapid onset reaching full effect after 15 minutes of continuous infusion and it has a half-life of 10 minutes.[4]

Fenoldopam should be used with caution in patients with glaucoma, as it has been shown to raise intraocular pressure. Like other vasodilating agents, it can also cause tachycardia and headaches.

Phenylephrine

Phenylephrine is a synthetic sympathomimetic agent that exhibits potent vasoconstriction activity via α_1 receptor activation. Its hemodynamic effects are seen almost immediately after IV administration, and these effects persist for up to 15 minutes. At very high doses, it may activate β receptors but at commonly used doses only the α effects are seen. These effects include a rise in systemic blood pressure and reflex bradycardia.

Phenylephrine is indicated for use in patients with hypotension due to vasodilation. It must be used cautiously in patients with poor left ventricular function as cardiac output may be further decreased by the increased peripheral vascular resistance caused by phenylephrine.

Ephedrine

Ephedrine is a sympathomimetic that has both direct α and β activity. Its effects are similar to epinephrine, although ephedrine is much less potent and has a longer duration of action. Ephedrine exhibits indirect activity as well due to its ability to release norepinephrine from presynaptic nerve terminals. Ephedrine can be used for the short-term treatment of vasodilatory hypotension and is often the first choice among vasoconstrictors to counteract the vasodilation associated with spinal or epidural anesthesia. Its effects on hemodynamics are seen almost immediately after IV administration, and these effects last for up to 10 minutes. The effects may last for up to 1 hour after IM or subcutaneous administration. Ephedrine is metabolized by hepatic enzymes as well as excreted unchanged in the urine.

Ephedrine has become the preferred vasoconstrictor in obstetric patients because it is believed to cause less reduction in uterine blood flow when compared to phenylephrine.[5,6]

BETA AGONISTS

Dobutamine

Dobutamine is a synthetic analog of dopamine and has predominantly β_1 effects. Hemodynamic effects occur immediately after IV administration, and peak effects occur with 10 minutes after starting a continuous infusion. It has a half-life of 2 minutes and is primarily cleared by hepatic metabolism. In healthy patients, dobutamine has been shown to increase cardiac output in a linear fashion. At low doses (2.5 mcg/kg/min) cardiac output rises due to increased stroke volume. At higher doses the stroke volume is unchanged, and the increased heart rate accounts for the continued rise in cardiac output.[7]

Dobutamine has the ability to increase cardiac output without the vasoconstriction and tachycardia associated with other agents. This has made it particularly useful in the treatment of congestive heart failure. It is also useful for improving ventricular function after cardiopulmonary bypass or acute myocardial infarction when the cardiac output is low but may recover within hours to days after the injury.

Isoproterenol

Isoproterenol is a nonselective β agonist and causes vasodilation, tachycardia, and increased cardiac output. It is a very short-acting medication after IV bolus dosing, with effects lasting only a few minutes. The availability of β_1-selective agents has limited its use, but it can be used in situations where increased inotropy and chronopy are desirable. It may also be useful in treating symptomatic bradycardia when atropine has failed. Isoproterenol may also be considered in the treatment of overdosage of β blockers and calcium channel blockers.[8] It can also be used to treat acute bronchospasm during general anesthesia.[9]

ADRENERGIC RECEPTOR BLOCKERS

Selective α receptor blocking agents are used in the treatment of hypertension, benign prostatic hyperplasia, and preoperatively to decrease the effects of pheochromocytoma. The only agent with a parenteral formulation is phentolamine. Phentolamine is a competitive antagonist at both α_1 and α_2 receptors and is used to counteract the effects of excessive catecholamine secretion seen in patients with pheochromocytoma. Phentolamine is given as an IM or intravenous dose of 5 to 15 mg. It has an onset of action of 1 to 2 minutes and a duration of 10 to 30 minutes.[10] It is typically dosed every 1 to 2 hours for the treatment of acute hypertension due to pheochromocytoma. It can also be used when a vasoconstrictive agent is inadvertently infused into tissue rather than the circulation. Phentolamine diluted to 0.5 to 1.0 mg/mL can be injected directly into the affected tissue and may restore enough circulation to limit or prevent tissue necrosis.[11]

Agents that block β-adrenergic receptors are used in the treatment of hypertension and tachycardia. Propranolol is a nonselective β blocker in that it blocks both β_1 and β_2 receptors. Atenolol, esmolol, and metoprolol are β_1-selective agents. They have much less activity at β_2 receptors compared to β_1, but they still activate β_2 receptors to a small degree.

Nonselective β agonists are contraindicated in patients with reactive airway disease or chronic obstructive pulmonary disease as β_2 blockade may cause symptomatic bronchoconstriction in these patients. β_1-selective agents may still exhibit activity at β_2 receptors, so these agents should be used cautiously in this patient group as well.

Propranolol

IV propranolol is indicated for the treatment of life-threatening supraventricular dysrhythmias. It may be given as a 1- to 3-mg bolus dose. It has an immediate onset of action and a duration of action of less than 5 minutes.

Esmolol

Esmolol has an onset of action of 1 minute and a half-life of approximately 9 minutes. It is rapidly metabolized by erythrocyte esterases, so its effect may be prolonged in anemic patients. It can be used as a bolus dose or continuous infusion to rapidly control hypertension or tachycardia. It can also be given as a bolus to determine if β blockade will have the desired effect, such as determining if slowing the heart rate will cause unacceptable hypotension. This information can aid in deciding if using a longer acting β antagonist is appropriate.

Metoprolol

Metoprolol is indicated for the control ventricular heart rate in supraventricular tachycardias, including atrial fibrillation. It is dosed at 2.5 to 5 mg IV every 2 to 5 minutes as needed to achieve heart rate control, up to a maximum dose of 15 mg IV.

β Antagonists should not be administered to patients with high levels of circulating α agonists (pheochromocytoma, accidental α agonist overdose) as the combination of decreased inotropy and arterial vasoconstriction may cause acute left ventricular failure. β Antagonists may be administered to patients with pheochromocytoma after α antagonist therapy has been initiated.

Labetalol

Labetalol is a nonselective β blocker that also blocks α_1 receptors. It has an α-to-β activity ratio of 1:7 after IV administration. Labetalol can be bolus dosed at 20 to 80 mg IV. It has on onset of action of 2 to 5 minutes and a duration of 2 to 4 hours after multiple bolus doses are used to achieve a desired blood pressure.[10] Labetalol may be associated with higher cardiac output when compared to other agents as its negative inotropic effects are counterbalanced by vasodilation.

PHOSPHODIESTERASE INHIBITORS

Milrinone and inamrinone are IV formulations of phosphodiesterase (PDE) inhibitors approved for patient use. Inamrinone was originally named amrinone but was renamed to avoid confusion with the antidysrhythmic drug amiodarone. Both milrinone and inamrinone are selective inhibitors of PDE_3, an intracellular enzyme responsible for the degradation of cyclic adenosine monophosphate (cAMP). In cardiac tissue, elevated levels of cAMP lead to increased inotropy while causing vasodilation in vascular tissue. These properties make the agents useful in the treatment of ventricular failure. Their vasodilator effects may cause significant hypotension and limit their use in patients with low systemic blood pressure. Milrinone is the most preferred of the the 2 available agents. It has a shorter half-life (30–60 minutes compared to 2–3 hours for inamrinone) and does not have the 10% incidence of thrombocytopenia that is associated with inamrinone. It can be administered as a loading dose of 50 mcg/kg IV given over 10 minutes, followed by a continuous infusion of 0.375 to 75 mcg/kg/min.

There is some evidence that milrinone may cause more pulmonary vasodilation than dobutamine.[12] This could make milrinone a better choice in patients with right ventricular dysfunction, but milrinone has not been proven to improve outcomes in these patients when compared to dobutamine.

Sildenafil is a PDE inhibitor widely used for erectile dysfunction. More recently, it has been found to have a role in the treatment of right heart failure by virtue of its dilation of the pulmonary vasculature. It and similar drugs may enhance right heart function immediately after cardiopulmonary bypass, particularly after heart transplantation, although more research is needed to determine if treatment will improve outcomes. Drugs in this class are also used to lower pulmonary arterial pressures in patients with mild to moderate pulmonary hypertension.[13]

CALCIUM CHANNEL BLOCKERS

Calcium channel blockers cause a decrease in systemic blood pressure by decreasing intracellular calcium levels and impeding smooth muscle contraction. They also decrease calcium in myocardial cells, thereby decreasing inotropy. At therapeutic doses their effect is most pronounced in arteriolar smooth muscle; they lower blood pressure primarily by vasodilation. Some agents (verapamil, diltiazem) also have a negative chronotropic effect by slowing conduction through the atrioventricular node. Parenteral formulations are available for verapamil, diltiazem, nicardipine, and clevidipine. IV infusions of verapamil and diltiazem are indicated for heart rate control in atrial flutter or fibrillation as well as conversion of supraventricular tachycardias.

Nicardipine

Nicardipine infusion is indicated for control of severe hypertension and perioperative hypertension. It may also replace oral calcium channel blocker therapy when enteral administration is not appropriate. It is given as a continuous infusion with a dose range of 5 to 15 mg/h. It is cleared by hepatic and renal mechanisms and will have prolonged effects in patients with dysfunction of these organ systems.

Clevidipine

Clevidipine is a dihydropyridine calcium channel blocker. It is metabolized by blood esterases, so its clearance is not dependent on liver or renal function. It has a half-life of 1 minute.[14] It is given as a continuous infusion starting at 5 to 15 mg/h. The dose can be doubled every 90 seconds until the desired blood pressure effect is seen. The medication is an injectable emulsion, so it cannot be easily diluted and must be used within 4 hours after the vial is punctured.

ANGIOTENSIN-CONVERTING ENZYME INHIBITORS

Angiotensin-converting enzyme (ACE) inhibitors control blood pressure by inhibiting the conversion of angiotensin I to angiotensin II (ATII). ATII causes vasoconstriction, particularly in the renal and splanchnic vascular beds. ATII also causes sodium retention in the kidneys. Enalaprilat is an ACE inhibitor in parenteral formulation. It is indicated for the treatment of hypertension when it is not appropriate to administer these agents orally. The recommended dose range is 0.625 to 1.25 mg every 6 hours. A clinical response to the agent can be seen 15 to 30 minutes after administration. The peak effect may not occur for up to 4 hours after the first dose, and the duration of action is 12 to 24 hours.[10] It is generally not recommended for hypertensive emergencies because its long duration of action makes it difficult to titrate.

NITRIC OXIDE MODULATORS

The release of nitric oxide (NO) by vascular endothelial cells leads to relaxation of vascular smooth muscle. NO is rapidly inactivated in the blood, giving it a half-life of only a few seconds. Nitroglycerin and sodium nitroprusside are vasodilating agents that act by releasing NO into the vascular endothelium. Inhaled NO may also have a role in the perioperative period.

Nitroglycerin

Nitroglycerin (NTG) can be used in the treatment of perioperative hypertension, hypertensive emergency, and unstable angina. NTG has an onset of action in less than 5 minutes and a duration of less than 10 minutes, making it rapidly titratable as a continuous infusion. At lower doses venodilation predominates, causing decreased left ventricular filling. At higher doses arterial dilation becomes more pronounced, and the combination of reduced preload and afterload can decrease myocardial oxygen demand. NTG is contraindicated in patients with elevated intracranial pressure (ICP) as the vasodilation of intracranial vessels may cause a further increase in ICP.

Sodium Nitroprusside

Sodium nitroprusside (SNP) also causes the release of NO. Unlike NTG, SNP dilates arterial and venous vessels equally. SNP causes only a minimal increase in heart rate and usually causes a decrease in myocardial oxygen demand due to decreased afterload. Blood pressure can begin to decrease within 30 seconds after an IV dose, and the effects will dissipate within 3 minutes after stopping an infusion. A typical dose range is 0.3 to 2.0 mcg/kg/min (see Table 14–1).

A breakdown product of SNP is cyanide, which can impair cellular oxygen utilization. Cyanide toxicity is very rare and associated with extremely high SNP doses (> 30 mcg/kg/min).[15] Cyanide is converted to thiocyanate in the liver and then excreted in the urine, so patients with hepatic or renal dysfunction are at higher risk for accumulating cyanide and developing toxic effects.

SNP can also counteract hypoxic pulmonary vasoconstriction. This can increase intrapulmonary blood flow to nonventilated regions of the lungs and may cause hypoxemia in patients with poor pulmonary function.

INHALED VASOACTIVE AGENTS

Nitric Oxide

Inhaled NO has been used to increase oxygenation by causing vasodilation of the pulmonary vasculature. This causes increased blood flow to lung tissue, particularly to areas that are ventilated and thus exposed to the NO. It is broken down by hemoglobin and has a half-life of only a few seconds. Because it is broken down before it reaches the systemic circulation, inhaled NO has no clinically significant effect on the systemic blood pressure. Inhaled NO has been found to transiently raise blood oxygen levels in patients with acute respiratory distress syndrome but has not been shown to decrease mortality in these patients.[16] It has also been used immediately after cardiopulmonary bypass to improve right ventricular function.[17] The administration of inhaled NO requires a dedicated delivery system and personnel trained in its use to ensure the correct dosing.

Prostacyclin

Prostacyclins cause smooth muscle relaxation and have been used to treat pulmonary hypertension. Inhaled prostacyclins have also been used to improve right ventricular output in critically ill patients without the side effects of systemic administration. Iloprost is a prostacyclin with a half-life of 20 to 30 minutes that has been approved for treatment of pulmonary hypertension via inhalation. In trials in patients with acute respiratory distress syndrome, inhaled iloprost was found to improve oxygenation. However, like inhaled NO, it has not been found to improve survival. It has been shown to decrease pulmonary arterial pressures and improve cardiac index after cardiopulmonary bypass[18] and heart transplantation.[17]

VASOACTIVE AGENTS

Hydralazine

Hydralazine is an arteriolar vasodilator, but its exact mechanism of action has not been clearly defined. It can cause reflex tachycardia and should be used with caution in patients who may not tolerate an increase in myocardial oxygen demand. It has been used safely in the treatment of severe hypotension associated with preeclampsia. It can cause a lupus-like syndrome in patients who have received the drug for at least 6 months.

Vasopressin

Vasopressin, also called antidiuretic hormone, is a polypeptide secreted by the hypothalamus. As a hormone it plays a significant role in maintaining serum osmolality, but it has found clinical use for its vasoconstrictive properties. It is mentioned in cardiopulmonary resuscitation guidelines as a bolus dose of 40 units to be used in place of the first or second dose of epinephrine in adult cardiac arrest.[8] Vasopressin is recommended as second-line therapy in septic shock if norepinephrine alone does not produce the desired rise in blood pressure.[3] Vasopressin is less likely to cause dysrhythmias than other direct-acting adrenergic agonists and therefore may be a better choice in those patients who cannot tolerate the hemodynamic effects of such

TABLE 14–1 Recommended dosing of vasoactive drugs.

Drug	Intravenous Bolus Dosing	Intravenous Infusion Dosing	Duration of Action
Vasogenic Hypertension			
Dopamine	—	2–20 mcg/kg/min	10 min
Ephedrine	5–10 mg		10 min
Epinephrine	Mild hypotension: 5–10 mcg Severe hypotension: up to 1000 mcg	0.02–2 mcg/kg/min	3–5 min
Norepinephrine	—	0.01–3 mcg/kg/min	3–5 min
Phenylephrine	50–200 mcg	0.5–3 mcg/kg/min	10 min
Vasopressin[19]	Mild hypotension: 1 unit Severe hypotension: up to 40 units	0.01–0.04 units/min	
Cardiogenic Hypotension			
Dobutamine	—	2–20 mcg/kg/min	10 min
Epinephrine	50–1000 mcg	0.02–2 mcg/kg/min	3–5 min
Levosimendan[20]	5–20 mcg/kg	0.1–0.2 mcg/kg/min	45 min
Milrinone	—	0.375–0.75 mcg/kg/min	45 min
Isoproterenol[9]	0.02–0.2 mg	0.5–5 mcg/min	
Urgent or Emergent Hypertension			
Clevidipine[21]		1–20 mg/min	1 min
Enalaprilat[10]	0.625–1.25 mg		12 h
Esmolol[10]	0.5–1 mg/kg	50–300 mcg/kg/min	9 min
Fenoldopam[22]		0.1–1.5 mcg/kg/min	10–30 min
Hydralazine[10]	10–20 mg		4–6 h
Labetalol[10]	20–80 mg		2–4 h
Nicardipine[23]		5–15 mg/h	Up to 3 h
Nitroglycerin[10]	25–50 mcg	5–200 mcg/min	10 min
Nitroprusside[24]		0.1–5.0 mcg/kg/min	2–3 min
Propranolol[25]	1–5 mg		4 h
Supraventricular Tachycardia			
Diltiazem[8]	15–25 mg	5–15 mg/h	1–3 h
Esmolol[8]	0.5 mg/kg	50 mcg/kg/min	10 min
Metoprolol[8]	5 mg		5 h
Verapamil[8]	2.5–10 mg		30 min

dysrhythmias. Vasopressin is typically dosed at 0.01 to 0.04 units/min in septic shock (Table 14-1), but doses up to 1 unit/min have been recommended when used to cause mesenteric vasoconstriction in patients with gastrointestinal bleeding.

Methylene Blue

Methylene blue is a dye that may have use in treating acute vasoplegia associated with cardiopulmonary bypass. Methylene blue blocks cyclic guanosine monophosphate (cGMP) formation. This monophosphate mediates vasodilation caused by NO, so inhibiting cGMP formation may inhibit the vasodilation caused by NO. Methylene blue has been used after separation from cardiopulmonary bypass to treat severe hypotension unresponsive to other pressors, but its use has not been validated by any large clinical studies.

Levosimendan

Levosimendan is a calcium-sensitizing agent. It makes troponin more sensitive to intracellular calcium and also inhibits PDE_3. Clinically, it causes an increase in myocardial contractility without increasing myocardial oxygen demand. It also causes a decrease in afterload. These effects make it useful in the treatment of biventricular failure. No difference in outcomes was found when levosimendan was compared to dobutamine for treatment of acute heart failure.[26]

CASE DISCUSSION

A 51-year-old man is undergoing débridement of necrotizing fasciitis of his lower abdominal wall. His height is 172 cm and his weight is 153 kg. His medical history is significant for diabetes mellitus, hypertension with baseline blood pressure of 155/90 mm Hg, obstructive sleep apnea, and hypercholesterolemia. An echocardiogram performed 1 month prior was notable for a mildly dilated right atrium, estimated pulmonary arterial pressure of 65/35 mm Hg, a left ventricular ejection fraction of 50%, and no wall motion abnormalities.

Four minutes after induction of anesthesia with propofol, the patient's blood pressure is 82/54 mm Hg. How could this hypotension be managed?

Hypotension after a bolus dose of a sedative–hypnotic agent is a common occurrence. Most often, it is primarily due to vasodilation and decreased blood return to the left ventricle. The effect often lasts less than 10 minutes but frequently requires pharmacologic intervention. Bolus dosing of a short-acting agent with primarily α-adrenergic activity (50–100 mcg of phenylephrine) may cause enough vasoconstriction to improve venous return and raise arterial blood pressure to an acceptable level. Similarly, low doses of short-acting agents with direct or indirect α and β activity may also be appropriate (eg, ephedrine 5–10 mg or epinephrine 10–20 mcg). If vasodilating anesthetic agents will continue to be administered during the procedure, an IV fluid bolus may also be considered and may provide a longer duration with desirable blood pressure.

The patient responds to a single bolus dose of pressor and stabilizes at an acceptable blood pressure. Thirty minutes later and after débridement has begun, the patient has progressively become hypotensive to 78/40 mm Hg and tachycardic. How could this be managed?

Likely causes of hypotension in this circumstance include hypovolemia, sepsis, or ventricular failure. The use of a vasoactive drug should be considered a temporizing measure, and treatment of the cause of hypotension should begin at the same time. If hypovolemia is suspected and the hypotension does not resolve quickly with fluid resuscitation, a vasoactive drug with activity at α_1 receptors could be administered. The goal should be to raise blood pressure and provide adequate organ perfusion while continuing to treat the hypovolemia. Norepinephrine should be considered if sepsis seems to be the most likely cause of hypotension. If ventricular failure is the presumed cause, epinephrine or high-dose dopamine may the agent of choice to provide both increased inotropy as well as vasoconstriction during a hypotensive event.

While a PDE inhibitor would also increase inotropy, its vasodilating properties would likely cause exacerbate the hypotension.

The presumed cause of hypotension is sepsis. An IV fluid bolus is started, but the patient remains hypotensive and tachycardic. The patient responds to a 50 mcg bolus dose of epinephrine, but before a norepinephrine infusion can be prepared, his blood pressure falls to 60/20 mm Hg. How could this be managed?

The immediate goal should be to maintain adequate organ perfusion, particularly to the brain and heart. A second larger bolus dose of epinephrine or a bolus dose of vasopressin could be considered. A rapid fluid infusion may also produce the desired hemodynamic response. Initiation of cardiopulmonary resuscitation should be considered if the blood pressure falls further or is believed to be inadequate for cerebral and coronary perfusion. If available, echocardiographic evaluation could provide information about ventricular function and filling. This may direct therapy toward inotropic support, fluid resuscitation, or both.

Twenty-four hours postoperatively, the patient has responded to treatment for sepsis. He has received 8 L of crystalloid and remains on a norepinephrine infusion. He is now becoming progressively hypotensive due to right ventricular volume overload and failure. How could this be managed?

A PDE inhibitor might be the agent of choice due to its ability to increase inotropy and cause vasodilation, including vasodilation of the pulmonary vasculature. This may increase right ventricular stroke volume. A selective β agonist such as dobutamine might also be a reasonable choice to improve ventricular function.

REFERENCES

1. Rollerston HD. The Goulstonian Lectures on the Suprarenal Bodies Delivered before the Royal College of Physicians of London. *Br Med J*. 1895;1(1788):745-748.
2. Simons FER, Gu X, Simons KJ. Epinephrine absorption in adults: intramuscular versus subcutaneous injection. *J Allergy Clin Immunol*. 2001;108:871-873.
3. Dellinger RP, Levy MM, Rhodes A, et al. Surviving Sepsis Campaign: International guidelines for management of severe sepsis and septic shock: 2012. *Crit Care Med*. 2013;41:580-637.
4. Weber RR. Pharmacokinetics and pharmacodynamic properties of intravenous fenoldapam. *Br J Clin Pharmacol*. 1988;25:17-21.
5. Tong C, Eisenbach JC. The vascular mechanism of ephedrine's beneficial effect on uterine perfusion during pregnancy. *Anesthesiology*. 1992.76:792-798.
6. James FM III, Greiss FC Jr, Kemp RA. The evaluation of vasopressor therapy for maternal hypotension during spinal anesthesia. *Anesthesiology*. 1970; 33(1):25-34.
7. Ahonen J, Aranko K, Livanainen A, et al. Pharmacokinetic-pharmacodynamic relationship of dobutamine and heart rate, stroke volume and cardiac output in healthy volunteers. *Clin Drug Invest*. 2008; 28(2):121-127.
8. Neumar RW, Otto CW, Link MS, et al. Part 8: Adult advanced cardiovascular life support: 2010 American Heart Association Guidelines for Cardiopulmonary Resuscitation and Emergency Cardiovascular Care. *Circulation*. 2010;122:S729-S767.
9. Isuprel (Isoproterenol hydrochloride injection USP). Lake Forest, IL: Hospira; 2004.
10. Rhoney D, Peacock WF. Intravenous therapy for hypertensive emergencies, part 1. *Am J Health-Syst Pharm*. 2009;66:1343-1352.
11. Phentolamine mesylate package insert. Beford, OH: Bedford Laboratories; 1999.
12. Jenkins IR, Dolman J, O'Connor JP, Ansley DM. Amrinone versus dobutamine in cardiac surgical patients with severe pulmonary hypertension after cardiopulmonary bypass: a prospective, randomized double-blinded trial. *Anaesth Intensive Care*. 1997; 25(3):245-249.
13. Archer SL, Michelakis ED. Phosphodiesterase type 5 inhibitors for pulmonary arterial hypertension. *N Engl J Med*. 2009;361(19):1864-1871.
14. Singla N, Warltier DC, Gandhi SD, et al. Treatment of acute postoperative hypertension in cardiac surgery patients: an efficacy study of clevidipine assessing its postoperative antihypertensive effect in cardiac surgery-2 (ESCAPE-2), a randomized, double-blind, placebo-controlled trial. *Anesth Analg*. 2008; 107(1): 59-67.
15. Friederich JA, Butterworth JF. Sodium nitroprusside: twenty years and counting. *Anesth Analg*. 1995;81: 152-162.
16. Afshari A, Brok J, Møller AM, Wetterslev J. Inhaled nitric oxide for acute respiratory distress syndrome

(ARDS) and acute lung injury in children and adults. *Cochrane Database Syst Rev*. 2010;(7):CD002787.
17. Khan TA, Schnickel G, Ross D, et al. A prospective, randomized, crossover pilot study of inhaled nitric oxide versus inhaled prostacyclin in heart transplant and lung transplant recipients. *J Thorac Cardiovasc Surg*. 2009;138(6):1417-1424.
18. Winterhalter M, Simon A, Fischer S, et al. Comparison of inhaled iloprost and nitric oxide in patients with pulmonary hypertension during weaning from cardiopulmonary bypass in cardiac surgery: a prospective randomized trial. *J Cardiothorac Vasc Anesth*. 2008;22(3):406-413.
19. Maybauer MO, Walley KR. Best vasopressor for advanced vasodilatory shock: should vasopressin be part of the mix? *Intensive Care Med*. 2010;36(9):1484-1487.
20. Figgitt D, Gillies PS, Goa KL. Levosimendan. *Drugs*. 2001;61(5):613-627.
21. Erickson AL, DeGrado JR, Fanikos JR. Clevidipine: a short-acting intravenous dihydropyridine calcium channel blocker for the management of hypertension. *Pharmacotherapy*. 2010;30(5):515-528.
22. Murphy MB, Murray C, Shorten GD. Fenoldopam–a selective peripheral dopamine receptor agonist for the treatment of severe hypertension. *N Engl J Med*. 2001;345(21):1548-1557.
23. Sorkin EM, Clissold SP. Nicardipine: a review of its pharmacodynamic and pharmacokinetic properties, and therapeutic efficacy, in the treatment of angina pectoris, hypertension and related cardiovascular disorders. *Drugs*. 1987;33(4):296-345.
24. American Heart Association (AHA). 2005 AHA Guidelines for Cardiopulmonary Resuscitation and Emergency Cardiovascular Care. Part 7.4. Monitoring and medications. *Circulation*. 2005;112(suppl 1): IV78-IV83.
25. Propranolol hydrochloride injection prescribing information. Beford, OH: Bedford Laboratories; 2008.
26. Mebazaa A, Nieminen MS, Packer M, et al. Levosimendan vs dobutamine for patients with acute decompensated heart failure: the SURVIVE randomized trial. *JAMA*. 2007;297(17):1883-1891.

CHAPTER

15

Antiemetics

Amy K. Manchester, MD, and Tong J. Gan, MD

INTRODUCTION

Postoperative nausea and vomiting (PONV) is the most common complication associated with anesthesia and surgery, occurring in approximately one-third of all patients and up to 70% of "high-risk" patients.[1] PONV is a cause of great distress for patients, and in addition to creating a highly unpleasant experience of discomfort, it can lead to a variety of unintended consequences such as delayed discharge, wound dehiscence, dehydration, tearing of sutures, and potential pulmonary aspiration, all of which serve to greatly increase medical costs.[2] Understanding the various mechanisms involved in PONV is critical for optimizing the prophylaxis and treatment of this unwanted side effect of anesthesia.

RISK FACTORS

There are numerous risk factors associated with the development of PONV, and these can be divided into patient specific risk factors, anesthesia-related factors, and surgery-related factors (Table 15–1). By careful evaluation of an individual's risk factors for the development of PONV, those who will most likely benefit from prophylactic antiemetic therapy can be more easily identified.

PHYSIOLOGIC MECHANISM OF EMESIS

The physiologic process of vomiting (emesis) involves a series of autonomic changes that operate in the brainstem at the level of the medulla oblongata. Within this region of the hindbrain, various afferent sources of emetic input are received by the area postrema, known as the chemoreceptor trigger zone (CTZ), and the vomiting center located in the nucleus tractus solitarius (NTS).[3] The signals received by the CTZ and the vomiting center are mediated primarily by major neurotransmitter receptor systems. The major neurotransmitters and receptors that supply signals to the CTZ and vomiting center are serotonin (5-HT3), dopamine (D_2), histamine (H_1), muscarinic acetylcholine, and neurokinin (Figure 15–1). Pharmacologic antiemetic agents that work to block the neurotransmitters involved in the development of emesis have long been the mainstay of prophylaxis and treatment of PONV.

ANTIEMETIC PHARMACOLOGIC THERAPY

Serotonergic Receptor Antagonists

Serotonin is found in high levels peripherally in the enterochromaffin cells of the gastrointestinal tract as well as in the central nervous system (CNS). In response to noxious or mechanical stimuli, serotonin is released and stimulates vagal afferent neurons that in turn activate the CTZ and vomiting center of the NTS.[4] The most important serotonin receptor involved in PONV is the 5-HT3 subtype. Antagonism of the 5-HT3 receptor effectively blocks the nausea and vomiting cascade mediated by serotonin, and 5-HT3 antagonists have been proven to be safe and widely used for both prophylaxis and treatment of PONV.

Ondansetron was the first of the 5-HT3 antiemetic drugs to be marketed in the United States, and most of the research available regarding 5-HT3 antagonists involves ondansetron. The recommended effective dose of ondansetron is 4 mg

TABLE 15–1 Risk factors for postoperative nausea and vomiting (PONV) in adults.

Type of Risk Factor	Specific Factor Associated With Increased PONV
Patient-specific	Female gender
	Nonsmoking
	Previous history of PONV
	History of motion sickness
Anesthesia-related	Use of volatile agents
	Use of nitrous oxide
	Use of perioperative opioids
	High doses of neostigmine (> 2.5 mg)
Surgery-related	Lengthy surgical procedure
	Intra-abdominal surgery
	Gynecologic surgery
	Laparoscopic procedures
	Major breast surgery
	Neurologic surgery
	Ear, nose, and/or throat surgery
	Strabismus repair

intravenously (IV) for adults, and it has been found to be most efficacious when given at the end of surgery. Ondansetron has been shown to be somewhat more effective at preventing vomiting than preventing nausea, with a number needed to treat (NNT) of 6 for the prevention of vomiting within the first 24 hours postsurgery and an antinausea NNT of 7.[5]

Other 5-HT3 antagonists include dolasetron, granisetron, ramosetron, and tropisetron (ramosetron and tropisetron are not available in the United States). If given at their optimal doses, there is no evidence to support a difference in efficacy between the various 5-HT3 receptor antagonists.[6] The choice then usually is made based on availability and cost. Ondansetron, which is now available in generic form, is substantially less expensive than other drugs in this class, making it the preferred drug of choice. Most 5-HT3 antagonists are most effective during the early phase of PONV (0–24 hours postsurgery) and are less effective during the late phase. Palonosetron is a novel 5-HT3 antagonist with unique pharmacologic properties, and initial studies have shown a single dose of 0.075 mg IV to be effective at preventing PONV for as long as 3 days postsurgery.[7]

All 5-HT3 receptor antagonists are metabolized by cytochrome P450 in the liver. Ondansetron as well as most other 5-HT3 antagonists are specifically metabolized by the CYP2D6 isoform. Genetic polymorphism of the CYP2D6 isoform influences the metabolism and efficacy of ondansetron, as patients with CYP2D6 deficiency display poor metabolism of the drug (leading to accumulation in the body) and patients with increased CYP2D6 have ultrarapid metabolism that leads to increased incidence of ondansetron prophylaxis failure.[8,9] The 5-HT3 antagonists are a popular and widely used choice for antiemetic therapy because of their favorable side effect profile. 5-HT3 antagonists have been found to cause constipation, headache, elevated liver enzymes, and asymptomatic QT prolongation, but the number needed to harm (NNH) associated with these side effects is high at 23, 36, and 31 respectively, thus making 5-HT3 antagonists a safe choice for PONV treatment and prevention.[5]

Dopaminergic Receptor Antagonists

D_2 receptor antagonists are a useful class of antiemetics; they successfully block D_2 receptors located in the CTZ. Among the subtypes of D_2 antagonists are the phenothiazines (eg, promethazine, prochlorperazine, chlorpromazine), butyrophenones (eg, droperidol, haloperidol), and benzamides (eg, metoclopramide, domperidone).[4]

The phenothiazines have historically been widely used for the treatment of PONV. Prochlorperazine given at 5 to 10 mg IV/intramuscularly (IM) and promethazine given at 12.5 to 25 mg IV have both been shown to be effective at reducing PONV. Optimal timing of administration for prochlorperazine is at the end of surgery and for promethazine at induction of anesthesia.[10,11] Low-dose promethazine (6.25 mg) has also been shown to be more effective than repeat dosing of ondansetron after failed

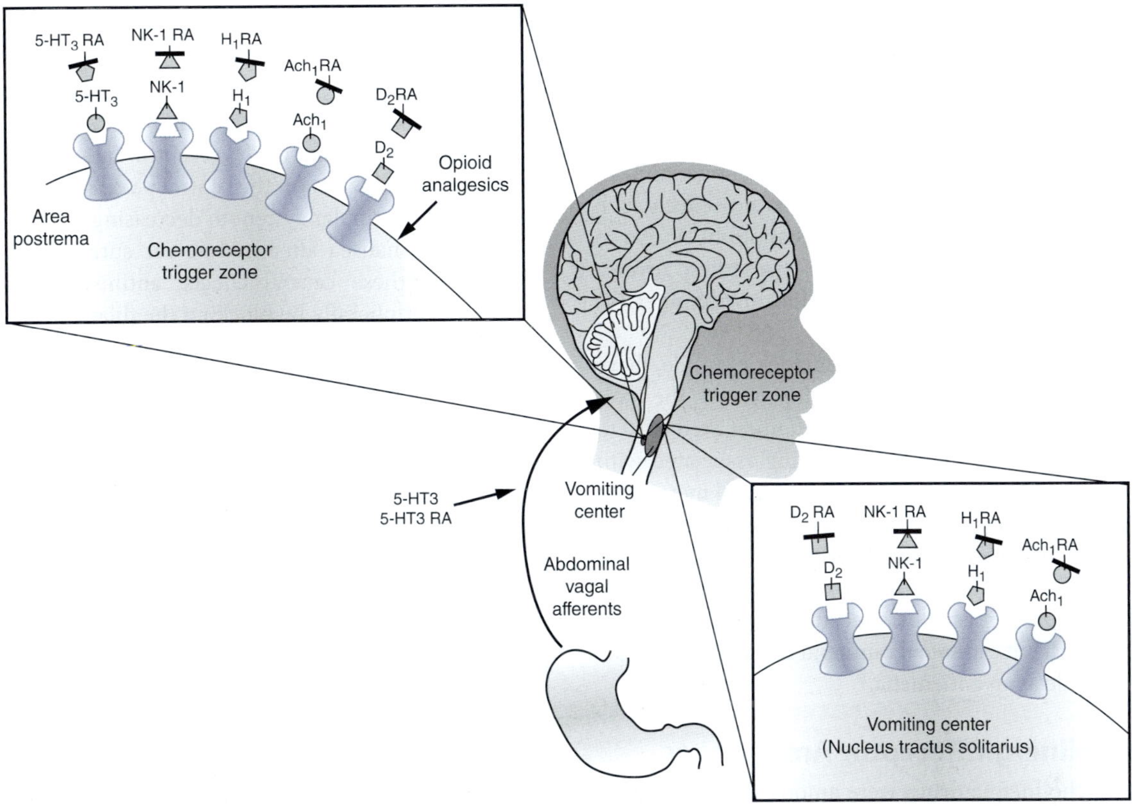

FIGURE 15–1 Receptor sites, receptor agonists, and receptor antagonists involved in the prophylaxis and/or treatment of postoperative nausea and vomiting. Ach, acetylcholine; D, dopamine; H, histamine; 5-HT3, serotonin; NK-1, neurokinin; RA, receptor antagonist. Numbers indicate receptor types (H_1 is histamine receptor type 1).

ondansetron prophylaxis.[12] These drugs have significant side effects that limit their usefulness as first-line agents due to the high incidence of lethargy and sedation associated with them, although this may be dose dependent in nature. In addition, clinically significant respiratory depression may occur when phenothiazines are used in conjunction with postoperative opioids for pain control. Promethazine can also cause severe tissue injury including gangrene with perivascular extravasation from an infiltrated IV catheter or inadvertent arterial injection of the drug. In 2009, the Food and Drug Administration (FDA) issued a black box warning for promethazine delineating these risks.

Butyrophenones such as droperidol are effective antiemetics that have been used as single agents or in conjunction with 5-HT3 receptor antagonists. Droperidol has been found to be effective for both early and late PONV, likely because of its long duration of action (up to 24 hours postadministration) despite its relatively short half-life. The recommended dosing for droperidol with a NNT of 7 has been found to be 1.25 mg.[13] However, the widespread clinical use of this drug has significantly decreased as a result of the "black box warning" issued by the FDA in 2001. The "black box warning" was issued because of the association between droperidol administration and prolonged QT interval leading to fatal cardiac dysrhythmias.[14] (See Update: QT prolongation associated with many antiemetics at the end of the chapter for more information on this topic.) Given the decreased use of droperidol after the FDA issued the "black box warning," haloperidol started to gain clinical use as an alternative butyrophenone for PONV. Low doses of 0.5 to 2 mg IV/IM have been shown to be effective in the treatment of PONV (NNT of 4–6), although there is insufficient evidence to support its role in the prophylaxis of PONV.[15] Its label has recently been revised to highlight the risk of QT prolongation with administration and other untoward side effects such as sedation and extrapyramidal symptoms similar to droperidol. Especially in higher doses, these adverse side effects have limited the clinical usefulness of haloperidol as an antiemetic.

Benzamides such as metoclopramide have also been used as a treatment for PONV. The typical antiemetic dose of metoclopramide used is 10 to 20 mg IV, with higher doses being associated with significant unwanted side effects. Several meta-analyses have been conducted to evaluate the efficacy of metoclopramide in the treatment of PONV. They have concluded that it has no clinically relevant antiemetic properties; thus, a recent consensus panel has stated that it cannot recommend the use of metoclopramide as an antiemetic.[16]

Cholinergic Receptor Antagonists

Anticholinergic drugs were among those first used for the treatment of PONV. Their mechanism of action is to antagonize muscarinic cholinergic receptor sites located in the vomiting center as well as in the cerebral cortex and pons.[17] Scopolamine has been determined to be the anticholinergic drug with the most significant antiemetic properties. It is typically administered as a 1.5-mg transdermal patch, and it is best applied either the night prior to surgery or 4 hours before the end of surgery, since the clinical onset of the patch is not seen until 2 to 4 hours after its application. The NNT for PONV prophylaxis is 6, with its use as a rescue treatment being slightly less effective (NNT of 8). Scopolamine is also useful as an adjunct when used in conjunction with other drug modalities.[18] The common side effects of anticholinergics such as dry mouth, dizziness, visual disturbances, and drowsiness may pose a limit to its everyday use, especially in the elderly population. The main advantage of the scopolamine patch is its long duration of action; it can be left in place for up to 72 hours, making it a good choice for postdischarge PONV prophylaxis.

Histamine Receptor Antagonists

Antihistamines exert their antiemetic effect by successfully blocking H_1 receptors in the vomiting center of the NTS, and also by blocking acetylcholine in the vestibular apparatus. H_1 receptor-antagonists have been found to act on the central pattern generator and the vestibular system to decreasing motion sickness and nausea after middle ear surgery.[4] In addition to these central effects, antihistamines also work peripherally by blocking the dilation and increased permeability of capillaries as well as the contraction of smooth muscle caused by peripheral H_1 receptors. Commonly used antihistamines for PONV are cyclizine, meclizine, hydroxyzine, dimenhydrinate and diphenhydramine. In randomized controlled trials, dimenhydrinate given at 1 mg/kg IV was found to be a useful antiemetic with an efficacy similar to 5-HT3 receptor antagonists and droperidol.[19] Antihistamines have a variety of common adverse side effects such as dry mouth, constipation, sedation, urinary retention, confusion, and blurry vision.

Corticosteroids

Corticosteroids such as dexamethasone do not block specific neurotransmitter receptor sites, and although their specific mechanism of action for treating PONV is unknown, it is thought that they provide both peripheral and central membrane stabilization as well as anti-inflammatory properties.[4] They were first found to be effective in the prevention and treatment of chemotherapy-induced nausea and vomiting, prompting their evaluation in the management of PONV. The recommended dose of dexamethasone is 4 mg IV in adults, and it is most efficacious when administered at induction of anesthesia. Dexamethasone has a long duration of action, making it effective against early onset PONV as well as preventing late PONV, with a NNT of 4.[20] Corticosteroids can cause adverse side effects such as gastrointestinal distress, insomnia, anxiety, hyperglycemia, immunosuppression, and avascular necrosis of the femur. However, no dexamethasone-related adverse side effects have been reported when small antiemetic doses of dexamethasone (4 mg) have been given with an interval of at least 24 hours between doses. Although antiemetic doses can cause a transient increase in blood glucose levels in both diabetics and nondiabetics after a single dose, this transient effect resolves without treatment and causes no untoward effects.[21]

RECOMMENDED STRATEGIES FOR PREVENTION AND TREATMENT OF POSTOPERATIVE NAUSEA AND VOMITING

In determining the best way to approach prophylaxis and treatment of PONV given the large body of evidence on the subject and the various number of available drug choices, it is perhaps best to follow the practical and rational approach known as the *rule of three*: (1) correctly identify patients at risk, (2) keep the baseline risk low, and (3) use effective antiemetics and combine them when appropriate.[22] Current consensus guidelines recommend the following strategies to reduce the baseline risk of PONV[23]:

- Use of regional anesthesia when appropriate over general anesthesia
- Use of propofol for induction and maintenance of anesthesia (total intravenous anesthesia)
- Adequate hydration
- Avoidance of nitrous oxide and inhaled volatile agents
- Minimizing the use of neostigmine and postoperative opioids

For patients deemed low risk, no antiemetic therapy is necessary unless there is a risk of harmful medical sequelae from the development of PONV. For patients with moderate risk of PONV, single-agent therapy should be considered. For high-risk patients, combination therapy with either 2 or 3 agents from different classes should be used for prophylaxis. See Table 15–2 for dosing details. In general, combination therapy using agents with different mechanisms of action has been found to be more effective than monotherapy. The Society for Ambulatory Anesthesia (SAMBA) published the following consensus guidelines and treatment algorithm for the management of PONV in 2007 (Figure 15–2).[24]

CASE DISCUSSION

A 43-year-old female nonsmoker is scheduled for bilateral breast reconstruction following bilateral mastectomy for breast cancer. Past surgical history includes mastectomy, axillary lymph node dissection, and laparoscopic cholecystectomy. The patient reports severe, debilitating PONV following each surgical procedure. Multiple regimens, including the use of total intravenous anesthesia and combination pharmacologic therapy (ondansetron, scopolamine patch, and promethazine) have failed to prevent PONV in this patient.

What can be done when the standard approach to treating PONV fails?

A Look to the Future: Novel Antiemetic Therapies

NK-1 receptors are located in the CTZ and are thought to play an important role in modulating the development of PONV. Substance P is a tachykinin peptide and an endogenous NK-1 receptor ligand in the CTZ. It also acts as an important neurotransmitter for the vagal afferent neural transmission of emesis; it is released from enterochromaffin cells of the gastrointestinal tract.[25] Numerous NK-1 receptor antagonists are in various stages of development. There has been a considerable amount of recent interest in the development of these novel agents, as they appear to be effective in the prevention of both acute and delayed emesis. This is highly desirable given that the current mainstay of PONV treatment, 5-HT3 antagonists, is most effective only against the prevention of early PONV. Currently, there are no meta-analyses available for NK-1 antagonists and their effectiveness in prophylaxis and treatment of PONV. Of the currently NK-1 antagonists in development, aprepitant is the most studied compound. At a dose of 40 mg orally, aprepitant was found to be equally as effective as ondansetron 4 mg IV at preventing PONV within the first 24 hours postoperatively and significantly more effective than ondansetron at preventing late PONV (0–48 hours).[26] This improved efficacy for delayed PONV is consistent with the long half-life of 9 to 12 hours for aprepitant.

TABLE 15–2 Antiemetic doses and timing for prevention of postoperative nausea and vomiting.

Antiemetic Class	Drug	Recommended Dose	Timing of Administration
5-HT3 Antagonist	Ondansetron	4–5 mg IV	End of surgery
	Dolasetron	12.5 mg IV	End of surgery
	Granisetron	0.35–1.0 mg IV	End of surgery
	Tropisetron	5 mg IV	End of surgery
	Palonosetron	0.075 mg IV	End of surgery
D2 Antagonist	Prochlorperazine	10 mg IV/IM	End of surgery
	Promethazine	6.25 mg IV	At induction
	Droperidol	0.625–1.25 mg IV	At induction
	Haloperidol	0.5–2 mg IV/IM	End of surgery
Anticholinergic	Scopolamine	1.5-mg transdermal patch	Prior evening or 4 hours before surgery
H1 Antagonist	Cyclizine	50 mg IV	End of surgery
	Dimenhydrinate	1 mg/kg IV	At induction
Corticosteroid	Dexamethasone	4–5 mg IV	At induction
NK-1 Antagonist	Aprepitant	40 mg PO	60–90 min before induction
Other	Ephedrine	0.5 μg/kg	End of surgery
	Naloxone	0.25 μg/kg/h	No data available

Increased commercial availability of aprepitant as well as other NK-1 antagonists (eg, casopitant and rolapitant) in development is expected in the near future, although the long-term tolerability of these agents is still undergoing investigation.

In addition to NK-1 antagonists, several other novel therapies have been studied, although there is limited evidence currently available of their efficacy in the treatment of PONV. Ephedrine at a dose of 0.5 mg/kg when administered at the end of surgery has been found in small studies to be an effective antiemetic.[27] Low-dose naloxone (0.25 mcg/kg/h), an opioid receptor antagonist, has also been shown to reduce PONV and the need for rescue medication.[28] Further research on these drugs is necessary before they can be recommended over more established antiemetics due to the paucity of data currently available for these novel therapeutics.

Update: QT Prolongation Associated With Many Antiemetics

QT interval prolongation is an adverse side effect most commonly associated with droperidol since the FDA issued its "black box warning" for the drug. Although droperidol is the most widely known antiemetic causing QT prolongation, it is important to note that practically all antiemetics currently available have an effect on the QT interval. This includes not only butyrophenones (droperidol), but also phenothiazines (promethazine), 5-HT3 antagonists (ondansetron), and H_1 antagonists (dimenhydrinate).[29] The FDA warning for

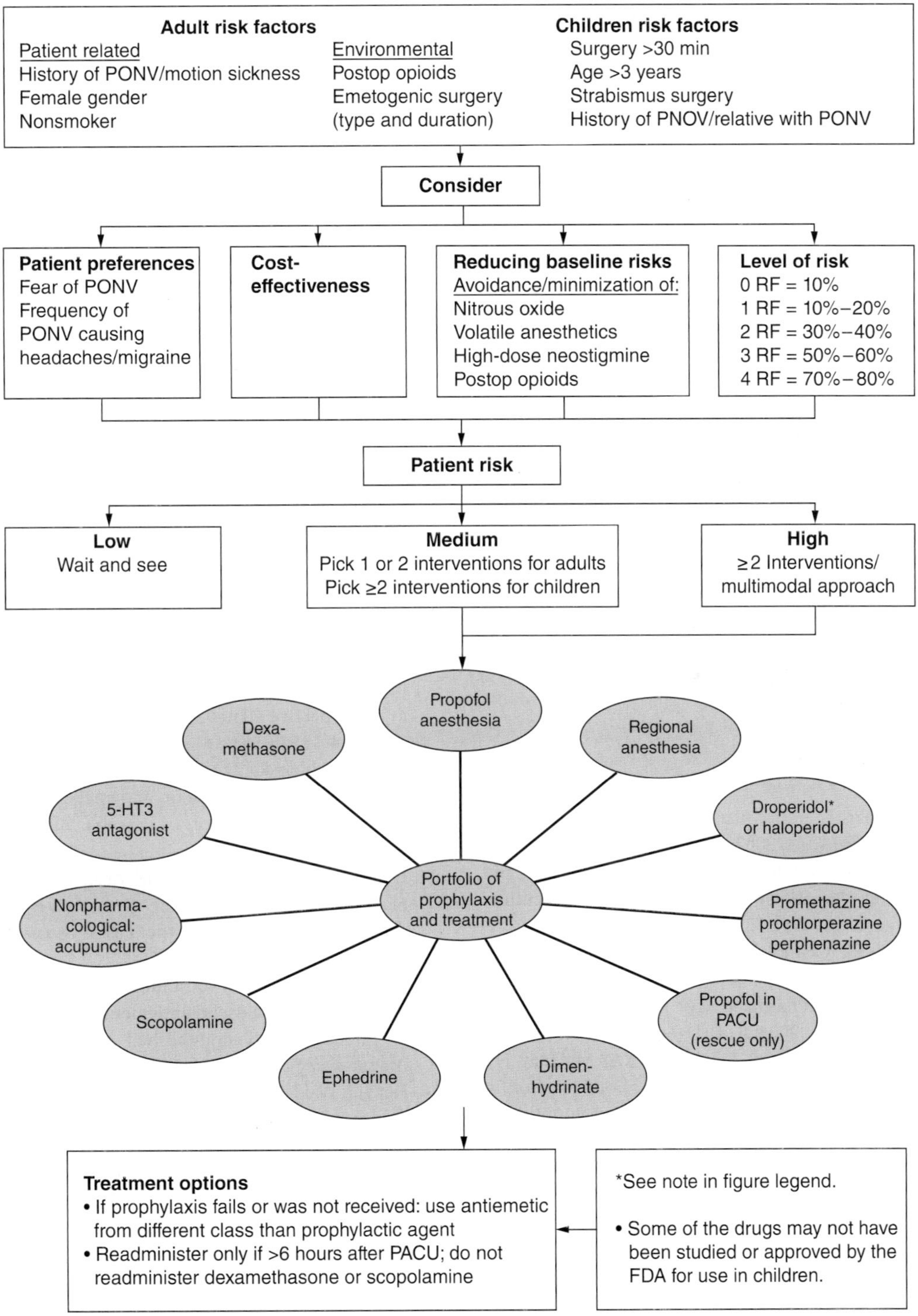

FIGURE 15–2 Treatment algorithm for the management of postoperative nausea and vomiting (PONV). Use droperidol in children only if other therapy has failed and the patient is being admitted to the hospital. FDA, Food and Drug Administration; PACU, postanesthesia care unit; postop, postoperative; RF, risk factors.

droperidol is based on a series of 273 case reports collected over 4 years, with the majority of deaths occurring at high doses of 25 to 50 mg, greater than 15 times the optimal dose used in treating PONV. In only 10 of these cases was 1.25 mg or less used. It is difficult to conclude from the evidence a cause-and-effect relationship between QT interval prolongation and fatal cardiac dysrhythmias, as the incidence of cardiac events following droperidol administration has been estimated at 74 in 11 million.[30] Despite the lack of convincing evidence that droperidol given at antiemetic doses increases the incidence of dysrhythmias, there is no doubt that it does cause a dose-dependent QT segment prolongation that usually occurs within 5 minutes of administration, with the prolongation effect diminishing after 10 minutes.[29] This amount of QT prolongation is similar to that caused by ondansetron, and recent studies have shown that when compared with placebo, there is no significant increase in the incidence of QT prolongation among patients receiving low-dose droperidol or ondansetron for prophylaxis of PONV.[29,31]

REFERENCES

1. Gan TJ. Postoperative nausea and vomiting—can it be eliminated? *JAMA*. 2002;287(10):1233-1236.
2. Watcha MF, White PF. Postoperative nausea and vomiting. Its etiology, treatment, and prevention. *Anesthesiology*. 1992;77(1):162-184.
3. Hornby PJ. Central neurocircuitry associated with emesis. *Am J Med*. 2001;111(suppl 8A):106S-112S.
4. Scuderi PE. Pharmacology of antiemetics. *Int Anesthesiol Clin*. 2003;41(4):41-66.
5. Tramer MR, Reynolds DJ, Moore RA, McQuay HJ. Efficacy, dose-response, and safety of ondansetron in prevention of postoperative nausea and vomiting: a quantitative systematic review of randomized placebo-controlled trials. *Anesthesiology*. 1997;87(6):1277-1289.
6. Kazemi-Kjellberg F, Henzi I, Tramer MR. Treatment of established postoperative nausea and vomiting: a quantitative systematic review. *BMC Anesthesiol*. 2001;1(1):2.
7. Candiotti KA, Kovac AL, Melson TI, Clerici G, Joo Gan T. A randomized, double-blind study to evaluate the efficacy and safety of three different doses of palonosetron versus placebo for preventing postoperative nausea and vomiting. *Anesth Analg*. 2008;107(2):445-451.
8. Janicki PK. Cytochrome P450 2D6 metabolism and 5-hydroxytryptamine type 3 receptor antagonists for postoperative nausea and vomiting. *Med Sci Monit*. 2005;11(10):RA322-RA328.
9. Candiotti KA, Birnbach DJ, Lubarsky DA, et al. The impact of pharmacogenomics on postoperative nausea and vomiting: do CYP2D6 allele copy number and polymorphisms affect the success or failure of ondansetron prophylaxis? *Anesthesiology*. 2005;102(3):543-549.
10. Khalil S, Philbrook L, Rabb M, et al. Ondansetron/promethazine combination or promethazine alone reduces nausea and vomiting after middle ear surgery. *J Clin Anesth*. 1999;11(7): 596-600.
11. Chen JJ, Frame DG, White TJ. Efficacy of ondansetron and prochlorperazine for the prevention of postoperative nausea and vomiting after total hip replacement or total knee replacement procedures: a randomized, double-blind, comparative trial. *Arch Intern Med*. 1998;158(19):2124-2128.
12. Habib AS, Reuveni J, Taguchi A, White WD, Gan TJ. A comparison of ondansetron with promethazine for treating postoperative nausea and vomiting in patients who received prophylaxis with ondansetron: a retrospective database analysis. *Anesth Analg*. 2007;104(3):548-551.
13. Hill RP, Lubarsky DA, Phillips-Bute B, et al. Cost-effectiveness of prophylactic antiemetic therapy with ondansetron, droperidol, or placebo. *Anesthesiology*. 2000;92(4):958-967.
14. Habib AS, Gan TJ. Food and drug administration black box warning on the perioperative use of droperidol: a review of the cases. *Anesth Analg*. 2003;96(5):1377-1379.
15. Buttner M, Walder B, von Elm E, Tramer MR. Is low-dose haloperidol a useful antiemetic?: A meta-analysis of published and unpublished randomized trials. *Anesthesiology*. 2004;101(6):1454-1463.
16. Henzi I, Walder B, Tramer MR. Metoclopramide in the prevention of postoperative nausea and vomiting: a quantitative systematic review of randomized, placebo-controlled studies. *Br J Anaesth*. 1999;83(5):761-771.
17. Habib AS, Gan TJ. Evidence-based management of postoperative nausea and vomiting: a review. *Can J Anaesth*. 2004;51(4):326-341.
18. Kranke P, Morin AM, Roewer N, Wulf H, Eberhart LH. The efficacy and safety of transdermal scopolamine for the prevention of postoperative nausea and vomiting: a quantitative systematic review. *Anesth Analg*. 2002;95(1): 133-143.

19. Kranke P, Morin AM, Roewer N, Eberhart LH. Dimenhydrinate for prophylaxis of postoperative nausea and vomiting: a meta-analysis of randomized controlled trials. *Acta Anaesthesiol Scand*. 2002;46(3): 238-244.
20. Liu K, Hsu CC, Chia YY. Effect of dexamethasone on postoperative emesis and pain. *Br J Anaesth*. 1998;80(1):85-86.
21. Henzi I, Walder B, Tramer MR. Dexamethasone for the prevention of postoperative nausea and vomiting: a quantitative systematic review. *Anesth Analg*. 2000;90(1): 186-194.
22. Tramer MR. Rational control of PONV—the rule of three. *Can J Anaesth*. 2004;51(4):283-285.
23. Gan TJ, Meyer T, Apfel CC, et al. Consensus guidelines for managing postoperative nausea and vomiting. *Anesth Analg*. 2003;97(1):62-71.
24. Gan TJ, Diemunsch P, Habib AS, et al. Consensus guidelines for the management of postoperative nausea and vomiting. *Anesth Analg*. 2014;118:85-113.
25. Saito R, Takano Y, Kamiya HO. Roles of substance P and NK(1) receptor in the brainstem in the development of emesis. *J Pharmacol Sci*. 2003;91(2):87-94.
26. Gan TJ, Apfel CC, Kovac A, et al. A randomized, double-blind comparison of the NK1 antagonist, aprepitant, versus ondansetron for the prevention of postoperative nausea and vomiting. *Anesth Analg*. 2007;104(5):1082-1089.
27. Rothenberg DM, Parnass SM, Litwack K, McCarthy RJ, Newman LM. Efficacy of ephedrine in the prevention of postoperative nausea and vomiting. *Anesth Analg*. 1991;72(1):58-61.
28. Gan TJ, Ginsberg B, Glass PS, Fortney J, Jhaveri R, Perno R. Opioid-sparing effects of a low-dose infusion of naloxone in patient-administered morphine sulfate. *Anesthesiology*. 1997;87(5):1075-1081.
29. Charbit B, Albaladejo B, Funck-Brentano C, et al. Prolongation of QTc interval after postoperative nausea and vomiting treatment by droperidol or ondansetron. *Anesthesiology*. 2005;102(6):1094-1100.
30. Gold BS, Kitz DS, Lecky JH, Neuhaus JM. Unanticipated admission to the hospital following ambulatory surgery. *JAMA*. 1989;262(21):3008-3010.
31. White PF, Song D, Abrao J, Klein KW, Navarette B. Effect of low-dose droperidol on the QT interval during and after general anesthesia: a placebo-controlled study. *Anesthesiology*. 2005;102(6):1101-1105.

CHAPTER 16

Anticoagulant and Antiplatelet Drugs

David N. Morgan, MD, and Jennifer J. Davis, MD

INTRODUCTION

Anticoagulants are widely used in the perioperative period. The anesthesia consultant must have an understanding of their pharmacology and the implications of their use in a myriad of clinical scenarios. Intricate and complex processes that influence coagulation and anticoagulation are always in a dynamic state of equilibrium. The balance is shifted one way or the other by various disease states, medications, or perioperative events (ie, hemodilution with aggressive resuscitation). Anesthesiologists are often called upon to find a reasonable balance between anticoagulation and hemostasis in a variety of circumstances, such as during procedures associated with blood loss in patients at risk for arterial thrombotic events or when managing postoperative neuraxial analgesia in patients at high risk for deep vein thrombosis. The focus of this chapter is on elements of anticoagulant clinical pharmacology that are important for anesthesiologists to understand. Anticoagulation drugs represent a rapidly expanding field, with many novel agents in various stages of testing and approval. However, this chapter will be confined to classes of anticoagulants and antiplatelets in clinical use. A summary of these drugs is presented in Table 16–1.

ANTICOAGULANTS

Antithrombin III Binding Agents

Heparin and Low-Molecular-Weight Heparin

Mechanism of Action Both unfractionated heparin (UH) and low-molecular-weight heparin (LMWH) produce anticoagulation indirectly by causing a conformational change in antithrombin III (ATIII), increasing its catalytic activity by 1000 fold.[1,2] ATIII primarily inhibits the actions of factor IIa, thrombin, and Xa, as well as factors IXa, XIa, and XIIa to a lesser extent.[3] There are 2 major factors that determine the activity of heparin: (1) polysaccharide chain length and (2) a specific 5-sugar (pentasaccharide) sequence within the heparin molecule.[4] In general, inhibition by ATIII of both factors IIa and Xa occurs in response to UH. Low-molecular-weight heparins will selectively inhibit factor Xa via ATIII.[1] The interaction with ATIII is mediated by a unique pentasaccharide sequence that is randomly distributed along the heparin molecule.[5] This pentasaccharide sequence is present in 30% of the chains of UH and 15% to 22% of the chains of LMWH.[1,6] Binding of the pentasaccharide sequence causes a conformational change in ATIII that accelerates its interaction with thrombin and activated factor X.

Heparin chain length partially determines the factors that ATIII inhibits. UH has chain lengths of 45 to 50 sugars, whereas LMWH has lengths of 13 to 22 sugars.[1,4] Any pentasaccharide-containing chain can catalyze the inhibition of factor Xa simply by binding to ATIII and causing a conformational change. In contrast, to inactivate thrombin, heparin must bind to both antithrombin and thrombin, forming a ternary complex (3 proteins bound together). This complex can be formed only by pentasaccharide-containing chains composed of at least 18 saccharide units.[6] Less than 50% of LMWH chains are of sufficient length to bind to both thrombin and ATIII. As a result, UH usually has an anti Xa-to-IIa ratio of 1:1, whereas LMWHs typically have a ratio of 2:1 to 4:1.[1,3] Both LMWH and UH are inactive against fibrin-bound thrombin, and neither agent inhibits factor Xa bound to platelets within the prothrombinase complex.[7]

TABLE 16–1 Anticoagulant and antiplatelet drugs.

	Route	Indications
ANTICOAGULANTS		
Antithrombin III Binding Agents		
Heparins		
Heparin.	IV, SC	DVT/PE prophylaxis Treatment for ACS, DVT, PE Anticoagulation for AF, CPB, ECHO Patency of indwelling venous catheters
Low-molecular-weight heparin		
Enoxaparin (Lovenox, Clexane, Xaprin)	SC	DVT/PE prophylaxis Treatment of DVT, ACS
Tinzaparin (Innohep)	IV, SC	DVT/PE prophylaxis (safe in pregnancy)
Fondaparinux (Arixtra)	SC	DVT/PE prophylaxis
Factor Xa Inhibitors		
Rivaroxaban (Xarelto)	Oral	DVT/PE prophylaxis Anticoagulation for nonvalvular AF Treatment for DVT/PE
Direct Thrombin Inhibitors		
Lepirudin (Refludan)	IV	Heparin alternative for HIT
Argatroban (Argatroban)	IV	DVT prophylaxis Treatment for DVT Heparin alternative for HIT
Bivalirudin (Angiomax, Angiox)	IV	Anticoagulation for PCA Heparin alternative for HIT
Dabigatran etexilate (Pradaxas, Pradax, Prazaxa)	Oral	CVA prevention in patients with AF
Clotting Factor Synthesis Inhibitor		
Warfarin (Coumadin, Jantoven, Marevan, Warfant)	Oral	DVT/PE prophylaxis Anticoagulation for AF, antiphospholipid syndrome, and mechanical heart valves
ANTIPLATELET AGENTS		
Cyclooxygenase Inhibitors		
Aspirin	Oral	MI and CVA prophylaxis
Nonsteroidal anti-inflammatory drugs	IV, Oral	

(*Continued*)

TABLE 16–1 Anticoagulant and antiplatelet drugs. (*Continued*)

	Route	Indications
Thienopyridines (Adenosine Diphosphate Inhibitors)		
Clopidogrel (Plavix) Oral	Oral	Clot prevention for coronary artery, peripheral artery, and cerebral artery vascular disease Treatment for ACS, PCI
Ticlopidine (Ticlid)	Oral	Similar to clopidogrel Associated with thrombotic thrombocytopenic purpura; supplanted by clopidogrel
Prasugrel (Effient)	Oral	Treatment for ACS, PCI
GpIIb/IIIa Inhibitors		
Abciximab (ReoPro)	IV, IC	Treatment for PCI
Eptifibatide (Integrilin)	IV	Treatment for PCI Treatment of acute myocardial ischemic events or unstable angina
Tirofiban (Aggrastat)	IV	Treatment for PCI Treatment of acute myocardial ischemic events or unstable angina

Drugs are listed by their generic names with trade names in parentheses.
ACS, acute coronary syndrome; AF, atrial fibrillation; CPB, cardiopulmonary bypass; CVA, cerebrovascular accident; DVT, deep vein thrombosis; ECMO, extracorporeal membrane oxygenation; Gp, glycoprotein; HIT, heparin-induced thrombocytopenia; IC, intracoronary; IV, intravenous; MI, myocardial infarct; PCA, percutaneous coronary angioplasty; PCI, percutaneous coronary intervention (stents); PE, pulmonary embolism; SC, subcutaneous.

Dosing UH is parenterally administered either intravenously or subcutaneously. There are a variety of clinical scenarios requiring different dosing regimens of UH.[8] Dosing is dependent upon the therapeutic goal. Primary uses of heparin include thrombosis prevention (lower doses) and anticoagulation (higher doses). Common dosing for thrombosis prophylaxis includes subcutaneous injection of 5000 to 7500 units every 8 to 12 hours. Higher doses are warranted (5000 units subcutaneously every 8 hours) in high-risk patients (eg, history of cancer, known hypercoagulopathy, anticipated prolonged postoperative course in a sedentary state). This may present a clinical conundrum in managing postoperative pain with indwelling epidural catheters (see Clinical Implications: Anticoagulants and Neuraxial Anesthesia).

Anesthesiologists are almost always called upon to administer heparin for cardiopulmonary bypass and frequently called upon to administer heparin for vascular and endovascular procedures. For cardiopulmonary bypass, a large bolus dose is administered (300 units/kg) to achieve an activated clotting time (ACT) greater than 400 seconds. Additional doses may be required to maintain the ACT at that level. For vascular procedures, even following consultation with surgical colleagues, a review of recent laboratory values for activated partial thromboplastin time (aPTT), international normalized ratio (INR), hemoglobin concentration, platelet count, consideration of the surgical procedure, and a careful review of the risk–benefit in this setting (eg, excessive blood loss versus vascular graft patency), intraoperative dosing is often variable.

Aspects of heparin use are perhaps beyond the scope of practice for anesthesiologists. Heparin is used to treat acute coronary syndromes, deep vein thromboses, pulmonary emboli, cerebrovascular accidents, and transient ischemic attacks. Initial dosing for acute coronary syndromes is a 60-unit/kg bolus followed immediately by a continuous infusion of 15 units/kg/min. Initial dosing for deep vein thromboses, pulmonary emboli, cerebrovascular accidents, and transient ischemic attacks is a

80-units/kg bolus followed immediately by an infusion of 18 units/kg/min.

UH is available in many concentrations ranging from 1 unit/mL to 10,000 units/mL. The wide variety in preparations makes it a high-risk medication, since significant harm may occur from either overdosing or underdosing.

Traditionally, a unit is defined as the amount needed to maintain 1 mL of citrated sheep's plasma liquid for 1 hour after recalcification. It is now defined based on a reference antifactor Xa activity. In 2009, the United States Pharmacopeia (USP) changed the reference standard and potency assay for UH. The USP unit is harmonized with the International Unit (IU). The result is that a unit of UH is 10% less potent than the traditional definition. With large boluses, a larger heparin dose may be required. End points in monitoring should remain the same. The new preparation has an "N" after the lot number. This change was made to deal with the contamination crisis in 2007-2008.[8]

Pharmacokinetics and Monitoring The kinetic profile of UH is unpredictable and dependent on multiple factors. Even with precise weight-based bolus and continuous infusion dosing, the extent of anticoagulation is variable. Some patients will be underdosed or overdosed, while others will be dosed appropriately.[9] There is a high degree of protein binding as well as binding to endothelium and macrophages. Polysaccharide chain length plays a key role in the function of heparin and LMWH. The smaller the chain length, the less affinity a molecule has for plasma proteins. Lack of protein binding translates into a more predictable anticoagulant response and reduces or completely eliminates the need for laboratory monitoring.[1]

The high degree of protein binding has been a major drawback of UH. Many of these proteins are acute-phase reactants and vary markedly between patients. Other proteins, such as platelet factor 4 (PF4) and von Willebrand factor, are released from platelets when they are activated by thrombin. High concentrations of PF4 and von Willebrand factor at sites of vascular injury can neutralize UH and lower its effectiveness in the vicinity of thrombus.[10,11] The high degree of protein binding of UH means that a loading dose is required to occupy these protein binding sites before effective anticoagulation through binding to ATIII can be achieved.[2] The anticoagulant effect of UH is dependent both on dose and molecular size. It is not linear and increases disproportionately with increasing doses. With its smaller chain size, LMWH has much less binding to plasma proteins and a more predictable anticoagulant response, largely eliminating the need for laboratory monitoring.[12]

Heparin resistance, in which much higher than normal doses are required to achieve the desired effect, is relatively common. This can be due to the effects of protein binding as described above, variations in potency, increased clearance, or acquired or congenital antithrombin deficiency. Because heparin is dependent on ATIII for its effect, antithrombin deficiency can produce heparin resistance. For instance, this occurs when a patient has had a prolonged exposure to heparin as when the patient is awaiting a coronary artery bypass graft or after having an acute coronary syndrome. Antithrombin deficiency can be treated by giving fresh-frozen plasma or, with less exposure to the risks of blood products, ATIII concentrates.[3]

Because the relationship between a given dose and the degree of anticoagulation is unpredictable, and the harm from inadequate or excessive anticoagulation potentially severe, therapy is tailored by monitoring anticoagulant effect. The effect of UH can be monitored using the aPTT or ACT. The aPTT is a very sensitive test of heparin effect suited to lower plasma concentrations of heparin as is used in treatment of venous thromboembolism or acute coronary syndrome. The target aPTTs when managing a venous thromboembolism or an acute coronary syndrome are 60 to 80 seconds and 50 to 70 seconds, respectively.[3] For much higher plasma concentrations used in cardiopulmonary bypass, the time required to measure a aPTT is excessive, so the ACT is used. An ACT of greater than 400 seconds is required prior to initiation of cardiopulmonary bypass.

In most instances, laboratory monitoring of LMWH is unnecessary because of a predictable antithrombotic response. In certain patients, however, monitoring of LMWH activity may be useful.

For example, patients with renal failure experience an enhanced response to LMWHs because of dependence on renal clearance.[1] LMWHs do not affect the traditional measures of clotting such as detected by the aPTT or prothrombin time (PT). The only available test to monitor LMWH activity is an anti-Xa level. Although anti-Xa is a reliable measure of antithrombotic effect, it is not a reliable measure of antihemostatic effect and is not predictive of bleeding risk.[13] At the present time, there is no reliable and practical laboratory assay that accurately measures bleeding risk.

Clearance and Reversal Clearance of UH is characterized as slower first-order kinetics, where mechanisms to break down heparin are quickly saturated. As the dose increases, the amount of available heparin to exert an effect increases in a nonlinear fashion. For example, for a dose of 25 U/kg the half-life is 25 minutes whereas for a dose of 400 U/kg the half-life is 150 minutes. The half-life of UH is reported as 60-90 minutes, but as the example suggests, the actual half-life is dose dependent. For smaller bolus doses, such as those often used in the operating room or interventional suite, the half-life is shorter. Bolus dosing may need to be repeated more frequently to achieve the desired effect.[3]

UH has the benefit of a rapid, reliable reversible agent in protamine sulfate. Protamine is a strong cationic substance derived from salmon sperm that interacts with the strong anionic substance, heparin, to form a stable salt. Each 100 units of heparin is neutralized by 1 mg of protamine. The dose required for reversing anticoagulation can be derived from the time course and dose of heparin but is more accurately accomplished with automated titration of the blood sample against different concentrations of protamine.

Protamine has a variety of potentially serious adverse effects, including systemic hypotension, elevations in pulmonary vascular resistance, and anaphylactoid reactions. In order to minimize the adverse effects as well as to match the slow return of protein-bound heparin to the circulation, it is recommended that protamine be given by slow intravenous infusion.

Protamine neutralizes the antithrombin activity of LMWH but only partially reverses (40%–70%) the antifactor-Xa activity. A dose of 1-mg protamine per 100 anti-Xa units reverses 90% of anti-IIa and 60% of anti-Xa activity. The clinical significance of the residual anti-Xa effect is unknown. Both anti-IIa and anti-Xa activity may return up to 3 hours after protamine reversal, which is thought to be due to release of additional LMWH from a tissue depot if administered subcutaneously.[4]

Heparin-Induced Thrombocytopenia Heparin-induced thrombocytopenia (HIT) is an antibody-mediated hypercoagulable state with formation of thromboses in the venous and arterial systems; HIT is associated with a high degree of morbidity and mortality. Heparin can cause a mild early non–immune-mediated drop in platelet count that is clinically unimportant (formerly called type I HIT). In some patients treated with heparin for more than 4 days, antibodies form to the complex of heparin and PF4 on the surface of platelets. In a subset of patients, the antibodies are functionally active, causing the degranulation of procoagulant substances, strong platelet activation and thrombin formation. HIT can occur with any type of heparin at any dose but is more commonly associated with unfractionated heparin, longer duration of exposure, surgical rather than medical patients and female gender.[14,15]

Diagnosis of HIT is based on clinical and laboratory criteria. Clinical criteria include thrombocytopenia, timing, thrombosis, and other causes of thrombocytopenia (known as the 4 Ts). HIT is suspected with (1) a drop in platelet count by 50% or more than 20×10^9 cells/L from baseline for heparin therapy that exceeds 5 to 10 days or (2) an immediate drop in platelets with a recent exposure to heparin. It is also suspected in the presence of venous or arterial thrombosis or skin necrosis or in the absence of a clear reason for a fall in platelets. Diagnostic testing is done with enzyme-linked immunosorbent assay (ELISA), for presence of the heparin–PF4 antibody, and platelet activation tests, which are highly sensitive and specific, respectively. The presence of an antibody can often be present without HIT, so a confirmatory functional test such as the serotonin release assay or platelet aggregation assay should be performed. Heparin/PF4 antibodies typically drop to minimal or undetectable levels after 100 days and require several days of heparin reexposure to become clinically significant.[16] When the diagnosis of HIT is made, all forms of heparin and LMWH at any dose should be discontinued. The patient has a coagulation risk in excess of the initial indication for heparin and requires another form of immediate-acting anticoagulation. This is usually accomplished with a direct thrombin inhibitor or anti-Xa medication. These agents will be discussed in a subsequent section of this chapter.

Clinical Implications: Cardiopulmonary Bypass in the Presence of Heparin-Induced Thrombocytopenia Safe cardiopulmonary bypass is dependent on a reliable, effective, and testable method of anticoagulation that can be returned to a normal state of coagulation within a reasonable time. UH is ideally suited to this application. Using UH may put the patient at risk, and this represents a unique anticoagulation challenge. There are circumstances in which a discreet reexposure to heparin has a favorable risk–benefit profile and other circumstances in which alternative strategies are preferred. The American College of Chest Physicians has published practice guidelines that provide an evidence-based approach to this difficult situation.

The immune response in HIT is not a typical anamnestic response (ie, a rapid production of antibody with reexposure to heparin). HIT antibodies are typically transient, disappearing or dropping to low levels by 100 days. When these patients are reexposed, the heparin/PF4 antibody does not reappear more quickly or at higher levels than with the initial exposure. The risk of thrombosis is not increased with a brief exposure to heparin followed by reversal. For patients who are HIT antibody negative, UH is recommended during cardiopulmonary bypass only and any preoperative or postoperative anticoagulation should be accomplished with a nonheparin anticoagulant. When the HIT antibody is still present but a functional assay is negative, the same strategy may be used. When possible, it is beneficial to postpone cardiac surgery until the antibody disappears to utilize the benefits of standard UH.

When cardiac surgery is necessary during acute HIT, other approaches to anticoagulation may be used. With its history of use, favorable pharmacokinetics and monitoring with the ACT, bivalirudin, a direct thrombin inhibitor, is the agent of choice for cardiopulmonary bypass. Some important considerations for its use in cardiopulmonary bypass include (1) it should not be allowed to stagnate within the pump reservoir or within the coronary circulation or grafts and (2) cardiotomy suction should not be returned to the pump. The dose for cardiopulmonary bypass is a 1-mg/kg bolus, 50 mg in the pump prime, followed by 2.5 mg/kg/h with 0.1- to 0.5-mg boluses to maintain the ACT. Other strategies that are less preferred but may be useful include UH plus epoprostenol or tirofiban, lepirudin, danaparoid, or argatroban.[16]

Fondaparinux

Fondaparinux is a selective ATIII-dependent inhibitor of factor Xa produced entirely by chemical synthesis.[17] It interrupts at the point where the intrinsic and extrinsic coagulation paths merge, the start of the common pathway for the coagulation cascade. It binds selectively and reversibly to ATIII, inducing a conformational change in the antithrombin molecule that increases the affinity for factor Xa by 300-fold.[17] Endogenous levels of ATIII are the rate-limiting factor for its anti-Xa activity. Each molecule of fondaparinux can bind to several molecules of ATIII, as its binding to ATIII is reversible.[18] Because it is only 5 saccharides in length, it is too short to bridge from antithrombin to thrombin. As a result, it has no direct inhibitory action against thrombin or other serine proteases.[19]

The clinical pharmacology of fondaparinux is highly predictable. It has 100% bioavailability after subcutaneous or intravenous injection, and its pharmacokinetic parameters are the same for either route of administration. It does not bind to plasma proteins, and age has minimal effect on its pharmacokinetics.[17] Fondaparinux has no effect on platelet function or aggregation and because it does not interact with platelets or PF4, it is unlikely to produce HIT.[20] Thrombocytopenia can occur with fondaparinux, but it does not appear to be antibody mediated. Due to the linear and dose-dependent pharmacokinetic profile, which provides a highly predictable anticoagulant response, no laboratory monitoring should be necessary.[17] If laboratory monitoring is required in a clinical scenario such as bleeding or overdose, anti-factor Xa levels can be checked, but fondaparinux does not prolong the PT or aPTT. Its use is contraindicated in patients with severe renal insufficiency (creatinine clearance <30 mL/min). Clearance of fondaparinux is decreased by 25% in patients older than 75 years and by 30% in patients weighing less than 50 kg. Currently, there is no reversal agent for fondaparinux. Recombinant factor VIIa and prothrombin complex concentrates have been investigated as possible options.[21]

Factor Xa Inhibitor

Rivaroxaban

Rivaroxaban is an oral medication that acts by a direct inhibition of factor Xa rather than indirectly through antithrombins such as heparin, LMWH, and fondaparinux. Free factor Xa is inhibited as well as Xa within the prothrombinase complex. Rivaroxaban has been approved for venous thromboembolism prevention after total knee and hip arthroplasty. It has been extensively studied for the prevention of stroke with atrial fibrillation and will likely be used for this purpose in the future.[22] It has predictable pharmacokinetics and dynamics and does not require coagulation monitoring. Rivaroxaban has 80% oral bioavailability and peaks 2 to 3 hours after administration. The half-life is 7 to 11 hours. One-third of the drug is cleared unchanged in the urine, with the rest metabolized and eliminated through urine and feces.[23,24]

DIRECT THROMBIN INHIBITORS

Direct thrombin inhibitors inactivate fibrin-bound as well as circulating thrombin. They offer several advantages over heparin. Fibrin-bound thrombin is protected from inhibition by heparin but remains enzymatically active promoting thrombus growth and activation of platelets.[25] Unlike heparins, direct thrombin inhibitors do not bind to plasma proteins, so they produce a more predictable anticoagulant response relative to UH. They do not interact with PF4 and therefore eliminate the risk of HIT. All of these drugs prolong PT, aPTT, and thrombin clotting time.[26]

Intravenous Thrombin Inhibitors

In the United States, the Food and Drug Administration (FDA) has approved 3 parenteral direct thrombins for treatment of patients with HIT: hirudin, lepirudin, and argatroban. Bivalirudin is approved as a heparin substitute in patients undergoing coronary angioplasty.

There are no specific reversal agents for the direct thrombin inhibitors. Factor VIIa may be able to reverse the anticoagulant effect. Monitoring anticoagulant effect is accomplished using aPTT and ACT. However, the correlation is less reliable than with UH, and the possibility exists for excess anticoagulation at a given ACT. Ecarin clotting time has a better correlation with the degree of anticoagulation but is less available.[3]

Lepirudin, a recombinant form of hirudin, is the substance naturally found in leech saliva. Lepirudin forms an irreversible complex with thrombin. When used in HIT, it is dosed at 0.15 mg/kg/h with or without a 0.4-mg/kg bolus to achieve an aPTT of 1.5 to 2.5 times normal. The half-life is 60 minutes when given intravenously. It is renally cleared, thus the dose should be decreased for renal insufficiency; the drug is contraindicated in renal failure. Lepirudin can generate antibody formation with the potential for anaphylaxis with reexposure.[3,23]

Argatroban is a competitive inhibitor of thrombin, which forms a reversible complex. It is used for prevention of HIT thrombosis and percutaneous interventions, dosed at 2 mcg/kg/min. It is metabolized by the liver with a half-life of 45 minutes and is more suitable for renal failure patients.[3,23]

Bivalirudin is a synthetic analog of hirudin and forms a complex with thrombin, which is reversible by proteolytic cleavage of bivalirudin. Thrombin can regain its activity when bivalirudin is cleaved. This may occur in static environments such as with cardiopulmonary bypass circuit reservoirs or cell-saver reservoirs. To avoid this problem, blood should be kept moving. The dose of bivalirudin is 0.75-mg/kg bolus followed by 1.75 mg/kg/h for interventional procedures and a 1-mg/kg bolus, 2.5 mg/kg/h for cardiopulmonary bypass as above. Its half-life is 24 minutes with return of thrombin function, which is of great benefit. It has the additional benefits of minimal renal elimination and nonimmunogenicity.[3,23]

Oral Thrombin Inhibitor

Dabigatran etexilate is an oral direct thrombin inhibitor approved by the FDA specifically for decreasing stroke risk in atrial fibrillation. Like intravenous direct thrombin inhibitors, it is able to inactivate fibrin-bound thrombin as well as free thrombin. It does not bind to plasma proteins and thus has a predicable response without the need for laboratory monitoring. It has minimal food and drug interactions. Elimination is primarily through the kidney, with 80% of the drug unchanged in the urine. Doses are adjusted in patients with moderate renal impairment, and it is not recommended in patients with a creatinine clearance less than 30 ml/min. In healthy patients, the half-life is approximately 14 to 17 hours unless there is renal dysfunction, in which case it may be longer.[23,24]

These new oral anticoagulants, dabigatran etexilate and the factor Xa inhibitor rivaroxaban, have the potential for widespread use in the future. These medications were initially approved for prevention of venous thromboembolism following total joint replacement, but data from several large studies have shown that they are equally or more effective than warfarin at preventing embolic stroke due to atrial fibrillation. These agents have the advantage of more predictable dose responses and, because of this, do not require regular coagulation monitoring. The risk of bleeding appears to be no worse and possibly better than warfarin.[22] This may make these drugs potentially very appealing to patients who require long-term anticoagulation. The striking disadvantages of these medications are the lack of a reliable reversal agent and long half-lives, which have implications for the perioperative setting.

Clotting Factor Synthesis Inhibitor

Warfarin

Warfarin inhibits the synthesis of vitamin K–dependent post-translational γ-carboxylation of procoagulant factors II, VII, IX, and X and the anticoagulant proteins C and S.[2] Thus, it affects both the intrinsic and extrinsic arms of the coagulation cascade. In order to use warfarin safely and effectively, practitioners should understand the mechanism of action and pharmacokinetics of warfarin. This includes understanding the correlation between the various vitamin K–dependent coagulation factors and INR.

Anticoagulation The effects of warfarin are not apparent until a significant amount of biologically inactive factors are synthesized. PT and INR are most responsive to activities of factors VII and X and relatively insensitive to factor II.[27] Since factor VII has a short half-life (6–8 hours), the PT may be therapeutically prolonged within 24 to 36 hours, predominantly reflecting the reduction in factor VII activity.[2] However, adequate anticoagulation is not achieved until the levels of biologically active factors II and X are sufficiently depressed.[28] Because of the longer half-lives of factors II (50–80 hours) and X (25–60 hours), adequate anticoagulation requires 4 to 6 days.[29] In general, a prolongation of INR to greater than 1.2 reflects a factor VII activity of 55% of baseline, whereas an INR of 1.5 corresponds to a factor VII level of 40% of baseline. Clinical experience in patients with congenital deficiencies in factors II, IX, and X suggests that a factor level of 40% is associated with normal or near-normal hemostasis. Therefore, an INR of less than 1.5 is associated with normal hemostasis.[27]

Many drugs interact with warfarin and if taken concomitantly, may increase bleeding risk in patients using warfarin. Factors associated with increased sensitivity to warfarin include age greater than 65 years; female gender; weight less than 100 pounds; excessive surgical blood loss; liver, cardiac, and renal disease; and Asian ancestry. Warfarin has a narrow therapeutic window and large interpatient variability. Because of the unpredictable response to warfarin, PT/INR should be monitored.

Recovery of Normal Hemostasis Recovery of normal hemostasis parallels the development of anticoagulation in reverse. Factor II and X activities are the slowest to return to normal after cessation of therapy. Therefore, an INR of 1.4 in a patient who has recently discontinued warfarin therapy does not guarantee normal coagulation.[30] The INR, primarily determined by factor VII, may be normalized although levels of factor II and X are still depleted. Adequate levels of all vitamin K–dependent factors are typically present when INR has returned to normal range.[31]

Management of the patient on warfarin who requires surgery sooner than coagulation factors recover on their own is dependent on the urgency of the procedure. If surgery is urgent but can be delayed 18 to 24 hours, reversal can be accomplished with vitamin K (phytonadione) 2.5 to 5 mg orally or by slow intravenous infusion. The intravenous route carries a black box warning because of the possibility of reactions resembling anaphylaxis as well as cardiac and respiratory arrest, and the treatment should be reserved for urgent situations and when other routes are not feasible. When the invasive procedure is emergent and cannot be delayed, fresh-frozen plasma can be administered. Administration of fresh frozen plasma in this scenario should be accompanied by vitamin K since the procoagulant effects of exogenous factors will only last 4 to 6 hours.[31]

Clinical Implications: Anticoagulants and Neuraxial Anesthesia The subject of neuraxial anesthesia in the setting of anticoagulant therapy is a complex and nuanced topic that warrants a more extensive discussion than can be provided here. Below is a brief overview and summary of the American Society of Regional Anesthesia and Pain Medicine (ASRA) guidelines from its Third Consensus Conference on Regional Anesthesia and Anticoagulation.[27] The recommendations are based on expert opinion and evidence derived from case series, case reports, closed claims, and the pharmacology of the agents evaluated. Because of the rarity of neuraxial hematoma, no clinical study is powered to adequately define the optimal management of perioperative anticoagulation in the setting of neuraxial anesthesia. The reader is referred to the original document for background and rationale for these guidelines.

One of the notable differences from prior ASRA guidelines are changes in recommendations regarding the use of UH for venous thromboembolism prophylaxis. The differences are based on recommendations found in the 2008 practice guidelines of the American College of Chest Physicians. The use of UH 5000 units 3 times a day is now recommended for venous thromboembolism prophylaxis unless there is high risk of bleeding. This differs from typical 2 times a day dosing in the past, for which there is no contraindication to neuraxial anesthesia, other than it be avoided when UH levels are peaking 2 to 4 hours after administration. Three times a day UH is associated with increased bleeding in both medical and surgical patients. Some portion of patients will have an elevated aPTT, but the degree of prolongation is highly variable. The risk of spinal hematoma with neuraxial anesthesia is unknown but raises some concerns. The guidelines are appropriately vague in their recommendation that risks and benefits be assessed on an individual basis. Although not recommended explicitly, it seems reasonable to check an aPTT prior to needle placement or catheter removal. When using neuraxial technique for vascular procedures, heparin administration should be delayed for at least 1 hour.

The use of LMWH for thromboprophylaxis and therapy has added complexity. For patients receiving preoperative LMWH, needle placement should not occur until 12 hours after the last dose for daily prophylactic dosing or 24 hours after the last dose for 2 times a day dosing or therapeutic dosing. The extended interval for 2 times a day dosing is due to a higher trough level compared to daily dosing. General surgery patients who receive LMWH 2 hours prior to surgery should not receive a neuraxial block, since this is when the LMWH activity peaks. For patients who receive LMWH postoperatively, no other hemostasis-altering medications should be given. Two times a day dosing caries a higher risk of spinal hematoma, and the first dose should occur no earlier than 24 hours postoperatively and 4 hours after catheter removal if one was used. Once-daily prophylactic dosing is acceptable with indwelling catheters, with the first dose no sooner than 8 hours postoperatively and no less than 24 hours until the next dose. Caution should be used with this strategy, since much of the data in the recommendations comes from the experience in Europe, where a high proportion of neuroaxial interventions are a single-shot spinal technique versus an indwelling epidural catheter.

As discussed above, in the first 1 to 3 days after warfarin discontinuation, the INR may decrease but the patient may still be more anticoagulated than is reflected because of persistently low factor II and X levels. Neuraxial block should not be attempted until 4 to 5 days after discontinuation and an INR less than 1.5 has been confirmed. Use of other anticoagulants with warfarin is a contraindication to neuraxial technique even if the INR is in the reference range, since the bleeding risk is elevated and not reflected in the test. While an epidural catheter is in place, the INR should be monitored daily and the catheter should only be removed when it is less than 1.5.

Nonsteroidal anti-inflammatory drugs (NSAIDs), including aspirin, are not a contraindication to neuraxial anesthesia. However, this neuraxial should be avoided if aspirin/NSAIDS are taken with other anticoagulants or their use is anticipated perioperatively. The neuraxial technique should be deferred until 7 days after the last dose of clopidogrel. For glycoprotein IIb/IIIa inhibitors, neuraxial block should be avoided until 48 hours after abciximab and 8 hours for eptifibatide or tirofiban. Testing of platelet function and bleeding risk in patients on antiplatelet therapy is unreliable. Attention should be paid to clinical factors such as easy bruising or bleeding, advanced age and female gender.[32]

ANTIPLATELET AGENTS

Platelets exist in a quiescent state when traversing intact vessels. Disruption of endothelium exposes thrombogenic subendothelial vessel wall constituents (von Willebrand factor, collagen, and fibrinogen). Platelets adhere to these thrombogenic substances to form a hemostatic plug. Adhesion begins a cascade of intracellular reactions that lead to platelet activation.[33] There are multiple platelet activators, many of which have been the target of antiplatelet drugs. Platelet activators include thrombin (the most potent platelet agonist), adenosine diphosphate (ADP), thromboxane A2 (TXA2), epinephrine, and serotonin.[34] Platelet activation causes a conformational change in glycoprotein IIb/IIIa receptors and an increase in their number on the surface of platelets.[35] The vitamin K–dependent IIb/IIIa receptors are essential for platelet aggregation, enabling platelet-to-platelet bridging by fibrinogen (**Figure 16–1**).

Cyclooxygenase Inhibitors

Aspirin

Aspirin irreversibly acetylates and inactivates cyclooxygenase, with a 10-fold higher affinity for platelet cyclooxygenase as compared to the cyclooxygenase of other cells.[36] This inhibition of cyclooxygenase prevents formation of prostaglandin endoperoxides and TXA2. This inhibition is transient in most cells because the plasma half-life of aspirin is short (15–20 minutes), but this inhibition is irreversible in enucleated platelets, which lack the ability to regenerate the enzyme.[37]

Aspirin affects the balance between TXA2, a potent vasoconstrictor and platelet aggregation stimulator, and prostacyclin, a potent vasodilator and platelet aggregation inhibitor. Platelet cyclooxygenase is preferentially inhibited at lower doses of aspirin (30–300 mg), mainly impeding TXA2 production.[36] Prostacyclin production in vascular endothelium is much less influenced as it requires higher aspirin doses (1.5–2.0 g) daily to be inhibited. Therefore, lower doses of aspirin have a predominant antithrombotic effect, while larger doses of aspirin shift the balance toward prostacyclin inhibition, favoring platelet aggregation.[37]

The inhibition of TXA2 formation partially inhibits platelet aggregation by blocking a single metabolic pathway. Aspirin and NSAIDs still allow normal platelet adherence to subendothelium and formation of a primary hemostatic plug. Platelet aggregation in response to other stimuli that induce platelet release (thrombin, sheer stress) are not impaired by aspirin.[33] In addition, alternative pathways exist for the production of TXA2, which can limit the effectiveness of aspirin.[38] Therefore, the inhibitory effects of aspirin on platelet function are only partial because they are limited to one of several intracellular signaling pathways.

Effects of aspirin are seen in 30 minutes from a single dose as low as 81 mg.[39] In contrast, it can take up to 3 to 4 hours to reach peak plasma concentrations after the administration of enteric-coated aspirin. Plasma half-life of aspirin is short, but because of the anuclear state of platelets, the inhibitory effect lasts for the 7- to 10-day lifespan of platelets. For example, 5 to 6 days after the last aspirin dose, 50% of circulating platelets function normally.

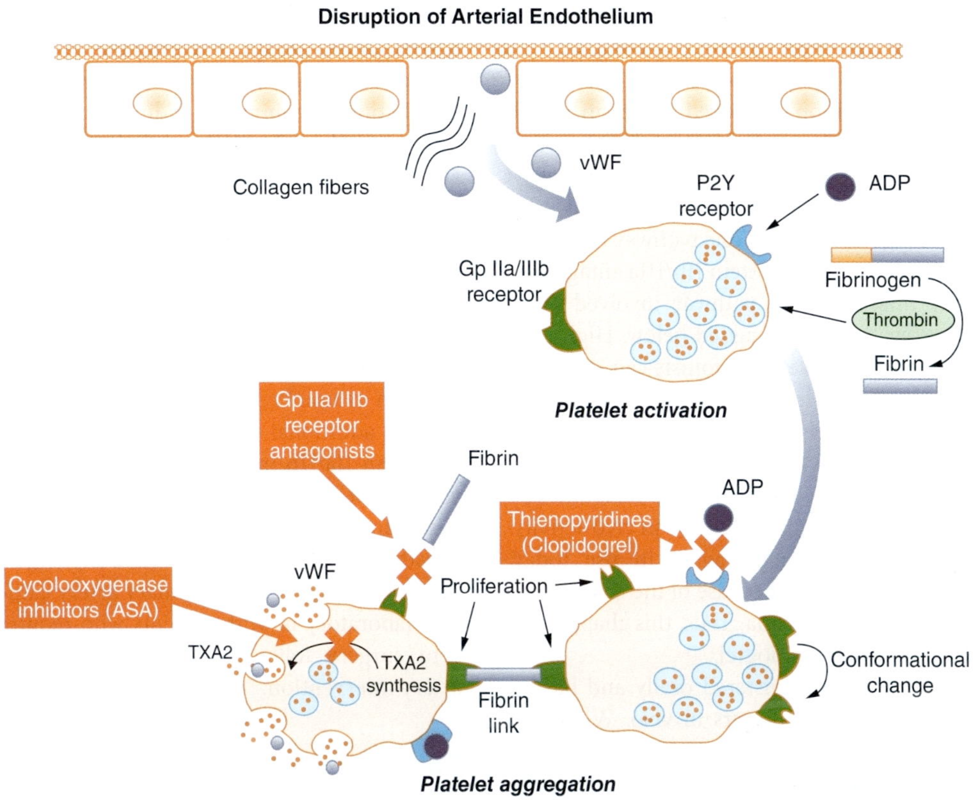

FIGURE 16–1 Schematic presentation of mechanisms of antiplatelet drugs. Substances associated with platelet activation include collagen, von Willebrand factor (vWF), adenosine diphosphate (ADP), thromboxane A2 (TXA2), and thrombin, among others. Activation causes a proliferation and conformational change in the glycoprotein IIb/IIIa receptor complex (Gp IIa/IIb), synthesis of TXA2, and degranulation with release of vWF and TXA2. Gp IIa/IIIb receptors bind to other platelets via fibrin. Cyclooxygenase inhibitors such as aspirin (acetylsalicylic acid; ASA) block synthesis of TXA2. Thienopyridines block the binding of ADP to purinergic (P2Y) receptors. Gp IIa/IIIb receptor antagonists block these receptors from binding to fibrin. (Schematic drawn using figures from Motifolio, Inc., Ellicot City, MD, with permission.)

Ten percent of the platelet pool is turned over each day, so once-a-day dosing of aspirin is sufficient to maintain complete inhibition of TXA2 production through inhibition of cyclooxygenase. The inhibition of cyclooxygenase-dependent inflammation and hyperalgesia requires larger and more frequent dosing of aspirin because of the decreased sensitivity of nonplatelet cyclooxygenase to aspirin and the ability of nucleated cells to resynthesize the enzyme.[40]

Nonsteroidal Anti-inflammatory Drugs

NSAIDs reversibly inhibit platelet cyclooxygenase. At conventional doses, platelet cyclooxygenase activity is only partially inhibited (70%—85% inhibition). Platelet function usually returns to normal within 72 hours after the last dose. Therapeutic efficacy requires maintenance of high plasma levels and multiple daily dosing.[41]

Thienopyridines

Thienopyridines are a class of ADP antagonists that exert antiplatelet action by irreversibly inhibiting the binding of ADP to P2Y receptors, a protein found on platelet cell membranes. This antagonism prevents ADP-induced platelet aggregation and ADP-mediated amplification of other platelet agonists.

In addition, these agents reduce the ADP-induced activation of the glycoprotein IIb/IIIa complex.[42] By comparison, these agents produce a moderate levels of platelet inhibition compared to aspirin, which produces a lesser degree of platelet inhibition, and glycoprotein IIb/IIIa inhibitors, which produce a greater degree of platelet inhibition.[43] Both aspirin and ADP antagonists inhibit one pathway in platelet activation, whereas glycoprotein IIb/IIIa antagonists inhibit the final common pathway involved in all platelet aggregation, as discussed below. High concentrations of strong platelet agonists can still overcome the inhibitory effects of ADP antagonists.[44]

Both clopidogrel and ticlopidine are ADP antagonists. They are inactive in vitro and require breakdown to an active metabolite or metabolites by hepatic biotransformation to achieve in vivo activity. Clopidogrel is the primary agent in use today. Ticlopidine is rarely used because of the risk of neutropenia and aplastic anemia. Thus, this chapter will focus discussion on clopidogrel.

Clopidogrel is administered orally and has an elimination half-life of 8 hours in vivo. Without a loading dose, maximal inhibition of ADP-induced aggregation takes 3 to 7 days to achieve, but significant inhibition is present after 2 to 3 days.[40] After a loading dose of 375 to 400 mg, maximal inhibition of ADP-induced platelet aggregation is seen in as little as 2 to 5 hours.[45] At steady state, the average level of platelet inhibition is 40% to 60% with a dose of 75 mg of clopidogrel per day.[46] The antiplatelet effect induced by this agent is irreversible. Therefore, the inhibitory action persists for 7 to 10 days after discontinuing therapy, consistent with the lifetime of platelets in the circulation. Several studies have shown that concomitant aspirin use results in synergistic platelet inhibition.[47]

Dose adjustments are not required in the elderly or patients with renal impairment. The manufacturer does recommend that the drug be used with caution in patients with severe hepatic disease.

The use of clopidogrel is complicated by a high degree of resistance to its effect due to pharmacogenomic variability. Clopidogrel is administered as a prodrug that requires oxidation by 2 enzymes in the cytochrome P450 system, specifically CYP2C19 and CYP3A4, to form the active compound. There is considerable variation in the enzymes' activity across ethnic groups. For example, 30% of whites, 40% of blacks, and 55% of Asians have a loss of function in one of their alleles coding for these enzymes. Those who have limited metabolism of clopidogrel (ie, the prodrug is not converted to its active form) have higher rates of death from cardiovascular causes, myocardial infarction, stroke, and in-stent thrombosis. The newer thienopyridine, prasugrel, requires metabolism in only one step to become active, therefore its activity should be more consistent. However, there have been higher rates of bleeding with its use.[48]

An additional class of antiplatelet drugs is glycoprotein IIa/IIb inhibitors. These are short-acting agents that are primarily used during and just after percutaneous coronary artery interventions. Thus, anesthesiologists may have limited exposure to these drugs other than in the coronary artery catheterization laboratory or with patients who require emergent surgery following a percutaneous coronary artery intervention.

Clinical Implications: Perioperative Antiplatelet management for Inpatients With Coronary Stents

The perioperative management of antiplatelet therapy for patients with bare-metal or drug-eluting coronary artery stents is an important topic that every anesthesia consultant caring for adults is certain to face. About 5% of patients in whom coronary stents are placed will need surgery within 12 months of placement.[49] Dual antiplatelet therapy, usually consisting of aspirin and a thienopyridine, is maintained for varying periods of time after stent placement. This therapy prevents thrombosis on the foreign material and disrupted endothelium of the coronary artery until the stent lumen has endothelialized. Thrombosis within the stent is potentially catastrophic, presenting as myocardial infarction or death in the vast majority of cases.[50] This risk and the need for antiplatelet therapy decreases as the stent becomes more endothelialized, which may take a significant length of time in the case of drug-eluting stents.

The optimal duration of dual therapy remains to be determined for drug-eluting stents. The guidelines for percutaneous coronary intervention from 2005 recommend clopidogrel for a minimum of 1 month for bare-metal stents, 3 months for sirolimus-eluting stents, and 6 months for paclitaxel-eluting stents. It should be noted that these recommendations are for on-label uses in low-risk patients with low-risk lesions. Two-thirds of all stents are currently placed in off-label situations.[48] Risk factors for late-stent thrombosis include many off-label uses, such as diabetes mellitus, low ejection fraction, renal failure, and lesions that require complex stenting—long, overlapping, ostial, and bifurcating lesions. The prevalence of late-stent thrombosis has led to revised recommendations for dual therapy of 1 month for bare-metal stents and 12 months for drug-eluting stents in all patients with stents. When the hypercoagulable, inflammatory state induced by surgery is present, management may become more complicated.

In 2007, the American Heart Association, American College of Cardiology, Society for Cardiovascular Angiography and Interventions, American College of Surgeons, and American Diabetes Association issued a science advisory on prevention of premature discontinuation of dual antiplatelet therapy with recommendations for the perioperative period. These recommendations are based on expert opinion and are supported by the 2007 American College of Cardiology/American Heart Association guidelines on perioperative cardiovascular evaluation and care after noncardiac surgery. These guidelines state that elective surgery is not recommended within 4 to 6 weeks of bare-metal coronary stent implantation and within 12 months of drug-eluting coronary stent implantation in patients in whom thienopyridine therapy or aspirin and thienopyridine therapy will need to be discontinued perioperatively. If surgery cannot be deferred and thienopyridine must be stopped, it is reasonable to continue aspirin if possible and restart thienopyridine therapy as soon as possible. In patients with drug-eluting stents who are more than 12 months from implantation, consideration should be given to continuing aspirin perioperatively and continuing dual antiplatelet therapy when the risk is high.[51]

Decisions about when and under what circumstances elective surgery will proceed should be determined jointly and collaboratively with the patient's anesthesiologist, surgeon, cardiologist, and primary care provider.

REFERENCES

1. Weitz JI. Low-molecular-weight heparins. *N Engl J Med.* 1997;337(10):688-698.
2. Majerus PW, Tollefsen DM. Oral anticoagulants. 10th ed. In: Hardman JG, Lee Limbird, Gilman AG, eds. *Goodman and Gilman's The Pharmacological Basis of Therapeutics.* New York: McGraw-Hill; 2001:1519-1538.
3. Hirsh J, Bauer KA, Donati MB, Gould M, Samama MM, Weitz JI. Parenteral anticoagulants: American College of Chest Physicians Evidence-Based Clinical Practice Guidelines (8th edition). *Chest.* 2008;133(6 suppl): 141S-159S.
4. Horlocker TT, Heit JA. Low molecular weight heparin: biochemistry, pharmacology, perioperative prophylaxis regimens, and guidelines for regional anesthetic management. *Anesth Analg.* 1997;85(4):874-885.
5. Quader MA, Stump LS, Sumpio BE. Low molecular weight heparins: current use and indications. *J Am Coll Surg.* 1998;187(6):641-658.
6. Harenberg J, Wurzner B, Zimmermann R, Schettler G. Bioavailability and antagonization of the low molecular weight heparin CY 216 in man. *Thromb Res.* 1986;44(4):549-554.
7. Weitz JI, Hudoba M, Massel D, Maraganore J, Hirsh J. Clot-bound thrombin is protected from inhibition by heparin-antithrombin III but is susceptible to inactivation by antithrombin III-independent inhibitors. *J Clin Invest.* 1990;86(2):385-391.
8. Holbrook A, Schulman S, Witt DM, et al. Evidence-based management of anticoagulant therapy: Antithrombotic Therapy and Prevention of Thrombosis, 9th ed: American College of Chest Physicians Evidence-Based Clinical Practice Guidelines. *Chest.* 2012;141 (2 suppl):e152S-e184S.
9. Cheng S, Morrow DA, Sloan S, Antman EM, Sabatine MS. Predictors of initial nontherapeutic anticoagulation with unfractionated heparin in ST-segment elevation myocardial infarction. *Circulation.* 2009;119(9):1195-1202.
10. Young E, Prins M, Levine MN, Hirsh J. Heparin binding to plasma proteins, an important mechanism for heparin resistance. *Thromb Haemost.* 1992;67(6): 639-643.
11. Heit JA. Low-molecular-weight heparin: biochemistry, pharmacology, and concurrent drug precautions. *Reg Anesth Pain Med.* 1998;23(6 suppl 2):135-139.

12. Hirsh J, Raschke R, Warkentin TE, Dalen JE, Deykin D, Poller L. Heparin: mechanism of action, pharmacokinetics, dosing considerations, monitoring, efficacy, and safety. *Chest.* 1995;108(4 suppl): 258S-275S.
13. Horlocker TT, Wedel DJ. Neuraxial block and low-molecular-weight heparin: balancing perioperative analgesia and thromboprophylaxis. *Reg Anesth Pain Med.* 1998;23(6 suppl 2):164-177.
14. Shantsila E, Lip GY, Chong BH. Heparin-induced thrombocytopenia. A contemporary clinical approach to diagnosis and management. *Chest.* 2009;135(6): 1651-1664.
15. Arepally GM, Ortel TL. Clinical practice. Heparin-induced thrombocytopenia. *N Engl J Med.* 2006;355(8): 809-817.
16. Warkentin TE, Greinacher A, Koster A, Lincoff AM. Treatment and prevention of heparin-induced thrombocytopenia: American College of Chest Physicians Evidence-Based Clinical Practice Guidelines (8th edition). *Chest.* 2008;133(6 suppl):340S-380S.
17. Samama MM, Gerotziafas GT, Elalamy I, Horellou MH, Conard J. Biochemistry and clinical pharmacology of new anticoagulant agents. *Pathophysiol Haemost Thromb.* 2002;32(5-6):218-224.
18. Comp PC. Selective factor Xa inhibition improves efficacy of venous thromboembolism prophylaxis in orthopedic surgery. *Pharmacotherapy.* 2003;23(6): 772-787.
19. Weitz JI, Hirsh J, Samama MM. New anticoagulant drugs: the Seventh ACCP Conference on Antithrombotic and Thrombolytic Therapy. *Chest.* 2004;126(3 suppl):265S-286S.
20. Elalamy I, Lecrubier C, Potevin F, et al. Absence of in vitro cross-reaction of pentasaccharide with the plasma heparin-dependent factor of twenty-five patients with heparin-associated thrombocytopenia. *Thromb Haemost.* 1995;74(5):1384-1385.
21. Bijsterveld NR, Moons AH, Boekholdt SM, et al. Ability of recombinant factor VIIa to reverse the anticoagulant effect of the pentasaccharide fondaparinux in healthy volunteers. *Circulation.* 2002;106(20):2550-2554.
22. Katsnelson M, Sacco RL, Moscucci M. Progress for stroke prevention with atrial fibrillation: emergence of alternative oral anticoagulants. *Stroke.* 2012;43(4): 1179-1185.
23. Levy JH, Key NS, Azran MS. Novel oral anticoagulants: implications in the perioperative setting. *Anesthesiology.* 2010;113(3):726-745.
24. Weitz JI, Eikelboom JW, Samama MM. New antithrombotic drugs: Antithrombotic Therapy and Prevention of Thrombosis, 9th ed: American College of Chest Physicians Evidence-Based Clinical Practice Guidelines. *Chest.* 2012;141(2 suppl):e120S-151S.
25. Weitz JI, Crowther M. Direct thrombin inhibitors. *Thromb Res.* 2002;106(3):V275-284.
26. Weitz JI, Hirsh J. New anticoagulant drugs. *Chest.* 2001;119(1 suppl):95S-107S.
27. Horlocker TT, Wedel DJ, Benzon H, et al. Regional anesthesia in the anticoagulated patient: defining the risks (the second ASRA Consensus Conference on Neuraxial Anesthesia and Anticoagulation). *Reg Anesth Pain Med.* 2003;28(3):172-197.
28. Zivelin A, Rao LV, Rapaport SI. Mechanism of the anticoagulant effect of warfarin as evaluated in rabbits by selective depression of individual procoagulant vitamin K-dependent clotting factors. *J Clin Invest.* 1993;92(5):2131-2140.
29. Horlocker TT, Wedel DJ, Schlichting JL. Postoperative epidural analgesia and oral anticoagulant therapy. *Anesth Analg.* 1994;79(1):89-93.
30. Enneking FK, Benzon H. Oral anticoagulants and regional anesthesia: a perspective. *Reg Anesth Pain Med.* 1998;23(6 suppl 2):140-145.
31. Douketis JD, Berger PB, Dunn AS, et al. The perioperative management of antithrombotic therapy: American College of Chest Physicians Evidence-Based Clinical Practice Guidelines (8th edition). *Chest.* 2008;133(6 suppl):299S-339S.
32. Horlocker TT, Wedel DJ, Rowlingson JC, Enneking FK. Executive summary: regional anesthesia in the patient receiving antithrombotic or thrombolytic therapy: American Society of Regional Anesthesia and Pain Medicine Evidence-Based Guidelines (3rd edition). *Reg Anesth Pain Med.* 2010;35(1):102-105.
33. Schafer AI. Antiplatelet therapy. *Am J Med.* 1996;101(2):199-209.
34. Bennett JS. Novel platelet inhibitors. *Annu Rev Med.* 2001;52:161-184.
35. Ferguson JJ, Waly HM, Wilson JM. Fundamentals of coagulation and glycoprotein IIb/IIIa receptor inhibition. *Eur Heart J.* 1998;19(suppl D):D3-D9.
36. Roth GJ, Calverley DC. Aspirin, platelets, and thrombosis: theory and practice. *Blood.* 1994;83(4): 885-898.
37. Patrono C, Coller B, FitzGerald GA, Hirsh J, Roth G. Platelet-active drugs: the relationships among dose, effectiveness, and side effects: the Seventh ACCP Conference on Antithrombotic and Thrombolytic Therapy. *Chest.* 2004;126(3 suppl):234S-264S.
38. Theroux P. Oral inhibitors of platelet membrane receptor glycoprotein IIb/IIIa in clinical cardiology:

issues and opportunities. *Am Heart J*. 1998;135(5 Pt 2 suppl):S107-S112.

39. Dabaghi SF, Kamat SG, Payne J, et al. Effects of low-dose aspirin on in vitro platelet aggregation in the early minutes after ingestion in normal subjects. *Am J Cardiol*. 1994;74(7):720-723.
40. Patrono C, Coller B, Dalen JE, et al. Platelet-active drugs: the relationships among dose, effectiveness, and side effects. *Chest*. 2001;119(1 suppl):39S-63S.
41. Calverley DC, Roth GJ. Antiplatelet therapy. Aspirin, ticlopidine/clopidogrel, and anti-integrin agents. *Hematol Oncol Clin North Am*. 1998;12(6):1231-1249, vi.
42. Jarvis B, Simpson K. Clopidogrel: a review of its use in the prevention of atherothrombosis. Drugs. 2000;60(2):347-377.
43. Sharis PJ, Cannon CP, Loscalzo J. The antiplatelet effects of ticlopidine and clopidogrel. *Ann Intern Med*. 1998;129(5):394-405.
44. Quinn MJ, Fitzgerald DJ. Ticlopidine and clopidogrel. *Circulation*. 1999;100(15):1667-1672.
45. Savcic M, Hauert J, Bachmann F, Wyld PJ, Geudelin B, Cariou R. Clopidogrel loading dose regimens: kinetic profile of pharmacodynamic response in healthy subjects. *Semin Thromb Hemost*. 1999;25(suppl 2): 15-19.
46. Plavix (clopidogrel bisulfate) prescribing information. New York: Sanofi-Synthelabo/Bristol-Myers Squibb; 2000.
47. Uchiyama S, Sone R, Nagayama T, et al. Combination therapy with low-dose aspirin and ticlopidine in cerebral ischemia. *Stroke*. 1989;20(12):1643-1647.
48. Barash P, Akhtar S. Coronary stents: factors contributing to perioperative major adverse cardiovascular events. *Br J Anaesth*. 2010;105(suppl 1):i3-15.
49. Vicenzi MN, Meislitzer T, Heitzinger B, Halaj M, Fleisher LA, Metzler H. Coronary artery stenting and non-cardiac surgery—a prospective outcome study. *Br J Anaesth*. 200696(6):686-693.
50. Sharma AK, Ajani AE, Hamwi SM, et al. Major noncardiac surgery following coronary stenting: when is it safe to operate? *Catheter Cardiovasc Interv*. 2004;63(2):141-145.
51. Grines CL, Bonow RO, Casey DE Jr, et al. Prevention of premature discontinuation of dual anti-platelet therapy in patients with coronary artery stents: a science advisory from the American Heart Association, American College of Cardiology, Society for Cardiovascular Angiography and Interventions, American College of Surgeons, and American Dental Association, with representation from the American College of Physicians. *Circulation*. 2007;115(6):813-818.

CHAPTER 17

Anticonvulsants in Anesthesia

Natalie Winter, MD

INTRODUCTION

For anesthesiologists, a working knowledge of antiepileptic mechanisms of action is helpful when caring for patients with known or suspected seizure disorders. This chapter provides a brief overview of how antiepileptics work and how to use them when managing a seizure in the perioperative period.

HISTORY OF DEVELOPMENT

Although potassium bromide was the original antiepileptic drug discovered in 1857, treatment of epilepsy began in earnest with the discovery of the anticonvulsant effects of phenobarbital. Although barbiturates had been first synthesized in 1864, Alfred Hauptmann, a young resident psychiatrist in 1912, was often awoken at night when epileptic patients fell out of bed while having tonic-clonic seizures. He administered phenobarbital, thinking it was a sedative, so patients would sleep through the night. He discovered that they had fewer seizures during the night and into the next day.

Although effective, phenobarbital often oversedated patients. In 1936, phenytoin was introduced as a nonsedating alternative to phenobarbital. Some 30 years later, phenytoin was followed by carbamazepine, diazepam, and valproate, all introduced in the mid-1960s. All were found to be effective in treating seizures.

In 1975, the Anticonvulsant Drug Development Program was initiated in the United States and sparked the discovery of 28,000 new drugs for the treatment of epilepsy. Most of these had similar mechanisms of action, and only those with novel mechanisms, improved efficacy, and fewer side effects have been evaluated.[1] Some of the older medications have proven efficacy and are familiar to prescribers, but the newer medications have additional benefits. There is a reduction in the amount of refractory seizures, improved efficacy, and decreased side effects. Research continues on finding better drugs for the treatment of seizures.

MECHANISM OF ACTION

Seizures result when the electrical balance along neuronal cell membranes renders them hyperexcitable within the central nervous system.[2] Treatment focuses on either augmenting inhibitory or inhibiting excitatory processes. Multiple sites may contribute to seizure activity. One postulated mechanism is an inherited change in sodium channel proteins, which makes the channel hyperexcitable. Elevated levels of glutamate and calcium may also be causes for epileptic activity. A decrease in inhibition may also result in epilepsy; for example, mutations leading to ineffective γ-aminobutyric acid (GABA) may be a possible cause. These causes of seizure activity are common targets for pharmacologic intervention.

Several groups of medications, each group with a different mechanism of action, can be used to increase seizure thresholds. Selected groups and their associated mechanism of action are presented (Figure 17–1). More than one medication may be required to control seizures; up to 50% of epilepsy patients do not have adequate control with one medication.[3] To improve efficacy, multiple sodium channel blocking agents can be used simultaneously.[2,4]

Sodium Channel Blockers

Conductance of neuronal action potentials is via voltage-gated sodium channels embedded in axon

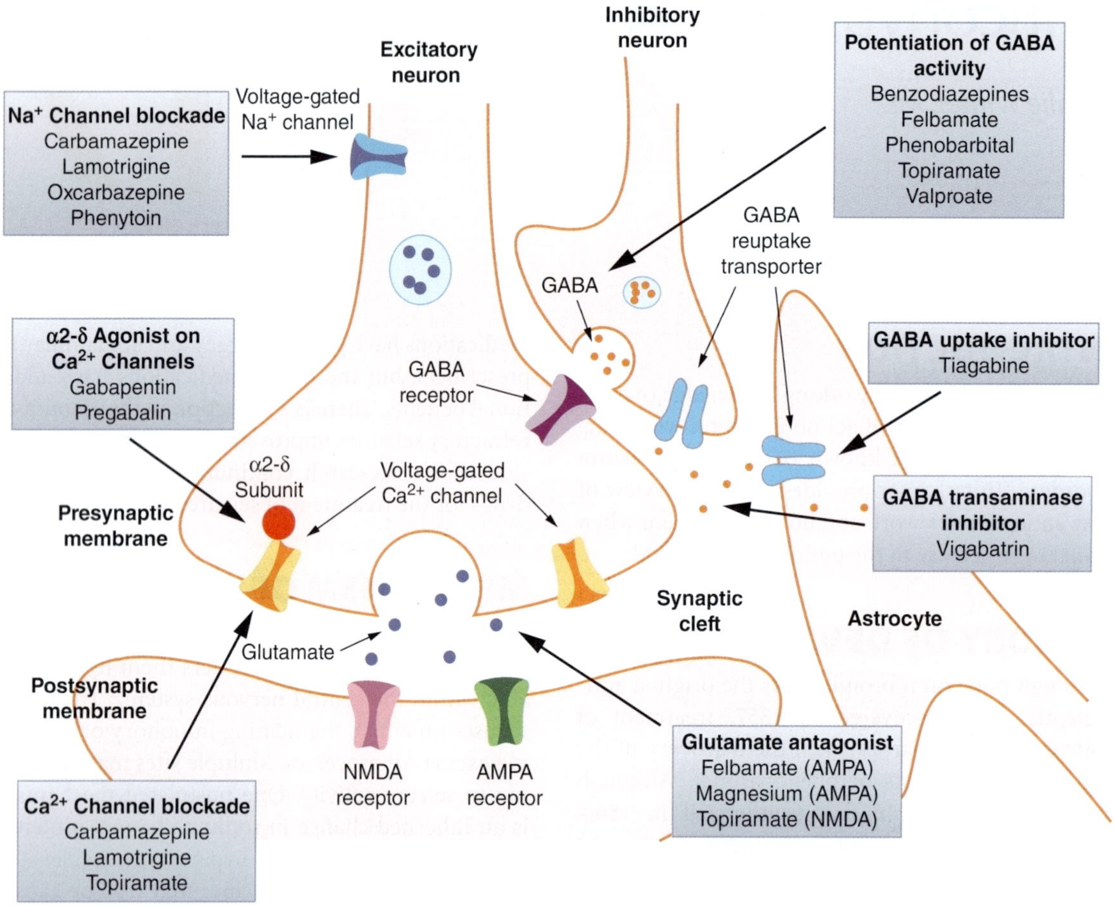

FIGURE 17–1 Mechanisms of action for selected antiepileptic drugs. AMP, α-amino-hydroxy-5-methylisoxazole-4-propionic acid; GABA, γ-aminobutyric acid; NMDA, *N*-methyl-D-aspartate.

membranes. Antiepileptic drugs bind to the inactive configuration of sodium channels and keep them closed, decreasing conductance of action potentials. Partial seizures and tonic-clonic seizures respond to antagonism of sodium channels. Common sodium channel blocking antiepileptic drugs include carbamazepine and phenytoin. Newer blockers include lamotrigine and oxcarbazepine.

Lidocaine is also a sodium channel blocker, which has been investigated in treatment of seizures. It is thought to be both proconvulsant as well as anticonvulsant. This is dose dependent. At toxic levels, lidocaine blocks the inhibitory cortical neurons, thereby increasing cortical irritability, and it ultimately results in seizure activity prior to coma. At therapeutic doses (0.5–5.0 mg/kg), lidocaine may be an effective treatment for seizures because of its activity on the sodium channel of excitatory neruons.[5]

Calcium Channel Blockers

Voltage-gated calcium channels are found throughout neural tissue and stabilize normal rhythmic brain activity. There are several types in neural tissue; some include L-, N-, and T-type. T and L stand for "transient" and "long," respectively, referring to the length of activation. N stands for neural or non-L. Calcium channels consist of 5 protein subunits.[6]

The α_1 subunit determines the channel type. It is sensitive to membrane voltage changes and contains the ion pore that facilitates movement of calcium ions. Several calcium channel blockers are used as antiepileptics. Lamotrigine, gabapentin, pregabalin, carbamazepine, and topiramate inactivate L-type channels. Ethosuximide, a prototype drug, inactivates T-type channels. Antagonism of T-type calcium channels is an effective treatment of absence seizures.

Both gabapentin and pregabalin work on the calcium channels by way of binding to the $\alpha_2\delta$ ligand on the calcium channel. This results in similar action to these other medications that block the calcium channel. Both drugs are now more commonly used in the treatment of neuropathic pain but are also appropriate treatments of epilepsy.

γ-Aminobutyric Acid Receptor Agonist/Reuptake Inhibitors

GABA is a naturally occurring inhibitory neurotransmitter that regulates neuronal excitability throughout the central nervous system. GABA exerts an effect through receptors embedded in nerve cell membranes in the presynaptic and postsynaptic regions of a synaptic cleft. GABA receptors allow negatively charged chloride ions to flow into cells and positively charged potassium ions to flow out of cells. This ion flux hyperpolarizes neurons decreasing their ability to reach an action potential. GABA is cleared from the synaptic cleft by transport proteins and is then either recycled or metabolized by GABA-transaminase.[2,3]

Several antiepileptic drugs exert their action on the GABA system. GABA agonists include benzodiazepines and phenobarbital. Benzodiazepines mimic GABA and increase the frequency, whereas phenobarbital increases the duration of GABA ion channel opening. Topiramate and felbamate activate the GABA receptors with similar effects. Tiagabine blocks transporter proteins, reducing GABA reuptake. Vigabatrin prevents GABA metabolism by antagonizing GABA-transaminase. Both of these processes thereby increase the amount of GABA available for activity. Although not well understood, gabapentin, lamotrigine, and valproate all increase GABA concentrations via unknown mechanism.[2,6]

Reduction in Glutamate-Mediated Excitation

The most important excitatory neurotransmitters include glutamate and aspartate. Excitation occurs by glutamate binding to glutamate receptors, resulting in an increase of sodium and calcium into and potassium out of neural cells. Glutamate can be targeted either by reducing its release from synaptic vesicles or blocking its action at the ligand-gated ion channel it binds. There are 5 binding sites on glutamate receptors, and 2 of these are α-amino-hydroxy-5-methylisoxazole-4-propionic acid (AMPA) and *N*-methyl-D-aspartate (NMDA).[2] Antiepileptic drugs inhibit glutamate activity via the AMPA binding site (topiramate) and the NMDA binding site (felbamate and magnesium).[3]

Ketamine is a common anesthetic used for the management of pain in the operating room. It is a known NMDA antagonist. The data about its effects in epilepsy are conflicting.

Other Mechanisms of Action

Newer drugs have unique mechanisms of action. For example, pregabalin, like gabapentin, is structurally related to GABA and originally thought to mimic GABA. However, these agents do not influence the GABAergic system. They bind to a subunit of calcium channels, the $\alpha_2\delta$ site, reducing calcium influx and decreasing release of excitatory neurotransmitters.[3] Another example is levetiracetam, which binds to a specific synaptic vesicle protein. It has little effect on normal neural function but effectively suppresses epilepsy.[2]

DOSING REGIMENS

Dosing regimens for common antiepileptic medications are presented in Table 17–1.[2] This table includes medications used to treat chronic epilepsy and to treat seizures perioperatively.

Dosing oral antiepileptic drugs is often determined by half-life. For half-lives greater than 24 hours, once-a-day dosing is used. Some of the antiepileptic drugs have a high affinity for their binding site in the brain and will have a longer half-life for its activity than what is seen in the serum.

TABLE 17–1 Dosing information for common antiepileptics.

Antiepileptic	Dose	Route	Notes
Benzodiazepines			Rapid onset effective at subduing seizure activity Continuous infusions may be required following bolus dosing to maintain antiseizure activity. Large doses or continuous infusions may lead to respiratory depression that requires tracheal intubation and mechanical ventilation.[7-9]
Midazolam	Bolus: 0.03 mg/kg Infusion: 0.25–1 mcg/kg/min	IV	
Lorazepam	Bolus: 0.05 mg/kg Infusion: 2 mg/min	IV	
Diazepam	Bolus: 0.2 mg/kg Infusion: 5 mg/min	IV	Painful with injection
Propofol	Bolus: 1 mg/kg over 5 min Infusion: 30–70 mcg/kg/min	IV	Doses necessary to treat seizures may render unconsciousness and respiratory depression that requires ventilatory assistance.[10]
Phenytoin (Dilantin)	PO dose: 100–300 mg/d Loading dose: 18 mg/kg Infusion: no greater than 50 mg/min	PO IV	Adverse effects: hypotension and dysrhythmias Therapeutic level: 10–20 mcg/mL
Barbiturate			Uncommon because of excessive sedation, hypotension, and dysrhythmias
Phenobarbital	Loading dose: 20 mg/kg Infusion: no greater than 100 mg/min	IV	Highly sedating, respiratory depressant Will likely need controlled ventilation Therapeutic level: 15–35 mcg/mL
Valproate	Loading dose: 20 mg/kg Infusion: 20–50 mg/min	IV	As effective as phenytoin for long-term treatment of status epilepticus Few side effects Stable hemodynamic profile Therapeutic level: 50–100 mcg/mL
Levetiracetam (Keppra)	500–1000 mg	PO IV	Not approved for treatment of status epilepticus; useful for prophylaxis Preliminary retrospective studies suggest it is effective. Commonly administered for perioperative seizure prophylaxis Attractive safety profile Less sedating Minimal interactions with anesthetics; no monitoring of serum concentrations necessary[10,11] Reduce dose in patients with renal failure.

Intravenous antiepileptics provide rapid onset compared to their enteral counterparts and can be administered perioperatively.[7] Some oral drugs have intravenous formulations, such as fosphenytoin, sodium valproate, lamotrigine, and levetiracetam. Fosphenytoin is a prodrug for phenytoin. It is easier to formulate than phenytoin because it does not require propylene glycol and high alkalinity to bring it into solution. Fosphenytoin is rapidly absorbed after intramuscular or intravenous administration.

Intravenous fosphenytoin produces fewer local side effects than intravenous phenytoin and has not been associated with serious cardiovascular adverse events. Fosphenytoin has become an appropriate intravenous replacement for phenytoin. Carbamazepine is insoluble, yet adding it to a cyclodextrin derivative (as with etomidate) allows for an intravenous preparation.[12]

PHARMACOKINETICS

Pharmacokinetic properties for several antiepileptics are presented in Table 17–2. Most antiepileptic drugs have linear kinetics; as dose increases, so do plasma concentrations. Phenytoin, carbamazepine, and lamotrigine, however, have nonlinear kinetics and can be difficult to titrate to steady-state conditions. Phenytoin is highly protein bound. Phenytoin plasma concentrations and the percentage of unbound drug increase disproportionately more than increases in dose. This makes it difficult to achieve appropriate therapeutic levels.[2] For carbamazepine, there is great variability in drug levels due to autoinduction of its own metabolism. Over time, there is an increase in clearance, resulting in much less active drug after the first few weeks of therapy. There are also significant interindividual differences in drug metabolism.[2,3,13,14]

Most antiepileptic drugs undergo hepatic biotransformation via various cytochrome isoenzymes into water-soluble compounds that are excreted by the kidneys. Some drugs, such as gabapentin, levetiracetam, and topiramate, undergo little biotransformation and are largely excreted unchanged by the kidneys. Patients in renal failure may require dosing adjustments.[2] Levetiracetam is one of the safest antiepileptic medications as it has minimal side effects. It also undergoes little hepatic metabolism and has little effect on cytochrome P450 enzymes.

CLINICAL APPLICATIONS

Pharmacologic Management of Status Epilepticus

Several drugs are available to anesthesiologists to treat seizures in the perioperative period (see Table 17–1). A common approach is start with a fast-acting benzodiazepine administered intravenously followed by a longer acting antiepileptic

TABLE 17–2 Pharmacokinetic features of antiepileptic agents.

Drug	Elimination Half Life ($t_{1/2}$) (h)	Steady-State Concentration time (d)	Protein Binding (%)	Therapeutic Drug Concentration (mcg/mL)	Renal Elimination (%)
Carbamazepine	14–27	3–4	66–69	4–12	1
Clonazepam	20–40		86	0.02–0.08	< 5
Gabapentin	5–7		0	12–20	100
Lamotrigine	30		55	3–14	10
Levetiracetam	6–8		< 10	10–40	100
Oxcarbazepine	9		40	3–40	1
Phenobarbital	40–136	12–21	40–60	10–40	25
Phenytoin	12–36	7–28	69–96	10–20	5
Topiramate	20–30		15	5–25	65
Valproate	6–15	1–2	80–95	50–150	2

(phenytoin) to provide continued antiseizure therapy. Diazepam has a rapid onset, but its clinical effectiveness is limited to 20 to 30 minutes because of rapid distribution. Lorazepam also has a slower onset, but it has a slower distribution. It is 89% effective in stopping a seizure within 10 minutes.[1,15,16] If conventional therapy fails, general anesthesia can be used. Most anesthetics have predominantly antiepileptic properties but may have some proconvulsant properties (Table 17–3).[10,16]

Epilepsy patients are often on chronic antiepileptic therapy. The incidence of status epilepticus in patients with a known seizure disorder during the perioperative period is low; one study reported an incidence of 3.4%.[8] Seizures that occur while on chronic antiepileptic therapy may be due to prolonged nothing-by-mouth status without the use of intravenous antiepileptics, noncompliance with antiepileptic medications, sleep deprivation, or changes in gastrointestinal motility.

TABLE 17–3 Proconvulsant and anticonvulsant features for selected anesthetics.

Anesthetic	Proconvulsant	Anticonvulsant
Nitrous oxide	+	–
Isoflurane	++	+++
Sevoflurane	++	
Desflurane	++	–––
Thiopental	++	+++
Methohexital	+++	+++
Etomidate	+++	+++
Benzodiazepines	–––	+++
Ketamine	++	++
Propofol	++	++
Opioids	+++	

Positive studies (+): isolated case (++); several cases (+++); reproducible, controlled study, or many cases.
Negative studies (–): isolated case (––); several cases (–––); reproducible, controlled study, or many cases.

Electroconvulsive Therapy

Choice of anesthetic agents for electroconvulsive therapy (ECT) is a balance between providing a general anesthetic with rapid onset and recovery and allowing a seizure to occur for as long as possible given that the effectiveness of ECT is a function of seizure duration. Unlike other barbiturates, methohexital has proconvulsant features, a rapid onset, and a brief duration of effect when administered as a bolus. For patients who cannot tolerate barbiturates, etomidate is a reasonable alternative. It also has proconvulsant effects. Studies have shown that propofol and etomidate do not result in quicker emergence from anesthesia than methohexital, so methohexital remains the preferred agent. If there are no contraindications to barbiturates, methohexital should be used.[17]

ADVERSE EFFECTS

Drug Interactions

Some of the common antiepileptics significantly influence hepatic drug metabolism by either inducing or inhibiting selected cytochrome P450 isoenzymes (Table 17–4). Anesthetics, as substrates for these isoenzymes, may be metabolized more quickly or slowly altering plasma concentrations and the duration of effect. For example, phenytoin induces CYP3A4, an important isoenzyme in the metabolism of midazolam and fentanyl. This may lead to a more rapid elimination than anticipated. This is also quite commonly noted when using neuromuscular blockers. Patients receiving phenytoin or carbamazepine exhibit resistance to nondepolarizing neuromuscular blockers. Carbamazepine will result in enzyme induction in 1 month; phenytoin takes a few days to weeks. The amount of induction is dose-dependent. Carbamazepine and phenytoin also induce metabolism of each other and can result in lower blood concentrations, although this interaction can be quite complex and variable. By contrast, valproate inhibits the isoenzyme CYP2D6, which metabolizes methadone. This may lead to slower elimination of methadone than anticipated. Other antiepileptics (lamotrigine, tiagabine, and zonisamide) have no effect on cytochrome P450 isoenzymes, but they are susceptible to increased

TABLE 17–4 Antiepileptic drugs that induce or inhibit selected cytochrome p450 isoenzymes and selected anesthetics and perioperative medications that serve as substrates to these isoenzymes.

Antiepileptic	Isoenzyme	Anesthetics as Substrates	Perioperative Medications as Substrates
Inducers			
Phenobarbital Carbamazepine Phenytoin	CYP3A4	Benzodiazepines Buprenorphine Fentanyl Meperidine Methadone	Codeine Hydrocodone Tramadol Trazodone Antidysrhythmics β Blockers Statins (except pravastatin and rosuvastatin) Oral contraceptives
Phenobarbital Valproate Carbamazepine Phenytoin	CYP2C19	Diazepam	Proton pump inhibitors
Phenobarbital	CYP2B6	Methadone	
Inhibitors			
Valproate	CYP2D6	Methadone	

metabolism if coadministered with antiepileptics that alter hepatic microsomal enzymes.[10,13]

Although induction or inhibition of microsomal enzymes by selected antiepileptics is well established, how this phenomenon actually influences the behavior of anesthetics in terms of their onset and duration of effect is not well described. As an example, consider fentanyl; if its metabolism is markedly accelerated in a patient that chronically consumes phenytoin, what changes if any should be taken in bolus or continuous infusion dosing? Unfortunately, answers to these questions are largely unknown, and it is left to clinicians to use their experience and judgment to identify the proper dose.

Hypothetically, factors that influence the onset and duration of a fentanyl bolus are largely unrelated to its elimination and more influenced by its volume of distribution and subsequent redistribution. Only once the plasma concentration has dropped by 85% does elimination play a role in the decline of plasma concentrations. By contrast, the behavior of a continuous fentanyl infusion is influenced by its elimination. One of the drawbacks to fentanyl is that it accumulates with prolonged infusions. For example, with an infusion rate of 3 mcg/kg/h, plasma concentrations continue to climb even after 12 hours. This may not occur in patients who consume phenytoin.

Neurologic, Psychologic, and Hemodynamic Adverse Side Effects

Numerous adverse side effects are associated with antiepileptics (Table 17–5[3,18]). Central nervous system effects may include dizziness, ataxia, headache, vision changes, and tremor. Psychologic changes may include depression and sedation. Systemic side effects may include abdominal pain, nausea, and weight changes.

Teratogenic or Postdelivery Effects

Many anticonvulsants are teratogenic. For example, prenatal exposure to valproate is associated with neural tube defects, craniofacial anomalies,

TABLE 17–5 Adverse effects associated with antiepileptics.

	Ataxia	Dizziness	Fatigue	Headache	Nausea	Sedation	Tremor	Other
Carbamazepine		X				X		Skin rash Stevens-Johnson syndrome Toxic epidermal necrolysis Agranulocytosis
Gabapentin	X	X	X			X	X	Weight gain
Lamotrigine	X	X	X	X	X			Diplopia Mild skin rashes Stevens-Johnson syndrome
Levetiracetam		X				X	X	Emotional instability Anorexia
Oxcarbazepine	X	X	X		X	X		Hyponatremia Mild skin rashes Serious hypersensitivity reactions
Phenytoin	X	X					X	Giddiness Lupus Nystagmus Megaloblastic anemia Rash
Topiramate		X	X			X		Mental slowing Paresthesias Anorexia Nephrolithiasis Metabolic acidosis Weight loss
Valproate	X	X		X			X	Confusion Thrombocytopenia Anorexia

limb abnormalities, and cardiovascular anomalies. Neonatal exposure is associated with hepatotoxicity, coagulopathies, and hypoglycemia. Carbamazepine is associated with a fetal syndrome characterized by facial dysmorphism and fingernail hypoplasia. There is also the potential for neural tube defects and other developmental anomalies. Recent work suggests that the teratogenic rate may be lower than previously reported and carbamazepine may be reasonable therapy during pregnancy. Lamotrigine is associated with cleft palate. Phenytoin is associated with craniofacial abnormalities, inhibited growth, and mental disabilities. Newer antiepileptics are theoretically better during pregnancy, but definitive studies confirming their safety profile have yet to be completed. Studies do suggest that monotherapy with the lowest dose are associated with less risk.[19,20]

In order to reduce risk to the fetus, it is recommended to avoid polytherapy, avoid high-risk drugs, choose newer agents, and administer folate concomitantly. Valproate, carbamazepine, and phenobarbital have the highest risk. The newer agents—gabapentin, oxcarbazepine, levetiracetam, topiramate—are safer for the fetus and are viable choices during pregnancy. Dosing should be closely monitored as blood levels may decrease during pregnancy.[21]

Benzodiazepines can also be used acutely for controlling seizures, but the infant should be monitored closely initially for acute intoxication. In chronic exposure, neonates may be at risk for withdrawal.

REFERENCES

1. Brodie MJ. Antiepileptic drug therapy the story so far. *Seizure*. 2010;19:650-655.
2. Guimaraes J, Ribeiro JA. Pharmacology of antiepileptic drugs in clinical practice. *Neurologist*. 2010;16:353-357.
3. Stefan H, Feuerstein TJ. Novel anticonvulsant drugs. *Pharmacol Ther*. 2007;113:165-183.
4. LaRoche SM, Helmers SL. The new antiepileptic drugs: clinical applications. *JAMA*. 2004;291:615-620.
5. DeToledo JC, Minagar A, Lowe MR. Lidocaine-induced seizures in patients with history of epilepsy: effect of antiepileptic drugs. *Anesthesiology*. 2002;97: 737-739.
6. Rose MA, Kam PC. Gabapentin: pharmacology and its use in pain management. *Anaesthesia*. 2002;57: 451-462.
7. Millikan D, Rice B, Silbergleit R. Emergency treatment of status epilepticus: current thinking. *Emerg Med Clin North Am*. 2009;27:101-113, ix.
8. Niesen AD, Jacob AK, Aho LE, et al. Perioperative seizures in patients with a history of a seizure disorder. *Anesth Analg*. 2010;111:729-735.
9. Trinka E: What is the relative value of the standard anticonvulsants: phenytoin and fosphenytoin, phenobarbital, valproate, and levetiracetam? *Epilepsia*. 2009;50(suppl 12):40-43.
10. Kofke WA, Tempelhoff R, Dasheiff RM. Anesthetic implications of epilepsy, status epilepticus, and epilepsy surgery. *J Neurosurg Anesthesiol*. 1997;9:349-372.
11. Usery JB, Michael LM II, Sills AK, Finch CK. A prospective evaluation and literature review of levetiracetam use in patients with brain tumors and seizures. *J Neurooncol*. 2010;99:251-260.
12. Bialer M. Clinical pharmacology of parenteral use of antiepileptic drugs. *Epilepsia*. 2007;48(suppl 8):46-48.
13. Browne TR. Pharmacokinetics of antiepileptic drugs. *Neurology*. 1998;51:S2-S7.
14. Gatti G, Bonomi I, Jannuzzi G, Perucca E. The new antiepileptic drugs: pharmacological and clinical aspects. *Curr Pharm Des*. 2000;6:839-860.
15. Leppik IE, Derivan AT, Homan RW, Walker J, Ramsay RE, Patrick B. Double-blind study of lorazepam and diazepam in status epilepticus. *JAMA*. 1983;249:1452-1454.
16. Voss LJ, Sleigh JW, Barnard JP, Kirsch HE. The howling cortex: seizures and general anesthetic drugs. *Anesth Analg*. 2008;107:1689-1703.
17. Ding Z, White PF. Anesthesia for electroconvulsive therapy. *Anesth Analg*. 2002;94:1351-1364.
18. French JA, Pedley TA. Clinical practice. Initial management of epilepsy. *N Engl J Med*. 2008;359:166-176.
19. Tomson T, Battino D. Teratogenic effects of antiepileptic medications. *Neurol Clin*. 2009;27:993-1002.
20. Tomson T, Hiilesmaa V. Epilepsy in pregnancy. *BMJ*. 2007;35:769-773.
21. Sethi NK, Wasterlain A, Harden CL. Pregnancy and epilepsy—when you're managing both. *J Fam Pract*. 2010;59:675-679.

CHAPTER

18

Drugs That Influence Renal Function

John Farr, MD

OVERVIEW

Kidneys perform a number of essential physiologic functions, including water management, electrolyte homeostasis, acid–base balance, and several neurohumoral and hormonal functions. Anesthesiologists are often called upon to (1) assess and manage perioperative oliguria (Table 18–1); (2) provide renal protection; and (3) use renal function to achieve goals not directly related to urine output, such as decreasing brain swelling or decreasing accumulation of fluid in lung alveoli.

This chapter will briefly discuss drugs used to preserve or manipulate renal function. In general, several drugs are effective diuretics but less effective at providing renal protection.

FUROSEMIDE

Furosemide was first approved for human use in the United States by the Food and Drug Administration, in July of 1982. It subsequently became a common treatment for congestive heart failure in the late 1980s. Its most common uses are in the treatment of hypertension; mobilization of edema fluid due to renal, hepatic, or cardiac dysfunction; treatment of increased intracranial pressure; and in the differential diagnosis of acute oliguria. Interestingly, furosemide has also long been used in veterinary medicine to prevent thoroughbred racehorses from bleeding through the nose during races.

Mechanism of Action

Furosemide exerts its diuretic effect by inhibiting the reabsorption of sodium and chloride, primarily in the medullary portions of the ascending limb of the loop of Henle. Protein-bound drug is secreted into the renal tubules and specifically acts on the sodium-chloride-potassium cotransporters on the intraluminal side of the loops of Henle (Figure 18–1). The accumulation of ions inside the lumen of renal tubules that occurs after furosemide administration inhibits the passive reabsorption of potassium, calcium, and magnesium. This results in urinary losses of these ions. Furosemide also stimulates renal production of prostaglandins, resulting in renal vasodilation and increased renal blood flow.

Dosing Regimen

Furosemide is effective when administered orally or intravenously. Oral dosing is 0.75 to 3.0 mg/kg and intravenous (IV) dosing is 0.1 to 1.0 mg/kg. If IV furosemide is used to replace oral furosemide, only half of the oral dose is required due to greater bioavailability. IV furosemide is approximately twice as potent and is faster than oral furosemide in inducing diuresis.[1] IV furosemide can be given as a bolus or as a continuous infusion.

Onset and Duration of Action

With oral administration, onset is within 1 hour and the duration is approximately 6 to 8 hours. With IV administration, onset is in 5 minutes and the duration is approximately 2 hours.

Pharmacokinetics

Furosemide is a weak organic acid. It is predominantly cleared by the kidneys (85%). Approximately half is metabolized and half is secreted in an unchanged form by organic acid transporters in the proximal tubules. Greater than 98% of furosemide is protein bound, and only a very small fraction of the drug is filtered through the glomerulus. However, it

TABLE 18–1 Sources of perioperative oliguria.

Category	Description
Preexisting renal insufficiency	Decreased glomerular filtration rate[a] Decreased renal reserve Increased sensitivity to any renal insult
Conditions associated with chronic renal insufficiency	Coronary artery disease Congestive heart failure Hypertension Diabetes Peripheral vascular disease Liver failure Sepsis Advanced age
Nephrotoxic drugs	Acetaminophen Angiotensin-converting enzyme Inhibitors Aminoglycosides Cephalosporins Cimetidine Metoclopramide Nonsteroidal anti-inflammatory drugs Penicillins Sulfonamides
Procedures associated with acute renal failure	Biliary surgery Thermal injuries Cardiac surgery Genitourinary surgery Organ transplant surgery Trauma Vascular surgery (especially with a suprarenal aortic cross-clamp) Prolonged intraoperative hypovolemia
Anesthetic effects	Decreased glomerular filtration rate Hypoperfusion (MABP < 70–80 mm Hg in healthy adults) Urinary retention
Mechanical causes	Kinked or obstructed urinary catheter

MABP, mean arterial blood pressure,

is the protein-bound drug, secreted into the renal tubules, that facilitates its diuretic effect.[2] In the setting of hypoalbuminemia, or in the presence of another highly protein-bound drug, tubular secretion of furosemide, and therefore its diuretic effect, is decreased.[1]

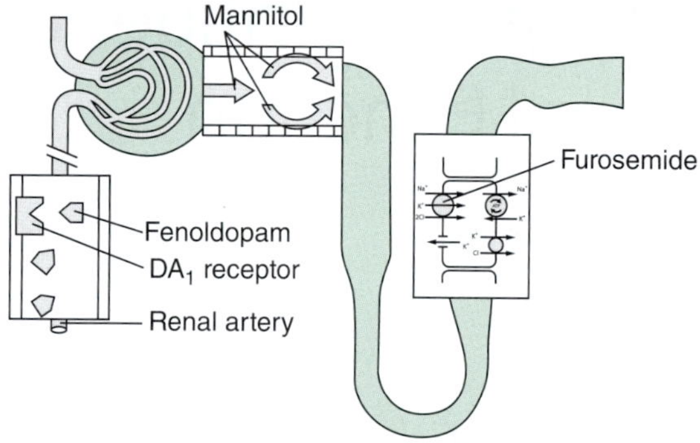

FIGURE 18–1 Location and mechanisms of action for furosemide, mannitol, and fenoldopam. The image shown represents the renal artery, glomerulus, and the descending and ascending loop of Henle. Each box shows a magnified representation of the underlying structure. DA_1, dopaminergic receptor.

Plasma clearance of furosemide is prolonged in neonates when compared to adults. The fraction of renal versus nonrenal clearance, and plasma half-life, are higher in neonates. This is attributed to a volume of distribution in infants that is approximately twice that of adults. Administration of furosemide to low-birth-weight neonates and premature infants should be done with caution due to the risk of drug accumulation and potential toxic effects.[3]

Clinical Applications

Anesthesiologists should have a healthy respect for furosemide. Perioperative oliguria may tempt a provider to administer a potent diuretic; however, the indications for furosemide therapy are more selective than poor urine output. Furosemide is used to treat a variety of pathologic conditions (Table 18–2) but should be administered only under euvolemic or hypervolemic conditions. Furosemide therapy in patients who are oliguric secondary to hypovolemia may cause hypotension and renal ischemic injury.

Furosemide is commonly used in critically ill patients with acute renal failure, but its clinical efficacy remains uncertain. In a recent meta-analysis, loop diuretics were not associated with improved

TABLE 18–2 Clinical uses of furosemide.

Disease Condition	Notes
Sodium retention	Common with congestive heart failure, renal failure, and cirrhosis
Hypercalcemia	An effective inhibitor of calcium reabsorption
Elevated intracranial pressure	An effective means of decreasing cerebrospinal fluid production by interfering with sodium ion transport in glial tissue, and by resolving cerebral edema. Not as effective as mannitol[4]
Hyperkalemia	Promotes kaliuresis in a dose-dependent fashion
Hypermyoglobinuria Hyperhemoglobinuria	Used in combination with sodium bicarbonate to keep large myoglobin or hemoglobin molecules from precipitating in nephrons by keeping the glomerular filtration rate high and myoglobin in solution
Pulmonary edema	Diuretic effect promotes alveolar fluid resorption to improve gas exchange. Aggressive use may lead to hypovolemia and poor lung perfusion.

mortality or rate of independence from renal replacement therapy, but loop diuretics were associated with a shorter duration of renal replacement therapy and with increased urine output.[5] Similarly, despite extensive study, furosemide has not been found to consistently provide a renal protective effect.

Adverse Effects

The most common side effects associated with furosemide therapy are abnormalities of fluid and electrolyte balance. Hypokalemia is the most common imbalance, but hyponatremia, hypocalcemia, and hypomagnesemia are also often seen. Furosemide can deplete myocardial potassium stores, making digitalis toxicity more likely. In addition, renal tissue concentrations of aminoglycosides are increased with furosemide therapy, enhancing the possible nephrotoxic effects of these antibiotics. Acute hypovolemia may result from administration of loop diuretics to hypovolemic patients, which may result in hypotension and ischemic renal injury.

IV furosemide at doses of 1 mg/kg or greater enhances neuromuscular blockade produced by nondepolarizing neuromuscular blocking drugs. This is most likely caused by inhibition of cyclic adenosine monophosphate production, leading to decreased prejunctional acetylcholine.[6]

Ototoxicity, manifested as deafness, is a rare dose-dependent complication of furosemide. Ototoxicity is most likely to occur with prolonged increases in the plasma concentration of furosemide in the presence of other ototoxic drugs (eg, gentamicin, cisplatin, meloxicam), and can be transient or permanent.

MANNITOL

Mannitol is a 6-carbon alcohol and was originally isolated from the secretions of the flowering ash tree in southern Europe, called manna after their resemblance to the biblical food. Clinical interest in mannitol began in 1940 when Smith and associates[7] demonstrated that mannitol clearance closely reflected the glomerular filtration rate in humans, and it was first used as a treatment for intracranial hypertension in 1961.[8]

Mechanism of Action

Mannitol is freely filtered through the glomerulus and poorly reabsorbed in renal tubules. This exerts a diuretic effect by increasing the osmotic pressure of the glomerular filtrate, which inhibits the reabsorption of tubular water and electrolytes, leading to increased urine output. In addition to its osmotic actions, mannitol has other features that are not as well defined, including oxygen free radical scavenging. Oxygen free radicals are associated with ischemia–reperfusion injury, which can be seen in many organs, including the heart and kidneys. However, the potential benefits of mannitol administration in this setting are ill defined.[9-11]

Dosing Regimen

When using mannitol, a few basic practices apply: (1) a test dose should always be given when administering to an oliguric patient, (2) urine output should always be monitored, and (3) if urine output decreases, consider discontinuing mannitol therapy.

- Mannitol is available in multiple different percent solutions and should be dosed on a gram per kilogram basis.
- For treatment of cerebral edema, mannitol 0.25 to 2.0 g/kg is administered intravenously over 30 minutes. This can be repeated every 6 to 8 hours.
- For increased intraocular pressure, a dose of 0.25 to 2.0 g/kg is indicated. When used preoperatively, the dose should be given 60 to 90 minutes before surgery to achieve maximal reduction of intraocular pressure.
- Studies supporting the use of mannitol in renal transplantation used a single dose of 250 mL of 20% mannitol. Other protocols for this indication dictate a dose of 1 g/kg, to be given just prior to arterial cross-clamp release.

Onset and Duration of Action

Time of onset of diuresis is typically within 15 to 30 minutes of administration. A reduction in intracranial pressure from mannitol administration should be seen within approximately 15 to 30 minutes and often is seen sooner. Reduction of intraocular pressure typically occurs within 30 to 60 minutes.

Pharmacokinetics

Mannitol distributes almost entirely into the extracellular space and is virtually inert. The liver metabolizes only 7% to 10%; the rest is filtered by glomeruli and excreted in the urine. Approximately 7% excreted in the urine is reabsorbed by the renal tubules. With normal kidney function, the half-life of plasma mannitol following a single bolus is 15 minutes. Approximately 95% of an injected dose is recovered in the urine after 24 hours.[12]

Clinical Applications

Anesthesiologists may administer mannitol for 1 of 5 main indications: (1) prophylaxis against acute renal failure, (2) treatment of increased intracranial pressure, (3) treatment of increased intraocular pressure, (4) prevention of acute renal failure in the transplanted kidney, and (5) as a tool in a differential diagnosis of acute oliguria.

Not all of these uses of mannitol are supported by evidence. Mannitol is often given as part of prophylactic renal protection protocols during cardiovascular surgery, extensive trauma, or in nephrotoxic conditions. Under these conditions, there is little data to support its efficacy.[13,14] Mannitol administration during and after infrarenal aortic cross-clamping does not prevent transient renal dysfunction if hemodynamic stability is maintained.[13] Mannitol administered during cardiovascular surgery reliably leads to diuresis, but there is no evidence this is renal protective. By contrast, mannitol in the cardiopulmonary bypass priming solution can lead to hypovolemia and hypokalemia postoperatively.

Mannitol is indicated in the treatment of increased intracranial pressure. Mannitol reduces brain volume by drawing free water out of the brain tissue and into the circulation, where it is subsequently excreted by the kidneys, thus dehydrating brain parenchyma.[15] When used to decrease intracranial pressure, mannitol has some important considerations that merit review.

- First, if the blood-brain barrier is not intact (eg, Alzheimer disease, multiple sclerosis flare, meningitis), mannitol will enter the brain and pull fluid with it, causing a rebound cerebral edema.
- Second, mannitol becomes less effective with chronic use as the brain adapts to high plasma osmolality. Additionally, administration of mannitol for longer than 24 hours can induce significant increases in cerebrospinal fluid osmolarity in patients with subarachnoid hemorrhage or severe head injury. This is undesirable and potentially dangerous. Cerebrospinal fluid osmolarity should be measured regularly in all patients receiving mannitol for longer than 24 hours. If cerebrospinal fluid osmolarity increases, discontinuation or tapering of mannitol therapy should be considered.[16]
- Third, mannitol is a cranial vessel vasodilator. Administration should be slow over 10 to 30 minutes to prevent a transient initial increase in intracranial pressure.

Mannitol may be given to reduce intraocular pressure. When administered for this indication, the dose should be given 60 to 90 minutes before surgery to achieve maximal reduction of intraocular pressure.

Mannitol is beneficial in renal transplantation. Several studies have demonstrated a significantly decreased incidence of acute renal failure and acute tubular necrosis after cadaveric renal transplantation when 250 mL of 20% mannitol was administered immediately before arterial clamp removal, in addition to moderate fluid therapy, compared to fluid therapy alone.[17,18]

Adverse Effects

The most common adverse effects associated with mannitol therapy are fluid and electrolyte imbalance. Water losses associated with mannitol therapy can result in hypovolemia and severe hypernatremia.[6] If mannitol, as a hypertonic solution, is poorly excreted because of renal failure or excessive doses, plasma osmolality will rise. Increased plasma osmolality will recruit intracellular fluid into the extravascular space. This will lead to hypervolemia, hyponatremia, hyperkalemia, and a metabolic acidosis.[19,20] This fluid overloaded state could also potentially cause congestive heart failure, leading to hypotension and tachycardia, pulmonary congestion, headache, and thrombophlebitis.

FENOLDOPAM

Fenoldopam is a selective dopaminergic agonist. It is primarily used as an antihypertensive agent for rapid short-term management of severe hypertension. It has the unique advantage of lowering blood pressure while preserving renal blood flow. It also has been used to treat oliguria.

Mechanism of Action

Fenoldopam activates the dopaminergic 1 (DA_1) receptor, which is a potent vasodilator found throughout the body. It causes arterial/arteriolar vasodilation in renal, mesenteric, and coronary arteries. In the kidney, DA_1 receptors within the nephron also promote sodium excretion. When compared to dopamine, fenoldopam has no α or β effects.

Dopamine receptors are present along the nephron in the kidney, with proximal tubule epithelial cells showing the highest density. IV fenoldopam has direct natriuretic and diuretic properties and promotes an increase in creatinine clearance. During administration of fenoldopam renal blood flow can be preserved or augmented, even though the primary effect of the drug is blood pressure reduction.

Dosing Regimen

Infusion doses range from 0.1 to 0.8 mcg/kg/min. It has recently been shown that improvement of renal perfusion in patients undergoing cardiac surgery begins at a dose of 0.1 mcg/kg/min, and the highest renal flow increase was seen at a dose of 0.3 mcg/kg/min.[21] Infusion rates below 0.1 mcg/kg/min have modest effects. Aggressive dosing may lead to reflex tachycardia. Fifteen minutes are required for infusion rate changes to reach near steady state; therefore, doses may be titrated every 15 minutes.

Ampules of fenoldopam should be diluted in normal saline or 5% dextrose and given as an infusion. Bolus dosing can easily precipitate hypotension.

Onset and Duration of Action

Fenoldopam has a rapid onset and offset (5 minutes). Steady-state levels are attained in approximately 15 minutes and are proportional to the infusion rate. Approximately 90% of the infused dose is eliminated in the urine and 10% in feces. About 4% is excreted unchanged.

Clinical Applications

The preservation of renal blood flow during periods of low blood pressure may be of use during many perioperative situations, including cardiothoracic and major vascular surgeries, and may also provide protection against radiocontrast-induced nephropathy. Human studies have shown that fenoldopam is a potent direct renal vasodilator and promotes increased urine output. The role of fenoldopam in preventing renal dysfunction is still debatable due to conflicting results in different studies.[22-24] However, recent data seem promising. In a meta-analysis of 1059 patients undergoing cardiovascular surgery, pooled from 13 randomized and case-matched studies, fenoldopam consistently and significantly reduced the need for renal replacement therapy (odds ratio. 0.37 [0.23–0.59]; $P < .001$) and in-hospital death (odds ratio, 0.46 [0.29–0.75]; $P = .01$).[25]

Fenoldopam has been compared to dopamine and sodium nitroprusside for renal protection and hemodynamic control in patients undergoing cross-clamping of the abdominal aorta. The occurrence of hypotension, maximum systolic blood pressure, need for additional antihypertensive drugs, and all indices of renal function were not different between the groups. The authors concluded that fenoldopam has no therapeutic advantage compared with similar therapies in patients undergoing major vascular surgery involving cross-clamping of the aorta.[26]

Fenoldopam can be used in treating acute hypertension and offers advantages in the acute resolution of severe hypertension compared to sodium nitroprusside, particularly if the patient has preexisting renal disease.[27]

Adverse Effects

The most common adverse effects of fenoldopam are related to the vasodilation that is precipitated, and they include hypotension, flushing, dizziness, headache, tachycardia, and nausea. Fenoldopam is also associated with hypokalemia. It should be used with extreme caution in patients with glaucoma, as it can produce increased intraocular pressure.

RENAL DOSE DOPAMINE

Dopamine is a vasoactive amine that has dominant effects at different concentrations. At high doses, greater than 10 mcg/kg/min, the predominant effect is α-adrenergic receptor activation, which increases systemic vascular resistance. At doses between 5 and 10 mcg/kg/min, dopamine stimulates β-adrenergic receptors and increases cardiac output. Low, or "renal-dose," dopamine, at 1 to 3 mcg/kg/min, acts on dopaminergic receptors in the renal and mesenteric vasculature, causing vasodilation and increased blood flow. Data has been published both in favor of and against the efficacy of low-dose dopamine for renal protection. A recent meta-analysis reviewing this topic included 61 studies that randomly assigned 3359 patients. This analysis showed no effect of low-dose dopamine on mortality or need for renal

Summary of selected drugs that influence renal function.

Drug	Mechanism of Action	Dosing	Onset and Duration	Possible Indications
Furosemide	Inhibits reabsorption of sodium and chloride in the loop of Henle; stimulates prostaglandin production; increases renal blood flow	Oral dosing: 0.75–3.0 mg/kg IV dosing: 0.1–1.0 mg/kg	Oral onset: 1 h; duration: 6–8 h IV onset: 5 min; duration: 2 h	Third spacing Congestive heart failure Renal failure Cirrhosis Hypercalcemia Hyperkalemia Elevated intracranial pressure
Mannitol	Increases osmotic pressure of glomerular filtrate, inhibiting reabsorption of tubular water and electrolytes, increasing urine output	0.25–1.0 g/kg of 15% to 20% solution IV over 30 min	ICP reduction within 15–30 min Diuresis within 1–3 h	Elevated intracranial pressure Elevated intraocular pressure Renal transplant Differential diagnosis of acute oliguria
Fenoldopam	Binds to dopaminergic 1 receptors, causing arterial and arteriolar vasodilation, leading to decrease in blood pressure	IV infusion 0.1–0.8 mcg/kg/min; titrate every 15 min	Onset of action: 5 min Quickly reversible	Severe hypertension with preexisting renal disease Intra-operative renal cross-clamping Renal protection during coronary artery bypass

replacement therapy. Additionally, although low-dose dopamine increased urine output by 24% after 1 day of therapy, there was no significant difference in serum creatinine levels or measured creatinine clearance.[28] Dopamine augments renal blood flow in class III/IV heart failure patients,[29] providing a mechanistic understanding of the natriuretic effect of low-dose dopamine. However, this does not seem to make a difference in meaningful outcomes.

CLINICAL DISCUSSION

Intraoperative Oliguria

A 58-year-old, 100-kg male with no significant past medical history is under general anesthesia for a multilevel posterior spinal fusion with instrumentation in the prone position. By the fourth hour of the surgery, urine output is 25 mL. Volume resuscitation with crystalloid has been adequate. Assuming possible persistent intravascular volume depletion despite adequate resuscitation, an additional 500-mL bolus of normal saline was administered. No change in urine output was observed. Preoperative transthoracic echocardiogram showed no evidence of congestive heart failure (CHF), normal systolic and diastolic function, and euvolemia. Intraoperative transesophageal echocardiography is unattainable with the patient in the prone position. Mean arterial blood pressures have been 70 to 80 mm Hg throughout. The urinary catheter appears patent.

Diagnostic Studies

Fractional excretion of sodium and blood urea nitrogen to creatinine ratio is helpful in differentiating between prerenal and intrinsic renal compromise. There is adequate volume resuscitation, no history of CHF, and no known reason for intrinsic renal failure; the time required to collect and process them may make them impractical for acute management. Right and left heart filling pressures via central venous or pulmonary artery catheter monitoring may be considered to guide intravascular expansion.

Medical Management

In a euvolemic or hypervolemic patient, both mannitol and furosemide may help oliguria. In addition, furosemide may also be useful in treating oliguria associated with diminished effective circulating volume from left ventricular failure/congestive heart failure, liver cirrhosis, or nephrotic syndrome. In the absence of these diagnoses, the perioperative use of diuretics is controversial. With persistent oliguria despite a fluid challenge, furosemide administration should be considered with caution. Conventional management includes obtaining a measure of right- and/or left-sided filling pressures and continued volume resuscitation as needed.

Although controversial, some authors recommend a furosemide drip (10–40 mg/h).[30] If urinary output fails to increase within 1 to 2 hours, the dose may be doubled. If there is no response, furosemide is discontinued. If there is a response in urine output, serial measurements of volume status, hemodynamics, and electrolytes are required.[31]

Another approach is to administer a renal function test dose of mannitol, 0.2 g/kg IV over 3 to 5 minutes. Urine output should increase to 30 to 50 mL/h. If responsive to the test dose, a one-time full dose of 0.3 to 0.4 g/kg up to 100 g may be administered. Reevaluation is warranted if urine output does not increase with the test dose. Additional mannitol is not indicated with persistent oliguria.

Prone Positioning and Urine Output

Although anecdotally urine output is decreased in the prone position, available evidence supporting this perception is not well established. One small study showed that prolonged prone positioning in patients with acute lung injury had no change on urine output or renal blood flow.[32] An additional study showed that children with acute respiratory failure placed in the prone position for 12-hour periods had significantly increased urine output.[33] Explanations other than positioning should be sought after in prone patients who are oliguric.

In summary, with a failed response to a crystalloid fluid challenge, additional volume resuscitation should be considered. When appropriate during or shortly after the surgical procedure, invasive or sonographic monitoring of atrial filling pressures should be employed to guide fluid administration. Diuresis in this setting may lead to unwanted intravascular volume depletion. Although controversial, some authors recommend using furosemide or mannitol to treat oliguria not responsive to volume expansion. Additional work is warranted to verify the clinical value of these recommendations.

REFERENCES

1. Ho KM, Power BM. Benefits and risks of furosemide in acute kidney injury. *Anaesthesia.* 2010;65(3):283-293.
2. Pichette V, Geadah D, du Souich P. Role of plasma protein binding on renal metabolism and dynamics of furosemide in the rabbit. *Drug Metab Dispos.* 1999; 27(1):81-85.
3. Prandota J. Clinical pharmacology of furosemide in children: a supplement. *Am J Ther.* 2001;8:275-289.
4. Cottrell JE, Robustelli A, Post K, et al. Furosemide and mannitol-induced changes in intracranial pressure and serum osmolarity and electrolytes. *Anesthesiology.* 1977;47:28-30.
5. Bagshaw SM, Delaney A, Haase M, et al. Loop diuretics in the management of acute renal failure: a systematic review and meta-analysis. *Crit Care Resusc.* 2007;9(1):60-68.
6. Stoelting RK, Hillier SC. *Pharmacology and Physiology in Anesthetic Practice.* 4th ed. Philadelphia: Lippincott Williams & Wilkins; 2006:225.
7. Smith WW, Finkelstein N, Smith HW. Renal excretion of hexitols and their derivatives and of endogenous creatinine-like chromogen in dog and man. *J Biol Chem.* 1940;135:231-250.
8. Wise BL, Chater N. The value of hypertonic mannitol solution in decreasing brain mass and lowering cerebrospinal fluid pressure. *J Neurosurg.* 1962;19: 1038-1043.
9. Larsen M, Webb G, Kennington S, et al. Mannitol in cardioplegia as an oxygen free radical scavenger measured by malondialdehyde. *Perfusion.* 2002;17(1): 51-55.
10. Shim JK, Choi SH, Oh YJ, et al. The effect of mannitol on oxygenation and creatine kinase MB release in patients undergoing multivessel off-pump coronary artery bypass surgery. *J Thorac Cardiovasc Surg.* 2007;133(3):704-709.
11. Wijnen MH, Vader HL, Van Den Wall Bake AW, et al. Can renal dysfunction after infra-renal aortic aneurysm repair be modified by multi-antioxidant supplementation? *J Cardiovasc Surg (Torino).* 2002;43(4):483-438.
12. Nissenson AR, Weston RE, Kleeman CR. Mannitol. *West J Med.* 1979;131:277-284.
13. Joannidis M, Druml W, Forni LG, et al. Prevention of acute kidney injury and protection of renal function in the intensive care unit. Expert opinion of the Working Group for Nephrology, ESICM. *Intensive Care Med.* 2010;36(3):392-411.
14. Karajala V Mansour W, Kellum JA. Diuretics in acute kidney injury. *Minerva Anestesiol.* 2009;75(5):251-257.
15. Paczynski RP. Osmotherapy. Basic concepts and controversies. *Crit Care Clin.* 1997;13:105.
16. Polderman KH, van de Kraats G. Increases in spinal fluid osmolarity induced by mannitol. *Crit Care Med.* 2003;31(2):584-590.
17. Van Valenberg PL, Hoitsma AJ, Tiggeler RG, et al. Mannitol as an indispensable constituent of an intraoperative hydration protocol for the prevention of acute renal failure after renal cadaveric transplantation. *Transplantation.* 1987;44(6):784-788.
18. Tiggeler RG, Berden JH, Holtsma AJ, Koene RA. Prevention of acute tubular necrosis in cadaveric kidney transplantation by the combined use of mannitol and moderate hydration. *Ann Surg.* 1985;201(2):246-251.
19. Gipstein RM, Boyle JD. Hypernatremia complicating prolonged mannitol diuresis. *N Eng J Med.* 1965;272: 1116-1117.
20. Oster JR, Singer I. Hyponatremia, hyposmolality, and hypotonicity: tables and fables. *Arch Intern Med.* 1999;159:333.
21. Meco M, Cirri S. The effect of various fenoldopam doses on renal perfusion in patients undergoing cardiac surgery. *Ann Thorac Surg.* 2010;89(2):497-503.
22. Stone GW, McCullough PA, Tumlin JA, et al. Fenoldopam mesylate for the prevention of contrast-induced nephropathy: a randomized controlled trial. *JAMA.* 2003;290:2284.
23. Zacharias M, Gilmore IC, Herbison GP, et al. Interventions for protecting renal function in the perioperative period. *Cochrane Database Syst Rev.* 2005:CD003590.
24. Landoni G, Biondi-Zoccai GG, Tumlin JA, et al. Beneficial impact of fenoldopam in critically ill patients with or at risk for acute renal failure: a meta-analysis of randomized controlled trials. *Am J Kidney Dis.* 2007:49:56.
25. Landoni G, Biondi-Zoccai GG, Marino G, et al. Fenoldopam reduces the need for renal replacement

therapy and in-hospital death in cardiovascular surgery: a meta-analysis. *J Cardithorac Vasc Anesth.* 2008;22(1):27-33.

26. Oliver WC, Nuttall GA, Cherry KJ, et al. A comparison of fenoldopam with dopamine and sodium nitroprusside in patients undergoing cross-clamping of the abdominal aorta. *Anesth Analg.* 2006;103(4):833-840.
27. Feneck R. Drugs for the perioperative control of hypertension: current issues and future directions. *Drugs.* 2007;67:2023.
28. Friedrich JO, Adhikari N, Herridge MS, Beyene J. Meta-analysis: low-dose dopamine increases urine output but does not prevent renal dysfunction or death. *Ann Intern Med.* 2005;142(7):510-524.
29. Uri Elkayam, Ng MH, Hatamizadeh P, et al. Renal vasodilatory action of dopamine in patients with heart failure. magnitude of effect and site of action. *Circulation.* 2008;117(2):200-205.
30. Majumbdar S, Kjellstrand CM. Why do we use diuretics in acute renal failure? *Semin Dial.* 1996;9:454-459.
31. Klahr S, Miller SB. Acute oliguria. *N Engl J Med.* 1998;338(10):671-675.
32. Hering R, Wrigge H, Vorwerk R, et al. The effects of prone positioning on intraabdominal pressure and cardiovascular and renal function in patients with acute lung injury. *Anesth Analg.* 2001;92(5):1226-1231.
33. Kornecki A, Frndova H, Coates AL, Shemie SD. A randomized trial of prolonged prone positioning in children with acute respiratory failure. *Chest.* 2001; 119(1):211-218.

CHAPTER 19

Perioperative Assessment of Diabetes

Jennifer DeCou, MD

INTRODUCTION

Diabetes is a condition of elevated blood glucose caused by a number of factors and affects approximately 8% of the population.[1] There are 2 types: type 1, which refers to an absolute deficiency, and type 2, which refers to a relative deficiency of insulin. Diabetes is the leading cause of kidney failure and blindness in adults, as well as a major cause of heart disease and stroke. Diabetic patients are challenging to anesthesiologists and often present with comorbidities and complications, including obesity, neurologic disease, kidney disease, cardiovascular disease, and metabolic abnormalities. Perioperative assessment should focus on prevention of complications that occur in higher frequency in diabetic patients. These include postoperative infections and cardiovascular events such as stroke, myocardial ischemia, and heart failure.[2-4] The cornerstone of prevention is perioperative glucose control.[5-7]

DIAGNOSIS OF DIABETES

In the United States, the Centers for Disease Control and Prevention and the American Diabetes Association estimate that 25% of diabetic patients are unaware that they have the disease. Preoperative glucose testing confirms this finding. Diabetic complications such as retinopathy, nephropathy, neuropathy, or cardiovascular disease may be present before a diagnosis of diabetes is made. A fasting blood glucose obtained in preoperative clinic or on the day of surgery provides an important opportunity to screen patients with suspected or known diabetes.[8]

Perhaps a better measure of glycemic history in diabetic patients is the hemoglobin A1C (presented as the percent of glycosylated hemoglobin). Over the life span of a red blood cell (up to 3 months), glucose will attach to hemoglobin and provide an estimate of average blood glucose levels over several months. In general, ideal hemoglobin A1C levels should be below 8%. More aggressive glucose control to a percentage less than 8% may lead to frequent episodes of hypoglycemia. Criteria used to distinguish normal categories of hyperglycemia are presented in Table 19–1.[9]

Perioperatively, other conditions can increase blood glucose levels including surgical stress, infections, corticosteroid use, total parenteral nutrition, kidney or liver disease, or pregnancy. Perioperative hyperglycemia is associated with increased length of stay, complications, and mortality in surgical and hospitalized patients, even in those without a history of diabetes.[10,11]

HEALTH RISKS OF DIABETES

Cardiovascular Problems

Cardiovascular risk is substantial in diabetic patients and is of significant importance to the perioperative physician. There is mounting evidence that glucose control is important to prevent adverse outcomes in hospitalized patients and in critical care settings, although how tightly blood glucose levels should be maintained is still a matter of debate.[12] In general, there is a direct relationship between fasting blood glucose concentration and the risk of having a cardiovascular event, such as sudden cardiac death, acute myocardial infarction, or stroke. Fasting plasma glucose levels greater than 110 mg/dL are associated with substantial cardiovascular risk.[13] Among patients who have had a

TABLE 19–1 Diagnostic criteria for prediabetes and diabetes.

	Normal	Prediabetes (impaired glucose tolerance or impaired fasting glucose)	Diabetes
Fasting glucose (mg/dL)	< 100	100–125	> 126
2-hour glucose (mg/dL) after 75 g OGTT	< 140	140–199	> 200
Hemoglobin A1C (%)	< 5.7	5.7–6.4	> 6.4

hemoglobin A1C, glycosylated hemoglobin; OGTT, oral glucose tolerance test.

myocardial infarction, diabetes is an independent risk factor for increased morbidity and mortality.[14] Other studies demonstrate that those with the highest glucose values at the time of an acute myocardial infarction also have the highest mortality rates.[15]

Neuropathy

Peripheral neuropathy can lead to heel ulceration, poor wound healing, and increased rates of perioperative infection. Preoperatively, clinicians should evaluate for pressure ulcers and protect lower extremities from pressure intraoperatively. Perioperative glycemic control will decrease these complications.

Autonomic neuropathy may be detected by the presence of orthostatic hypotension, resting tachycardia, and loss of heart rate variability. This may signal intraoperative difficulties. Gastroparesis may increase the risk of aspiration. Consider a prokinetic agent if appropriate (metoclopramide).

Nephropathy

Nephropathy or renal insufficiency may be present. Pretreat for contrast-induced nephropathy and decrease the use of nephrotoxic drugs such as aminoglycosides and nonsteroidal anti-inflammatory drugs. If contrast is being used, metformin should be discontinued prior to surgery and for 48 hours after the use of contrast.[16] Consider checking a creatinine prior to restarting metformin.

Retinopathy

Retinopathy is often a late complication of diabetes. Optimize blood pressure and glycemic control perioperatively to decrease the risk of further damage. Maintain proper eye protection.

Airway Problems

Airway concerns are always a special consideration in diabetics, as "stiff joint syndrome" may be present affecting temporomandibular and cervical spine mobility, particularly in type 1 diabetics. An inability to approximate the palmar surfaces while pressing the hands together (a positive "prayer sign") is associated with cervical spine immobility and a potential difficult intubation.

PREOPERATIVE MANAGEMENT

In the preoperative clinic, diabetic patients should be screened for cardiovascular risk factors, including a family history of heart disease or stroke and a history of smoking, as well as hypertension and hyperlipidemia. Standard electrocardiogram screening may not be useful in predicting occult heart disease.[17] There should be a low threshold for screening for cardiac disease with more definitive testing such as an exercise stress test, resting echocardiogram, dipyridamole thallium scintigraphy, or a dobutamine stress echocardiogram. Consulting the American College of Cardiology and American Heart Association guidelines to characterize perioperative cardiac risk is recommended.[18] In addition, consideration should be given to perioperative β blockers,[19] lipid-lowering therapy, and antiplatelet agents as appropriate.

Crucial to reducing the patient's morbidity and mortality is perioperative glucose control. The fasting blood glucose threshold at which a surgical

TABLE 19–2 Preoperative insulin management by insulin type.

Insulins	Preoperative Management	
Short and rapid acting Regular insulin (Humulin R, Novolin R) Lispro (Humalog) Aspart (NovoLog) Glulisine (Apidra)	Hold dose on morning of procedure.	Resume usual dose when eating.
Intermediate acting NPH (Humulin N, Novolin N) Zinc insulin (Lente) Extended zinc insulin (Ultralente)	Take half of usual dose morning of procedure.	Resume usual dose when eating.
Long acting Glargine (Lantus) Detemir (Levemir)	Decrease usual dose by 20% morning of surgery or night before surgery.	Resume usual dose after procedure.
Mixed insulins	Hold on morning of procedure.	Resume usual schedule when eating.
Subcutaneous insulin infusion pumps	Consider a discussion with patient and/or endocrinologist. In general, basal rate can be continued at usual dose, and mealtime corrections can be discontinued until patient is eating.	

procedure should be delayed or cancelled to optimize blood glucose concentrations is at the discretion of perioperative physicians (anesthesiologists in consultation with surgical colleagues) and based on the patient's chronic glucose control and the nature and urgency of the surgery. When the fasting glucose is more than 300 mg/dL, it is reasonable to rule out diabetic ketoacidosis, particularly in type 1 diabetics who may require volume resuscitation and correction of acid–base and electrolyte disturbances prior to elective surgery.[20] Although tight preoperative control of glucose seems ideal, there are no definitive data in the literature that define an ideal range or duration of glucose control prior to surgery.

Other special considerations include the microvascular complications associated with diabetes. Postoperative hyperglycemia is associated with an increased risk of infection and renal and pulmonary complications, as well as mortality. Tighter glycemic control has been shown to have a profound effect on reducing the incidence of these complications.[21]

Recommended preoperative management for oral, intravenous, and subcutaneous administration of diabetic medications are presented in Tables 19–2, and 19–3.[22-25]

PERIOPERATIVE MANAGEMENT

Several protocols for perioperative glucose management in diabetic patients exist, with no succinct evidence to suggest that one is better than another. However, a few guiding principles are important to consider.

First, the type of diabetes, technique used for glycemic control, the effectiveness of that technique, and the surgical procedure should be taken into account.[26]

Second, management should include insulin therapy and frequent (eg, every hour) blood glucose monitoring. Type 1 diabetics are more susceptible to developing ketoacidosis or hyperosmolar hyperglycemic nonketotic syndrome. Type 2 diabetics who use insulin may also require similar management.

Third, the primary medications for glycemic management are short-acting and rapid-acting insulins (see Table 19–2). Routes of administration include intravenous, as a bolus or continuous infusion, and subcutaneous. Glucose- and potassium-containing solutions may be required to address hypoglycemia and/or hypokalemia.

TABLE 19–3 Non-insulin antidiabetic agents.

Drug Class	Examples	Mechanism of Action	Anesthetic Risks and Considerations	Recommendations
Incretins or GLP-1 mimetics	Exenatide (Byetta) Liraglutide (Victoza)	↑ Insulin production in pancreatic beta cells ↓ Glucagon secretion; slows gastric emptying	These drugs are short-acting *injections* taken with meals. Decreased gastric emptying may increase aspiration.	Do not take on day of surgery. Resume when eating.
Synthetic amylin analogs	Pramlintide (Symlin)	Peptide hormone secreted in response to meals. Acts to: ↓ Glucagon secretion ↓ Gastric emptying ↑ Satiety	Subcutaneous *injection* taken before meals with a rapid onset and duration of action Hypoglycemia can occur.	Do not take on day of surgery. Resume when eating.
Biguanides	Metformin (Fortamet, Glucophage)	↓ Hepatic gluconeogenesis Improves insulin sensitivity	Lactic acidosis is a potential concern. Does not cause hypoglycemia	If no renal or liver dysfunction, healthy patient, and low-risk surgery, continue to take. Otherwise, do not take on day of surgery. Restart as soon as possible. Hold for 48 hours if receiving contrast agents.
Dipeptidyl peptidase-4 (DPP-4) inhibitors	Sitagliptin (Januvia) Saxagliptin (Onglyza) Linagliptin (Tradjenta)	DPP-4 enzyme inactivates incretins These drugs lead to: ↑ Effect of GLP-1 ↑ Release of insulin ↓ Release of glucose from the liver	Side effects include ↑ blood pressure, neurogenic inflammation, and immunological reactions	Do not take the day of surgery or the night before surgery. Resume when eating.
Thiazolidinediones	Rosiglitazone (Avandia) Pioglitazone (Actos)	Enhance insulin sensitivity (mainly in adipose and muscle tissue) by increasing the efficiency of glucose transporters	May cause new or worsen peripheral edema and potentially worsen heart failure Possible risk of myocardial ischemia When administered by itself, does not cause hypoglycemia	Evaluate for signs of heart failure. Hold on day of surgery. Resume when eating.
Sulphonylureas	Glipizide (Glucotrol) Glyburide (DiaBeta, Glynase, Micronase) Glimepiride (Amaryl) Glipizide XL (Glucotrol XL)	Stimulate insulin release from the beta cells of the pancreas	Potential risk of hypoglycemia Controversy regarding cardiovascular risk	Hold on day of surgery or the evening prior to surgery. Resume when eating.

(*Continued*)

TABLE 19–3 Non-insulin antidiabetic agents. (*Continued*)

Drug Class	Examples	Mechanism of Action	Anesthetic Risks and Considerations	Recommendations
Meglitinides	Repaglinide (Prandin) Nateglinide (Starlix)	Secretagogues that stimulate rapid insulin production by the pancreas	Risk of hypoglycemia Metabolized by the liver, so can be used with impaired renal function	Hold on day of surgery. Resume when eating.
α-glucosidase inhibitors	Acarbose (Precose, Glucobay, Prandase) Miglitol (Glyset)	Works in the small intestine by blocking or delaying the absorption of glucose	Taken before carbohydrate-containing meals and not used when not eating No hypoglycemia	Hold on day of surgery. Resume when eating.
Sodium-glucose co-transporter 2 (SGLT2) inhibitors	Invokana (canaglifozin)	Blocks reabsorption of glucose by the proximal tubule of the kidney Increases glucose excretion in the urine	Possible hypotension due to hypovolemia, osmotic diuresis effect Possible hypoglycemia Cardiovascular risk unknown, currently being studied	Hold on day of surgery; resume usual dose when eating

GLP-1, glucagon-like peptide.
Vouyiouklis, MD. Canagliflozin: *Improving Diabetes by making urine sweet*. Cleveland Clinic Journal of Medicine, November 2013. Vol 80:11 (683-687).

Fourth, the stress of surgery is associated with insulin resistance, and additional insulin may be necessary to maintain normal blood sugar concentrations. The mechanism of insulin resistance is not well defined but thought to be related to an increase in adrenergic agonists and inflammatory cytokines as well as alterations in muscle and adipose cell activity, all of which substantially alter intracellular utilization of insulin.[7] The time course of insulin resistance can be up to 5 days. Work by Thorell et al demonstrated insulin resistance in as soon as 2 hours following intermediate-risk surgery of moderate duration. and decreased insulin sensitivity remains 50% of normal for 5 days, returning to normal levels in the following 2 to 3 weeks.[27]

Fifth, numerous retrospective studies have suggested that tight perioperative glycemic control (ie, blood sugar levels between 70 and 110 mg/dL) reduces the risk of adverse events (eg, death, stroke, myocardial infarction). However, there are no randomized prospective studies supporting tight perioperative glycemic control. There is, however, a concern for episodes of harmful hypoglycemia in debilitated patients.[7] In fact, findings from the Normoglycemia in Intensive Care Evaluation–Survival Using Glucose Algorithm Regulation (NICE-SUGAR) trial, an international study exploring the value of tight glycemic control in intensive care unit patients, revealed an increased mortality in patients receiving tight glycemic control.[28]

In summary, although addressing hyperglycemia in the perioperative period is of paramount importance, tight perioperative glycemic control (between 70 and 110 mg/dL) may be harmful. Until definitive studies identify best practices, maintaining blood sugar levels below 180 mg/dL using intravenous insulin and close glucose monitoring is advised.

REFERENCES

1. Centers for Disease Control and Prevention. National diabetes fact sheet: national estimates and general information on diabetes and prediabetes in the United States, 2011. Atlanta, GA: US Department of Health and Human Services, Centers for Disease Control and Prevention, 2011.
2. Szekely A, Levin J, Miao Y, et al. Impact of hyperglycemia on perioperative mortality after coronary artery bypass graft surgery. *J Thorac Cardiovasc Surg*. 2011;142(2):430-437, e431.

3. Frisch A, Chandra P, Smiley D, et al. Prevalence and clinical outcome of hyperglycemia in the perioperative period in noncardiac surgery. *Diabetes Care.* 2010;33(8):1783-1788.
4. Debing E, Aerden D, Van den Brande P. Diabetes mellitus is a predictor for early adverse outcome after carotid endarterectomy. *Vasc Endovasc Surg.* 2011;45(1):28-32.
5. Kadoi Y. Perioperative considerations in diabetic patients. *Curr Diabetes Rev.* 2010;6(4):236-246.
6. Dhinsa BS, Khan WS, Puri A. Management of the patient with diabetes in the perioperative period. *J Perioper Pract.* 2010;20(10):364-367.
7. Akhtar S, Barash PG, Inzucchi SE. Scientific principles and clinical implications of perioperative glucose regulation and control. *Anesth Analg.* 2010;110(2):478-497.
8. Hatzakorzian R, Bui H, Carvalho G, Shan WL, Sidhu S, Schricker T. Fasting blood glucose levels in patients presenting for elective surgery. *Nutrition.* 2011;27(3):298-301.
9. ADA. Diagnosis and classification of diabetes mellitus. *Diabetes Care.* 2012;35(35):S64-71.
10. Kaukinen S, Salmi J, Marttinen A, Koivula T. Postoperative hyperglycaemia—are the patients diabetic? *Exp Clin Endocrinol.* 1992;100(3):85-89.
11. Capes SE, Hunt D, Malmberg K, Gerstein HC. Stress hyperglycaemia and increased risk of death after myocardial infarction in patients with and without diabetes: a systematic overview. *Lancet.* 2000;355(9206):773-778.
12. Lipshutz AK, Gropper MA. Perioperative glycemic control: an evidence-based review. *Anesthesiology.* 2009;110(2):408-421.
13. Goldberg RB, Mellies MJ, Sacks FM, et al. Cardiovascular events and their reduction with pravastatin in diabetic and glucose-intolerant myocardial infarction survivors with average cholesterol levels: subgroup analyses in the cholesterol and recurrent events (CARE) trial. The Care Investigators. *Circulation.* 1998;98(23):2513-2519.
14. Malmberg K, Ryden L. Myocardial infarction in patients with diabetes mellitus. *Eur Heart J.* 1988;9(3):259-264.
15. Soler NG, Frank S. Value of glycosylated hemoglobin measurements after acute myocardial infarction. *JAMA.* 1981;246(15):1690-1693.
16. Chen D, Lee SL, Peterfreund RA. New therapeutic agents for diabetes mellitus: implications for anesthetic management. *Anesth Analg.* 2009;108(6):1803-1810.
17. Mantha S, Roizen MF, Barnard J, Thisted RA, Ellis JE, Foss J. Relative effectiveness of four preoperative tests for predicting adverse cardiac outcomes after vascular surgery: a meta-analysis. *Anesth Analg.* 1994;79(3):422-433.
18. Fleisher LA, Beckman JA, Brown KA, et al. ACC/AHA 2006 guideline update on perioperative cardiovascular evaluation for noncardiac surgery: focused update on perioperative beta-blocker therapy—a report of the American College of Cardiology/American Heart Association Task Force on Practice Guidelines (Writing Committee to Update the 2002 Guidelines on Perioperative Cardiovascular Evaluation for Noncardiac Surgery). *Anesth Analg.* 2007;104(1):15-26.
19. American College of Cardiology Foundation/American Heart Association Task Force on Practice Guidelines, American Society of Echocardiology, American Society of Nuclear Cardiology, et al. 2009 ACCF/AHA focused update on perioperative beta blockade incorporated into the ACC/AHA 2007 guidelines on perioperative cardiovascular evaluation and care for noncardiac surgery. *J Am Coll Cardiol.* 2009;54(22):e13-e118.
20. Tridgell DM, Tridgell AH, Hirsch IB. Inpatient management of adults and children with type 1 diabetes. *Endocrinol Metab Clin North Am.* 2010;39(3):595-608.
21. Lazar HL, Chipkin SR, Fitzgerald CA, Bao Y, Cabral H, Apstein CS. Tight glycemic control in diabetic coronary artery bypass graft patients improves perioperative outcomes and decreases recurrent ischemic events. *Circulation.* 2004;109(12):1497-1502.
22. Nicholson G, Hall GM. Diabetes mellitus: new drugs for a new epidemic. *Br J Anaesth.* 2011;107(1):65-73.
23. Nassar AA, Boyle ME, Seifert KM, et al. Insulin pump therapy in patients with diabetes undergoing surgery. *Endocr Pract.* 2012;18(1):49-55.
24. Joshi GP, Chung F, Vann MA, et al. Society for Ambulatory Anesthesia consensus statement on perioperative blood glucose management in diabetic patients undergoing ambulatory surgery. *Anesth Analg.* 2010;111(6):1378-1387.
25. Killen J, Tonks K, Greenfield JR, Story DA. New insulin analogues and perioperative care of patients with type 1 diabetes. *Anaesth Intensive Care.* 2010;38(2):244-249.
26. Dagogo-Jack S. Preventing diabetes-related morbidity and mortality in the primary care setting. *J Natl Med Assoc.* 2002;94(7):549-560.
27. Thorell A, Efendic S, Gutniak M, Haggmark T, Ljungqvist O. Insulin resistance after abdominal surgery. *Br J Surg.* 1994;81(1):59-63.
28. NICE-SUGAR Study Investigators. Hypoglycemia and risk of death in critically ill patients. *N Engl J Med.* 2012;367(12):1108-1118.

CHAPTER 20

Implications of Obesity on Anesthetic Drug Behavior

Elizabeth M. Thackeray, MD, MPH, Lara Brewer, PhD, and Ken B. Johnson, MD

INTRODUCTION

Adverse physiologic changes in obese patients (Table 20-1) present multiple challenges in the operating room, including intravenous line placement, airway management, positioning, surgical exposure, and blood glucose control.[10] Perhaps most important is determining the appropriate dose of anesthetic, as it will impact airway management and extubation and pain management. Although manufacturer's dosing recommendations are weight-normalized (mg/kg), obese patients are often excluded from clinical trials during drug development.[9] Anesthesiologists rarely use total body weight (TBW) when programming an infusion pump or administering an induction dose for fear of an overdose; they often use something less than TBW to get "close enough" to the desired effect while avoiding significant adverse effects.[11,12]

A popular method of administering intravenous anesthetics is as a continuous infusion. To improve the accuracy of infusion delivery, computerized infusion pumps that use pharmacokinetic models have been developed to quickly achieve and maintain desired target effect-site concentrations. This delivery technique, known as target-controlled infusions (TCI), has become popular worldwide. Unfortunately, neither have models used to drive TCI been validated in obese patients nor has agreement regarding the correct weight to input been identified. Most models were developed with normal-sized patients or volunteers and extrapolated for use in larger patients. The main limitation is that the composition of normal size and obese patients is not the same; hence, kinetic model predictions are likely to be less accurate in the obese.

To address these issues and others, clinical pharmacologists have put forth various "scaled weights" for dosing anesthetics and recommended modified or improved kinetic models to drive TCI pumps for selected anesthetics (ie, propofol and remifentanil). For most anesthetics, however, dosing recommendations are extrapolated and not based on studies in obese patients, making them difficult to reliably use.

DOSING "WEIGHTS" FOR OBESE PATIENTS

A simple approach when formulating a dose in obese patients is to use TBW. This approach assumes that the volume of distribution and clearance are the same in all patients, lean or obese.[11] This holds true if drugs are highly soluble and distributed throughout all tissue *and* if drug clearance is the same regardless of body habitus. For anesthetics, the assumptions of ubiquitous drug distribution and clearance regardless of body habits are wrong,[1] and dosing to TBW can often lead to a significant overdose.

To get beyond the limitations of TBW, various estimates of body habitus have been adapted for dosing anesthetic drugs.[1,2,9,10] Some of these include ideal body weight (IBW), lean body weight (LBW), and fat-free mass (FFM). Each makes assumptions and has limitations (Table 20-2), but none enjoys applicability across all anesthetic drugs. Table 20-3 presents dosing weights for lean and obese females,

TABLE 20–1 Adverse effects of obesity by organ system.

Organ System	Adverse Effects
Cardiovascular	Increased vascular volume and cardiac output[1-3] Decreased myocardial compliance[3] Hypertension and left ventricular hypertrophy[1]
Respiratory	Decreased lung compliance and functional residual activity[4] Restrictive lung disease[5] Rapid oxygen desaturation following apnea[4] Increased risk of sleep apnea[6] High airway pressures required to achieve adequate ventilation[4]
Airway	Increased likelihood of difficult ventilation and tracheal intubation[6]
Hepatic	Minimal effect on drug metabolism. Drug clearance: variable cytochrome P450 enzyme activity with altered drug binding to α_1 glycoprotein but not albumin[7,8]
Renal	Glomerular filtration and creatinine clearance may exhibit no change, an increase, or decrease[8,9]

both 155 cm tall, using various dosing scalars. A key point is that using many of these scalars, especially LBW, may substantially under dose anesthetics.

Besides under dosing, LBW has an additional issue. As TBW approaches morbid obesity, LBW starts to decrease in size (Figure 20–1) for 2 reasons: (1) estimates of LBW are based on a quadratic equation fit to old population height–weight data, when morbid obesity was rare, and (2) there was little need to predict LBW for a body mass index (BMI) greater than 45 kg/m^2.

To achieve a more appropriate (larger) dosing weight, authors have also put forth dosing scalars that not only account for the lean or fat free mass, but a component of fat mass as well.[18,19] Methods have been developed to estimate normal and excessive amounts of fat. Dosing weights for patients with a BMI greater than 30 kg/m^2 have been devised that include lean body and normal fat mass.[19]

Empirical approximations of this approach have been successfully used to dose anesthetics.[16,17] One approximation used by Cortinez et al, modified fat-free mass (MFFM), is defined as FFM + fat mass × (TBW – FFM), where fat mass is a parameter that accounts for the different types of fat with a range from 0 (some combination of normal and excessive fat) to 1 (normal fat only). Prior work has used a fat mass of 0.4 to dose propofol in obese patients[16] but is likely to vary for different anesthetic drugs and the extent of obesity. For simulation purposes, the fat mass will be assumed to be 0.5.

DOSING CONSIDERATIONS FOR SELECTED ANESTHETICS

Sedative–Hypnotics

Propofol

Dosing Scalars Propofol is difficult to characterize in obese patients for several reasons. Plasma propofol concentrations are highly sensitive to cardiac output[20]; obese individuals often have an increased cardiac output compared to their lean counterparts.[1] In terms of distribution, propofol is lipophilic and rapidly moves from the plasma to the peripheral tissues,[10] suggesting that distribution is a function of body habitus (ie, with more adipose tissue, more propofol can leave the plasma). Propofol clearance, unlike distribution, is independent of body habitus and correlates well with TBW.[16] Both distribution and clearance influence drug concentration changes over time; distribution influences concentration peaks with bolus dosing, and clearance influences concentrations during and following infusions. Authors have put forth recommendations consistent with these observations to include LBM[21] for induction and TBW or MFFM for infusions.[16,22] One concern with using TBW to drive propofol infusions in obese patients is drug accumulation that may lead to prolonged drug effect and delayed emergence. Prior work using TBW compared to other scaled weights has not supported this concern.[16]

Simulations of a bolus followed by an infusion using various weight scalars (Table 20–3) are presented in Figure 20–2. The simulations present the predicted propofol effect-site concentrations from a

TABLE 20–2 Metrics of body habitus used to dose anesthetics.

Name	Equations	Advantages	Disadvantages
Ideal body weight	Male: 50 kg + 2.3 kg for each 2.54 cm (1") over 152 cm (5 ft) Female: 45.5 kg + 2.3 kg for each 2.54 cm over 152 cm	Accounts for gender and height	May under dose[a] Does not account for body habitus[b]
Lean body mass	Male: $1.1 \times TBW - 128 \times (TBW/Ht)^2$ Female: $1.07 \times TBW - 148 \times (TBW/Ht)^2$	Accounts for gender and body habitus (height and weight)	May under dose[a] For a BMI > 35 kg/m^2, LBM becomes smaller than for lower BMIs
Fat-free mass[13]	Male: $(9.27 \times 10^3 \times TBW)/(6.68 \times 10^3 + 216 \times BMI)$ Female: $(9.27 \times 10^3 \times TBW)/(8.78 \times 10^3 + 244 \times BMI)$	Accounts for gender and body habitus (height and weight)	May underdose[a]
Pharmacokinetic mass[14,15]	$52/[1 + (196.4 \cdot e^{-0.025\,TBW} - 53.66)/100]$	Correlates well with measured fentanyl concentrations	Does not account for gender or height
Modified fat-free mass[16,17]	FFM + 0.5*(TBW – FFM)	Accounts for gender and body habitus (height, LBW, and adipose weight).	Empirically derived

[a]The dose/kg using IBW, TBW, or FFM in an obese person are all less than the dose/kg using TBW in a nonobese patient.
BMI, body mass index; FFM, fat-free mass; Ht, height in centimeters; IBW, ideal body weight; LBM, lean body mass; TBW, total body weight in kg.
[b]Lean body mass increases with increasing weight; however, the IBW dosing scalar is constant for height and gender and does not account for the increased LBM in obese patients.

TABLE 20–3 Dosing weights based on various dosing scalars.

	155 cm (5'1") Female	
	60 kg BMI = 25 kg/m^2	140 kg BMI = 58 kg/m^2
Dosing Scalar	Dosing Weight (kg)	Dosing Weight (kg)
Total body weight	60	140
Ideal body weight	48	48
Lean body mass	42	29
Fat-free mass	37	56
Modified fat -free mass	49	98

BMI, body mass index.

bolus (2 mg/kg) and 1-hour infusion (150 mcg/kg/min) in a 155 cm (5'1") obese (140 kg) and lean (60 kg) female. If dosed according to TBW, plasma concentrations in a lean and obese individual are similar; their respective peak propofol concentrations are approximately 7 and 8 mcg/mL (gray and black lines). The probability of unresponsiveness is also similar during the bolus and infusions, but the obese individual has a prolonged duration of effect once the 1-hour infusion is terminated. The time required to reach less than a 5% probability of unresponsiveness once the infusion is terminated is 18 and 26 minutes for a lean and obese individual, respectively.

Of note, dosing according to IBW, LBM, and FFM all lead to effect-site concentrations that are substantially lower than those dosed to TBW and are likely to yield inadequate effect, especially during the infusion. The most worrisome of these 3 weight scalars is LBM. The obese patient from Table 20-3

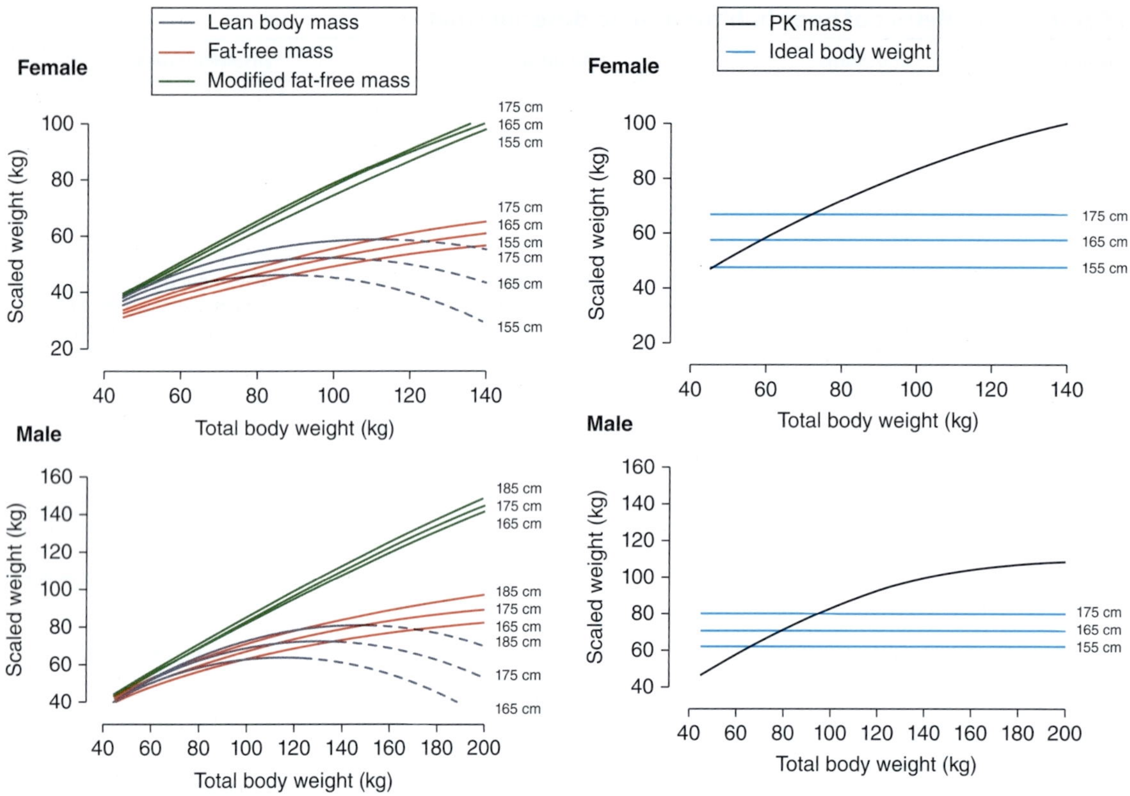

FIGURE 20–1 Predictions of scaled weight based on lean body mass, fat-free mass,[13] modified fat-free mass,[16,17] ideal body weight, and pharmacokinetic (PK) mass[14,15] are presented for female and male individuals of various heights over a range of total body weights. At a total body weight of 90 kg for the female and 130 kg for the male, the lean body mass predictions start to decrease for increasing total body weight represented with a dashed blue line. The ideal body weight remains the same regardless of total body weight (red line). PK mass remains the same regardless of height and gender (black line).

dosed using LBM would be given an induction dose of 2 mg/kg, or 58 mg, in contrast to the induction dose of 120 mg given to her lean counterpart.

A reasonable dosing scalar for propofol is the MFFM. When using this scalar, plasma concentrations are similar but somewhat lower to what is achieved when dosing a lean individual to TBW (green versus gray lines in Figure 20–2). Following the bolus dose, the probability of unresponsiveness does drop below 80%, making this dosing scalar perhaps unattractive if propofol is used as the sole anesthetic.

Kinetic Models for Target-Controlled Infusions
Several kinetic models of propofol are available for TCI and have been used with obese patients with varied results. Perhaps the 2 most widely used models are those published by Marsh et al and Schnider et al.[24,25] The Marsh model was built from data collected in a pediatric population. Although it is useful, it may have limited application in obese patients. Using the Marsh model, researchers have explored different dosing weights for propofol in morbidly obese patients when coadministered with remifentanil.[22,26] Results have been variable. Although TCI using TBW may better predict measured plasma concentrations in this population than the corrected weight used by Servin et al,[16] authors recommend that TCI using the Marsh model should be titrated to target processed electroencephalogram (EEG) values[22] in this patient group regardless of weight is used.

The Schnider model was built from data collected in adults over a range of weights, heights, and

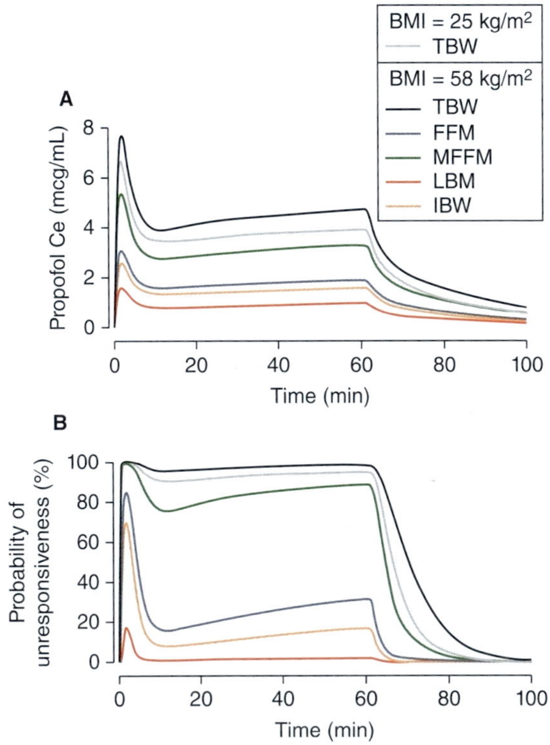

FIGURE 20–2 **(A)** Simulation of propofol effect-site concentrations (Ce) that result from a bolus (2 mg/kg) and 1-hour infusion (150 mcg/kg/min) for a 53-year-old 155-cm (5′1″) female. **(B)** Simulation of probability of unresponsiveness after a 2 mg/kg bolus and 1 hour infusion (150 mcg/kg/min) for a 53-year-old 155-cm (5′1″) female. Simulations include 2 dosing weights: (1) total body weight (TBW) of 60 kg with a body mass index (BMI) of 25 kg/m² and (2) 140 kg with a BMI of 58 kg/m². Simulations also include several weight scalars for the 140-kg weight: FFM, fat-free mass; MFFM, modified fat-free mass; LBM, lean body mass; and IBW, ideal body weight. Estimates of propofol Ce levels were made using pharmacokinetic parameters published by Cortinez et al.[17] Predictions of loss of responsiveness were made using the pharmacodynamic model published by Kern et al.[23]

age, but it did not specifically include obese patients. It uses LBM as described above and so may have limited application in morbidly obese patients.[27] By way of comparison, researchers have explored dosing requirements needed for induction of anesthesia using either the Marsh or the Schnider model on morbidly obese patients. They concluded that either model works when dosing to TBW but that the target concentrations should be different for each model; they reported a target effect-site concentration to achieve a 95% probability of effect of 4.2 and 5.5 mcg/mL for the Marsh and Schnider models, respectively.[28]

Cortinez et al developed a model based on measured propofol concentrations in obese patients specifically designed to administer propofol TCI.[17] The authors took advantage of an international data repository called "Open TCI" (http://www.opentci.org) to build a model using propofol concentrations from a wide range of body weights. They published model parameters that scaled normal size to obese individuals using an empirically derived formula. The formula uses TBW and accounts for differences in distribution volumes and clearances in obese patients; TBW is divided by a standard patient size (70 kg) and raised to the power of 1 for distribution volumes and by the power of 0.75 for clearances.

A simulation of 90-minute propofol target controlled infusion using each of these models[17,24,25] is presented in Figure 20–3 for a 155-cm, 140-kg female.

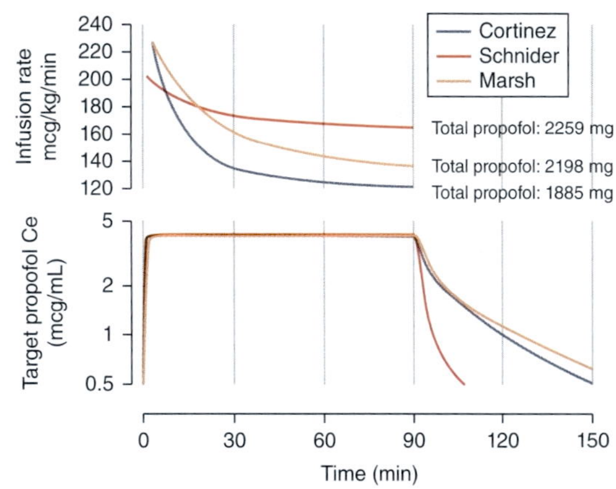

FIGURE 20–3 Simulations of a 90-minute propofol target controlled infusion set to achieve and maintain a target effect-site concentration (Ce) of 4 mcg/mL using 3 different pharmacokinetic models for a 53-year-old 140-kg, 155-cm (5′1″) female, with a body mass index of 58 kg/m². The pharmacokinetic models include parameters published by Marsh et al,[24], Schnider et al,[25] and Cortinez et al.[17] The top panel presents the propofol infusion rates for each model. Not shown are the initial bolus doses, which include 1000 mg, 1200 mg, and 1300 mg for the Cortinez, Schnider, and Marsh models, respectively. The bottom panel presents the propofol effect-site concentrations as predicted by each model.

Of note is the difference in the total amount of propofol delivered using each model to maintain a plasma propofol concentration at 4 mcg/mL. Driving the infusion with the Cortinez model used less propofol than the others. The difference is substantial—up to 374 mg less propofol over 90 minutes—indicating that model choice can impact clinical performance of TCIs. By comparison, a 2-mg/kg bolus followed by a 150-mcg/kg/min infusion dosed to TBW for 90 minutes requires 2170 mg, yielding predicted effect-site concentrations just above 4 mcg/mL, a total dose similar to what is delivered when using the Marsh model to drive the TCI. Each model also makes different predictions about how quickly propofol plasma concentrations and drug effect (ie, loss of responsiveness) will dissipate. Once the infusion is stopped, the Schnider model predicts a rapid decline in propofol concentrations compared to the others.

In summary, the Cortinez model may be best suited for TCI in this patient group. It was derived from data collected in obese patients and delivers less propofol by weight compared to other models. This model, however, is not yet available in many commercial TCI pumps, leaving clinicians to use techniques described above with the Marsh or Schnider models. It is important to remember that differences between models may be overshadowed by substantial interindividual variability and using any one of the three models may yield similar clinical results, especially when titrated to effect with processed EEG monitoring.

Other Sedatives Unlike propofol, the behavior of many other sedatives (ie, etomidate, ketamine, barbiturates, and midazolam) is not as well characterized in obese people. One study, however, has compared midazolam pharmacokinetics in obese and normal size volunteers with interesting results.[29] They found the volume of distribution, even when normalized to weight (ie, L/kg) was larger in obese patients. These results suggest that adipose tissue may take up more midazolam than other lean tissues. Hence, the volume of distribution of midazolam has a linear relationship with TBW; as patient size increases, so does the volume of distribution. They also found that the rate of drug elimination is the same in obese and lean volunteers. These results suggest that regardless of the amount of midazolam administered, the hepatic biotransformation of midazolam is fixed, meaning that the larger volume of drug distribution in the obese will require more time for elimination. However, despite the larger volume of distribution, peak plasma drug concentrations of midazolam and time to peak concentration were the same in obese and lean volunteers given the same dose.

Although these findings have not been clinically validated in obese patients, they may have important dosing considerations. Given that the volume of distribution was larger in the obese population, the authors concluded that bolus doses should be scaled to TBW (ie, 0.03 mg/kg). If other dosing scalars are used (ie, IBW), the authors postulated that midazolam may not achieve its desired effect (ie, anxiolysis or sedation). By contrast, since midazolam clearance is proportional to IBW, continuous infusion rates should use IBW for dosing purposes.[29]

Opioids

It is well known that opioids cause worrisome respiratory depression and diminished ventilatory response to elevated $PaCO_2$ levels in obese patients.[30] With the high incidence of obstructive sleep apnea in this population, identifying the appropriate opioid dose is particularly relevant.[31] Unfortunately, with the exception of remifentanil, minimal work has described the kinetic and dynamic behavior of opioids in obese individuals.

Remifentanil

Dosing Scalars The kinetic profile of remifentanil is not substantially altered by body habitus, due to the metabolism of remifentanil by plasma esterases. The volume of distribution and clearance are similar in lean and obese patients. To illustrate these features, consider the simulations presented in Figure 20–4. Similar to the simulations with propofol above, these simulations presents the predicted remifentanil effect-site concentrations from a bolus (1 mcg/kg) and 1-hour infusion (0.15 mcg/kg/min) in two 155-cm (5′1″) females, one obese (140 kg), and one lean (60 kg). Again, for the obese individual, dosing is scaled by weights presented in Table 20–3.

If dosed according to TBW, what leads to reasonable plasma concentrations in a lean individual is excessive in an obese individual. For example, the

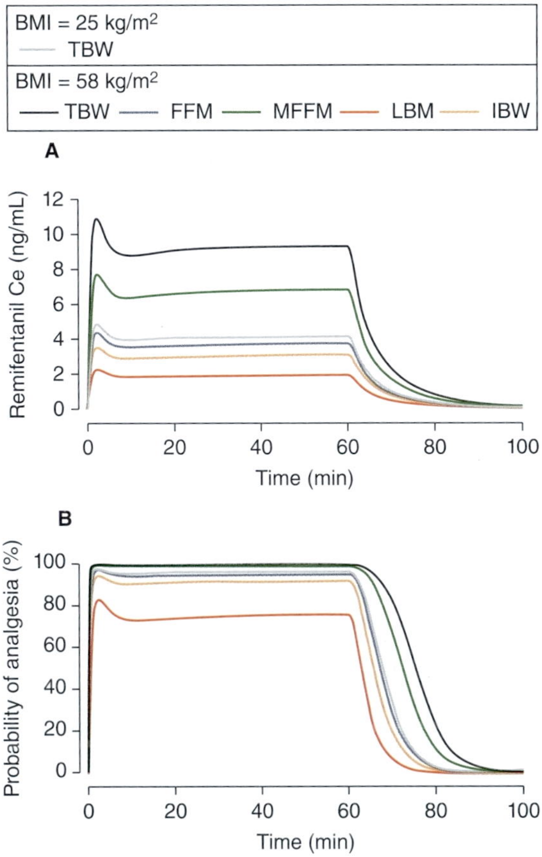

FIGURE 20–4 **(A)** Simulation of remifentanil effect-site concentrations (Ce) that result from a bolus (1 mcg/kg) and 1-hour infusion (0.15 mcg/kg/min) for a 53-year-old 155-cm (5′1″) female. **(B)** Simulation of the probability of analgesia after a bolus (1 mcg/kg) and 1-hour infusion (0.15 mcg/kg/min) for a 155-cm (5′1″) female. Simulations include 2 dosing weights: total body weight (TBW) of (1) 60 kg with a body mass index (BMI) of 25 kg/m^2 and (2) 140 kg with a BMI of 58 kg/m^2. Simulations also include several weight scalars for the 140-kg female: FFM, fat-free mass; MFFM, = modified fat-free mass; LBM, lean body mass; and IBW, ideal body weight. Estimates of remifentanil Ce level were made using pharmacokinetic parameters published by Minto et al.[32] Predictions of analgesia were made using a pharmacodynamic model published by Johnson.[33] Analgesia was defined as loss of response to 30 pounds per square inch of pressure on the anterior tibia in healthy volunteers. Of note, predicted remifentanil Ce levels when dosed using pharmacokinetic mass were similar to those when dosed using MFFM.

peak concentrations are 5 and 11 ng/mL for the lean and obese individual (gray and black lines, respectively). Analgesic effect is also prolonged in the obese individual. Once the infusion has ended, the time required to reach less than a 5% probability of analgesic effect is 18 and 27 minutes for the lean and obese individual, respectively.

To avoid this overdosing problem, Egan et al. advocate IBW or LBM as a dosing scalar for remifentanil.[34] As with propofol, LBM has limited application in morbidly obese patients (see Figure 20–1) as with excessive body weights, calculated LBM becomes smaller as TBW increases. As illustrated in Figure 20–4, dosing remifentanil to LBM leads to plasma concentrations yielding a lower probability (75%–80%) of effect rather than the greater than 95% probability of effect seen when the other dosing scalars are used.

Computer simulations suggest that dosing remifentanil on FFM may overcome this limitation. Dosing remifentanil to FFM (blue line) leads to concentrations and effect that are similar to those achieved by dosing the lean individual to TBW. With remifentanil, dosing to MFFM (green line), unlike propofol, actually leads to higher plasma concentrations when compared to levels achieved when doing to TBW in a lean individual. This may lead to pronounce and prolonged effect.

Kinetic Models for Target-Controlled Infusions Only one pharmacokinetic model, developed by Minto et al, is available to drive a target-controlled infusion (TCI). The Minto model was built from data collected in adults over a range of weights, heights, and age but did not specifically target obese patients. Like the Schnider model for propofol, many of the model parameters are scaled to LBM; hence, the model may have limited application in morbidly obese patients. The Minto model is currently the only kinetic model commercially available for remifentanil TCIs.

To get around this limitation, La Colla et al introduced a weight-adjusted height to use when programming a TCI pump for delivery of remifentanil to morbidly obese.[35] The aim of the adjusted height is to counter the inaccurate influence of LBM on model predictions of plasma remifentanil concentrations used to drive the infusion pump. This fictitious weight adjusted height (h_f) uses metrics of body habitus (actual height and weight) to estimate a new height (ie, taller) that will cause the Minto model to provide more remifentanil via TCI in a morbidly obese patient (Equations 20–1 and 20–2). For example, with a 155-cm, 140-kg 53-year-old female, the adjusted fictitious height is 176 cm.

$$h_{fmen} = \text{sqrt}[(128 * TBW * (6680 + 216 * BMI)) / (-1922 + (1.1 * 216 * BMI))] \quad \text{Eq. 20–1}$$

$$h_{fwomen} = \text{sqrt}[(148 * TBW * (8780 + 244 * BMI)) / (124.6 + (1.07 * 1.07 * BMI))] \quad \text{Eq. 20–2}$$

Other investigators have developed a new remifentanil kinetic model for obese patients. In collaboration with other researchers, Egan and Obara used measured remifentanil concentrations from several different studies, many of which included obese and morbidly obese individuals, to create a new model.[36]

A simulation of 90-minute propofol target controlled infusion using each of these models[32,35,36] is presented in Figure 20–5. Of note is the difference in the total amount of remifentanil delivered using each model to maintain a plasma propofol concentration at 3 ng/mL. Driving the infusion with the Obara model used more remifentanil than the others (up to 250 mcg more). Similar to propofol, it appears that model choice can impact clinical performance of remifentanil target controlled infusions. Each model also makes different predictions about how quickly remifentanil plasma concentrations and drug effect (ie, analgesia) will dissipate. Once the infusion is stopped, all models predict a rapid decline in remifentanil concentrations.

In summary, both available models (Minto or the La Colla modified Minto model) are appropriate for TCI in this patient group. The Obara model shows promise in this patient group, but it warrants further investigation before it is suitable for use in remifentanil TCI.

Fentanyl

The pharmacokinetics and pharmacodynamics of fentanyl are well characterized[37,38] but have not been specifically described in the obese population. As with intravenous anesthetics, using TBW for bolus dosing or weight-based continuous infusions may lead to high drug concentrations and prolonged

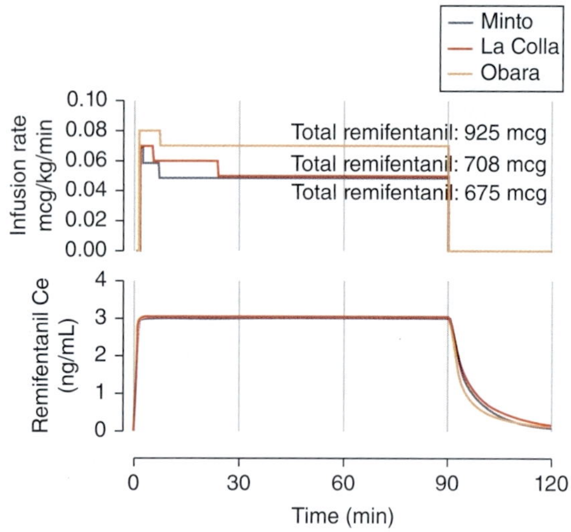

FIGURE 20–5 Simulations of a 90-minute remifentanil target-controlled infusion set to achieve and maintain a target effect-site concentration (Ce) of 3 ng/mL using 3 different pharmacokinetic models for a 53-year-old, 140-kg, 155-cm (5′1″) female, with a body mass index of 58 kg/m^2. The pharmacokinetic models include parameters published by Minto et al,[32] La Colla et al,[35], and Egan and Obara.[36] The top panel presents the remifentanil infusion rates for each model. Not shown are the initial bolus doses, which are 48 mcg, 54 mcg, and 49 mcg for the Minto, La Colla, and Obara models, respectively. The bottom panel presents the remifentanil effect site concentrations as predicted by each model.

drug effect. Researchers have used previously published fentanyl concentrations[14,15] in lean (BMI < 30 kg/m^2) and obese (BMI > 30 kg/m^2) patients to identify a unique weight scalar for use when dosing fentanyl. They found that existing kinetic models overestimate plasma concentrations of fentanyl as TBW increases, suggesting that fentanyl's volume of distribution does not linearly increase with TBW. They proposed dosing fentanyl to "pharmacokinetic (PK) mass" (see Figure 20–1). Like the other scaled weights, PK mass is greater than IBW but less than TBW and when used to predict fentanyl plasma concentrations was better than TBW. Although PK mass provided better predicted plasma concentrations than TBW in previously published data, it does not account for patient height. This may make it difficult to use in patients of the same weight who are different heights (ie, weight of 100 kg but heights of 155 cm and 190 cm). It is likely that the kinetic profile in each of these patients would be different, yet the PK mass would be equivalent in both.

Other Opioids

Minimal dosing information in obese patients is available for other opioids such as morphine, meperidine, methadone, and alfentanil. Some literature does explore the behavior of sufentanil in obese patients. Researchers have found that sufentanil's volume of distribution increased linearly with TBW[39] and suggest that this may be a function of the high lipid solubility. They also found that the clearance was similar between the obese and lean patients but did report a prolonged elimination rate in the obese. Based on these findings, they suggest that loading doses (ie, a bolus) should use TBW but that maintenance doses are "prudently reduced." No suggested scaled weight is available for sufentanil. With regard to TCI, using a previously published mode of sufentanil kinetics by Gepts et al,[40] Slepchenko et al found model estimates of sufentanil concentrations accurately predicted measured concentrations in morbidly obese patients.[41] Of note, the kinetic model they used was built from observations in patients with a weight range of 47 to 94 kg. The authors concluded that the Gepts model is suitable for sufentanil TCI in the obese.

Neuromuscular Blocking Agents

Succinylcholine

Obese patients have numerous comorbidities, such as a large neck circumference, presence of sleep apnea with a potential risk for difficult mask ventilation or tracheal intubation, and a large abdomen with an increased risk of aspiration.[42-44] A rapid-sequence induction may help ameliorate the risk of intubation in patients with these conditions. Succinylcholine has kinetic features that make it attractive to use in this patient group.

As with other intravenous anesthetics, researchers have explored how to dose neuromuscular agents in obese patients with varied results. Although a succinylcholine dose of 1 mg/kg results in excellent intubating conditions in almost all patients, 95% of average weight patients have satisfactory intubating conditions with only 0.6 mg/kg of succinylcholine.[45] Lemmens and Brodsky evaluated intubating conditions in obese patients (BMI > 40 kg/m^2) after doses of succinylcholine of 1 mg/kg based on IBW, LBW, and TBW. Excellent intubation conditions were defined as no response to laryngoscopy and tracheal intubation, open vocal cords, and a relaxed jaw. Poor conditions were defined as a response to laryngoscopy and tracheal intubation (limb movement), closed vocal cords, and poor jaw relaxation. The dose based on TBW resulted in 87% with "excellent" and 0% having "poor" intubating conditions. In contrast, the group dosed on IBW (the smallest dose) resulted in only 27% with "excellent" and 30% "poor" conditions.

A potential drawback to increasing the dose of succinylcholine is that it increases the duration of action; if difficulty with mask ventilation or intubation is encountered, a prolonged return to spontaneous ventilation may have grave consequences. Duration of action is determined by the amount of pseudocholinesterase activity and the volume of extracellular fluid, both of which are increased in obesity.[46] In obese adults, effective preoxygenation/denitrogenation provides on average less than 3 to 4 minutes of apneic oxygenation.[47] Unfortunately, the duration of action of even 1 mg/kg of succinylcholine dosed to IBW will prevent the return of spontaneous ventilation beyond 3 minutes.[45] When dosed by IBW, there is 10% recovery of neuromuscular function at 4 minutes and 90% recovery at 7 minutes without assurance of optimal intubating conditions. Given this conundrum, clinicians may consider dosing succinylcholine at 1 mg/kg of TBW to ensure ideal intubating conditions or choose an alternative approach to the airway if deemed to difficult to secure within 3 to 4 minutes.

To illustrate the importance of preoxygenation when using succinylcholine in an obese patient, consider the simulation presented in Figure 20–6 (see also Table 20–4). The figure presents the predicted effect-site concentrations and drug effects (loss of train-of-four and loss of responsiveness) in a 30-year, 170-cm, 124-kg male (BMI = 43 kg/m^2). It also presents the predicted lung oxygen uptake and dissipation and time course of oxygen saturation during preoxygenation and following the onset of apnea.

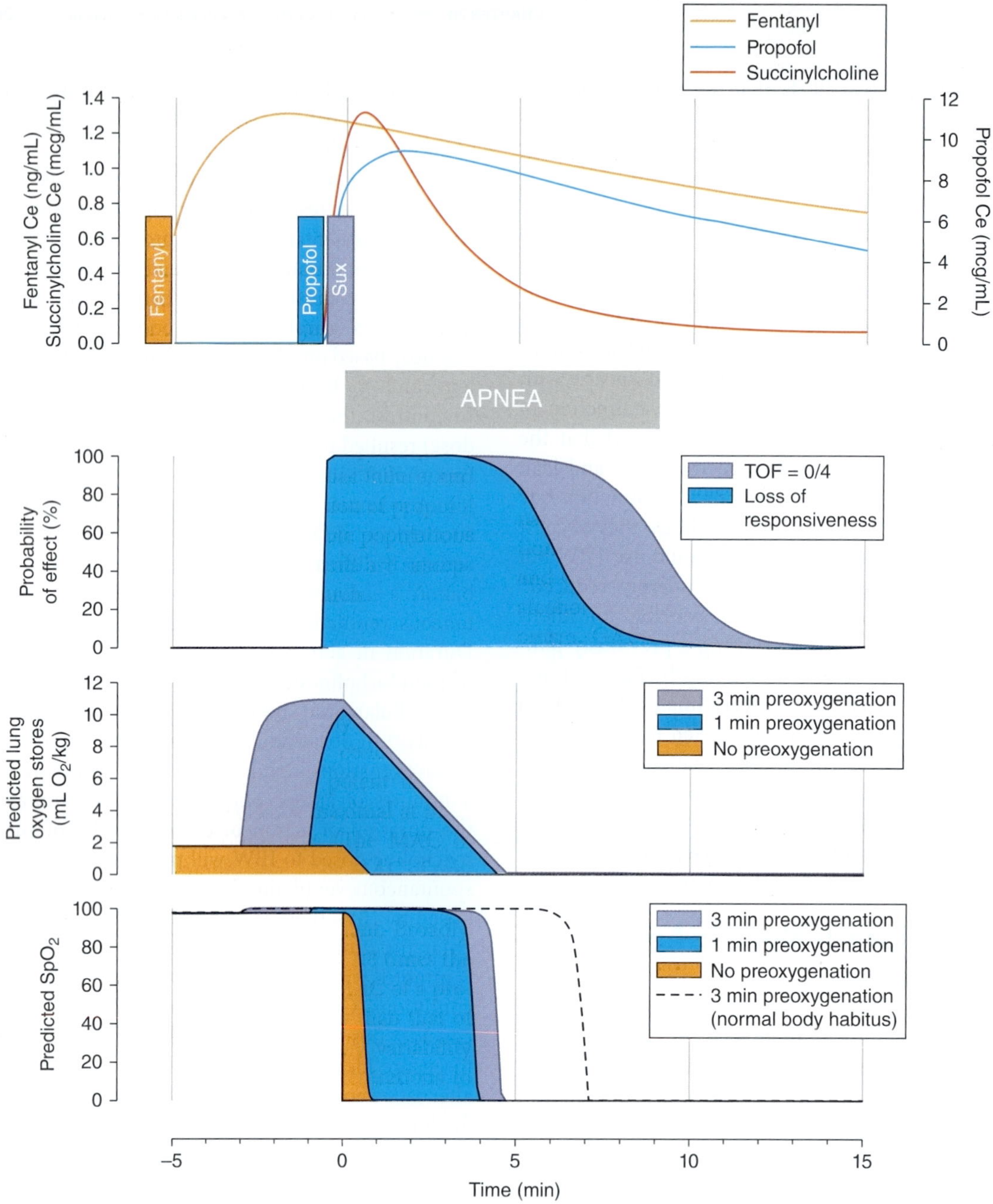

FIGURE 20–6 Simulation of effect-site concentrations (Ce) resulting from a fentanyl bolus (140 mcg) followed 5 minutes later by propofol (2 mg/kg) and succinylcholine (Sux; 1 mg/kg) boluses are presented in the top plot. Estimates of fentanyl, propofol, and succinylcholine Ce levels were made using published pharmacokinetic parameters.[17,38,48] Corresponding drug effects, probability of loss of responsiveness, and loss of train-of-four (TOF) are presented in the upper middle plot. The gray bar indicates the period of time where the probability of loss of TOF is greater than 50% (approximately 9 minutes). Predictions of drug effect were made based on published pharmacodynamic models.[23,48] Predicted lung oxygen stores following 0, 1, and 3 minutes of preoxygenation, assuming a FiO_2 of 0.8 and normal respiratory function, are presented in the lower middle plot. Predicted oxygen saturation (SpO_2) levels for the associated lung oxygen stores are presented in the bottom plot. For comparison, predicted SpO_2 for a normal body habitus individual preoxygenated for 3 minutes is also presented in the bottom plot. Assumption and limitations of these simulations are presented in Table 20–4.

TABLE 20–4 Assumptions and limitations of predicting oxygen saturation during apnea.

Assumptions
Preoxygenation with a well-sealed face mask on an anesthesia machine yields an inspired oxygen level (FiO_2) of 0.8.
Spontaneous respiratory rate is 10 breaths/min.
For each breath, the tidal volume is 7 mL/kg, anatomic dead space is 2.2 mL/kg, and alveolar tidal volume is 4.8 mL/kg.
Lung volumes are weight normalized to ideal body weight.
Cardiac output, hemoglobin concentration, arterial pH, arterial carbon dioxide, and temperature are within normal limits.
Exponential oxygen wash-in[49]
Estimates of oxygen consumption assume the basal metabolic rate,[50] resting energy expenditure, and respiratory quotient are all within normal limits.[51]
The Harris–Benedict formula estimates of basal metabolic are reasonable in morbidly obese individuals.[52]
The functional residual capacity in obese individuals is reduced.[53]
Increased alveolar–arterial oxygen gradient[54]
Estimates of SpO_2 can be made from arterial oxygen tension levels.[55]
Limitations
Ventilatory response to elevated arterial carbon dioxide levels may be decreased in obese individuals.
Values for cardiac output and arterial carbon dioxide levels are likely to be abnormal in obese individuals.

Two key points are visualized in this simulation. First, the duration of action (ie, loss of train-of-four) for this dose of succinylcholine is 9 minutes, and this is longer than both the duration of loss of responsiveness from propofol combined with fentanyl and the duration of oxygen saturation remaining above 90% even when preoxygenated for 3 minutes. For comparison, the estimated duration of oxygen saturation for a normal body habitus individual preoxygenated for 3 minutes is also presented. It remains above 90% for nearly as long as the duration of the effect from succinylcholine. Second, with decreased lung volumes (assumed in this simulation), the amount of oxygen that can be stored in the lungs is limited. Preoxygenation for longer than 3 minutes may provide some improvement, but the reduced oxygen-storage capacity of the lung is nearly full after 3 minutes. In summary, for obese patients where securing the airway is anticipated to take longer than 3 minutes and effective mask ventilation is potentially difficult, caution should be used when administering succinylcholine at 1 mg/kg of TBW.

Rocuronium

Unlike succinylcholine, intubating conditions are not improved by dosing rocuronium to TBW over IBW and as expected, dosing to TBW prolongs neuromuscular blockade.[56,57] Researchers have also explored kinetic and drug effect differences of rocuronium between obese (BMI > 28 kg/m²) and normal body habitus patients and found no difference in onset, duration, and spontaneous recovery.[58] Accordingly, dosing rocuronium to IBW in obese patients appears adequate.

Vecuronium

As with rocuronium, dosing obese patients to TBW prolongs neuromuscular blockade when compared with normal-weight patients.[59,60] Researchers have found that %IBW and BMI correlate well to duration of action,[61] but data clarifying whether dosing to IBW or TBW improves intubating conditions are not available. Given the paucity of available data, dosing vecuronium to IBW appears to be reasonable.

Atracurium

Kirkegaard-Nielsen et al found that the duration of action of atracurium correlated well with TBW and BMI over a range of normal to obese weights.[62] The authors proposed a dosing scheme where the standard dose (0.5 mg/kg) of atracurium be decreased by 2.3 mg for every 10 kg TBW over 70 kg. For example, a patient with TBW of 110 kg would be dosed as (0.5 mg/kg * 110 kg) – (2.3 mg * 40/10) = 45.8 mg. This proposed dosing scheme has not been clinically validated.

Cisatracurium

Prior work suggests that no adjustments are required in obese patients when dosing cisatracurium.[63]

Schmith et al explored whether age, weight, or gender influenced the kinetic and dynamic behavior of cisatracurium.[64] They found small changes in selected kinetic parameters (such as compartmental clearance and k_{e0}), but the clinical relevance of these were negligible. Based on these results, they concluded that no dose adjustment is needed in obesity. Similarly, Leykin and colleagues noted good to excellent intubating conditions in obese patients dosed on TBW or on IBW; although onset was shorter and the duration of effect was longer when dosed to TBW.[65] Hence, dosing to TBW may be more advantageous if onset time is more important than a prolonged duration, and dosing on IBW may be more appropriate if rapid recovery is more important than rapid onset.

A summary of the dosing weight scalars for each of the intravenous agents discussed is presented in Table 20–5.

TABLE 20–5 Summary of dosing scalars and pharmacokinetic models to drive target controlled infusions in obese individuals for selected intravenous anesthetic agents.

Agent	Dosing Scalar	Kinetic Model
Sedative–hypnotics		
Propofol bolus[21]	LBM, consider FFM for BMI > 40 kg/m²	
Propofol infusion[16,17,26]	TBW or MFFM	
Propofol TCI[24,25]		Marsh or Schnider; titrate with processed EEG.[a]
Midazolam[29]	TBW	
Etomidate[10]	LBM	
Opioids		
Remifentanil infusion[35]	IBW or FFM; LBW may underdose in the morbidly obese	
Remifentanil TCI[35,36]		Minto or La Colla (modified Minto) model[b]
Fentanyl[14,15]	PK mass	
Sufentanil bolus[39]	TBW	
Sufentanil infusion	Not available	
Sufentanil TCI[41]		Gepts
Neuromuscular blockers		
Succinylcholine[45]	TBW	
Rocuronium[56,57]	IBW	
Vecuronium[58,59]	IBW	
Atracurium[62,63]	Unique weight scalar (see text)	
Cisatracurium[65]	TBW	

[a]For propofol TCI, consider the Cortinez model if available.
[b]May consider Obara model.
EEG, electroencephalogram; FFM, fat-free mass; IBW, ideal body weight; LBM, lean body mass; MFFM, modified fat-free mass; PK, pharmacokinetic; TBW, total body weight; TCI, target-controlled infusion.

Inhalational Anesthetics

Drug Accumulation in the Obese Versus Nonobese

Anesthetic uptake, or the rate of increase of volatile anesthetic in the alveoli, is a function of tissue blood flow, and blood–gas and fat–blood partition coefficients (anesthetic solubility). A widely held perception of potent inhaled agents is that obese patients accumulate more agent that normal body habitus patients and require more time to emerge from anesthesia. Blood flow per kg of adipose tissue, however, *decreases* with increasing obesity,[66] and the time required to fill adipose tissue with inhaled agent is quite long (up to days).[67,68] For example, the time constant, or time to reach 63% of equilibrium within adipose tissue, of isoflurane and desflurane, are more than 35 and 22 hours, respectively. Given the decreased fat perfusion and prolonged time constants, the scientific foundation behind the perception of prolonged emergence in obese patients is not well defined and in fact may not be true.[69]

Isoflurane

Pharmacologists have explored the influence of body habitus on uptake and emergence for selected potent inhaled anesthetics. Lemmens et al administered a general anesthetic technique consisting of

0.6 minimum alveolar concentration (MAC) isoflurane, 50% nitrous oxide, and fentanyl as needed to obese (BMI > 30 kg/m^2) and nonobese patients for surgical procedures lasting 2.5 to 4 hours. They observed small differences in uptake but no difference in time to response to verbal command once the anesthetic was discontinued (mean of 7 minutes in both obese and nonobese patients). They suggested that the minor differences in uptake could be due to the increase in LBW seen in obesity or by intertissue diffusion to fat from adjacent well-perfused tissue.[70]

Desflurane

Using the same technique as with isoflurane, Lemmens et al investigated the behavior of desflurane in obese and nonobese patients. The researchers found that for general anesthetics lasting 2 to 4 hours at less than 1 MAC desflurane, obese and nonobese patients respond to command equally rapidly—about 4 minutes after discontinuing the anesthetic.[70,71] Emergence from anesthesia was shorter with desflurane than isoflurane regardless of body habitus. Similar results were reported by La Colla et al, where the kinetic and recovery profiles of desflurane are similar in obese and nonobese patients.[71]

Sevoflurane

Similar to isoflurane and desflurane, no evidence supports the hypothesis that obesity prolongs induction or emergence with sevoflurane. Cortinez et al studied the onset and offset of sevoflurane in obese and normal-weight patients and found no difference in sevoflurane pharmacokinetics.[69] Researchers have described short-term kinetic differences, but they are of minimal clinical relevance. For example, Casati et al found that sevoflurane wash-out kinetics are slightly slower in obese patients compared with nonobese patients for the first 3 minutes after discontinuation, but then the difference dissipates. They conclude that emergence time is minimally affected if at all, since at 5 minutes after discontinuing the sevoflurane, no differences were observed between obese and nonobese patients.[72]

Comparisons Between Potent Inhaled Agents

As with normal body habitus individuals, pharmacologic differences between common potent inhaled agents persist in obese patients. Anesthetic uptake and washout increases from desflurane to sevoflurane to isoflurane.[73] Researchers have found that decreasing the dose of sevoflurane or desflurane just prior to the end of surgery eliminated the emergence time difference between sevoflurane and desflurane in the obese (Table 20-6); however, if no titration occurs, emergence times are longer with sevoflurane than desflurane.[74]

For example, Strum et al found that in obese patients, emergence from desflurane was accomplished in less time than sevoflurane after anesthetic times of greater than 3 hours at 1 MAC.[74] The investigators also reported that obese patients anesthetized with desflurane arrived in the recovery room with higher modified Aldrete scores (a score used to assess how well patients are recovering from anesthesia) and greater oxyhemoglobin saturations than those anesthetized with sevoflurane. Similarly, De Baerdemaeker et al investigating an "inhalational bolus" technique in obese patients, noted more rapid recovery from desflurane than from sevoflurane. It is important to point out that in both of these studies, the anesthetic technique did not involve tapering of the anesthetic prior to the end of surgery.[75]

By contrast, Arain et al found that obese patients emerged equally rapidly after more than 2 hours of sevoflurane or desflurane, when inhaled anesthetic was titrated to Bispectral Index Scale of 45 to 50, and a Bispectral Index Scale of 60 was targeted during the last 15 minutes of surgery.[76] Similarly, Vallejo et al observed no difference in time to eye opening or extubation in obese patients given sevoflurane or desflurane at 1 MAC, decreased to 0.5 MAC during surgical closure.[77]

Desflurane Versus Total Intravenous Anesthesia

One concern with a propofol-based total intravenous anesthesia in obese patients is that it may decrease upper airway tone and lead to more airway obstruction than with inhaled agents. Researchers explored the effects of propofol and desflurane on oximetry and spirometry on obese patients (BMI = 25–35 kg/m^2) undergoing elective 2-hour procedures. They found forced expired volume in 1 second was 1.6 versus 2.1 L 30 minutes after surgery and pulse oximetry was 91% versus 92% immediately following surgery for

TABLE 20–6 Summary of literature comparing emergence times in obese patients receiving sevoflurane or desflurane.

Author	De Baerdemaeker et al[75]	Strum et al[74]	Arain et al[76]	Vallejo et al[77]
Time to eye opening (min)				
Desflurane	5	10	5	5
Sevoflurane	7[a]	18[a]	5	6
Time to extubation (min)				
Desflurane	8	14	7	6
Sevoflurane	9[a]	25[a]	6	8
Average BMI				
Desflurane	41	53	38	47
Sevoflurane	41	54	38	48
Average duration of anesthetic (min)				
Desflurane	112	275	216	150
Sevoflurane	112	258	211	151
Anesthetic technique	Titrate to BIS of 45–55	Titrate to 1 MAC	Titrate to BIS of 45–50	Titrate to 1 MAC
Taper technique	None	None	BIS of 60 during last 15 min	Taper to 0.5 MAC during skin closure

[a]Indicates a *P* value < 0.05 for comparisons between desflurane and sevoflurane.
BMI, body mass index; BIS, Bispectral Index Scale; MAC, minimum alveolar concentration; min, minutes—times are reported to the nearest minute.

the propofol and desflurane groups. The small differences in SpO_2 persisted for up to 2 hours after surgery and most of the spirometry effects persisted up to 24 hours after surgery.[78] These small changes may impact drug choice when managing obese patients in an ambulatory setting.

CASE DISCUSSION

Ulnar Nerve Transposition in a Morbidly Obese Patient

A 40-year-old, 175-cm, 135-kg male (BMI = 44 kg/m^2) presents for a left ulnar nerve transposition and left carpal tunnel release. Anticipated operating time is 45 minutes. The surgeon would prefer no neuromuscular blockade. Past medical history is significant for hypertension and type 2 diabetes. Preoperative blood glucose level is 165 mg/dL. Preoperative evaluation suggests obstructive sleep apnea. Past anesthetic history is significant for severe postoperative nausea and vomiting. The patient is anxious, refuses regional anesthesia, and has an intravenous catheter in place. Airway and physical examination are unremarkable. The plan is a general total intravenous anesthetic with endotracheal intubation.

Premedication

Consider an anxiolytic; use should be deliberate, rather than routine. Prolonged midazolam effect may affect discharge readiness. Consider antacid as needed. Consider preoperative oral administration of pregabalin, celecoxib, and/or tramadol with a sip of water to decrease perioperative opioid requirements.

Induction

Following more than 3 minutes of preoxygenation, administer fentanyl 2 mcg/kg using PK mass. Based on Figure 20–1, the PK mass for this individual is 98 kg; the total fentanyl dose is 190 mcg. Administer fentanyl 3 to 5 minutes prior to propofol so it reaches peak effect-site concentrations at laryngoscopy. Administer propofol 2 mg/kg using FFM. Based on Figure 20–1, the FFM is 77 kg; the total propofol dose is 154 mg. FFM was selected instead of LBM since the BMI is more than 40 kg/m^2. Administer succinylcholine 1 mg/kg using TBW (135 mg).

Maintenance

The total intravenous anesthetic will include propofol and remifentanil infusions and intermittent fentanyl boluses. The propofol infusion (100 mcg/kg/min) is dosed to TBW. The remifentanil infusion (0.2 mcg/kg/min) is dosed to FFM (as above, 77 kg). Fentanyl is dosed at 1 to 2 mcg/kg using PK mass (98 kg). Consider adjuncts such as intravenous paracetamol, ketorolac, ketamine, and local anesthetic infiltration of surgical wound to improve analgesia without promoting airway obstruction.[79-81] Consider administering dexamethasone and ondansetron.

Emergence

Extubation of a morbidly obese person should be planned as carefully as intubation. Preparation of an induction drug, muscle relaxant, and airway management devices allows a prompt response should respiratory distress occur after extubation. Obese patients are poor candidates for deep extubation, as the risk of upper airway obstruction is high.[82] Consider extubating the obese patient in a seated or semirecumbent position on the operating room table, with standard American Society of Anesthesiologists (ASA) monitors in place. This position will attenuate upper airway obstruction, while leaving the patient on the operating table fully monitored will facilitate mask ventilation or reintubation if necessary.

Simulation

A summary of this technique, a total intravenous anesthetic with propofol, fentanyl, remifentanil, and succinylcholine, is presented in Figure 20–7. It simulates premedication with fentanyl 2 mcg/kg scaled to PK mass, propofol 2 mg/kg scaled to FFM, succinylcholine 1 mg/kg scaled to TBW, remifentanil infusion 0.2 mcg/kg/min scaled to FFM, and propofol infusion 100 mcg/kg/min scaled to TBW. Fentanyl was administered 5 minutes prior to induction. The propofol and remifentanil infusions were run for 48 minutes.

Several points merit discussion. First, the propofol infusion rate may seem inadequate. Administration of 100 mcg/kg/min, by itself, does not achieve concentrations that will provide reliable loss of responsiveness. Shortly after induction, if only administering propofol, the probability of unresponsiveness drops below 70% and remains uncomfortably low for the rest of the procedure (dashed blue line in upper middle plot). The opioid and propofol, however, synergistically interact to provide a cumulative effect; the probability of no response is above 95% throughout the procedure (solid blue line). As dosed, once the infusions are terminated, 9 and 25 minutes are required to reach a 50% and 5% probability of unresponsiveness, a time window when the patient is likely to emerge. Clinicians may find this too long and choose to reduce the propofol infusion rate or administer less or no fentanyl prior to the end of the anesthetic.

Second, this technique provides adequate analgesia for laryngoscopy and tracheal intubation, likely the most stimulating part of this procedure (bottom middle plot, pink line). For moderately painful stimuli, a fentanyl bolus 10 minutes prior to terminating the anesthetic provides a long window of analgesia following termination of the remifentanil and propofol infusions. The probability of no response to a moderately painful stimulus drops below 50% and 5% between 50 and 90 minutes, a time period where the patient may begin to complain of pain.

Third, this technique leads to a brief period where ventilatory depression (defined as a respiratory rate less than 4 breaths/min in an unstimulated state) may be of concern following termination

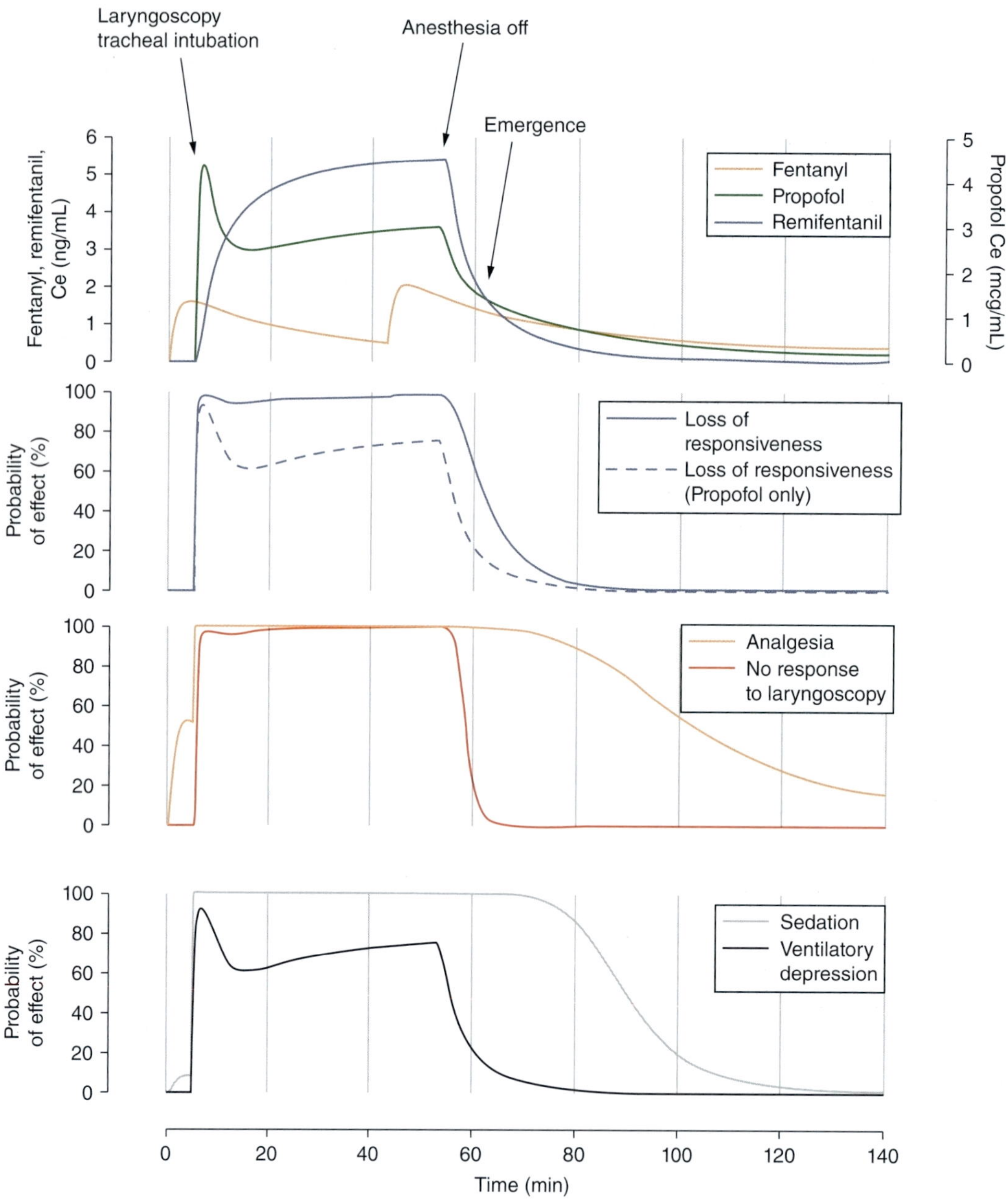

FIGURE 20–7 Simulation of effect-site concentrations (Ce) that result from two fentanyl boluses (2 mcg/kg) weight adjusted to pharmacokinetic mass (total fentanyl 190 mcg each), a propofol bolus (2 mg/kg) weight adjusted to fat-free mass, a remifentanil infusion (0.2 mcg/kg/min) weight adjusted to fat-free mass, and a propofol infusion (100 mcg/kg/min) weight adjusted to total body weight. Estimates of fentanyl, remifentanil, and propofol Ce levels were made using published pharmacokinetic parameters[17,32,38] and are presented in the top plot. Corresponding drug effects, probability of loss of responsiveness, loss of response to laryngoscopy, loss of response to a moderately painful stimulus, sedation, and ventilatory depression are presented in the remaining 3 plots. Predictions of drug effect were made based on published pharmacodynamic models.[23,24,83,84]

of the infusion rates (bottom plot, black line). If the patient is responsive, he would likely respond to a prompt to take a deep breath. The probability of ventilatory depression drops below 50% and 5% between 2 and 18 minutes. It is likely that the patient would be unresponsive and still intubated for most of this time; however, there may be a few minutes where worrisome ventilatory depression is present just after extubation if the man is left in an unstimulated state. These simulations emphasize the importance of vigilance in closely monitoring obese patients known to have upper airway obstruction and limited oxygen reserves where ventilatory depression can be especially harmful.

Fourth, this technique leads to prolonged postoperative sedation. The probability of sedation (defined as resting comfortably, but responsive when name is called) drops from 50% to 5% over 27 to 62 minutes. Prolonged sedation may be important to consider if the patient requires additional medications that have known sedating side effect.

Of particular interest in this simulation is how would a premedication dose of midazolam (ie, 2 mg) influence the duration of drug effects, especially during emergence. Although midazolam is quick acting, its effect dissipates slowly. It may continue to continue to exert some effect and influence time to emergence, duration of ventilatory depression and postoperative sedation. From a simulation standpoint, no models exist that characterize the interaction between (1) midazolam and propofol and (2) midazolam and opioids. Authors have suggested that the interactions are synergistic.[83–87]

In summary, this simulation presents a dosing approach to providing a total intravenous general anesthetic to a morbidly obese patient for a procedure associated with moderate postoperative pain. It presents predicted effects when using recommended dosing weight scalars found in the literature; they appear to provide an adequate anesthetic. As recommended by many authors, processed EEG monitoring is useful to guide dosing when using this technique in obese individuals. Finally, it is important to point out that this simulation and suggested technique have not been validated in obese patients; many assumptions and inherent inaccuracies could lead to varied clinical results.

REFERENCES

1. Abel ED, Litwin SE, Sweeney G. Cardiac remodeling in obesity. *Physiolog Rev*. 2008;88(2):389-419.
2. Kenchaiah S, Evans JC, Levy D, et al. Obesity and the risk of heart failure. *N Engl J Med*. 2002;347(5):305-313.
3. de Divitiis O, Fazio S, Petitto M, Maddalena G, Contaldo F, Mancini M. Obesity and cardiac function. *Circulation*. 1981;64(3):477-482.
4. Pelosi P, Croci M, Ravagnan I, Vicardi P, Gattinoni L. Total respiratory system, lung, and chest wall mechanics in sedated-paralyzed postoperative morbidly obese patients. *Chest*. 1996;109(1):144-151.
5. Biring MS, Lewis MI, Liu JT, Mohsenifar Z. Pulmonary physiologic changes of morbid obesity. *Am J Med Sci*. 1999;318(5):293-297.
6. Bird M. Acute pain management: a new area of liability for anesthesiologists. *ASA Newsletter*. 2007;71(8):7-9.
7. Cheymol G. Effects of obesity on pharmacokinetics implications for drug therapy. *Clin Pharmacokinet*. 2000;39(3):215-231.
8. Blouin RA, Warren GW. Pharmacokinetic considerations in obesity. *J Pharm Sci*. 1999;88(1):1-7.
9. Hanley MJ, Abernethy DR, Greenblatt DJ. Effect of obesity on the pharmacokinetics of drugs in humans. *Clin Pharmacokinet*. 2010;49(2):71-87.
10. Ingrande J, Lemmens HJ. Dose adjustment of anaesthetics in the morbidly obese. *Br J Anaesth*. 2010;105 (suppl 1):i16-i23.
11. Green B, McLeay SC. Anesthetizing the obese. *Anesth Analg*.. 2011;113(1):1-3.
12. Bouillon T, Shafer SL. Does size matter? *Anesthesiology*. 1998;89(3):557-560.
13. Janmahasatian S, Duffull SB, Ash S, Ward LC, Byrne NM, Green B. Quantification of lean bodyweight. *Clin Pharmacokinet*. 2005;44(10):1051-1065.
14. Shibutani K, Inchiosa MA Jr, Sawada K, Bairamian M. Accuracy of pharmacokinetic models for predicting plasma fentanyl concentrations in lean and obese surgical patients: derivation of dosing weight ("pharmacokinetic mass"). *Anesthesiology*. 2004;101(3):603-613.
15. Shibutani K, Inchiosa MA Jr, Sawada K, Bairamian M. Pharmacokinetic mass of fentanyl for postoperative analgesia in lean and obese patients. *Br J Anaesth*. 2005; 95(3):377-383.
16. Servin F, Farinotti R, Haberer JP, Desmonts JM. Propofol infusion for maintenance of anesthesia in morbidly obese patients receiving nitrous oxide. A clinical and pharmacokinetic study. *Anesthesiology*. 1993;78(4):657-665.
17. Cortinez LI, Anderson BJ, Penna A, et al. Influence of obesity on propofol pharmacokinetics: derivation of

a pharmacokinetic model. *Br J Anaesth*. 2010;105(4): 448-456.

18. Anderson BJ, Holford NHG. Mechanistic basis of using body size and maturation to predict clearance in humans. *Drug Metab Pharmacokinet*. 2009,24(1): 25–36.
19. Duffull SB, Dooley MJ, Green B, Poole SG, Kirkpatrick CMJ. A standard weight descriptor for dose adjustment in the obese patient. *Clin Pharmacokinet*. 2004;43(15): 1167-1178.
20. Upton RN, Ludbrook GL, Grant C, Martinez AM. Cardiac output is a determinant of the initial concentrations of propofol after short-infusion administration. *Anesth Analg*. 1999;89(3):545-552.
21. Ingrande J, Brodsky JB, Lemmens HJ. Lean body weight scalar for the anesthetic induction dose of propofol in morbidly obese subjects. *Anesth Analg*. 2011;113(1):57-62.
22. La Colla L, Albertin A, La Colla G, et al. No adjustment vs. adjustment formula as input weight for propofol target-controlled infusion in morbidly obese patients. *Eur J Anaesthesiol*. 2009;26(5):362-369.
23. Kern SE, Xie G, White JL, Egan TD. A response surface analysis of propofol-remifentanil pharmacodynamic interaction in volunteers. *Anesthesiology*. 2004;100(6): 1373-1381.
24. Marsh B, White M, Morton N, Kenny GN. Pharmacokinetic model driven infusion of propofol in children. *Br J Anaesth*. 1991;67(1):41-48.
25. Schnider TW, Minto CF, Gambus PL, et al. The influence of method of administration and covariates on the pharmacokinetics of propofol in adult volunteers. *Anesthesiology*. 1998;88(5):1170-1182.
26. Albertin A, Poli D, La Colla L, et al. Predictive performance of 'Servin's formula' during BIS-guided propofol-remifentanil target-controlled infusion in morbidly obese patients. *Br J Anaesth*. 2007;98(1):66-75.
27. Coetzee JF. Allometric or lean body mass scaling of propofol pharmacokinetics: towards simplifying parameter sets for target-controlled infusions. *Clin Pharmacokinet*. 2012;51(3):137-145.
28. Echevarría GC, Elgueta MF, Donoso MT, Bugedo DA, Cortínez LI, Muñoz HR. The effective effect-site propofol concentration for induction and intubation with two pharmacokinetic models in morbidly obese patients using total body weight. *Anesth Analg*. 2012; 115(4):823-829.
29. Greenblatt DJ, Abernethy DR, Locniskar A, Harmatz JS, Limjuco RA, Shader RI. Effect of age, gender, and obesity on midazolam kinetics. *Anesthesiology*. 1984;61(1):27-35.
30. Berkenbosch A, Teppema LJ, Olievier CN, Dahan A. Influences of morphine on the ventilatory response to isocapnic hypoxia. *Anesthesiology*. 1997;86(6): 1342-1349.
31. Benumof JL. Obesity, sleep apnea, the airway and anesthesia. *Curr Opin Anaesthesiol*. 2004;17(1):21-30.
32. Minto CF, Schnider TW, Egan TD, et al. Influence of age and gender on the pharmacokinetics and pharmacodynamics of remifentanil. I. Model development. *Anesthesiology*. 1997;86(1):10-23.
33. Johnson KB, Syroid ND, Gupta DK, et al. An evaluation of remifentanil propofol response surfaces for loss of responsiveness, loss of response to surrogates of painful stimuli and laryngoscopy in patients undergoing elective surgery. *Anesth Analg*. 2008;106(2):471-479.
34. Egan TD, Huizinga B, Gupta SK, et al. Remifentanil pharmacokinetics in obese versus lean patients. *Anesthesiology*. 1998;89(3):562-573.
35. La Colla L, Albertin A, La Colla G, et al. Predictive performance of the 'Minto' remifentanil pharmacokinetic parameter set in morbidly obese patients ensuing from a new method for calculating lean body mass. *Clin Pharmacokinet*. 2010;49(2):131-139.
36. Egan T, Obara S. Improving the performance of the "Minto" remifentanil pharmacokientic model by incorporating data from obese subjects. Abstract #17, presented at the annual meeting of the International Society of Anesthetic Pharmacology, 2011.
37. Scott JC, Stanski DR. Decreased fentanyl and alfentanil dose requirements with age. A simultaneous pharmacokinetic and pharmacodynamic evaluation. *J Pharmacol Exp Ther*. 1987;240(1):159-166.
38. Shafer SL, Varvel JR, Aziz N, Scott JC. Pharmacokinetics of fentanyl administered by computer-controlled infusion pump. *Anesthesiology*. 1990;73(6):1091-1102.
39. Schwartz AE, Matteo RS, Ornstein E, Young WL, Myers KJ. Pharmacokinetics of sufentanil in obese patients. *Anesth Analg*. 1991;73(6):790-793.
40. Gepts E, Shafer SL, Camu F, et al. Linearity of pharmacokinetics and model estimation of sufentanil. *Anesthesiology*. 1995;83(6):1194-1204.
41. Slepchenko G, Simon N, Goubaux B, Levron JC, Le Moing JP, Raucoules-Aime M. Performance of target-controlled sufentanil infusion in obese patients. *Anesthesiology*. 2003;98(1):65-73.
42. Brodsky JB, Lemmens HJ, Brock-Utne JG, Vierra M, Saidman LJ. Morbid obesity and tracheal intubation. *Anesth Analg*. 2002;94(3):732-736.
43. Ezri T, Gewurtz G, Sessler DI, et al. Prediction of difficult laryngoscopy in obese patients by ultrasound quantification of anterior neck soft tissue. *Anaesthesia*. 2003;58(11):1111-1114.

44. Ezri T, Medalion B, Weisenberg M, Szmuk P, Warters RD, Charuzi I. Increased body mass index per se is not a predictor of difficult laryngoscopy. *Can J Anaesth.* 2003;50(2):179-183.
45. Lemmens HJ, Brodsky JB. The dose of succinylcholine in morbid obesity. *Anesth Analg.* 2006;102(2):438-442.
46. Bentley JB, Borel JD, Vaughan RW, Gandolfi AJ. Weight, pseudocholinesterase activity, and succinylcholine requirement. *Anesthesiology.* 1982;57(1):48-49.
47. Jense HG, Dubin SA, Silverstein PI, O'Leary-Escolas U. Effect of obesity on safe duration of apnea in anesthetized humans. *Anesth Analg.* 1991;72(1):89-93.
48. Roy JJ, Donati F, Boismenu D, Varin F. Concentration-effect relation of succinylcholine chloride during propofol anesthesia. *Anesthesiology.* 2002;97:1082-1092.
49. Hardman JG, Wills JS, Aitkenhead AR. Factors determining the onset and course of hypoxemia during apnea: an investigation using physiological modelling. *Anesth Analg.* 2000;90(3):6190-6294.
50. Harris JA, Benedict FG. A biometric study of human basal metabolism. *Proc Natl Acad Sci.* 1918;4:370-373.
51. Weir JB. New methods for calculating metabolic rate with special reference to protein metabolism. *J Physiol.* 1949;109:1-9.
52. Müller B, Merk S, Bürgi U, Diem P. Calculating the basal metabolic rate and severe and morbid obesity. *Praxis (Bern 1994).* 2001;90(45):1955-1963.
53. Jones RL, Nzekwu MM. The effects of body mass index on lung volumes. *Chest.* 2006;130(3):827-833.
54. Taylor R. Kelly TM, Elliot GC, Jensen RL, Jones SB. Hypoxemia after gastric bypass surgery for morbid obesity. *Arch Surg.* 1985;120(11):1298–1302.
55. Kelman GR. Digital computer subroutine for the conversion of oxygen tension into saturation. *J Appl Physiol.* 1966;21(4):1375-1376.
56. Leykin Y, Pellis T, Lucca M, Lomangino G, Marzano B, Gullo A. The pharmacodynamic effects of rocuronium when dosed according to real body weight or ideal body weight in morbidly obese patients. *Anesth Analg.* 2004;99(4):1086-1089.
57. Meyhoff CS, Lund J, Jenstrup MT, et al. Should dosing of rocuronium in obese patients be based on ideal or corrected body weight? *Anesth Analg.* 2009; 109(3):787-792.
58. Puhringer FK, Keller C, Kleinsasser A, Giesinger S, Benzer A. Pharmacokinetics of rocuronium bromide in obese female patients. *Eur J Anaesthesiol.* 1999;16(8):507-510.
59. Weinstein JA, Matteo RS, Ornstein E, Schwartz AE, Goldstoff M, Thal G. Pharmacodynamics of vecuronium and atracurium in the obese surgical patient. *Anesth Analg.* 1988;67(12):1149-1153.
60. Schwartz AE, Matteo RS, Ornstein E, Halevy JD, Diaz J. Pharmacokinetics and pharmacodynamics of vecuronium in the obese surgical patient. *Anesth Analg.* 1992;74(4):515-518.
61. Kirkegaard-Nielsen H, Helbo-Hansen HS, Toft P, Severinsen IK. Anthropometric variables as predictors for duration of action of vecuronium-induced neuromuscular block. *Anesth Analg.* 1994;79(5):1003-1006.
62. Kirkegaard-Nielsen H, Helbo-Hansen HS, Lindholm P, Severinsen IK, Pedersen HS. Anthropometric variables as predictors for duration of action of atracurium-induced neuromuscular block. *Anesth Analg.* 1996;83(5):1076-1080.
63. van Kralingen S, van de Garde EM, Knibbe CA, et al. Comparative evaluation of atracurium dosed on ideal body weight vs. total body weight in morbidly obese patients. *Br J Clin Pharmacol.* 2011;71(1):34-40.
64. Schmith VD, Fiedler-Kelly J, Phillips L, Grasela TH Jr. Prospective use of population pharmacokinetics/pharmacodynamics in the development of cisatracurium. *Pharm Res.* 1997;14(1):91-97.
65. Leykin Y, Pellis T, Lucca M, Lomangino G, Marzano B, Gullo A. The effects of cisatracurium on morbidly obese women. *Anesth Analg.* 2004;99(4):1090-1094.
66. Lesser GT, Deutsch S. Measurement of adipose tissue blood flow and perfusion in man by uptake of 85Kr. *J Appl Physiol.* 1967;23(5):621-630.
67. Eger EI II, Bahlman SH, Munson ES. The effect of age on the rate of increase of alveolar anesthetic concentration. *Anesthesiology.* 1971;35(4):365-372.
68. Wahrenbrock EA, Eger EI IInd, Laravuso RB, Maruschak G. Anesthetic uptake—of mice and men (and whales). *Anesthesiology.* 1974;40(1):19-23.
69. Cortinez LI, Gambus P, Troconiz IF, Echevarria G, Munoz HR. Obesity does not influence the onset and offset of sevoflurane effect as measured by the hysteresis between sevoflurane concentration and bispectral index. *Anesth Analg.* 2011;113(1):70-76.
70. Lemmens HJ, Saidman LJ, Eger EI II, Laster MJ. Obesity modestly affects inhaled anesthetic kinetics in humans. *Anesth Analg.* 2008;107(6):1864-1870.
71. La Colla G, La Colla L, Turi S, et al. Effect of morbid obesity on kinetic of desflurane: wash-in wash-out curves and recovery times. *Minerva Anestesiol.* 2007;73(5): 275-279.
72. Casati A, Marchetti C, Spreafico E, Mamo D. Effects of obesity on wash-in and wash-out kinetics of sevoflurane. *Eur J Anaesthesiol.* 2004;21(3):243-245.
73. Torri G, Casati A, Comotti L, Bignami E, Santorsola R, Scarioni M. Wash-in and wash-out curves of sevoflurane and isoflurane in morbidly obese patients. *Minerva Anestesiol.* 2002;68(6):523-527.

74. Strum EM, Szenohradszki J, Kaufman WA, Anthone GJ, Manz IL, Lumb PD. Emergence and recovery characteristics of desflurane versus sevoflurane in morbidly obese adult surgical patients: a prospective, randomized study. *Anesth Analg.* 2004;99(6):1848-1853.
75. De Baerdemaeker LE, Struys MM, Jacobs S, et al. Optimization of desflurane administration in morbidly obese patients: a comparison with sevoflurane using an 'inhalation bolus' technique. *Br J Anaesth.* 2003;91(5):638-650.
76. LaPierre CD, Johnson KB, Randall BR, White JL, Egan TD. An exploration of remifentanil-propofol combinations that lead to a loss of response to esophageal instrumentation, a loss of responsiveness, and/or onset of intolerable ventilatory depression. *Anesth Analg.* 2011;113(3):490-499.
77. Bouillon TW, Bruhn J, Radulescu L, et al. Pharmacodynamic interaction between propofol and remifentanil regarding hypnosis, tolerance of laryngoscopy, bispectral index, and electroencephalographic approximate entropy. *Anesthesiology.* 2004;100(6):1353-1372.
78. Zoremba M, Dette F, Hunecke T, Eberhart L, Braunecker S, Wulf H. A comparison of desflurane versus propofol: the effects on early postoperative lung function in overweight patients. *Anesth Analg.* 2011;113(1):63-69.
79. Jahr JS, Lee VK. Intravenous acetaminophen. *Anesthesiol Clin.* 2010;28(4):619-645.
80. Lee WH, Kramer WG, Granville GE. The effect of obesity on acetaminophen pharmacokinetics in man. *J Clin Pharmacol.* 1981;21(7):284-287.
81. Golembiewski JA. Postoperative pain management—is there a role for gabapentin or pregabalin? *J Perianesth Nurs.* 2007;22(2):136-138.
82. Daley MD, Norman PH, Coveler LA. Tracheal extubation of adult surgical patients while deeply anesthetized: a survey of United States anesthesiologists. *J Clin Anesth.* 1999;11(6):445-452.
83. Arain SR, Barth CD, Shankar H, Ebert TJ. Choice of volatile anesthetic for the morbidly obese patient: sevoflurane or desflurane. *J Clin Anesth.* 2005;17(6):413-419.
84. Vallejo MC, Sah N, Phelps AL, O'Donnell J, Romeo RC. Desflurane versus sevoflurane for laparoscopic gastroplasty in morbidly obese patients. *J Clin Anesth.* 2007;19(1):3-8.
85. Bailey PL, Pace NL, Ashburn MA, et al. Frequent hypoxemia and apnea after sedation with midazolam and fentanyl. *Anesthesiology.* 1990;73:826-830.
86. Short TG, Chui PT. Propofol and midazolam act synergistically in combination. *Br J Anaesth.* 1991;67:539-545.
87. McClune S, McKay AC, Wright PMC, et al. Synergistic interactions between midazolam and propofol. *Br J Anaesth.* 1992;69:240-245.

CHAPTER

21

Anesthetic Clinical Pharmacology in Pediatric Patients

Jeffrey K. Lu, MD

INTRODUCTION

A common misconception of dosing anesthetics in pediatric patients is that children are miniature adults. Although there are substantial physiologic changes with early development and maturation (Table 21–1; Figures 21–1 through 21–3),[1-6] they are not rigorously accounted for in published dosing guidelines for pediatric patients. Ideally, dosing recommendations would be based on studies in children at various phases of maturation and characterize drug kinetic and dynamic behavior as a function of age and body composition. Without a scientific basis, anesthesiologists are left to make assumptions and educated guesses when formulating a dosing regimen and then rely on the forgiving nature of most anesthetics that have a wide therapeutic margin.

A major reason for the paucity of data characterizing anesthetic drug behavior in pediatric patients is drug development cost. Pharmaceutical companies that market drugs in the United States seek approval from the Food and Drug Administration (FDA) for adults but do not pursue approval in children because of prohibitive costs (up to $800 million for one drug[7]). As a result, several anesthetics are administered to children "off label" with drug adult doses scaled to pediatric patients.

To address this void, the National Institute for Childhood Health and Human Development in the United States formed the Pediatric Pharmacology Research Unit Network in 1994. This network encouraged the inclusion of pediatric patients during drug development.[8] The 1997 FDA Modernization Act further provided an incentive to pediatric pharmacology research by requiring drugs frequently prescribed to children to have FDA approval and allowing additional 6 months of market exclusivity for approved drugs.[9]

Over the years, clinical pharmacologists have explored numerous approaches to more accurately dose pediatric patients with formulas that incorporate age, weight, body surface area (BSA), or allometric scaling (Table 21–2). Although an improvement, none of them account for maturation and development in early childhood.

For example, early approaches used age to scale adult doses to children. Although easy to calculate, they were highly unreliable because of the large variability in weight at a given age. For a 3-year-old male child, the 3rd to 97th percentile for weight ranges from 12.5 to 19 kg (a comparable range in an adult would be 70 to 106 kg). A single anesthetic dose administered to patients over this weight range would likely lead to overdosing or underdosing.

Weight-based dosing techniques are most common. Although easy to calculate, dosing normalized to weight assumes that (1) people of different sizes and age have the same body composition and similar metabolism and excretion, and that (2) drug effects are similar regardless of age. This may be acceptable in children 2 years of age and older. But for younger infants and neonates, the physiologic differences described in Table 21–1 can substantially alter drug behavior.

Another approach is to scale adult doses by BSA. BSA assumes physiologic processes are nearly constant when expressed per unit of body surface area.[12] Although BSA is used to estimate organ size and fluid compartment volumes,[10] physiologic processes are not the same in infants, toddlers, and young children. Dosing scaled to BSA may lead to

TABLE 21–1 Body composition, absorption, distribution, metabolism, and renal excretion in young children.[1-6]

Physiologic Function	Differences in Young Children
Absorption	
Gastric motility	Gastric emptying is delayed in newborn infants and approaches adult values by 6 to 8 months of age.[1]
Gastric pH	Neutral at birth and then reaches adult levels by age 2 years.[2] Important in absorption of acid-labile drugs.[3]
Body composition	
Total body water	Declines from 95% of total body weight in the premature infant to 60% in young adults.
Extracellular water	Declines from 60% in premature infants to 20% in young adults.
Intracellular water	Rises from 25% in premature infants to 45% in young adults (Figure 21–1).[4]
Percent body fat	Rises from infancy, peaks at age 1, then reaches adult percentages of 15% (Figure 21–2).[5]
Volume of distribution	Decreases up to 50% for water soluble drugs (eg, muscle relaxants).[3]
Metabolism	Hepatic microsomal enzymes: low concentrations at birth that reach adult levels by 6 to 12 months of age. Hepatic conjugation (glucuronidation and acetylation): low at birth that reaches adult functionality by 3 to 6 months of age.[3]
Renal excretion	Glomerular filtration rate rises from 11 in the premature infant to 20 mL/min/1.73 m^2 in the young adult (Figure 21–3).

larger doses than with weight-based approaches in certain age groups. As an example, consider dosing fentanyl for a 15-kg, 76-cm, 2-year-old (BSA = 0.56 m^2) according to weight versus BSA. With a 2-mcg/kg (150-mcg) dose for a 75-kg adult (BSA = 1.73 m^2), the weight- and BSA-scaled doses are 30 and 50 mcg, respectively (70% increase).

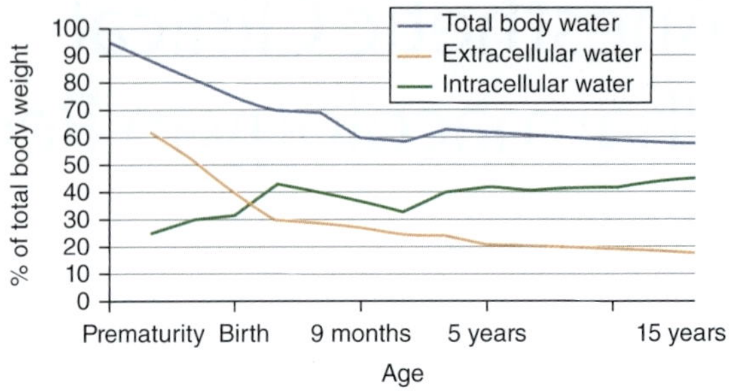

FIGURE 21–1 Estimated total, intracelluar, and extracelluar water as a percentage of total body weight by age.[1-6]

The clinical implications of differences between weight- and BSA-based dosing are not clear. Perhaps scaling to BSA better captures differences in body composition not accounted for by weight. By contrast, scaling to either BSA or weight may ignore important maturation processes as a function of age that directly influence drug clearance and lead to excessive dosing. A dramatic example of this involves the antimicrobial chloramphenicol. When dosed according to body weight, chloramphenicol caused cardiovascular collapse and "gray baby syndrome."[13,14] Newborn infants metabolize chloramphenicol by glucuronidation. This process is immature in newborns and proceeds at a slower rate than in adults—half life of 20 versus 4 hours.

An additional approach is allometric scaling. This technique scales clearance from adults to children as a function of body weight and assumes clearance is the same in young children and adults. Because of this assumption, it is limited to children

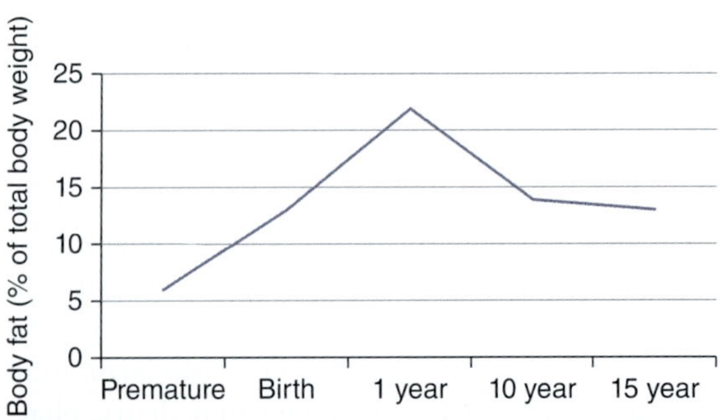

FIGURE 21–2 Body fat as a percentage of total body weight versus age.[1-6]

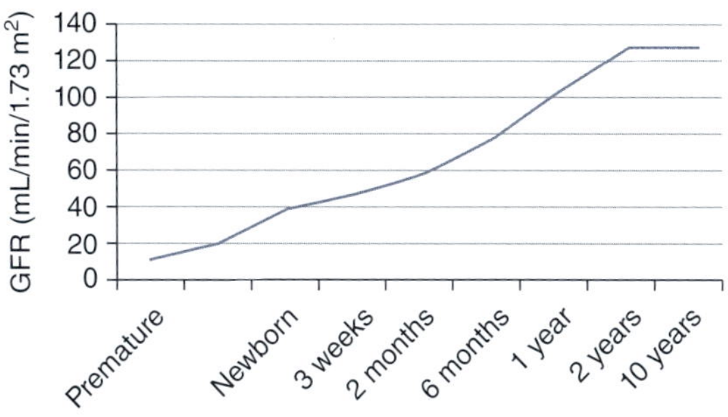

FIGURE 21–3 Glomerular filtration rate (GFR) as a function of age.[1-6]

8 years of age or older when clearance becomes similar to adults[15]; however, many researchers suggest that it should not be used at all.[16]

At present, most dosing recommendations for anesthetics in pediatric patients are simply weight based (ie, mg/kg), whereas some recommendations provide unique weight normalized dose for premature infants, neonates, toddlers, and children (Table 21–3). Selected anesthetics are discussed in more detail below.

MIDAZOLAM

Although 2-year-old children may approach pharmacologic maturity, they have not reached psychological, emotional, and intellectual maturity.

TABLE 21–2 Approaches to scaling adult doses to pediatric patients based on age, weight, and body surface area.[10]

Approach	Formulas
Age	1. Age/20 2. (4 × Age) + 20 3. Age/(Age + 12)
Weight	1. Wt/70 2. $Wt^{2/3}$ 3. (1.5 x Wt) + 10
Body surface area (BSA)[a]	$(Wt \times Ht)/3600^{1/2}$
Allometric scaling (clearance [CL]; in mL/min)	$CL_{child} = CL_{adult} \times (Wt_{child}/Wt_{adult})^{3/4}$

Pediatric doses are calculated as percentages of adult doses using each formula.
[a]There are numerous formulas for BSA (m²).[11]
Ht, height (cm); Wt, weight (kg).,

To minimize pain, fear, and separation anxiety, midazolam can be administered via several routes: intravenous, transmucosal (oral, sublingual, rectal, nasal), or intramuscular.

As a benzodiazepine, midazolam potentiates the neurotransmitter γ-aminobutyric acid (GABA). Central GABA receptor activation hyperpolarizes neuronal membranes inhibiting neural transmission resulting in sedation, anxiolysis, and amnesia.

An interesting feature of midazolam is that hepatic microenzymes (primarily CYP3A4) metabolizes midazolam into an active metabolite, α-hydroxy-midazolam, which is approximately as potent as midazolam. The pharmacokinetic profile of midazolam has been well established, but this is less true for its active metabolite. Combined pharmacokinetic–pharmacodynamic models that attempt to predict the onset and duration of effect (ie, sedation or anxiolysis) may underpredict the duration when not accounting for α-hydroxy-midazolam.

Intravenous bolus administration has an onset of sedation of 1 to 2 minutes. Kinetic models indicate that after a bolus, midazolam reaches a peak concentration within 9 minutes. When administered as an oral suspension, it has a slower onset of effect (20–30 minutes). Oral suspension doses of 0.25, 0.5, and 1 mg/kg[17] lead to plasma concentrations ranging from 68 to 161 ng/mL, 30 minutes after dosing. These plasma concentrations are consistent with satisfactory sedation scores and electroencephalographic effects known to occur during sedation.[18] Dose-finding studies recommend oral doses of 0.5 to 0.75 mg/kg administered 30 minutes before parental separation achieve adequate sedation for most children ages 1 to 10 years with minimal side effects.[19,20] Higher doses (0.75–1 mg/kg) may result in a 20% incidence of postoperative blurred vision, dysphoria, and ataxia.

KETAMINE

Ketamine is an *N*-methyl-D-aspartate (NMDA) receptor antagonist that inhibits neuronal calcium influx, blunting neuronal depolarization in the brain's limbic system, hypothalamus, and sensory cortex.[21] By disrupting the interplay between these areas of the brain responsible for emotions, sensory

TABLE 21–3 Dosages for common anesthetic drugs.

Drug	Premature	Neonate	Pediatric	Adult
Midazolam IV	0.02 mg/kg	0.02 mg/kg	0.04 mg/kg	0.2 mg/kg
Midazolam PO			0.5 mg/kg	
Propofol	2 mg/kg	2–3 mg/kg	3–4 mg/kg	2 mg/kg
Ketamine IV	2 mg/kg	2 mg/kg	2 mg/kg	2 mg/kg
Ketamine PO			5 mg/kg	5 mg/kg
Ketamine IM	2 mg/kg	2 mg/kg	2–4 mg/kg	3–5 mg/kg
Etomidate			0.02 mg/kg	0.02 mg/kg
Atropine	0.01 mg/kg	0.01 mg/kg	0.01 mg/kg	1 mg
Glycopyrollate	0.005 mg/kg	0.005 mg/kg	0.005 mg/kg	0.2 mg
Succinycholine	2 mg/kg	1–2 mg/kg	1–2 mg/kg	2 mg/kg
Rocuronium	0.8 mg/kg	0.6 mg/kg	0.6 mg/kg	0.6 mg/kg
Acetaminophen			15 mg/kg PR	
Sevoflurane		3.3%	2.6%	2.3%
Isoflurane	1.28%	1.69%	1.69%	1.27%
Desflurane		9.16%	8.62%	7.7%

perception, and memory, ketamine creates a “dissociative” anesthetic state. Patients entering or emerging from ketamine can experience vivid dreams, a floating sensation, and hallucinations.

Like midazolam, ketamine is administered as a premedicant using intravenous, transmucosal, or intramuscular delivery routes. It is metabolized by hepatic microsomal enzymes CYP3A4 and to a lesser extent 2B6 and 2C9 into pharmacologically active metabolites, norketamine and, to a lesser extent, dehydronorketamine. Norketamine has approximately one-third the potency of ketamine.[22]

Oral Administration

In adults, both ketamine and norketamine concentrations peak 45 minutes after administration. Because of the first-pass effect, norketamine levels are 5 times higher than ketamine,[23] and children produce significantly more norketamine than adults.[24]

Intramuscular Injection

In adults, ketamine concentrations peak 15 minutes after administration. With this route of administration, much of the drug bypasses the portal circulation, and ketamine concentrations are 5 times higher than the peak concentrations with equivalent oral doses. Norketamine concentrations peak 1 to 2 hours later and are substantially lower than ketamine concentrations. It is interesting to point out that plasma ketamine concentration associated with analgesia are 150 ng/mL following intramuscular injection versus 40 ng/mL following oral administration. Higher levels of norketamine with oral administration may explain this difference.[25]

Ketamine produces sedation and analgesia with minimal respiratory or cardiovascular depression. However, its side-effect profile is undesirable: excessive salivation and mucus production, dreaming, and dysphoria. Ketamine is often combined with an antisialagogue and a benzodiazepine to counter these side effects.[26]

A typical pediatric oral dose for anxious and upset children is ketamine 4 mg/kg, atropine 0.02 mg/kg, and midazolam 0.1 mg/kg mixed in cherry-flavored syrup. For children who reject oral medication, a typical intramuscular induction dose is ketamine 2 to 5 mg/kg, atropine 0.01 to 0.02 mg/kg, and midazolam 0.05 to 0.1 mg/kg. The average induction time is 4 minutes, although ketamine concentrations will likely continue to climb for another 10 minutes. The incidence of significant hypoxemia or respiratory depression is rare, but can occur, particularly in the neonates.[26] Ketamine as a premedication or induction agent in pediatric patients has a proven history of safety.

PROPOFOL

Unlike many other anesthetics, the kinetic behavior of propofol has been well characterized in neonates and children. For children, researchers have explored a wide range of bolus and continuous infusion dosing regimens and measured plasma propofol levels. These data have been used to build kinetic models and explore the ability of weight and BSA to improve model predictions. Weight-adjusted models significantly improved predictions, but BSA-adjusted models did not. Adjusting for age marginally improved model predictions. Thus, for propofol, weight-adjusted doses are best, whereas accounting for age and BSA is less helpful. When compared to adults, researchers have also found that children typically require more propofol. Suggested infusion rates are initially 50% to 100% higher in children than in adults for the first 30 minutes.[27]

Propofol pharmacokinetics have been studied in children. Kataria et al studied 53 children, aged 3 to 11 years, who underwent general anesthesia for superficial body surface surgery.[27] Twenty children received a single induction bolus of propofol, 3 mg/kg. The remaining 33 children received an induction bolus of propofol, 3.5 mg/kg, followed by a continuous propofol infusion. Following induction, 18 of these children received a continuous infusion of propofol, 150 mcg/kg/min; the remaining 15 children received a 30-minute continuous infusion of propofol, 200 mcg/kg/min, followed by a continuous infusion of 125 mcg/kg/min. After propofol administration, a total of 658 blood samples were collected from these children over time. These data were used to test 3 different pharmacokinetic models for best fit: standard 2-stage approach, naive pooled-data approach, and mixed-effects approach. The authors concluded that a 3-compartment model fit best for all of these models. The authors also found that the 3 modeling paradigms had comparable results.

Neonates undergoing chest tube removal were administered a single bolus of propofol, 3 mg/kg, prior to removal. Propofol concentrations were measured from blood samples collect over 24 hours and were fit to a 3-compartment pharmacokinetic model.

By comparison to children, propofol behaves differently in neonates. Neonates metabolize propofol more slowly, and propofol's volume of distribution is smaller than in older children. These differences disappear by approximately 3 months of postnatal life or 54 weeks postgestational age, when maturation of the propofol clearance mechanism is complete.[28]

Bartelink et al proposed guidelines for estimating pediatric doses in the absence of adequate pharmacologic data.[29] The researchers' algorithm selects doses based on either body weight or BSA. For drugs primarily excreted by the kidney, body weight or BSA is used depending on the age, volume of distribution, and glomerular filtration rate. For drugs metabolized by hepatic microsomal enzymes, pediatric doses are based on body weight; if not, they based on BSA.[12]

Propofol Infusion Syndrome

Long-term sedation with propofol in pediatric intensive care units is associated with propofol infusion syndrome (PRIS). Propofol infusion rates of greater than 4 mg/kg/h (67 mcg/kg/min) for more than 48 hours can result in refractory bradycardia and eventual asystole, in association with lactic acidosis, rhabdomyolysis, or hyperlipidemia. Although first reported in children, PRIS has also been reported in adults.[30,31] Two theories have been proposed as the cause of PRIS. The first theory proposes that propofol inhibits the mitochondrial respiratory chain, impairing electron transport and oxidative phosphorylation, eventually leading to cellular hypoxia and metabolic acidosis.[32] An alternative theory proposes that mitochondrial fatty acid metabolism is impaired, leading to a buildup of fatty acids. Excess serum fatty acids induce ventricular dysrhythmias.[33] Muscle and nerve cells heavily depend upon these pathways for energy. Disruption of mitochondrial oxidative phosphorylation or fatty acid metabolism results in rhabdomyolysis, heart failure, and neurologic injury.

Patients with mitochondrial myopathies develop symptoms similar to PRIS. When stressed (eg, infection), patients with mitochondrial myopathy are unable to metabolize lipids appropriately and develop severe rhabdomyolysis, cardiac failure, and hepatic failure.[34] The long-term infusion of propofol can lead to PRIS in certain susceptible populations of patients.[35] Identifying which patients are susceptible to PRIS is an active area of research.

INHALED ANESTHETICS

Inhaled anesthetic agents are a mainstay in the practice of anesthesiology and particularly in pediatric anesthesiology. Minimal alveolar concentration (MAC) changes with age. For all potent inhaled agents, except halothane, MAC is maximal at birth and gradually decreases with age. (The MAC of halothane peaks at 6 months age.) The MAC of premature infants is higher than in adults, but it is not as high as the MAC of a full-term infant. Broadly, the MAC of a full-term infant is 1.5 to 1.8 times the MAC of a 40-year-old adult, and the MAC of a premature infant is 1.2 to 1.6 times lower than that of a full-term infant.[36] Because interpatient variability is high, clinicians titrate inhaled concentrations to patient movement, hemodynamic stability, surgical stimulation, and pathophysiology, frequently combining them with opioids and other agents to achieve an optimum anesthetic state. In children, the required inhaled concentration of potent anesthetics will be higher than in adults.

Using a Bispectral Index Scale (BIS) monitor, Olofsen and Dahan et al measured the transport time between lung inhalation and the effect site for sevoflurane and isoflurane—3.5 and 3.2 minutes, respectively. Instead of MAC, they measured IC_{50}—the inhaled agent concentration that produces 50% BIS inhibition. They found that IC_{50} was maximal at birth and gradually declined with age, as with MAC.[37] The relationship between MAC and IC_{50} is not known.

ARE CERTAIN ANESTHETIC AGENTS BAD FOR CHILDREN?

Ikonomidou et al demonstrated that NMDA antagonism disrupted normal brain development in animal models by blocking glutamate action at the NMDA receptor.[38] The same group demonstrated that when alcohol (a known NMDA receptor antagonist) is administered to developing rats, they developed excessive programmed cell death, known as neuronal apoptosis. Their findings suggest a close connection between ethanol-induced NMDA antagonism and GABA, apoptotic neurodegeneration, and fetal alcohol syndrome.[39] Drugs that cause NMDA antagonism, GABA stimulation, or both, are associated with accelerated neuronal apoptosis and abnormal brain development. This mechanism has been confirmed in animal models, including primates.[40]

Most anesthetics, including benzodiazepines, barbiturates, ketamine, propofol, etomidate, and all inhaled anesthetic agents (such as nitrous oxide and xenon), possess either NMDA antagonist or GABA agonist properties (or both).[41] Therefore, all anesthetics are bad for the developing brain in animal models, including primates. Paule et al tested ketamine doses in newborn rhesus monkeys and found lower training scores and score lower than controls for at least 10 months after ketamine administration.[42] Can these troubling findings be generalized to children?

Currently, only retrospective studies suggest a connection between anesthesia and abnormal neurologic development in children. Wilder et al published a retrospective study of over 5357 children, with 593 undergoing anesthesia before age 4 years. The investigators found that 1 exposure to anesthesia was not a risk factor for learning disabilities but 2 or more anesthetics were. They also noted that risk for learning disabilities incrementally increased with the number of anesthetics administered.[43] While ongoing studies will yield more information about the risk of anesthesia to brain development in children, no firm conclusions may be drawn at the time of this writing.[44]

REFERENCES

1. Strolin Benedetti M, Baltes EL. Drug metabolism and disposition in children. *Fundam Clin Pharmacol.* 2003;17(3):281-299.
2. Rennie JM, Roberton NRC. *Roberton's Textbook of Neonatology*. 4th ed. Edinburgh: Elsevier/Churchill Livingstone; 2005.
3. Routledge PA. Pharmacokinetics in children. *J Antimicrob Chemother.* 1994;34(suppl A):19-24.
4. Friis-Hansen B. Water distribution in the foetus and newborn infant. *Acta Paediatr Scand Suppl.* 1983;305:7-11.
5. Bechard LJ, Wroe E, Ellis K. Body composition and growth (Chapter 4). In: Duggan C, Watkins JB, Walker WA, eds. *Nutrition in Pediatrics: Basic Science, Clinical Applications*. 4th ed. xvii. Hamilton, Ontario/Lewiston, NY: B.C. Decker; 2008.
6. Holliday MA, Barratt TM, Avner ED. *Pediatric Nephrology*. 3rd ed. Baltimore: Williams & Wilkins; 1994.
7. DiMasi JA, Hansen RW, Grabowski HG. The price of innovation: new estimates of drug development costs. *J Health Econ.* 2003;22(2):151-185.
8. National Institute for Childhood Health and Human Development: Pediatric Pharmacology Research Units (PPRU) Network. 2010.
9. Food and Drug Administration Modernization Act (FDAMA) of 1997.
10. Lack JA, Stuart-Taylor MA. Calculation of drug dosage and body surface area of children. *Br J Anaesth.* 1997;78:601-605.
11. Mosteller RD. Simplified calculation of body-surface area, *N Engl J Med* 1987;22;317(17):1098 (letter).
12. Crawford JD, Terry ME, Rourke GM. Simplification of drug dosage calculation by application of the surface area principle. *Pediatrics.* 1950;5(5):783-790.
13. Burns LE, Hodgman JE, Cass AB. Fatal circulatory collapse in premature infants receiving chloramphenicol. *N Engl J Med.* 1959;261:1318-1321.
14. McCracken GH, Jr. Pharmacological basis for antimicrobial therapy in newborn infants. *Am J Dis Child.* 1974;128(3):407-419.
15. Kearns GL, Abdel-Rahman SM, Alander SW, Blowey DL, Leeder JS, Kauffman RE. Developmental pharmacology–drug disposition, action, and therapy in infants and children. *N Engl J Med.* 2003;349(12):1157-1167.
16. Nagilla R, Ward KW. A comprehensive analysis of the role of correction factors in the allometric predictivity of clearance from rat, dog, and monkey to humans. *J Pharm Sci.* 2004;93(10):2522-2534.
17. Marshall J, Rodarte A, Blumer J, Khoo KC, Akbari B, Kearns G. Pediatric pharmacodynamics of midazolam oral syrup. Pediatric Pharmacology Research Unit Network. *J Clin Pharmacol.* 2000;40(6):578-589.
18. Mandema JW, Tuk B, van Steveninck AL, Breimer DD, Cohen AF, Danhof M. Pharmacokinetic-pharmacodynamic modeling of the central nervous system effects of midazolam and its main metabolite alpha-hydroxymidazolam in healthy volunteers. *Clin Pharmacol Ther.* 1992;51(6):715-728.
19. Feld LH, Negus JB, White PF. Oral midazolam preanesthetic medication in pediatric outpatients. *Anesthesiology.* 1990;73(5):831-834.
20. McMillan CO, Spahr-Schopfer IA, Sikich N, Hartley E, Lerman J. Premedication of children with oral midazolam. *Can J Anaesth.* 1992;39(6):545-550.
21. Bergman SA. Ketamine: review of its pharmacology and its use in pediatric anesthesia. *Anesth Prog.* 1999;46(1):10-20.
22. Ebert B, Mikkelsen S, Thorkildsen C, Borgbjerg FM. Norketamine, the main metabolite of ketamine, is a non-competitive NMDA receptor antagonist in the rat cortex and spinal cord. *Eur J Pharmacol.* 1997;333(1):99-104.
23. Grant IS, Nimmo WS, Clements JA. Pharmacokinetics and analgesic effects of i.m. and oral ketamine. *Br J Anaesth.* 1981;53(8):805-810.
24. Grant IS, Nimmo WS, McNicol LR, Clements JA. Ketamine disposition in children and adults. *Br J Anaesth.* 1983;55(11):1107-1111.
25. White PF, Way WL, Trevor AJ. Ketamine–its pharmacology and therapeutic uses. *Anesthesiology.* 1982;56(2):119-136.
26. Cotsen MR, Donaldson JS, Uejima T, Morello FP. Efficacy of ketamine hydrochloride sedation in children for interventional radiologic procedures. *AJR Am J Roentgenol.* 1997;169(4):1019-1022.
27. Kataria BK, Ved SA, Nicodemus HF, et al. The pharmacokinetics of propofol in children using three different data analysis approaches. *Anesthesiology.* 1994;80(1):104-122.
28. Allegaert K, de Hoon J, Verbesselt R, Naulaers G, Murat I. Maturational pharmacokinetics of single intravenous bolus of propofol. *Paediatr Anaesth.* 2007;17(11):1028-1034.
29. Bartelink IH, Rademaker CM, Schobben AF, van den Anker JN. Guidelines on paediatric dosing on the basis of developmental physiology and pharmacokinetic considerations. *Clin Pharmacokinet.* 2006;45(11):1077-1097.
30. Cremer OL, Moons KG, Bouman EA, Kruijswijk JE, de Smet AM, Kalkman CJ. Long-term propofol infusion

and cardiac failure in adult head-injured patients. *Lancet.* 2001;357(9250):117-118.
31. Parke TJ, Stevens JE, Rice AS, et al. Metabolic acidosis and fatal myocardial failure after propofol infusion in children: five case reports. *BMJ.* 1992;305(6854):613-616.
32. Schenkman KA, Yan S. Propofol impairment of mitochondrial respiration in isolated perfused guinea pig hearts determined by reflectance spectroscopy. *Crit Care Med.* 2000;28(1):172-177.
33. Wolf A, Weir P, Segar P, Stone J, Shield J. Impaired fatty acid oxidation in propofol infusion syndrome. *Lancet.* 2001;357(9256):606-607.
34. Walsh RJ, Amato AA. Toxic myopathies. *Neurol Clin.* 2005;23(2):397-428.
35. Kam PC, Cardone D. Propofol infusion syndrome. *Anaesthesia.* 2007;62(7):690-701.
36. Mazoit JX. Pharmacokinetic/pharmacodynamic modeling of anesthetics in children: therapeutic implications. *Paediatr Drugs.* 2006;8(3):139-150.
37. Olofsen E, Dahan A. The dynamic relationship between end-tidal sevoflurane and isoflurane concentrations and bispectral index and spectral edge frequency of the electroencephalogram. *Anesthesiology.* 1999;90(5):1345-1353.
38. Ikonomidou C, Bosch F, Miksa M, et al. Blockade of NMDA receptors and apoptotic neurodegeneration in the developing brain. *Science.* 1999;283(5398):70-74.
39. Ikonomidou C, Bittigau P, Ishimaru MJ, et al. Ethanol-induced apoptotic neurodegeneration and fetal alcohol syndrome. *Science.* 2000;287(5455):1056-1060.
40. Brambrink AM, Evers AS, Avidan MS, et al. Isoflurane-induced neuroapoptosis in the neonatal rhesus macaque brain. *Anesthesiology.* 2010;112(4):834-841.
41. Campagna JA, Miller KW, Forman SA. Mechanisms of actions of inhaled anesthetics. *N Engl J Med.* 2003;348(21):2110-2124.
42. Paule MG, Li M, Allen RR, et al. Ketamine anesthesia during the first week of life can cause long-lasting cognitive deficits in rhesus monkeys. *Neurotoxicol Teratol.* 2011;33:220-330.
43. Wilder RT, Flick RP, Sprung J, et al. Early exposure to anesthesia and learning disabilities in a population-based birth cohort. *Anesthesiology.* 2009;110(4):796-804.
44. Rappaport B, Mellon RD, Simone A, Woodcock J. Defining safe use of anesthesia in children. *N Engl J Med.* 2011;64:1387-1390.

CHAPTER

22

Anesthetic Implications of Poor Cardiac Function

Sonal Sharma, MD, and Marcel E. Durieux, MD, PhD

INTRODUCTION

Heart failure is increasingly being recognized as a growing health problem worldwide. It is estimated that the lifetime risk of developing heart failure is approximately 20% for patients older than 40 years.[1] Clinical anesthesiologists can therefore expect to see cases involving patients suffering from heart failure with increasing frequency. Symptomatic heart failure is associated with high risk of morbidity and mortality as a result of perioperative ischemia/infarction, dysrhythmias, worsening heart failure, postoperative cognitive dysfunction, and stroke.[2,3] Asymptomatic left ventricular dysfunction, which is considered a precursor of symptomatic heart failure and is assumed to have similar prevalence as symptomatic heart failure, is also associated with high perioperative mortality.[4] Since most anesthetics interfere with cardiovascular performance, either by direct myocardial depression or by depression of sympathetic activity, on which these patients rely, an appropriate anesthetic technique must be selected to minimize hemodynamic changes and maintain a near-normal physiologic status. This chapter discusses the aspects of dose reduction, titration of drugs, and the pharmacodynamic effects of each class of anesthetic drugs. As an example, the chapter provides a practical guide to the selection and use of general anesthetic agents in patients with poor cardiac function undergoing colectomy and discusses the pharmacologic management of acute cardiac deterioration.

HEART FAILURE: DEFINITION, PATHOPHYSIOLOGIC CHANGES, AND THEIR PHARMACOKINETIC IMPLICATIONS

Heart failure is a complex clinical syndrome, but the basic problem is the heart's inability to pump blood at a rate commensurate with the requirements of the metabolizing tissues or ability to do so only at elevated filling pressures. It can be broadly subdivided into 2 distinct forms. The first form, termed *diastolic dysfunction*, and is due to inadequate ventricular relaxation preventing adequate end-diastolic filling.[5,6] The second, termed *systolic dysfunction*, is due to inadequate force generation to eject blood normally. Therefore, it is important to be aware of the influence of anesthetics on both systolic and diastolic dysfunction.

In the failing ventricle, various adaptive mechanisms are initiated to help maintain arterial pressure and cardiac output (CO). The body activates several neurohumoral pathways to increase circulating blood volume. The sympathetic nervous system increases heart rate and contractility, causes arteriolar vasoconstriction in nonessential vascular beds, and stimulates secretion of renin from the juxtaglomerular apparatus of the kidney. Stimulation of the renin–angiotensin system results in further arteriolar vasoconstriction, sodium and water retention, and release of aldosterone. The increased aldosterone, in turn, also

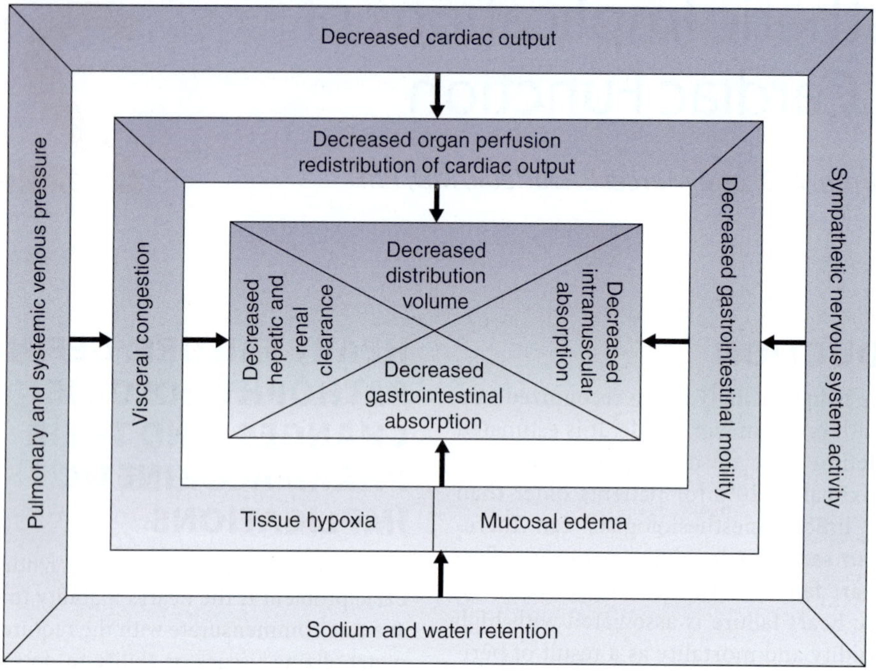

FIGURE 22–1 Pathophysiology of cardiac failure and its effects on pharmacokinetics. (Modified with permission from Benowitz NL, Meister W. Pharmacokinetics in patients with cardiac failure. *Clin Pharmacokinet* 1976;Nov-Dec:1(6):389-405.)

leads to sodium and water retention. Additionally, baroreceptor and osmotic stimuli lead to vasopressin release from the hypothalamus, causing reabsorption of water in the renal collecting duct. Although these neurohumoral pathways initially are beneficial, eventually they become deleterious and aggravate ischemia, potentiate dysrhythmias, cause endothelial dysfunction, promote cardiac remodeling, and are directly toxic to myocytes (Figure 22–1).

The pathophysiologic changes that occur in heart failure result in hepatic, gastrointestinal, and renal congestion, as well as hypoperfusion. These changes directly alter drug pharmacokinetics (absorption, distribution, metabolism, and excretion).[7]

Hepatic Metabolism

Liver function abnormalities are common. There is impairment of hepatic microsomal function, which affects drugs with low a hepatic extraction ratio, such as chlordiazepoxide, diazepam, lorazepam, methadone, and pentobarbital.

Renal Excretion

Activation of the renin–angiotensin system leads to vasoconstriction of the efferent arterioles, thereby maintaining glomerular capillary pressure and preserving glomerular filtration rate despite severe impairment of renal perfusion. Hepatic blood flow and enzymatic activity are more markedly reduced than renal function. Because anesthetic agents are primarily metabolized in the liver, drug toxicity with anesthetics occurs more readily in patients with heart failure.

Volume of Distribution

It might be expected that the volume of distribution of drugs is increased in congestive heart failure as the condition is associated with fluid retention. However, this is not the case, because excess fluid is retained interstitially and is not in direct communication with the cardiovascular system.[8] In fact, patients may have relative intravascular volume depletion resulting in higher drug concentrations after a loading dose of a drug.

Elimination Half-Life

Heart failure can lead to changes in the elimination half-life. The changes are a function of alterations in drug clearance and/or volume of distribution. Elimination half-life of agents that have a large volume of distribution and are highly cleared by the liver (ie, fentanyl, morphine, ketamine) may be twice as long in patients with heart failure compared to otherwise healthy patients. For example, in a simulation of fentanyl bolus (Figure 22–2), a doubling of the elimination half-life slows the decline in plasma and effect-site concentrations, prolonging the effect. As illustrated in the top plot, the duration of effect, assuming an analgesic threshold for fentanyl of 1 ng/mL is extended from 31 to 48 minutes for a 2-mcg/kg bolus. A slower elimination half-life has an even more pronounced impact on continuous fentanyl infusions. As illustrated in the bottom plot, the duration of effect is almost doubled, going from 48 to 90 minutes for a 1-hour fentanyl infusion dose at 3 mcg/kg/h. As with all simulations, they are based on mathematical equations and not measured drug concentrations. They are primarily used to illustrate a point, in this case decreased elimination. Estimates presented in these simulations are likely to have considerable variability in patients with poor cardiac function.

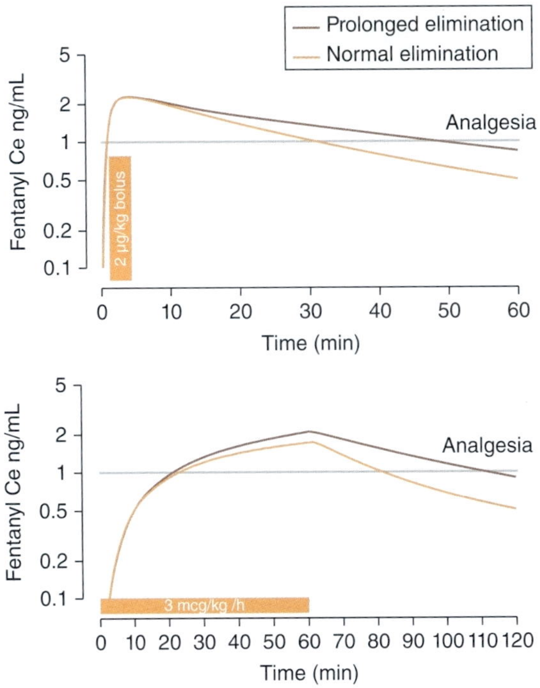

FIGURE 22–2 Simulations of a fentanyl bolus (top plot) and 1-hour infusion (bottom plot) administered to a 75-kg male with prolonged (dark red lines) and normal (red lines) elimination. Prolonged elimination was defined as a doubled elimination half-life. The gray line represents the effect-site concentration (Ce) threshold for analgesia.

INFLUENCE OF HEART FAILURE ON THE PHARMACOKINETICS OF INDIVIDUAL ANESTHETIC AGENTS

This section will describe the effects of the changes in pharmacokinetic parameters that result from cardiac failure on the clinical profiles of the most common anesthetic drugs. Effects of these drugs on the failing heart are described in the next section.

Inhalational Anesthetic Agents

Variation in CO has limited effect on the rate of rise of alveolar-to-inspired concentration ratio of the anesthetic (F_A/F_I) during the initial transfer of sparingly soluble agents (desflurane, sevoflurane, and nitrous oxide) as the rate of rise in F_A/F_I for these agents is not affected much by local alveolar perfusion. A decreased CO is likely to cause a concentrating effect[9] where a significant fraction of the inspired anesthetic is transported into the blood for soluble anesthetic agents (isoflurane, enflurane, and halothane). For example, consider the difference in the isoflurane, sevoflurane, and desflurane uptake for a CO of 6 L/min compared to 1.5 L/min during a 1-hour administration (Figure 22–3). These simulations illustrate how the more soluble agent (isoflurane) leads to a higher uptake over the duration of the 1-hour administration in comparison to less soluble agents (sevoflurane and desflurane).

In this case, arterial anesthetic partial pressure would be doubled. The doubling in anesthetic concentration would mean ultimately that the brain will "see" double the number of anesthetic molecules transferring in, and so there is a greater likelihood

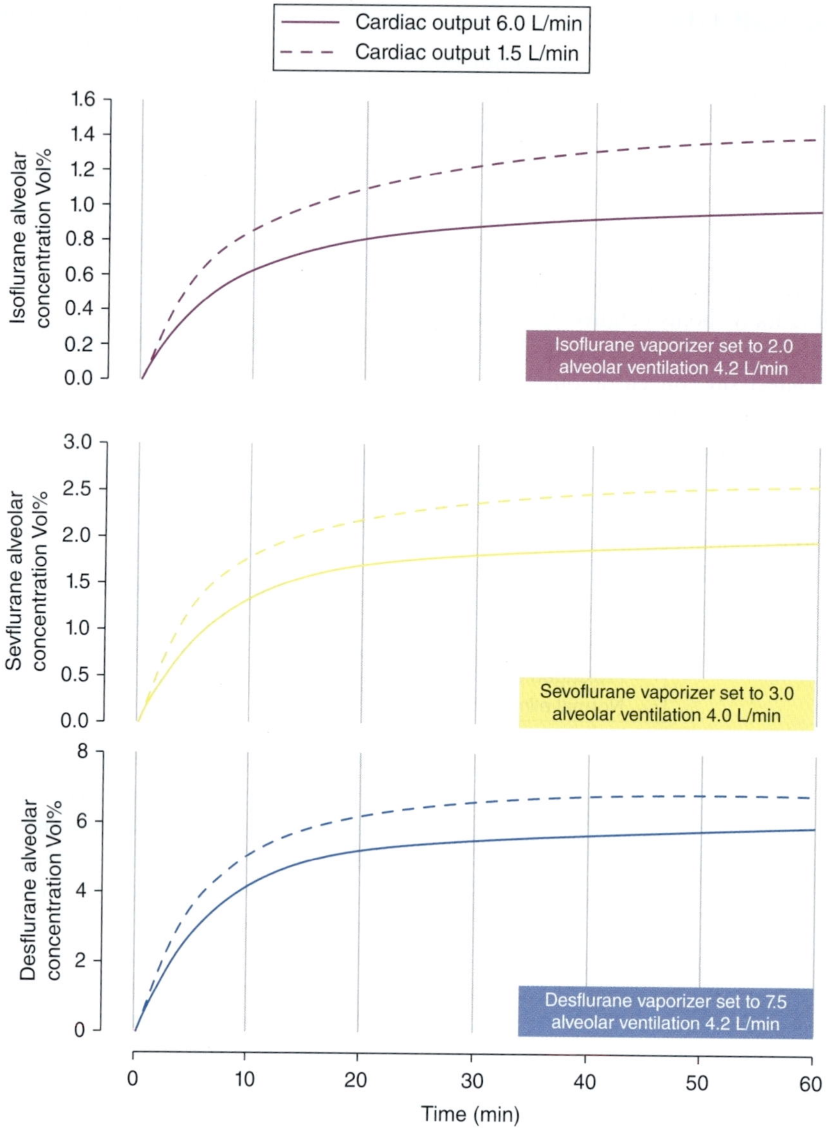

FIGURE 22–3 Anesthetic uptake for sevoflurane, desflurane, and isoflurane under normal and low cardiac output states. [With permission of the owner, James H. Philip, and the licensee, Med Man Simulations, Inc. (www.gasmanweb.com), a nonprofit charitable organization, PO Box 67160, Chestnut Hill MA 02467. Gas Man is a registered trademark of James H. Philip and Med Man Simulations, Inc., a nonprofit charitable organization.]

of anesthetic-mediated depression of the central nervous system. Also, the increase in anesthetic concentration causes further reduction in CO by depressing contractility and slowing the heart rate. An established vicious cycle can cause a potentially lethal increase in alveolar concentration. Therefore, in order to manage patients who exhibit ventricular dysfunction, agents with relatively low blood/gas solubility might be preferable, as the alveolar concentration of these agents would not be especially sensitive to cardiopulmonary changes. If more soluble agents are used, then they must be administered using gradual increments and their end-tidal concentrations should be monitored.

Intravenous Anesthetic Agents

Midazolam

The morphologic and functional liver changes caused by the reduced blood flow to the hepatocytes in patients with poor cardiac function lead to alterations in the pharmacokinetics of midazolam; these are reflected in the prolonged plasma half-life and increased serum levels of its metabolically active molecules as a result of the deceleration of its systemic clearance.[7] This deceleration results from a reduction in hydroxylation process which results in prolonged and more intense pharmacologic effects. Specifically, the half-life is prolonged by 50% and clearance is lowered by 32%.[10] Studies show that a 14.3% reduction in sedative dose of midazolam is required in patients with ejection fraction less than 55% to achieve the desired clinical effects without incurring toxic effects.[11]

Propofol

Although experimental evidence supports an influence of CO on kinetics, the number of drugs studied has been limited. Propofol is highly lipid soluble, has a very large volume of distribution, redistributes rapidly, and is eliminated via both hepatic and extrahepatic routes. In patients with ventricular dysfunction, the central volume of distribution is decreased, and both systemic and intercompartmental clearance is reduced. Thus, initial arterial concentration after intravenous bolus administration of propofol is particularly high, and greater adverse hemodynamic effects can be expected if a normal dose of propofol is injected into patients with a low CO.[12] Bolus doses should therefore be reduced when propofol is used for induction in patients with poor cardiac function. Also, the hemodynamic instability can be minimized if the bolus is given in a titrated manner over a longer period of time and laryngoscopy performed after reaching a pharmacodynamic end point, such as a bispectral index (BIS) less than 40.[13] However, this has been contradicted by a recent study, which found that the pharmacokinetic model significantly underestimates the plasma propofol concentration in patients with impaired left ventricular (LV) function. The predictive value of BIS for the desired level of sedation was insufficient in this patient cohort.[14] These findings suggest that widely used models of propofol kinetics are mis-specified when cardiac function is depressed, and in this setting they should not be used to formulate dosages or drive a target-controlled infusion pump.

Dose adjustments are also required during continuous infusion for the maintenance phase of an anesthetic; it has been shown in a swine model that a 42% decrease in CO from baseline results in 70% increase in propofol concentrations from baseline during a continuous infusion of propofol at 6 mg/kg/h.[15] This, combined with a prolonged context-sensitive half-time, can result in delayed emergence from anesthesia unless the dose is reduced during prolonged infusions.

Thiopental

Patients with poor cardiac function appear to have loss of eyelash reflex at a lower concentration of thiopental.[16,17] This increased sensitivity of patients with heart failure to thiopental is caused by a decreased central volume of distribution, resulting in higher effect-site concentration. In addition, the effect-site concentration of thiopental equilibrates faster with the arterial blood concentration. The faster rise observed in patients with low CO is a consequence of the slower distribution to the periphery. What is more worrisome is that the same would happen in the tissues of the cardiovascular system, leading to a more pronounced depression of the cardiovascular system in an already compromised patient. Therefore, extra caution should be exercised when inducing anesthesia with thiopental in such patients. The effect of thiopental is also prolonged because of slower elimination secondary to a decreased hepatic blood flow.

Opioids

When opioids are used as an integral part of anesthesia (rather than for postoperative analgesia), patients with significant myocardial dysfunction appear to require lower doses. Due to a decrease in liver blood flow consequent to decreased CO and reduced plasma clearance, these patients develop higher plasma and brain concentrations for a given loading dose or infusion rate than do patients with adequate ventricular function. This may lead to decreased sympathetic nervous system activity, on which these patients are dependent, and result in hypotension, which may be misinterpreted as hypovolemia. This is important because they can be erroneously given fluid to restore systemic blood pressure and subsequently accumulate extravascular water. As sympathetic tone and systemic vascular resistance (SVR) return toward normal in the postoperative period, they may then develop pulmonary edema.[18]

PHARMACODYNAMICS OF ANESTHETIC AGENTS IN HEART FAILURE

This section describes the cardiovascular effects of the most commonly used anesthetic drugs in the setting of cardiac failure.

Inhalational Anesthetic Agents

Early in vitro studies demonstrated that volatile anesthetics cause relatively greater decreases in contractility in failing versus normal isolated myocardium,[19-21] suggesting that patients with underlying contractile dysfunction may be more sensitive to the myocardial depressant properties of volatile anesthetics. However, further studies demonstrated that volatile anesthetics may affect LV function by producing favorable alterations in loading conditions and diastolic performance in the presence of LV dysfunction.[21-24] Isoflurane, but not halothane, improved indices of diastolic performance in dogs with pacing-induced LV dysfunction, despite producing simultaneous negative inotropic effects.[22] These findings were attributed to favorable reductions in LV preload and not to direct lusitropic effects.[22] They concluded that improvement of filling dynamics may partially offset the decrement in LV systolic function by isoflurane in the setting of LV dysfunction. Desflurane and sevoflurane were also shown to exhibit similar moderate beneficial actions on LV diastolic function, in the presence of severe abnormalities in systolic and diastolic functions during myocardial ischemia in dogs.[24,25]

Intravenous Anesthetic Agents

Etomidate

Etomidate is the intravenous anesthetic that causes the least cardiovascular depression and is a popular choice for induction of anesthesia in cardiac compromised patients. Although in humans, etomidate does produce a dose-dependent negative inotropic effect, it is significant only at concentrations considerably in excess of those occurring in clinical practice.[26] Etomidate has also been studied in cardiomyopathic hamsters, where similar negative inotropic effects were shown as in failing human ventricular muscles at supratherapeutic concentrations.[27,28] Another study has demonstrated that arterial pressure is maintained during etomidate anesthesia in the presence of preexisting pacing-induced LV dysfunction as a result of increases in total arterial resistance and aortic impedance and decreases in total arterial compliance. These adverse alterations in the determinants of LV afterload may further compromise LV systolic and diastolic performance in chronically instrumented dogs with LV failure.[29]

Ketamine

Ketamine, because it maintains hemodynamic stability, is often used for induction of anesthesia in high-risk patients. The favorable cardiovascular profile of ketamine is related to central sympathetic stimulation and inhibition of neuronal catecholamine uptake. These effects counteract the negative inotropic effect of ketamine on the myocardium. The net result in a healthy individual is a positive inotropic effect, with an increase in arterial blood pressure, heart rate, and CO. However, the failing myocardium has reduced ability to increase contractility when exposed to ketamine even in the presence of increased β-adrenergic stimulation.[30] In such patients and especially in the presence of adrenoceptor blockade, the negative inotropic effects may be unmasked, resulting in deterioration in cardiac performance and cardiovascular instability.[31] It has also been demonstrated to have negative lusitropic effect, decreasing diastolic compliance in states associated with depletion of catecholamines.[32] Similar effects have been observed when ketamine is used for long-term sedation in patients with catecholamine dependent heart failure.[33]

Midazolam

In patients who have elevated pulmonary capillary wedge pressure (PCWP) (> 18 mm Hg) and reduced cardiac index (CI) (< 2.0), induction with midazolam 0.2 mg/kg has been shown to be associated with a reduction in PCWP and a return of the CI to normal.[34] In these patients, a significant decrease in afterload allows the CO to remain unchanged despite a significant decrease in myocardial contractile performance by midazolam.[35] The effect of midazolam on LV filling in patients with LV diastolic dysfunction has been studied by Gare et al.[36] They reported that sedative doses of midazolam (≤ 0.1 mg/kg) do not adversely alter indices of diastolic performance in patients with preexisting diastolic dysfunction. The direct negative lusitropic effects are reported only with midazolam concentrations larger than 5 μM (achieved at doses > 0.3 mg/kg).[37]

Propofol

The hemodynamic effects of propofol in patients with mildly compromised LV function have been described as similar to those observed in patients with normal cardiac performance. The question arises, however, about the effects of propofol in patients with severe LV dysfunction. The experimental evidence in this area is conflicting, possibly reflecting different experimental set-ups and differences in the species studied, with some studies reporting direct negative inotropic effects[38-40] and others reporting no alteration in myocardial contractility in either failing or nonfailing hearts.[41-45]

The major hemodynamic consequences of propofol anesthesia in the setting of LV dysfunction due to cardiomyopathy are venodilatation and LV preload reduction, mediated primarily but not solely by its effects on the sympathetic nervous system. This results in a decrease in left ventricular end-diastolic pressure and a reduction in chamber dimensions. Such changes do not appear to compromise global LV performance and indeed may be beneficial as a result of decrease in myocardial oxygen consumption.[46] On the other hand, this sympathetic inhibition is amplified in patients with congestive heart failure, in whom sympathetic nervous system activity is high, and may lead to exaggerated hypotension as compared with healthy patients.[47] Propofol has also been shown to have no unfavorable effects on diastolic function in patients with preexisting diastolic dysfunction in a few studies.[36,48]

Animal studies suggest that the failing heart is susceptible to a more severe and prolonged reperfusion injury than the nonfailing heart.[49] In humans, baseline oxidant stress is shown to be greater in those with impaired cardiac function and cardiac failure and these patients may be prone to more severe reperfusion injury following a coronary artery bypass graft[50,51]; manifestations vary from transient ventricular dysfunction (stunning) to severe unresponsive cardiogenic shock, a result of impaired antioxidant reserve. The use of clinically relevant concentrations of propofol in patients with impaired myocardial function attenuates cardiac free radical–mediated injury by antioxidant action.[52] Whether this antioxidant action of propofol translates into a clinically important outcome such as improved postoperative myocardial function remains to be determined.

Thiopental

Induction doses of intravenously administered thiopental cause a fall in blood pressure and an elevation in heart rate. The hypotension is due to depression of the medullary vasomotor center, which dilates peripheral capacitance vessels, causes peripheral pooling of blood, and decreases venous return to the right atrium. The tachycardia is probably due to a central vagolytic effect. CO is often maintained by a rise in heart rate and increased myocardial contractility from compensatory baroreceptor reflexes. However, in the absence of an adequate baroreceptor response in patients with congestive heart failure, CO and arterial blood pressure may fall dramatically due to uncompensated peripheral pooling and unmasked direct myocardial depression.[53]

Opioids

Isolated heart or heart muscle studies have demonstrated dose-related negative inotropic effects for morphine, meperidine, fentanyl, and alfentanil.[54,55] However, these effects occurred at concentrations one hundred to several thousand times those found clinically. In fact, in canine hearts, the direct intracoronary injection of fentanyl in concentrations up to 240 ng/mL produced no changes in myocardial mechanical function.[56] The cardiovascular stability thus provided by opioids has become especially valuable for induction and maintenance of patients with severely impaired ventricular function.[27,57,58] A study demonstrating markedly decreased negative inotropic response to morphine in failing hearts suggested that opioid receptors do not play a part in this cardiac effect of morphine and could be due to interaction between opioid agonists and β-adrenergic receptors, which are down-regulated in heart failure.[59]

PHARMACOLOGIC MANAGEMENT OF PERIOPERATIVE ACUTE LEFT VENTRICULAR FAILURE

As stated previously, individuals with preexisting ventricular dysfunction who undergo surgical procedures are at higher risk of developing perioperative acute ventricular dysfunction.[2,3] Pharmacologic treatment of low CO and reduced oxygen delivery may be required. Inadequate treatment may lead to multiple organ failure, one of the main causes of prolonged hospital stays as well as postoperative morbidity and mortality. A wide range of inotropic agents is available. However, there is a paucity of comparative studies, evaluating the differential systemic and regional hemodynamic effects of various inotropes on CO in perioperative heart failure. Use of the following options, either alone or combined, should be considered.

- Among catecholamines, consider low to moderate doses of dobutamine and epinephrine: they both improve stroke volume and increase heart rate while PCWP is moderately decreased; however, they increase myocardial oxygen consumption at the same time.
- Milrinone decreases PCWP and SVR while increasing stroke volume and causes less tachycardia than dobutamine.
- Levosimendan, a calcium sensitizer, increases stroke volume and heart rate and decreases SVR.
- Norepinephrine should be used in case of low blood pressure due to vasoplegia in order to maintain an adequate perfusion pressure. Volume status should be repeatedly assessed to ensure that the patient is not hypovolemic while vasopressors are being administered.

PHARMACOLOGIC MANAGEMENT OF PERIOPERATIVE PULMONARY HYPERTENSION AND RIGHT VENTRICULAR FAILURE

In patients with chronic LV dysfunction, increased blood flow or pressure is transmitted to the pulmonary vasculature, leading to dysregulation of the vasoactive balance in the vasculature and endothelial damage.[60] These changes result in "secondary" pulmonary hypertension. Anesthetic management of these patients is challenging, because perioperative increases in PVR readily occur and the right ventricle is acutely sensitive to increases in PVR (afterload), it may provoke right-sided heart failure. Right ventricular dilatation that accompanies right ventricular failure can cause LV compression, further compromising systemic output.[61] Treatment of pulmonary hypertension predominantly focuses upon counteracting pulmonary vasoconstriction by use of pulmonary vasodilators (Table 22–1). If it is complicated by right-sided heart failure, concomitant inotropic support is also added. The β-adrenoceptor agonists isoproterenol and dobutamine are frequently used for right-sided heart failure treatment and are often used in combination with the phosphodiesterase inhibitor milrinone. Together these agents decrease PVR and have synergistic inotropic effects. Despite their usefulness, isoproterenol can cause tachycardia and both isoproterenol and milrinone may induce dysrhythmias. Additionally, these drugs can cause systemic vasodilatation, so systemic pressors may be required if large doses are used. If vasopressors are required, phenylephrine or norepinephrine can be used. Vasopressin can be used in refractory cases. It improves systemic pressures while keeping CO and PAP stable.[62] Levosimendan, because of its

TABLE 22–1 Agents used for the therapeutic management of pulmonary hypertension.

Agent	Dose	Advantages	Disadvantages
Calcium channel blockers		Decreases right ventricular afterload	May decrease right atrial contractility and cardiac output; should be used with caution in pulmonary hypertension with associated right-sided heart failure and avoided in hypotensive patients due to the risk of decreasing SVR
Inhaled nitric oxide	5–80 ppm continuous use	Does not significantly reduce SVR; beneficial in patients with pulmonary hypertension with associated right-sided heart failure	Expensive
Inhaled sodium nitroprusside, nitroglycerin, and nitric oxide precursor (citrulline)	Nitroglycerin: 2.5 mcg/kg over 10 min Citrulline: 150-mg/kg bolus followed by continuous infusion at 9 mg/kg/h up to 48 h	Decrease PAP and PVR without significant changes in heart rate, PCWP, or systemic arterial pressure	Citrulline is still experimental.
Prostaglandins and prostacyclins (epoprostenol, treprostinil, and iloprost)	Epoprostenol IV infusion: 1–50 ng/kg/min or continuous nebulization at 10–20 mcg/mL dilution Treprostinil: continuous infusion at 1.25 ng/kg/min or inhaled 18–54 µg qi.. Iloprost: continuous infusion of 1–5 ng/kg/min or inhaled 2.5–5.0 mcg, 6–9 times a day	Decreases PAP, PVR and inhibits smooth muscle proliferation; prevents long-term progression of pulmonary hypertension; can be administered IV or via inhalation Treprostinil may potentiate inotropic effects of catecholamines, contributing to benefit in patients with pulmonary hypertension with associated right-sided heart failure.	Inhaled epoprostenol and IV iloprost are not commercially available in United States.
Phosphodiesterase inhibitors (sildenafil, vardenafil, milrinone)	Milrinone: 50 mcg/kg over 10 min followed by 0.375–0.75 mcg/kg/min infusion or inhaled 60–90 mcg/kg bolus followed by 0.08–0.11 mcg/kg/min infusion Sildenafil: inhaled 10 mg in 20-mL buffer or oral 0.25–0.75 mg/kg every 4–6 h Vardenafil: oral 5 mg daily, then 5 mg bid. after 4 wk	Decrease PVR and PAP; increase exercise capacity, quality of life, and CI Milrinone also acts as a positive inotropic and can be administered via IV or inhalation.	Inhaled or IV sildenafil and inhaled milrinone are not available commercially.
Natriuretic peptides (nesiritide)	2-mcg/kg bolus followed by continual infusion of 0.01 mcg/kg/min	Decreases mean PAP, PCWP, RAP, and PVR	Lowers SVR
Endothelin receptor antagonists (Bosentan)	Oral 62.5–125 mg bid	Improves both total pulmonary resistance and CI	

bid, 2 times a day; CI, cardiac index; IV, intravenous; PAP, pulmonary artery pressure; PCWP, pulmonary capillary wedge pressure; PVR, pulmonary vascular resistance; qid, 4 times a day; RAP, right atrial pressure; SVR, systemic vascular resistance.

ability to decrease RV afterload and better restore ventricular–pulmonary arterial coupling in such cases, is being used frequently.[63,64] However, its use is still pending in the United States.

CASE DISCUSSION

Colectomy in a Patient With Congestive Heart Failure

In a patient with significant cardiac failure who presents for colectomy, the 2 principal cardiovascular parameters to control during anesthesia are myocardial depression and peripheral vasodilatation. Any changes in either of these variables should be minimized. Another factor to be considered is the prevention of ventricular dysrhythmias.

Preoperative Preparation

The preoperative preparation of these patients must be meticulous as they have minimal or no cardiac reserve (Table 22–2). Preoperatively, patients tend to be dehydrated (as most have received diuretics) and use angiotensin-converting enzyme (ACE) inhibitors or angiotensin-receptor blockers (ARBs), a further cause of hypotension during anesthesia. Preoperative hydration may not be desirable; it may lead to frank heart failure, making the fluid management critical. A vasopressor to mitigate the vasodilating effect of the anesthetic is a rational approach. A norepinephrine infusion of 4 to 8 mcg/min titrated to a systolic blood pressure above 90 to 100 mm Hg can be started preoperatively.

It is generally accepted that diuretics may be discontinued on the day of surgery. Maintaining β blocker therapy is essential to reduce perioperative morbidity and mortality. ACE inhibitors and ARBs are associated with profound hypotension upon anesthetic induction and should be discontinued the day before surgery. Antidysrhythmic medications including digoxin should be continued due to risk of ventricular dysrhythmias in the perioperative period. Some patients may already have an implantable cardioverter defibrillator implanted.

Hemoglobin should be maintained at an adequate level to optimize oxygen-carrying capacity. A level of 13 to 14 g/dL has been recommended, higher than in patients without cardiac failure.[65] Also, the results of recent renal function and liver function tests and the most recent electrocardiogram (ECG) and echocardiogram should be evaluated.

Finally, in a critically ill patient, an intra-aortic balloon pump may be placed preoperatively.

Intraoperative Monitoring and Anesthetic Management

In addition to pulse oximeter, ECG, and end-tidal carbon dioxide ($EtCO_2$), direct arterial blood pressure monitoring is required to identify abrupt hemodynamic changes. Transesophageal echocardiographic monitoring is also appropriate due to the complexity and the duration of surgery. It is useful in differentiating the cause of any hypotension as due to global hypokinesia, regional ischemic ventricular dysfunction, or hypovolemia. A pulmonary artery catheter may also be useful in evaluation of optimal fluid loading, but in patients with poor ventricular compliance, accurate assessment of LV end-diastolic volume may be quite difficult.

Although all types of general anesthetics have been successfully used in patients with heart failure, the doses need to be customized and titrated

TABLE 22–2 Preoperative assessment.

Volume status
Continue antidysrhythmic therapy, β blockers, and angiotensin-converting enzyme inhibitors. Discontinue diuretics and angiotensin receptor blockers.
Drug interactions with digoxin. Electrolytes–potassium/magnesium correction
Hemoglobin optimized. Recent liver function tests, renal function tests, electrocardiogram, and echocardiogram evaluated.
Implantable cardioverter defibrillator deactivation Inotropes (resistance to usual dose)
Intra-aortic balloon pump if necessary

to effect for those with an ejection fraction (EF) below 45%. Drugs such etomidate, opioids (fentanyl), and midazolam have minimal depressing effects on cardiac function and are particularly beneficial. It must be remembered, however, that addition of nitrous oxide to opioids or the combination of midazolam and opioids is associated with significant depression of CO and blood pressure. Administration of volatile anesthetic must be done cautiously in view of the dose-dependent cardiac depressant effects produced by these drugs. However, inhalation anesthesia at a low concentration (0.5–1 minimum alveolar concentration) with a low dose (2–3 mcg/kg) of fentanyl can be safely used without a decrease of cardiac contractile force. Use of vasoactive drugs like dobutamine and milrinone may be required frequently to counteract the negative effects of the anesthetics on cardiac function and increase EF.

Drug interactions in patients treated with digitalis should be anticipated. Sympathomimetics with β-agonist effects, as well as pancuronium, may increase the likelihood of cardiac dysrhythmias in patients treated with digitalis.[66] However, clinical experience does not support the occurrence of an increased incidence of cardiac dysrhythmias in patients treated with digitalis and receiving succinylcholine.[67]

Finally, the addition of positive end-expiratory pressure may be beneficial in decreasing pulmonary congestion and improving arterial oxygenation.

REFERENCES

1. Lloyd-Jones DM, Larson MG, Leip EP, et al. Lifetime risk for developing congestive heart failure: the Framingham Heart Study. *Circulation*. 2002;106:3068-3072.
2. Goldman L, Caldera DL, Nussbaum SR, et al. Multifactorial index of cardiac risk in noncardiac surgical procedures. *N Engl J Med*. 1977;297:845-850.
3. Howell SJ, Sear JW, Sear YM, Yeates D, Goldacre M, Foex P. Risk factors for cardiovascular death within 30 days after anaesthesia and urgent or emergency surgery: a nested case-control study. *Br J Anaesth*. 1999;82:679-684.
4. Flu WJ, van Kuijk JP, Hoeks SE, et al. Prognostic implications of asymptomatic left ventricular dysfunction in patients undergoing vascular surgery. *Anesthesiology*. 2010;112:1316-1324.
5. Hart CY, Redfield MM. Diastolic heart failure in the community. *Curr Cardiol Rep*. 2000;2:461.
6. Levine WC, Mehta V, Landesberg G. Anesthesia for the elderly: selected topics. *Curr Opin Anaesthesiol*. 2006;19:320-324.
7. Shammas FV, Dickstein K. Clinical pharmacokinetics in heart failure. An updated review. *Clin Pharmacokinet*. 1988;15:94-113.
8. Hepner GW, Vesell ES, Tantum KR. Reduced drug elimination in congestive heart failure. Studies using aminopyrine as a model drug. *Am J Med*. 1978;65:371.
9. Miller RD. *Miller's Anesthesia*. 7th ed. Edinburgh: Elsevier Churchill Livingstone; 2009.
10. Patel IH, Soni PP, Fukuda EK, Smith DF, Leier CV, Boudoulas H. The pharmacokinetics of midazolam in patients with congestive heart failure. *Br J Clin Pharmacol*. 1990;29:565-569.
11. Jose GM, Silva CE, Ferreira LD, et al. Effective dose of sedation in transesophageal echocardiography: relation to age, body surface area and left ventricle function. *Arq Bras Cardiol*. 2009;93:576.
12. Upton RN, Ludbrook GL, Grant C, Martinez AM. Cardiac output is a determinant of the initial concentrations of propofol after short-infusion administration. *Anesth Analg*. 1999;89:545.
13. Zheng D, Upton RN, Martinez AM, Grant C, Ludbrook GL. The influence of the bolus injection rate of propofol on its cardiovascular effects and peak blood concentrations in sheep. *Anesth Analg*. 1998;86:1109.
14. Keyl C, Trenk D, Laule S, et al. Predicted and measured plasma propofol concentration and bispectral index during deep sedation in patients with impaired left ventricular function. *J Cardiothorac Vasc Anesth*. 2009;23:182-187.
15. Kurita T, Morita K, Kazama T, Sato S. Influence of cardiac output on plasma propofol concentrations during constant infusion in swine. *Anesthesiology*. 2002;96:1498.
16. K Lim, T Lim, W Wong. *Pharmacokinetics of Thiopental in Patients with Cardiovascular Disease*. The Internet Journal of Anesthesiology. 2006; Volume 14 Number 1.
17. Wada DR, Bjorkman S, Ebling WF, Harashima H, Harapat SR, Stanski DR. Computer simulation of the effects of alterations in blood flows and body composition on thiopental pharmacokinetics in humans. *Anesthesiology*. 1997;87:884-899.

18. Wynands JE, Wong P, Whalley DG, Sprigge JS, Townsend GE, Patel YC. Oxygen-fentanyl anesthesia in patients with poor left ventricular function: hemodynamics and plasma fentanyl concentrations. *Anesth Analg*. 1983;62:476.
19. Kemmotsu O, Hashimoto Y, Shimosato S. The effects of fluroxene and enflurane on contractile performance of isolated papillary muscles from failing hearts. *Anesthesiology*. 1974;40:252.
20. Kemmotsu O, Hashimoto Y, Shimosato S. Inotropic effects of isoflurane on mechanics of contraction in isolated cat papillary muscles from normal and failing hearts. *Anesthesiology*. 1973;39:470-477.
21. Vivien B, Hanouz JL, Gueugniaud PY, Lecarpentier Y, Coriat P, Riou B. Myocardial effects of halothane and isoflurane in hamsters with hypertrophic cardiomyopathy. *Anesthesiology*. 1997;87:1406.
22. Pagel PS, Lowe D, Hettrick DA, et al. Isoflurane, but not halothane, improves indices of diastolic performance in dogs with rapid ventricular, pacing-induced cardiomyopathy. *Anesthesiology*. 1996;85:644.
23. Neuhauser C, Muller M, Welters I, Scholz S, Kwapisz MM. Effect of isoflurane on echocardiographic left-ventricular relaxation indices in patients with diastolic dysfunction due to concentric hypertrophy and ischemic heart disease. *J Cardiothorac Vasc Anesth*. 2006;20:509-514.
24. Sarkar S, GuhaBiswas R, Rupert E. Echocardiographic evaluation and comparison of the effects of isoflurane, sevoflurane and desflurane on left ventricular relaxation indices in patients with diastolic dysfunction. *Ann Card Anaesth*. 2010;13:130-137.
25. Vivien B, Hanouz JL, Gueugniaud PY, Lecarpentier Y, Coriat P, Riou B. Myocardial effects of desflurane in hamsters with hypertrophic cardiomyopathy. *Anesthesiology*. 1998;89:1191.
26. Sprung J, Ogletree-Hughes ML, Moravec CS. The effects of etomidate on the contractility of failing and nonfailing human heart muscle. *Anesth Analg*. 2000;91:68.
27. Rosow C. Remifentanil: a unique opioid analgesic. *Anesthesiology*. 1993;79:875-876.
28. Riou B, Lecarpentier Y, Viars P. Effects of etomidate on the cardiac papillary muscle of normal hamsters and those with cardiomyopathy. *Anesthesiology*. 1993;78:83.
29. Pagel PS, Hettrick DA, Kersten JR, Tessmer JP, Lowe D, Warltier DC. Etomidate adversely alters determinants of left ventricular afterload in dogs with dilated cardiomyopathy. *Anesth Analg*. 1998;86:932.
30. Sprung J, Schuetz SM, Stewart RW, Moravec CS. Effects of ketamine on the contractility of failing and nonfailing human heart muscles in vitro. *Anesthesiology*. 1998;88:1202.
31. Hanouz JL, Persehaye E, Zhu L, et al. The inotropic and lusitropic effects of ketamine in isolated human atrial myocardium: the effect of adrenoceptor blockade. *Anesth Analg*. 2004;99:1689-1695.
32. Pagel PS, Schmeling WT, Kampine JP, Warltier DC. Alteration of canine left ventricular diastolic function by intravenous anesthetics in vivo. Ketamine and propofol. *Anesthesiology*. 1992;76:419.
33. Christ G, Mundigler G, Merhaut C, et al. Adverse cardiovascular effects of ketamine infusion in patients with catecholamine-dependent heart failure. *Anaesth Intensive Care*. 1997;25:255.
34. Reves JG, Samuelson PN, Linnan M. Effects of midazolam maleate in patients with elevated pulmonary artery occluded pressure. In: Aldrete JA, Stanley TH, eds. *Trends in Intravenous Anesthesia*. Chicago: Yearbook Medical Publishers; 1980:253.
35. Messina AG, Paranicas M, Yao FS, et al. The effect of midazolam on left ventricular pump performance and contractility in anesthetized patients with coronary artery disease: effect of preoperative ejection fraction. *Anesth Analg*. 1995;81:793-799.
36. Gare M, Parail A, Milosavljevic D, Kersten JR, Warltier DC, Pagel PS. Conscious sedation with midazolam or propofol does not alter left ventricular diastolic performance in patients with preexisting diastolic dysfunction: a transmitral and tissue Doppler transthoracic echocardiography study. *Anesth Analg*. 2001;93:865.
37. Reves JG, Kissin I, Fournier S. Negative inotropic effects of midazolam. *Anesthesiology*. 1984;60:517.
38. Ouattara A, Langeron O, Souktani R, Mouren S, Coriat P, Riou B. Myocardial and coronary effects of propofol in rabbits with compensated cardiac hypertrophy. *Anesthesiology*. 2001;95:699-707.
39. Hebbar L, Dorman BH, Clair MJ, Roy RC, Spinale FG. Negative and selective effects of propofol on isolated swine myocyte contractile function in pacing-induced congestive heart failure. *Anesthesiology*. 1997;86:649.
40. Moravec CS, Schuetz SM, Stewart RW. Propofol exerts a direct negative inotropic effect on failing human ventricle. *Anesth Analg*. 1997;84:S108.
41. Riou B, Besse S, Lecarpentier Y, Viars P. In vitro effects of propofol on rat myocardium. *Anesthesiology*. 1992;76:609.
42. Riou B, Lejay M, Lecarpentier Y, Viars P. Myocardial effects of propofol in hamsters with hypertrophic cardiomyopathy. *Anesthesiology*. 1995;82:566-573.
43. Sprung J, Ogletree-Hughes ML, McConnell BK, Zakhary DR, Smolsky SM, Moravec CS. The effects of

propofol on the contractility of failing and nonfailing human heart muscles. *Anesth Analg.* 2001;93:550.

44. Bell J, Sartain J, Wilkinson GA, Sherry KM. Propofol and fentanyl anaesthesia for patients with low cardiac output state undergoing cardiac surgery: comparison with high-dose fentanyl anaesthesia. *Br J Anaesth.* 1994;73:162.
45. Hall RI, Murphy JT, Landymore R, Pollak PT, Doak G, Murray M. Myocardial metabolic and hemodynamic changes during propofol anesthesia for cardiac surgery in patients with reduced ventricular function. *Anesth Analg.* 1993;77:680-689.
46. Pagel PS, Hettrick DA, Kersten JR, Lowe D, Warltier DC. Cardiovascular effects of propofol in dogs with dilated cardiomyopathy. *Anesthesiology.* 1998;88:180.
47. Camci E, Koltka K, Sungur Z, et al. Implantable cardioverter-defibrillator placement in patients with mild-to- moderate left ventricular dysfunction: hemodynamics and recovery profile with two different anesthetics used during deep sedation. *J Cardiothorac Vasc Anesth.* 2003;17:613.
48. Filipovic M, Michaux I, Wang J, Hunziker P, Skarvan K, Seeberger M. Effects of sevoflurane and propofol on left ventricular diastolic function in patients with pre-existing diastolic dysfunction. *Br J Anaesth.* 2007;98:12-18.
49. Bril A, Forest MC, Gout B. Ischemia and reperfusion-induced arrhythmias in rabbits with chronic heart failure. *Am J Physiol.* 1991;261:H301.
50. Belch JJ, Bridges AB, Scott N, Chopra M. Oxygen free radicals and congestive heart failure. *Br Heart J.* 1991;65:245.
51. McMurray J, Chopra M, Abdullah I, Smith WE, Dargie HJ. Evidence of oxidative stress in chronic heart failure in humans. *Eur Heart J.* 1993;14:1493-1498.
52. Corcoran TB, Engel A, Sakamoto H, O'Shea A, O'Callaghan-Enright S, Shorten GD. The effects of propofol on neutrophil function, lipid preoxidation and inflammatory response during elective coronary artery bypass grafting in patients with impaired ventricular function. *Br J Anaesth.* 2006;97:825.
53. Traabadkar S, Kopriva CJ, Sreenivasan N, Leschovich F, Barash PG. Hemodynamic impact of induction in patients with decreased cardiac reserve. *Anesthesiology.* 1980;53:S43.
54. Zhang CC, Su JY, Calkins D. Effects of alfentanil on isolated cardiac tissues of the rabbit. *Anesth Analg.* 1990;71:268-274.
55. Strauer BE. Contractile responses to morphine, piritramide, meperidine, and fentanyl: a comparative study of effects on the isolated ventricular myocardium. *Anesthesiology.* 1972;37:304.
56. Kohno K, Takaki M, Ishioka K, et al. Effects of intracoronary fentanyl on left ventricular mechanoenergetics in the excised cross-circulated canine heart (revised publication). *Anesthesiology.* 1997; 87:658.
57. Wynands JE, Townsend GE, Wong P, Whalley DG, Srikant CB, Patel YC. Blood pressure response and plasma fentanyl concentrations during high- and very high-dose fentanyl anesthesia for coronary artery surgery. *Anesth Analg.* 1983;62:661-665.
58. Gutzke GE, Shah KB, Glisson SN, et al. Cardiac transplantation: a prospective comparison of ketamine and sufentanil for anesthetic induction. *J Cardiothorac Anesth.* 1989;3:389.
59. Llobel F, Laorden ML. Effects of morphine on atrial preparations obtained from nonfailing and failing human hearts. *Br J Anaesth.* 1996;76:106.
60. Moraes DL, Colucci WS, Givertz MM. Secondary pulmonary hypertension in chronic heart failure: the role of the endothelium in pathophysiology and management. *Circulation.* 2000;102:1718-1723.
61. Szabo G, Soos P, Bahrle S, et al. Adaptation of the right ventricle to an increased afterload in the chronically volume overloaded heart. *Ann Thorac Surg.* 2006;82:989.
62. Price LC, Forrest P, Sodhi V, et al. Use of vasopressin after Caesarean section in idiopathic pulmonary arterial hypertension. *Br J Anaesth.* 2007;99:552.
63. Poelzl G, Zwick RH, Grander W, et al. Safety and effectiveness of levosimendan in patients with predominant right heart failure. *Herz.* 2008;33:368-373.
64. Kerbaul F, Rondelet B, Demester JP, et al. Effects of levosimendan versus dobutamine on pressure load-induced right ventricular failure. *Crit Care Med.* 2006;34:2814.
65. Sharma R, Francis DP, Pitt B, Poole-Wilson PA, Coats AJ, Anker SD. Haemoglobin predicts survival in patients with chronic heart failure: a substudy of the ELITE II trial. *Eur Heart J.* 2004;25:1021-1028.
66. Cohen MC, Pierce ET, Bode RH, et al. Types of anesthesia and cardiovascular outcomes in patients with congestive heart failure undergoing vascular surgery. *Congest Heart Fail.* 1999;5:248-253.
67. Bartolone RS, Rao TL. Dysrhythmias following muscle relaxant administration in patients receiving digitalis. *Anesthesiology.* 1983;58:567-569.

CHAPTER 23

Implications of Blood Loss on Anesthetic Drugs

Ken B. Johnson, MD

INTRODUCTION

An interesting case report published in 2002 perhaps best sets the stage for understanding what anesthesiologists face when caring for a patient who suffers from severe blood loss while under an anesthetic.[1] In this case report, a 70-year-old woman is anesthetized using a total intravenous technique with propofol and alfentanil for an elective aortic abdominal aneurysm repair. Routine monitors and a Bispectral Index Scale (BIS) monitor were used. The patient was enrolled as a study subject exploring the antioxidant effects of propofol. The procedure and anesthetic were unremarkable until after the cross-clamp was removed; then, the BIS values dropped first (mid-30s to below 20) followed 7 minutes later by a blood pressure drop (systolic pressure fell from about 120 to about 60 mm Hg) (**Figure 23–1**). Results from the measured plasma propofol concentrations were also very compelling. At the time of cross-clamping, target and measured propofol concentrations were 5.0 and 4.7 mcg/mL, respectively. After the cross-clamp was removed, they were 3.0 and 7.2 mcg/mL, respectively. Thus, even though clinicians sought to decrease propofol dosing, plasma concentrations were more than double the desired level.

Dr. Halford, a surgeon, submitted a letter to the editor of *Anesthesiology* after caring for several trauma victims after the attack on Pearl Harbor in 1941. He noticed poor outcomes in patients anesthetized with intravenous anesthetic sodium pentothal. He commented: "Then let it be said that intravenous anesthesia is also an ideal form of euthanasia...With this heterogeneous mass of emergency anesthetists, it is necessary to choose an anesthetic involving the *widest margin of safety* for the patient ... Stick with *ether.*"[2]

Anesthesiologists recognize that (1) a full dose of certain anesthetics can lead to pronounced and often unwanted side effects with potentially disastrous consequences, (2) the need to be selective in choice of anesthetic, (3) and the need to incrementally dose their anesthetics for patients who have significant blood loss before or during surgery. The scientific basis for this practice, however, has not been well established. The main reason for this gap in anesthetic pharmacology research is that it is difficult and unethical to study how significant blood loss influences anesthetic in humans who suffer from hemorrhagic shock. As such, much of what drives clinical practice is based on research in animal models of hemorrhagic shock and limited observations in clinical practice, largely from case reports.

This chapter will review what is known about how blood loss and resuscitation influence the pharmacologic behavior of commonly used anesthetics (opioids, sedative–hypnotics, and inhalation agents) and the rational selection and dosing of these anesthetics when used for induction and/or maintenance of anesthesia. It will then formulate a set of key points targeted at improving patient safety.

INTRAVENOUS ANESTHETICS

Pharmacokinetics

Researchers have investigated how blood loss and hemorrhagic shock influence the behavior of numerous anesthetics that include sedative hypnotics,[3-9] benzodiazepines,[8,10] opioids,[11-14] and local anesthetics.[15] The most consistent finding is that equivalent dosing leads to higher drug concentrations in severe blood loss when compared with

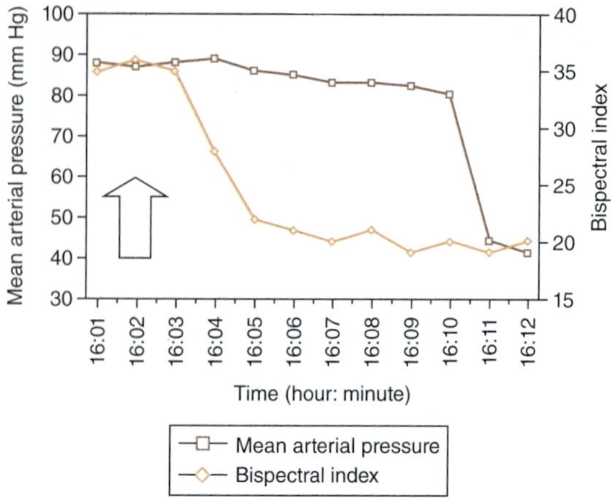

FIGURE 23–1 Changes in bispectral index and mean arterial blood pressure after declamping (arrow.).[1] (Reproduced with permission from Honan DM, Breen PJ, Boylan JF, McDonald NJ, Egan TD. Decrease in bispectral index preceding intraoperative hemodynamic crisis: evidence of acute alteration of propofol pharmacokinetics. *Anesthesiology* 2002;Nov;97(5):1303-5.)

normal hemodynamic conditions. Decreased blood volume and cardiac output[16,17] along with compensatory changes in vascular tone may explain these pharmacokinetic changes.

As an example, consider prior work exploring how moderate hemorrhage influences the pharmacokinetic profile of propofol.[5] This study included a series of pilot studies in swine to identify:

- The extent of blood loss (mL/kg) required to reach and maintain a target mean arterial blood pressure (MAP).
- The propofol infusion rate (mcg/kg/min) that would achieve near-maximal drug effect (ie, BIS near 0) but allow animal subjects to survive the study period.

Based on prior work with remifentanil,[13] an isobaric hemorrhage protocol (ie, blood removal to maintain a target pressure) removed a large volume of blood (48 mL/kg) over approximately 1 hour to maintain a MAP of 40 mm Hg. This was followed by a high remifentanil infusion of 10 mcg/kg/min for 10 minutes. This infusion rate is approximately 50- to 100-fold more than is used in clinical practice (0.1 to 0.2 mcg/kg/min). It is interesting to point out that when using this hemorrhage protocol and the high-dose remifentanil infusion, all animals survived.

When switching to propofol, in euvolemic control animals, a propofol infusion of 750 mcg/kg/min for 10 minutes was required to reach maximal effect (ie, BIS near 0). Using the same hemorrhage protocol used with remifentanil, a propofol infusion rate of 750 mcg/kg/min for 10 minutes was lethal. So were infusion rates of 500, 250, and 125 mcg/kg/min. Similar to what Dr. Halford experienced with sodium pentothal, it was clear that propofol's cardiovascular depressant properties were harmful in severe blood loss.

Unlike remifentanil, propofol infusion rates required to achieve maximal effect under euvolemic conditions were not tolerated after a 50% loss in blood volume. Key points from these pilot studies were:

- Selected sedative–hypnotics known to have cardiovascular depressant effects to include propofol and sodium pentothal are not well tolerated during or following moderate to severe blood loss.
- Even conventional doses can lead to cardiovascular collapse and death. If these drugs are to be used, doses should be markedly reduced to achieve desired clinical endpoints in sedation and hypnosis.
- By contrast, opioids, ketamine, and etomidate are better tolerated during or following moderate to severe hemorrhagic shock.

By conducting additional pilot studies, it was discovered that with moderate blood loss (30 mL/kg), animals would tolerate a low propofol infusion rate (200 mcg/kg/min). Although not nearly as severe as the blood loss tolerated with the remifentanil infusion, animals did exhibit hemodynamic signs and a metabolic profile consistent with hemorrhage shock (ie, tachycardia, low central venous pressure, low cardiac index [decreasing from 5.0 to 2.6 L/min/m^2], and lactic acidemia). The most important finding was that plasma propofol levels during and 3 hours following a brief 10-minute infusion were approximately 2-fold higher in the shock group (Figure 23–2). A pharmacokinetic analysis fitting a 3-compartment model to the propofol plasma concentrations over time for

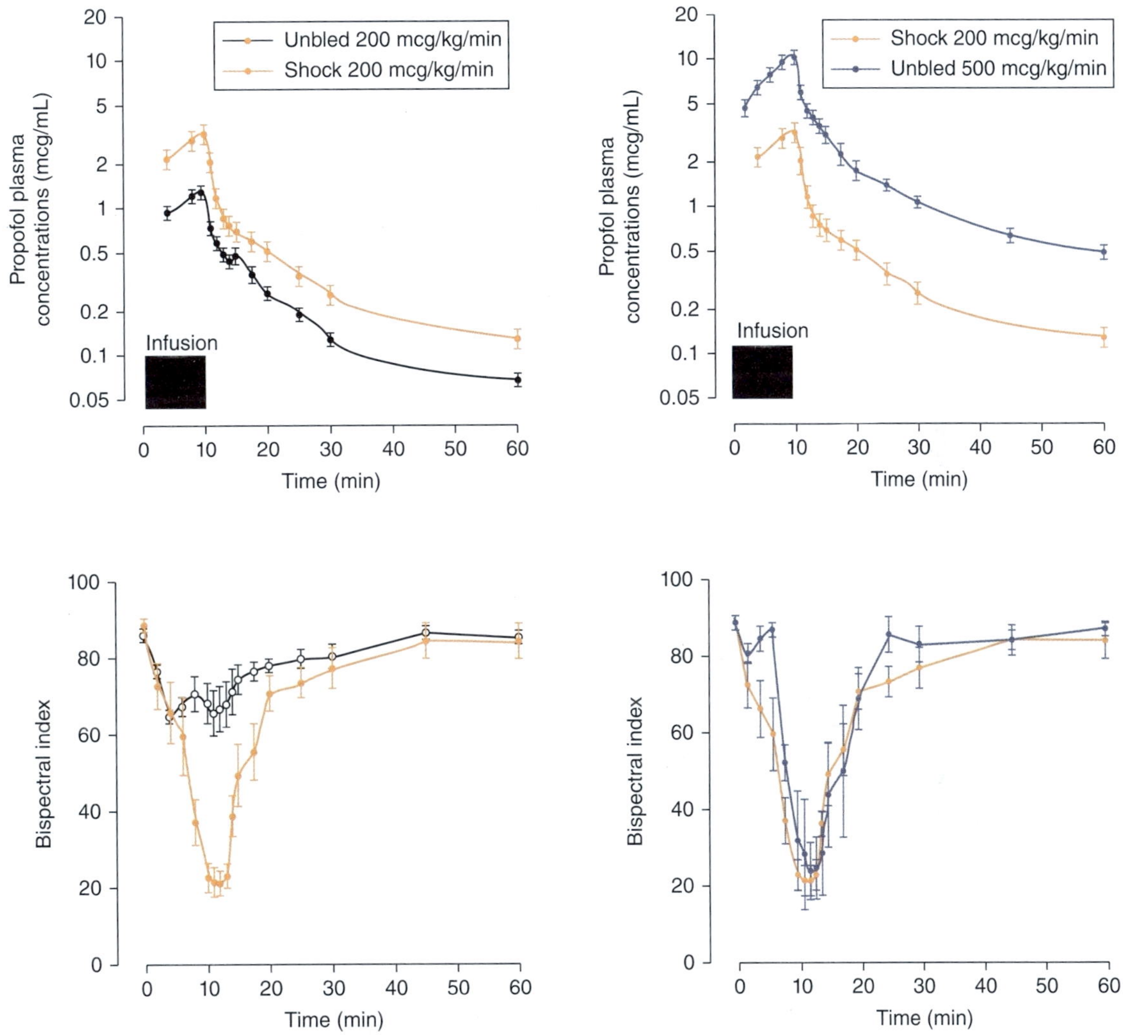

FIGURE 23–2 Presentation of measured plasma propofol concentrations and Bispectral Index Scale (BIS) levels in a swine hemorrhage model.[5] The top plots present the mean propofol plasma concentration versus time following an infusion of propofol. The left top plot presents the plasma concentrations from a 10-minute 200-mcg/kg/min infusion to bled (30 mL/kg) and euvolemic swine. The right top plot presents the plasma concentrations from a 10-minute 200-mcg/kg/min infusion to bled swine and a 500- mcg/kg/min infusion to euvolemic swine. The y-axis is on a log scale. The bottom plots represent the mean BIS levels in each group. Key points are:

- At an equivalent infusion rate (200 mcg/kg/min), propofol produces an effect (change in BIS) in bled animals but not euvolemic normotensive animals.
- When the infusion rate is increased 2.5-fold for euvolemic normotensive animals, the effect is near equivalent to what is observed in bled animals.

(Reproduced with permission from Johnson KB, Egan TD, Kern SE et al: The Influence of Hemorrhagic Shock on Propofol: A Pharmacokinetic and Pharmacodynamic Analysis, *Anesthesiology* 2003 Aug;99(2):409-420.)

euvolemic controls and the shock group revealed that compartment volumes were smaller and compartmental clearances were decreased in the shock group (Table 23–1).

Although compartment volumes and clearances do not represent true organ drug distribution and clearance, the changes do suggest that blood flow to peripheral tissues is markedly decreased such

TABLE 23–1 Summary of propofol pharmacokinetic parameter estimates by group.[5]

Parameter	Control Group	Shock Group
Volumes (L)		
Central compartment (V_1)	4.7	3.5
Rapidly equilibrating peripheral compartment (V_2)	16.7	7.4
Slowly equilibrating peripheral compartment (V_3)	232	165
Clearance (L/min)		
Elimination clearance (Cl_1)	1.6	0.8
Fast distribution clearance (Cl_2)	4.6	1.0
Slow distribution clearance (Cl_3)	1.9	0.9

Reproduced with permission from Johnson KB, Egan TD, Kern SE et al: The Influence of Hemorrhagic Shock on Propofol: A Pharmacokinetic and Pharmacodynamic Analysis, Anesthesiology 2003 Aug;99(2):409-420.

that intravenous anesthetics are essentially pumped straight to the brain in higher concentrations, leading to a more pronounced anesthetic effect.[18]

In this analysis, BIS was used as a surrogate measure of drug effect. In hypovolemic group, the propofol infusion produced a large decrease in the BIS that returned to baseline within 30 minutes of the infusion but had minimal effect in the euvolemic control group. To achieve a similar change in the BIS in the control group, the infusion rate had to be increased to 500 mcg/kg/min (see Figure 23–2).

Kurita et al recently studied the simultaneous infusion of propofol (100 mcg/kg/min) and remifentanil (0.5 mcg/kg/min) during compensated and uncompensated hemorrhagic shock in a swine model.[14] Plasma propofol and remifentanil concentrations increased during both compensated and uncompensated hemorrhagic shock, but the increase was more pronounced during uncompensated hemorrhagic shock. Uncompensated hemorrhagic shock was defined as the transition from increasing to decreasing systemic vascular resistance. In this study, 10% of estimated blood volume was removed every 30 minutes for 90 minutes followed by removal of 5% of estimated blood volume every 20 minutes until circulatory collapse. The onset of uncompensated hemorrhagic shock occurred within 3 to 4 hours at a point where 35% to 40% of the blood volume had been removed.

During the compensatory phase of this hemorrhage protocol, the rise in remifentanil and propofol concentrations as a percentage change from baseline concentrations prior to hemorrhage were different. Remifentanil plasma concentrations rose as a function of blood loss 3 times faster than propofol. The study results indicated that 30 minutes into the hemorrhage protocol, remifentanil concentrations increased by 95% over baseline. Propofol required 50 minutes to achieve the same percentage change over baseline. Once in the decompensatory phase, both remifentanil and propofol plasma concentrations rose at an even faster rate, with remifentanil out-pacing propofol until cardiovascular collapse.

The authors put forth several proposed mechanisms to describe their observations. They suggest that propofol concentrations were relatively insensitive to changes in cardiac output during the compensatory phase of hemorrhagic shock but became very sensitive during the uncompensated phase associated with a large decrease in cardiac output. Remifentanil was somewhat less sensitive to cardiac output changes. This may be because of remifentanil's metabolism by nonspecific esterases in peripheral tissues. This explains the large increase in remifentanil plasma concentrations once perfusion to peripheral tissues was decreased.[14]

Pharmacodynamics

Pharmacodynamics describes the concentration-effect relationship and parameters that describe a sigmoid curve (ie, effect-site concentration versus effect) to include E_{max} (a measure of the maximal effect), C_{50} (the effect-site concentration that produces 50% of the maximal effect), and γ (a measure of curve steepness) are used to characterize drug potency.

Prior work exploring changes in propofol pharmacodynamic parameters between euvolemic and hemorrhagic hypovolemic conditions in swine and

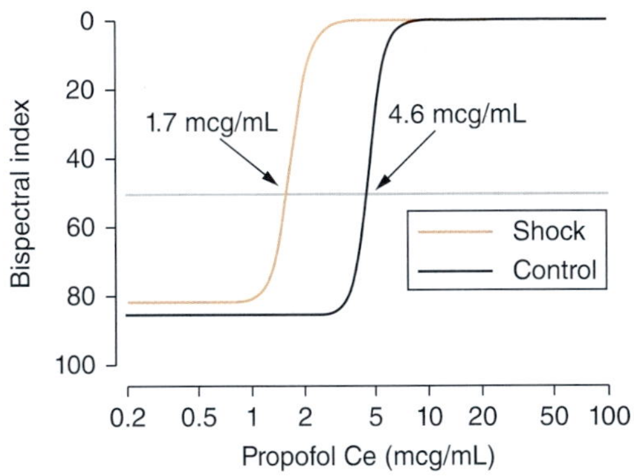

FIGURE 23–3 The concentration-effect relationship as characterized by the pharmacodynamic model. The black line represents the mean change in the Bispectral Index Scale (BIS) over a range of propofol effect-site concentration (Ce) levels for unbled controls. The orange lines represent the mean change in the BIS over a range of propofol Ce levels for bled animals. The black arrows illustrate the shift in the C_{50} between groups.[5]

rats has revealed that C_{50} was shifted to the left.[3,5] For example, in swine the C_{50} is 2.7-fold less in the shock group (4.6 versus 1.7 mcg/mL for the control and shock groups, respectively; Figure 23–3). The mechanism of how blood loss increases propofol potency is not clear but may be the result of a rise in circulating endorphins. The effects of propofol are known to synergistically interact with opioids.[19,20] Blood loss does lead to a rise in circulating β endorphins.[21-23] Hence, high levels of beta endorphins may interact synergistically with propofol to increase its potency. However, De Paepe et al[3] found that endorphin antagonism with naloxone did not influence end-organ sensitivity to propofol in a rodent hemorrhage shock model.

Other potential sources of increased propofol potency during or after hemorrhagic shock may include:

- An alteration in the end-organ response to propofol because of the lactic acidemia, hyperkalemia, tissue hypoxia, or other metabolic disturbances,
- An undetected increase in the fraction of unbound propofol because of decreased lipophilic binding sites within whole blood[24]

Clinical Implications

Perhaps the most dangerous implications of these results are during induction of anesthesia. After a propofol bolus, the concentration rapidly rises and then slowly decays, with effect-site concentrations lagging behind. This lag time represents the time required for a drug to diffuse from the bloodstream to the site of action and to exert an effect.

Prior work has explored propofol threshold effect-site concentrations associated with loss of responsiveness to various stimuli (ie, verbal or noxious).[25] By using these thresholds, simulations of the effect-site concentration over time can be used to predict the onset and the duration of analgesia and loss of responsiveness (Figure 23–4). The simulations show that the time to loss of response to verbal prompting occurs in approximately 1 minute followed by the loss of response to a noxious stimulus in 90 seconds. The duration of effect for loss of response to verbal stimuli and noxious stimuli are 5 and 3 minutes, respectively. It is important to point out that these times are for a propofol bolus only and perhaps does not reflect the routine practice of using an opioid and a sedative–hypnotic during the induction of anesthesia.

Figure 23–4 represents a simulation of the propofol effect-site concentration following a propofol bolus dose in a patient with an estimated blood loss of 35% of his or her blood volume. This simulation illustrates how pharmacokinetic *and* pharmacodynamic changes influence the duration of effect. This simulation accounts for the kinetic changes as manifest by an approximate 2.5-fold increase in the peak plasma propofol concentration and also the dynamic changes as manifest by a 2.7-fold decrease in the effect-site concentration required for loss of response to verbal and noxious stimuli. The onset of effect is accelerated by approximately 60 to 90 seconds, and the duration of effect for both stimuli is more than doubled (from 6 to 28 minutes for verbal stimuli and from 3 to 18 minutes for noxious stimuli).

Perhaps the most important consequence of blood loss on propofol behavior is the exaggerated hemodynamic response following a bolus dose. Propofol vasodilates peripheral vessels and suppresses contractility.[27-30] Based on the simulations

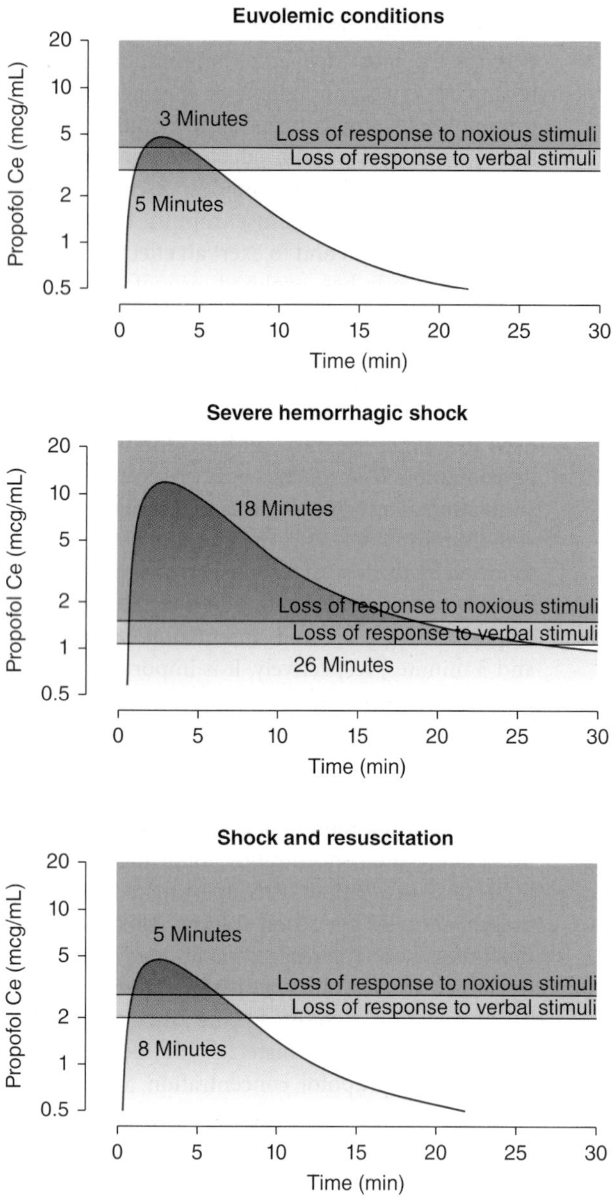

FIGURE 23–4 Illustration of how propofol may behave for 3 conditions: euvolemic normotension (top), hemorrhagic shock (middle), and hemorrhagic shock followed by resuscitation (bottom). This illustration uses simulations of a 2-mg/kg propofol bolus, which are based on the observed pharmacokinetic changes found to occur in swine models of moderate hemorrhage (30-mL/kg blood loss) and severe hemorrhage–partial resuscitation (42 mL/kg blood loss followed by 60 mL/kg of crystalloid).[5,26] Specifically, these changes include an approximate 2.5-fold increase in plasma propofol concentrations with moderate hemorrhage and minimal change with severe hemorrhage followed by partial resuscitation. The gray regions represent thresholds of predicted concentrations that lead to a loss of response to verbal prompting (light gray) and noxious stimuli (dark gray). These thresholds are based on previously reported observations in humans[25] and have been modified to account for the observed shifts in propofol C_{50} under each of these conditions (specifically, a 2.7-fold reduction with moderate hemorrhage and a 1.5 reduction with severe hemorrhage followed by partial resuscitation). These simulations predict the duration of effect (in minutes) for each condition. Key points are:

- The duration of each effect is relatively short with euvolemic conditions (top plot).
- Following moderate hemorrhage, the duration of each effect is markedly prolonged (middle plot).
- With severe hemorrhage and resuscitation, despite minimal changes in propofol kinetics, the duration of each effect is somewhat prolonged.

Ce, effect-site concentration. (Reproduced with permission from Smith CE: Trauma Anesthesia, 1st edition. New York, NY: Cambridge University Press, 2008.)

presented in Figure 23–4, of a propofol bolus dose leads to higher effect-site concentrations that remain elevated for a prolonged period of time, it is likely that they will amplify propofol's cardiovascular suppression. This may explain why Dr. Halford was so adamant about the dangers of intravenous anesthetic induction agents in victims of trauma at Pearl Harbor. With large blood loss, propofol should be used, if at all, with extreme caution! From these simulations, if we were to work backward and determine the appropriate dose for a person suffering from severe blood loss to render an equivalent effect in a euvolemic normotensive person, the propofol dose would be reduced 5-fold, to 0.4 mg/kg.

Resuscitation

Although interesting, the influence of severe blood loss on propofol does not reflect clinical practice where some degree of resuscitation has occurred before induction of anesthesia. Based on the premise that resuscitation will restore cardiac output and systemic blood flow, the shock-induced kinetic and dynamic changes may be reversed.

In a similar set of experiments, a comparison was made between unbled controls and bled and then resuscitated swine.[26] Blood loss was severe (42 mL/kg). Following hemorrhage, 59 mL/kg of lactated Ringer solution were infused over an hour to keep the MAP at 70 mm Hg. The plot in Figure 23–5 illustrates the time course of a 10-minute high-dose propofol infusion (750 mcg/kg/min). The propofol plasma concentrations were nearly identical. Resuscitation restored the shock-induced changes in propofol pharmacokinetics to near-baseline values (most likely due to a restoration in cardiac output, a major determinant of propofol kinetics with bolus administration). Distribution volumes and compartment clearances were nearly identical between groups.

The shock-induced increase in end-organ sensitivity to propofol after blood loss, however, was reduced but persisted with resuscitation. Although the propofol C_{50} increased from 2.7-fold following hemorrhage, it was still 1.5-fold higher following hemorrhage and resuscitation. Although the mechanism for this phenomenon is not well understood, increased end-organ sensitivity associated with severe blood loss persisted after resuscitation despite near normalization of the pharmacokinetics.

In this study, the hemorrhage protocol produced an estimated 60% decrease in blood volume. The resuscitation protocol replaced approximately 140% of the shed blood volume with lactated Ringer solution to maintain a near-normotensive MAP. The near-normal blood pressure was deceiving. The resuscitative effort was incomplete. Although the hemodynamic function appeared near normal, as manifest by a return of central venous pressure and cardiac index to baseline levels, the cardiovascular response to propofol remained exaggerated. During the propofol infusion, the cardiac index dropped 1.7 L/min/m^2 in the shock-resuscitation group but only 0.2 L/min/m^2 in the control group. The large hemodynamic changes in the shock-resuscitation group illustrate how propofol can lead to large cardiovascular changes despite a near-normal hemodynamic profile following partial resuscitation.

Figure 23–4 presents a simulation of the propofol effect-site concentration following a propofol bolus dose in a patient suffering from severe blood loss followed by partial resuscitation with crystalloid (1.5 mL of crystalloid per mL of estimated blood loss). This simulation accounts for the pharmacodynamic changes as manifest by a 1.5-fold decrease in the effect-site concentration required for loss of response to verbal and noxious stimuli. The onset of effect is accelerated by approximately 30 to 60 seconds, and the durations of effect for both stimuli are increased (from 6 to 8 minutes for verbal stimuli and from 3 to 6 minutes for noxious stimuli).

With partial crystalloid resuscitation, key points include:

- The exaggerated hemodynamic response to propofol is diminished but persists and may produce potentially dangerous cardiovascular depression.
- Shock-induced changes in propofol kinetics previously observed after hemorrhagic shock are restored to near baseline.
- Shock-induced changes in pharmacodynamics are diminished yet persist to a degree that conventional dosing can lead to a more pronounced drug effect.

A summary of the propofol bolus simulation (normal conditions, blood loss, and resuscitation following resuscitation) is presented in Table 23–2.

Opioids in Hemorrhagic Shock

Similar to propofol, opioids have an altered pharmacologic profile following severe blood loss. In experiments similar to those described for propofol, brief high-dose infusions led to plasma concentrations of opioid that were up to 2-fold higher in bled animals than unbled controls.[12,13] Both fentanyl and remifentanil exhibited pharmacokinetic changes to include a reduced volume of distribution and a decrease in drug clearance that were consistent with what has been observed with propofol[3,5] following blood loss.

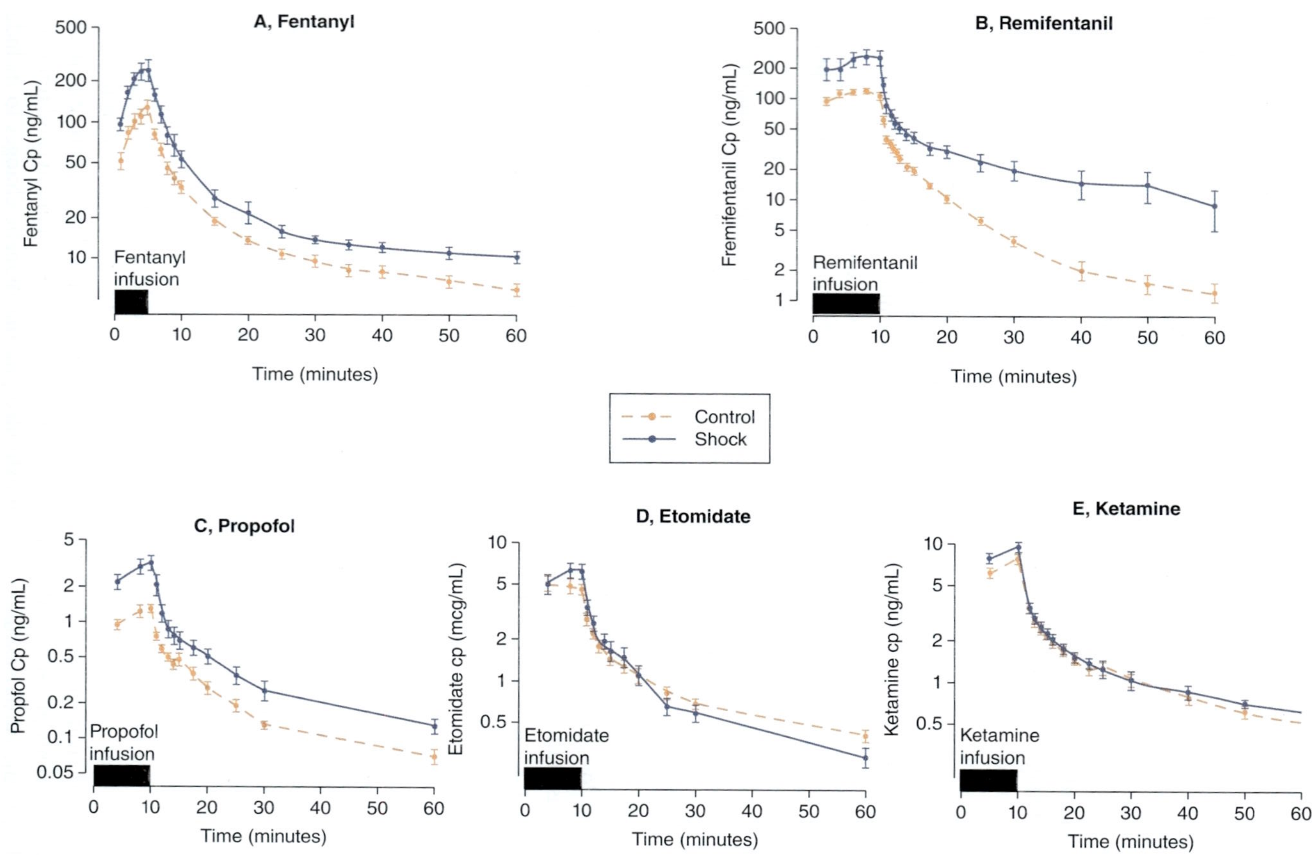

FIGURE 23–5 Plasma levels over time following brief infusions or bolus dosing for 5 intravenous anesthetics for euvolemic and hemorrhagic shock conditions (A–E). The solid and dashed lines represents unbled (control group) and bled (shock group) swine.[5,6,12,13,31] The y axis is on the log scale. Plasma ketamine levels represent the sum of the racemic ketamine enantiomers.[31] The key point is: plasma concentrations for euvolemic normotensive controls are near equivalent for etomidate and ketamine but not for remifentanil, fentanyl, and propofol when compared to hemorrhagic shock. Compiled from Johnson KB, Egan TD, Kern SE, White JL, McJames SW, Syroid N, et al. The Influence of Hemorrhagic Shock on Propofol: A Pharmacokinetic and Pharmacodynamic Analysis. Anesthesiology 2003;99(2):409-20; Johnson KB, Egan TD, Layman J, Kern SE, White JL, McJames SW. The influence of hemorrhagic shock on etomidate: a pharmacokinetic and pharmacodynamic analysis. Anesthesia and analgesia 2003;96(5):1360-8; Egan TD, Kuramkote S, Gong G, Zhang J, McJames SW, Bailey PL. Fentanyl pharmacokinetics in hemorrhagic shock: a porcine model. Anesthesiology 1999;91(1):156-66; Johnson KB, Kern SE, Hamber EA, McJames SW, Kohnstamm KM, Egan TD. Influence of hemorrhagic shock on remifentanil; a pharmacokinetic and pharmacodynamic analysis. Anesthesiology 2001;94(2):322-32; Black I, Grathwohl K, IB T, Martini W, Johnson K. The Influence of Hemorrhagic Shock on Ketamine: A Pharmacokinetic Analysis. Anesthesiology 2006;ASA Annual Meeting Abstracts:A203.

TABLE 23–2 Clinical implications of blood loss and resuscitation with a 2-mg/kg bolus of propofol: a summary of simulations exploring how pharmacokinetic and pharmacodynamic changes influence the pharmacologic behavior of propofol.

	Normal Euvolemia Normotensive	Blood Loss Hypovolemia Hypotensive	Resuscitation Following Blood Loss Mild Hypovolemia Normotensive
Propofol Ce for LOR to verbal stimuli	2.9 mcg/mL	1.1 mcg/mL	1.9 mcg/mL
Time to LOR to verbal stimuli	1 min	< 1 min	1 min
Duration of LOR to verbal stimuli	5 min	26 min	7 min
Propofol Ce for LOR to noxious stimuli	4.1 mcg/mL	1.5 mcg/mL	2.7 mcg/mL
Time to LOR to noxious stimuli	1 min	< 1 min	1 min
Duration of LOR to noxious stimuli	3 min	18 min	5 min

Simulations were performed using drug infusion simulation software (STANPUMP, Stanford University, Palo Alto, CA). Pharmacokinetic and pharmacodynamic parameters were adapted for simulation from Johnson et al.[5,26] Thresholds for LOR to verbal and noxious stimuli were adapted from work by Struys et al.[25]
Ce, effect-site concentration; LOR, loss of responsiveness.

These pharmacokinetic changes suggest that in the presence of moderate to severe blood loss, opioid dosing can be reduced by 50% to achieve a desired analgesic effect.

However, there are some important differences between the pharmacologic profile of opioids and propofol following hemorrhagic shock. When compared with propofol, the doses of opioid delivered following moderate to severe hemorrhage were, by contrast, much higher. For example, following a 30-mL/kg hemorrhage, swine would only tolerate a propofol dose of 200 mcg/kg/min for 10 minutes. This dose is notable for 3 reasons: (1) it was adequate to achieve the desired effect (near-maximal effect in the BIS), and higher doses were found to be lead to *irreversible* cardiovascular collapse; (2) it was 2.5-fold less than the dose required to achieve near-maximal effect in the unbled controls; and (3) this dose represents only a modest increase in what is typically administered to achieve sedation during a general anesthetic. By contrast, following a 25-mL/kg hemorrhage, swine tolerated a brief fentanyl infusion of 10 mcg/kg/min for 5 minutes.[12] This infusion rate represents a dose that is nearly 5- to 10-fold more than what is required to produce analgesia. The infusion was tolerated in *both* bled and unbled animal subjects. The cardiovascular depression from high-dose fentanyl in the presence of moderate blood loss was minimal. An important take-home message is that higher doses of fentanyl are better tolerated with less cardiovascular depression during hemorrhagic shock and demonstrate the wider therapeutic range of opioids when compared with propofol.

With regard to the influence of hemorrhagic shock on the pharmacodynamic profile of opioids, prior work has reported that the dynamics of remifentanil is relatively immune to the consequences of severe blood loss. This is again in stark contrast to what has been observed with propofol.

The Impact of Blood Loss on Etomidate and Ketamine

By comparison with propofol, both ketamine and etomidate have a higher degree of acceptance among clinicians caring for patients with significant blood loss. This is largely because the cardiovascular depression known to be exaggerated with propofol and sodium pentothal is not as apparent with etomidate—and even to a lesser extent with ketamine. For example, although etomidate is known to produce mild cardiovascular depression, prior work, surprisingly, has revealed minimal cardiovascular change following a high-dose, brief continuous etomidate infusion[10] during moderate hemorrhagic shock (30 mL/kg). As well, the kinetic and dynamic profile of etomidate following blood loss has also been found to be minimally influenced by blood loss.

Similar to etomidate, preliminary work has suggested that severe blood loss minimally influences the pharmacokinetic behavior of ketamine.[31] Ketamine is known to increase sympathetic tone, serve as a potent analgesic, and perform favorably in patients with poor cardiovascular function. During severe hemorrhage (39 mL/kg) in swine, equivalent dosing surprisingly led to near-equivalent plasma levels during and after a brief high-dose infusion. One disadvantage to studying ketamine is that it is difficult to characterize the influence of blood loss on the pharmacodynamic behavior. This is because it is difficult to identify and measure a surrogate of ketamine's sedative or analgesic effect (ie, BIS is not a reliable measure of ketamine's sedative effect).

Nevertheless, these preliminary results suggest that dosing requirements for ketamine and etomidate require minimal adjustment following moderate to severe blood loss and that these are important drugs to maintain in our pharmacologic armamentarium when caring for patients suffering from life-threatening blood loss.

INHALATION ANESTHETICS

Most work exploring the influence of hemorrhagic shock an inhalation anesthetic behavior has been done with isoflurane in various animal models.[32-37] The most important finding of this body of work is that inhalation agents behave much different during hemorrhagic shock and resuscitation than selected intravenous anesthetics. In fact, under conditions of moderate blood loss, the changes in isoflurane behavior were essentially negligible, suggesting they may be safer to use than propofol or sodium thiopental.

Kurita et al studied the influence of moderate hemorrhage (up to 30% of blood volume) in a swine model.[34] The researchers studied both the kinetic changes (the ratio of the end-tidal to inspired isoflurane concentrations over time in response to changes in vaporizer settings) and pharmacodynamic changes (the concentration-effect relationship using spectral edge from the electroencephalogram as a measure of drug effect). They found a subtle change in the ratio of expired-to-inspired isoflurane concentrations when comparing unbled controls to animals that had lost 20% and 30% of their blood volume. Namely under hypotensive conditions, the ratio changed more quickly. These changes were consistent with their observed changes in cardiac output. Moderate blood loss, however, did not shift the concentration-effect relationship.

Expanding their line of research, Kurita et al also explored the influence of severe blood loss leading to cardiovascular decompensation followed by resuscitation in a swine model.[33] In this protocol, blood loss was more severe (28 mL/kg, or 40% of the estimated blood volume) followed by resuscitation with 28 mL/kg of hydroxyethyl starch. Using the same tools to characterize changes in the kinetic and dynamic behavior of isoflurane, the study found that severe hemorrhage also slightly changed the ratio of inspired-to-expired isoflurane levels over time. Different from the findings with moderate hemorrhage, the researchers found a slight decrease in the concentration-effect relationship (C_{50} shift from 1.12% to 1%) with severe hemorrhage that did not improve with resuscitation. This concluded that the overall changes were minimal in comparison to several intravenous anesthetics.

In more recent work, the same group studied the influence of isoflurane during severe hemorrhage to an end point of a MAP of 10 mm Hg followed by cardiopulmonary resuscitation to include chest compressions, replacement of shed blood with hydroxyethyl starch, and intravenous epinephrine on BIS levels in a swine model.[33] They found that BIS levels did not change until the MAP dipped below 22 mm Hg, at which point the electroencephalogram became isoelectric. The C_{50} for isoflurane versus BIS at baseline, end of severe blood loss (40% of blood volume), and following cardiopulmonary resuscitation were 1.81, 1.69, and 1.54 vol% of isoflurane, respectively, indicating a small increase in isoflurane potency. The authors concluded that injury to brain tissue during severe hypotension may have contributed to the decrease in C_{50} following resuscitation.

SUMMARY

As anesthesiologists navigate patients suffering from blood loss through often perilous anesthetics, hemorrhage and even hemorrhage followed by resuscitation that appears to restore hemodynamic function to near normal can lead to dramatic alterations in the pharmacologic behavior of some anesthetics. Based on observations in animals studies, selected sedative–hypnotics (propofol, sodium pentothal, and perhaps midazolam[10]) are particularly dangerous. Other sedatives (etomidate and ketamine), isoflurane, fentanyl, and remifentanil appear to be less susceptible to potentially harmful changes in drug kinetics and dynamics with moderate to severe blood loss and resuscitation. Although there have been no data to support this assumption, it may be that other potent inhaled agents such as sevoflurane and desflurane and other fentanyl congeners such as alfentanil and sufentanil have a similar kinetic and dynamic profile under these conditions. A summary of how blood loss and resuscitation influence intravenous drug behavior is presented in Table 23–3.

TABLE 23–3 Summary of studies investigating the influence of blood loss and resuscitation on intravenous drug behavior.

Drug	PK Changes with BL	PD Changes with BL	PK Changes with BL and R	PD Changes with BL and R	Reference
Sedative–Hypnotics					
Propofol	+++	+++	+	+	De Paepe et al[3] Johnson et al[5] Johnson et al[30]
Sodium thiopental	+++	–	–	–	Halford[27] Weiskopf[12]
Etomidate	+	0	–	–	De Paepe et al[4] Johnson et al[6]
Ketamine	+	–	–	–	Black et al[31] Weiskopf et al[9]
Midazolam	++	–	–	–	Adams et al[10]
Opioids					
Morphine	++	–	–	–	De Paepe et al[11]
Fentanyl	+++	–	–	–	Egan et al[12]
Remifentanil	+++	0	–	–	Johnson et al[13]
Potent Inhaled Agents					
Isoflurane	+	0	+	+	Kurita et al[33,34,36]

+++, ++, +, 0 = large, moderate, small, and no change in parameters that lead to more pronounced and/or prolonged drug effect. An – indicates that no data are available.

BL, blood loss; PD, pharmacodynamic; PK, pharmacokinetic, R, resuscitation.

Reproduced with permission from Smith CE: Trauma Anesthesia, 1st edition. New York, NY: Cambridge University Press, 2008.

What remains unexplored is the influence of blood loss on drug behavior when sedatives and opioids are administered simultaneously, as is often done when providing a general anesthetic. It is well established that sedative–hypnotics and opioids have a synergistic relationship, but how that interaction behaves in the presence of intravascular volume depletion has not been described.

REFERENCES

1. Honan DM, Breen PJ, Boylan JF, McDonald NJ, Egan TD. Decrease in bispectral index preceding intraoperative hemodynamic crisis: evidence of acute alteration of propofol pharmacokinetics. *Anesthesiology.* 2002;97(5):1303-1305.
2. Halford F. A critique of intravenous anesthesia in war surgery. *Anesthesiology.* 1943;4:67-69.
3. De Paepe P, Belpaire FM, Rosseel MT, van Hoey G, Boon PA, Buylaert WA. Influence of hypovolemia on the pharmacokinetics and the electroencephalographic effect of propofol in the rat. *Anesthesiology.* 2000; 93(6):1482-1490.
4. De Paepe P, Belpaire FM, van Hoey G, Boon PA, Buylaert WA. Influence of hypovolemia on the pharmacokinetics and the electroencephalographic effect of etomidate in the rat. *J Pharmacol Exp Ther.* 1999; 290(3):1048-1053.
5. Johnson KB, Egan TD, Kern SE, et al. The influence of hemorrhagic shock on propofol: a pharmacokinetic and pharmacodynamic analysis. *Anesthesiology.* 2003; 99(2):409-420.
6. Johnson KB, Egan TD, Layman J, Kern SE, White JL, McJames SW. The influence of hemorrhagic shock on etomidate: a pharmacokinetic and pharmacodynamic analysis. *Anesth Analg.* 2003;96(5):1360-1368.
7. Kazama T, Kurita T, Morita K, Nakata J, Sato S. Influence of hemorrhage on propofol pseudo-steady state concentration. *Anesthesiology.* 2002;97(5):1156-1161.
8. Klockowski P, Levy G. Kinetics of drug action in disease states. XXV. Effect of experimental hypovolemia on the pharmacodynamics and pharmacokinetics of desmethyldiazepam. *J Pharmacol Exp Ther.* 1988;245(2): 508-512.
9. Weiskopf RB, Bogertz MS, Roizen MF, Reid IA. Cardiovascular and metabolic sequelae of inducing anesthesia with ketamine or thiopental in hypovolemic swine. *Anesthesiology.* 1984;60(3):214-219.
10. Adams P, Gelman S, Reves JG, Greenblatt DJ, Alvis M, Bradley E. Midazolam pharmacodynamics and pharmacokinetics during acute hypovolemia. *Anesthesiology.* 1985;63(2):140-146.
11. De Paepe P, Belpaire FM, Rosseel MT, Buylaert WA. The influence of hemorrhagic shock on the pharmacokinet and the analgesic effect of morphine in the rat. *Fundam Clin Pharmacol.* 1998;12(6):624-630.
12. Egan TD, Kuramkote S, Gong G, Zhang J, McJames SW, Bailey PL. Fentanyl pharmacokinetics in hemorrhagic shock: a porcine model. *Anesthesiology.* 1999;91(1):156-166.
13. Johnson KB, Kern SE, Hamber EA, McJames SW, Kohnstamm KM, Egan TD. Influence of hemorrhagic shock on remifentanil; a pharmacokinetic and pharmacodynamic analysis. *Anesthesiology.* 2001;94(2): 322-332.
14. Kurita T, Uraoka M, Morita K, Suzuki M, Morishima Y, Sato S. Influence of haemorrhage on the pseudo-steady-state remifentanil concentration in a swine model: a comparison with propofol and the effect of haemorrhagic shock stage. *Br J Anaesth.* 2011; 107(5):719-725.
15. Benowitz N, Forsyth RP, Melmon KL, Rowland M. Lidocaine disposition kinetics in monkey and man II. Effect of hemorrhage and sympathomimetic drug administration. *Clin Pharmacol Ther.* 1973;16(1): 99-109.
16. Kurita T, Morita K, Kazama T, Sato S. Influence of cardiac output on plasma propofol concentrations during constant infusion in swine. *Anesthesiology.* 2002; 96(6):1498-1503.
17. Upton RN, Ludbrook GL, Grant C, Martinez AM. Cardiac output is a determinant of the initial concentrations of propofol after short-infusion administration. *Anesth Analg.* 1999;89:545-552.
18. Shafer S. Shock Values. *Anesthesiology.* 2004;101: 568-570.
19. Kazama T, Ikeda K, Morita K. The pharmacodynamic interaction between propofol and fentanyl with respect to the supression of somatic or hemodynamic responses to skin incision, peritoneum incision, and wall retraction. *Anesthesiology.* 1998;89:894-906.
20. Pavlin DJ, Arends RH, Gunn HC, van Norman G, Koerschgen ME, Shen DD. Optimal propofol-alfentanil combinations for supplementing nitrous oxide for outpatient surgery. *Anesthesiology.* 1999;91:97-108.
21. McIntosh TK, Palter M, Grasberger R, et al. Endorphins in primate hemorrhagic shock:benificial action of opiate antagonists. *J Surg Res.* 1986;40(3):265-275.
22. Molina P. Opiate modulation of hemodynamic, hormonal, and cytokine response to hemorrhage. *Shock.* 2001;15(6):471-478.

23. Tuggle D, Horton J. Beta-endorphins in canine hemorrhagic shock. *Surg Gynecol Obstet.* 1986;163(2): 137-144.
24. Dutta S, Matsumoto, Yoshiaki, Ebling, William F. Propofol pharmacokinetics and pharmacodynamics assessed from a cremophor EL formulation. *J Pharm Sci.* 1997;86(8):967-979.
25. Struys MM, Vereecke H, Moerman A, et al. Ability of the bispectral index, autoregressive modelling with exogenous input-derived auditory evoked potentials, and predicted propofol concentrations to measure patient responsiveness during anesthesia with propofol and remifentanil. *Anesthesiology.* 2003;99(4):802-812.
26. Johnson K, Egan T, Kern S, McJames S, Cluff M, Pace N. Influence of hemorrhagic shock followed by crystalloid resuscitation on propofol: a pharmacokinetic and pharmacodynamic analysis. *Anesthesiology.* 2004;101:647-659..
27. Brussel T, Theissen JL, Vigfusson G, Lunkenheimer PP, van Aken H, Lawin P. Hemodynamic and cardiodynamic effects of propofol and etomidate: negative inotropic properties of propofol. *Anesth Analg.* 1989;69(1):35-40.
28. Goodchild C, Serrao J. Cardiovascular effects of propofol in the anaesthetized dog. *Br J Anesth.* 1989;63: 87-92.
29. Graham M, Thiessen D, Mutch W. Left ventricular systolic and diastolic function is unaltered during propofol infusion in newborn swine. *Anesth Analg.* 1998;86:717-723.
30. Pagel PS, Warltier DC. Negative inotropic effects of propofol as evaluated by the regional preload recruitable stroke work relationship in chronically instrumented dogs. *Anesthesiology.* 1993;78(1):100-108.
31. Black I, Grathwohl K, IB T, Martini W, Johnson K. The influence of hemorrhagic shock on ketamine: a pharmacokinetic analysis. *Anesthesiology.* ASA Annual Meeting, 2006; Abstract A203.
32. Haga H, Dolvik N. Evaluation of the bispectral index as an indicator of degree of central nervous system depression in isoflurane-anesthetized horses. *Am J Vet Res.* 2002;63(3):438-442.
33. Kurita T, Morita K, Fukuda K, et al. Influence of hemorrhagic shock and subsequent fluid resuscitation on the electroencephalographic effect of isoflurane in a swine model. *Anesthesiology.* 2005;103(6):1189-1194.
34. Kurita T, Morita K, Fukuda K, Uraoka M, Takata K, Sanjo Y, et al. Influence of hypovolemia on the electroencephalographic effect of isoflurane in a swine model. *Anesthesiology.* 2005;102(5):948-953.
35. Kurita T, Takata K, Uraoka M, et al. The influence of hemorrhagic shock on the minimum alveolar anesthetic concentration of isoflurane in a swine model. *Anesth Analg.* 2007;105(6):1639-1643.
36. Kurita T, Uraoka M, Morita K, Sato S. Influence of progressive hemorrhage and subsequent cardiopulmonary resuscitation on the bispectral index during isoflurane anesthesia in a swine model. *J Trauma Acute Care Surg.* 2012;72(6):1614-1619.
37. Samarska IV, van Meurs M, Buikema H, et al. Adjunct nitrous oxide normalizes vascular reactivity changes after hemorrhagic shock in mice under isoflurane anesthesia. *Anesthesiology.* 2009;111(3):600-608.

CHAPTER 24

Anesthetic Considerations in Cancer Patients

Marcel E. Durieux, MD, PhD

INTRODUCTION

Is it possible that particulars of perioperative anesthetic management (eg, using epidural local anesthetics during general anesthesia) might influence long-term recurrence risk after cancer surgery? Not too long ago, this would have been considered an impossibility, and at first glance, it does seem an unlikely proposition. How could a change in management during a procedure that lasts at most several hours lead to effects on cancer outcome years later? Yet, suggestive (though far from conclusive) retrospective clinical data indicate that there might be an effect, and even a significant one. Use of paravertebral blocks[1] or the addition of ketorolac[2] in breast cancer, or the addition of epidural anesthesia in prostate[3] or colon cancer[4] might reduce risk of recurrence. The story is far from clear, however, as other studies[5,6] do not indicate benefit. Prospective randomized trials are in progress, but it will be many years before the results of these will be known.

Much more data are available at the basic science level, and in this chapter we therefore will focus on some of this evidence, discussing, where possible, animal rather than cellular data. Before reviewing the effects of specific perioperative interventions, however, it is necessary to discuss briefly the mechanisms by which metastasis occurs in the perioperative period. Then we will describe the main effects of anesthetic drugs on these mechanisms. Although outside the domain of pharmacology, we will also briefly touch on potential effects on cancer recurrence of some other perioperative events, such as hypovolemia, anemia, transfusion, and hypothermia.

METASTASIS IN THE PERIOPERATIVE PERIOD

Why does cancer recurrence happen at all, after what was supposed to be curative surgery? This is a highly complex issue, and here we can provide only a brief and admittedly simplified description of the process.

Two main mechanisms explain why recurrence happens. The first mechanism is that cancer cells are released into the circulation during surgery. This is well documented,[7] unavoidable, and takes place even if a "no touch" technique is used for surgical resection. Pressure on the tumor will result in malignant cells being disseminated through the body. Tumor cell release into the circulation happens also in the absence of surgery, but the body has effective defense mechanisms that prevent (almost) all of these cells from surviving. Critical here are natural killer (NK) cells, which have the ability to recognize tumor cells and eliminate them.[8] It follows that decreases in the number or activity of NK cells induced by perioperative interventions might increase the number of cancer cells surviving in the body. Indeed, it has been shown for a variety of tumor types that low levels of NK cell activity predict worse outcome after cancer surgery. For example, NK cell activity levels less than 20% correlate with poor survival after "curative" colon cancer surgery.[9]

The second mechanism is the immune suppression induced by surgery, some drugs, and some perioperative events. The role of the immune system in cancer is exceedingly complex and only partially understood. Only the briefest of outlines can be given here. Even when seemingly a solitary tumor is identified by the best diagnostic imaging techniques, micrometastases are frequently present. These are small collections of tumor cells, and they are unable to grow into full metastases for 2 reasons. First, they are kept under control by the immune system, in a process known as "immune surveillance."[10] Second, their growth is limited by the absence of a supply of oxygen and nutrients. If a tumor is to grow beyond the millimeter stage, it can no longer depend on diffusion for its nutrient supply and has to "recruit" blood vessels from the surrounding tissue, inducing them to grow into the tumor stroma. In order for this to happen, angiogenic factors need to be released by the tumor. This would suggest that perioperative events that suppress immune functioning, or that are angiogenic, would lead to the "escape" of micrometastases and their development into larger tumors.

As we will see in subsequent sections, the hypotheses stated here are essentially correct. Decreases in NK cell number and activity, decreases in cellular immune functioning, and angiogenic stimulation appear to be the main pathways by which perioperative management influences cancer recurrence. NK cell number and activity assays are easily performed and can be done in humans. Animal studies allow further direct investigation. Animals can be subjected to surgery, and tumor cells can then be injected into the bloodstream and their fate assessed. If cells are labeled, retention in the lungs can be measured, as an indicator of the ability of tumor cells to survive in the blood stream and to migrate into tissues. Alternatively, investigators can let the animals survive for several weeks after tumor cell injection and then count the number of metastases as well as the total tumor load.

These are the main techniques used in the studies that will be described in the subsequent sections. They allow us to answer the question posed in the beginning of this chapter: "can perioperative management affect cancer recurrence?" The answer is an unequivocal "yes" – at least in animals. Figure 24–1 provides an example.[11] In this study, rats were subjected to laparotomy under halothane anesthesia, and MADB106 tumor cells were injected. As shown, the stress of surgery/anesthesia approximately tripled the number of metastases. So, the surgical setting itself is a major stimulus for cancer progression—and largely unavoidable. But other perioperative management also has significant impact. As shown, the combined administration of indomethacin and nadolol decreased the number of metastases almost by half.

DRUGS

In this section, we will review several classes of drugs used in the perioperative period for which evidence suggests a potential influence on tumor recurrence. These will include the typical anesthetic drugs, as well as some other compounds used commonly in the perioperative setting.

Induction Drugs

Thiopental, ketamine, and propofol are the main induction drugs for which data are available. Etomidate has not been studied in this setting, although its effects on steroid synthesis and the expected subsequent influence on the immune system suggest that it might be a worthwhile topic of investigation.

Of these drugs, propofol is by far the one used most commonly, and as it turns out, it is also likely to be the most beneficial drug in the setting of cancer surgery. Thiopental has immune suppressant effects and greatly reduces NK cell number and activity. Ketamine significantly increases lung retention of injected tumor cells.[12] Propofol showed fewer effects on NK cell number and activity than ketamine or thiopental and had no effect on lung tumor retention. In fact, when administered for longer periods of time, propofol may have protective actions in the setting of cancer. When mice received daily intraperitoneal injections with propofol for 3 days and were inoculated with tumor cells, their T cells showed increased tumor cell killing activity, and tumor load 28 days later was decreased by more than half as compared with animals who received saline injections.[13] The invasion ability of HeLa, HT1080, HOS, and RPMI-7951 cancer cell lines was reduced to negligible amounts by propofol 5 mcg/mL (which is approximately the upper concentration limit obtained in blood during propofol-induced general anesthesia), and continuous infusion of propofol

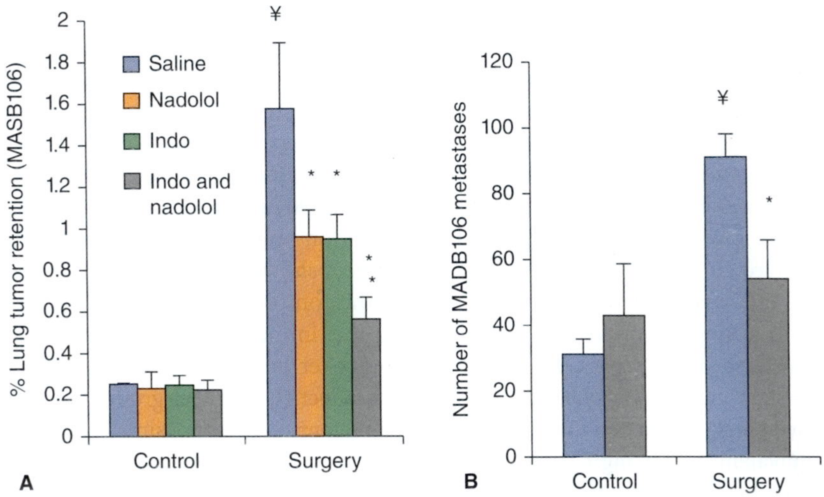

FIGURE 24–1 The effects of surgery and their attenuation by the β-adrenergic blocker nadolol, by the prostaglandin synthesis inhibitor indomethacin (Indo), and by the combined used of these drugs (Indo and nadolol) (mean ± standard error of the mean). Surgery increased lung tumor retention of the MADB106 tumor (A) and increased the number of experimental MADB106 lung metastases counted 3 weeks later (B). Each of the blockers attenuated these effects (A), and their combined use almost completely abolished them (A and B). ¥ indicates a significant effect of surgery (difference between the control saline and surgery saline groups), and * indicates a significant attenuation of this effect by drug treatment (difference between the surgery saline group and the surgery drug group). The combined treatment seen in A was significantly lower than each treatment alone (indicated by two *). A total of 105 and 57 male rats were used in A and B, respectively. Reproduced with permission from Melamed R, Rosenne E, Shakhar K, Schwartz Y, Abudarham N, Ben-Eliyahu S. Marginating pulmonary-NK activity and resistance to experimental tumor metastasis: suppression by surgery and the prophylactic use of a beta-adrenergic antagonist and a prostaglandin synthesis inhibitor. *Brain Behav Immun*. 2005;Mar19(2):114-26.

(40 mcg/kg/d for 4 weeks) in mice reduced by about 50% the metastatic load after inoculation with LM8 tumor cells.[14] Taken together, these data suggest that our usual choice of propofol as induction drug is appropriate in the setting of cancer surgery and that there may be potential additional benefits to longer-term propofol administration.

Volatile Anesthetics

For volatile drugs, unfortunately, the verdict is not as good. Although some variability exists between studies, the inhaled anesthetics generally have been found to increase tumor load in animal models. Halothane and isoflurane, for example, administered for 1.3 minimum alveolar concentration (MAC)-hour in mice, each more than doubled the number of metastases counted 21 days after intravenous administration of melanoma cells.[15] There are little data available on sevoflurane and desflurane. Nonetheless, the available basic science data suggest that of the compounds used routinely in anesthetic practice, the inhaled drugs may be some of the least appropriate in the setting of cancer surgery.

Muscle Relaxants

There are no data available on the ability of muscle relaxants to affect cancer recurrence. There also is no physiologic rationale as to why they would affect any of the parameters relevant to perioperative metastasis. It seems unlikely that muscle relaxants would significantly affect cancer recurrence.

Opiates

Opiates play a critical role in the treatment of cancer pain and in the treatment of postoperative pain after cancer surgery. Unfortunately, it now appears that these extremely useful drugs may well have some of the worst effects with regards to cancer recurrence. Two main mechanisms appear responsible for this effect. First, opiates are mitogenic stimulants. Morphine, for example, promotes cancer cell growth in several models.[16] Second, opiates are potent stimulants of tumor angiogenesis. As described above, for a tumor to grow beyond a minute size, it is dependent on the ingrowth of blood vessels in order to deliver nutrients and oxygen and to remove waste products. In addition, these blood vessels provide new pathways for metastasis of tumor cells. Opiates strongly promote such tumor vascularization. In animals treated for 1 week with morphine in a dose approximately equivalent to 50 mg/d in a 70-kg human and a further 2 weeks with a dose equivalent to 70 mg/d, tumor vascularity was approximately doubled.[17] Importantly, these effects can be blocked by opiate antagonists (such as the peripheral opiate receptor blocker methylnaltrexone.[18]

These findings would suggest that limiting opiates during and after cancer surgery would be beneficial, and circumstantial evidence suggests that this is indeed the case. Most of the retrospective clinical trials that demonstrated how changes in perioperative management could reduce cancer recurrence used approaches that would have resulted in a reduction in perioperative opiate load (paravertebral blocks[1] and epidural analgesia or administration of ketorolac[2]). Unfortunately, none of these studies measured actual opiate use. A recent study suggests that use of intraoperative sufentanil is associated with reduced biochemical recurrence-free survival rates after radical prostatectomy.[19]

Beta Blockers

The role of β blockade in the perioperative period continues to be debated, but so far only with regards to the cardiovascular effects of these drugs. Interesting data suggest that β blockers may have beneficial effects in the setting of cancer surgery as well. Epidemiologic studies have demonstrated a relationship between β blockers use and cancer recurrence in large populations. Patients with breast cancer, who used β blockers because of hypertension, showed significantly longer times before acquiring metastases and improved 10-year survival rates, as compared with nontreated patients.[20] Animal studies mimicking the perioperative period support these data and suggest that beneficial effects can be obtained with short-term treatment as well. Rats underwent laparotomy to induce a surgical stress response and were inoculated with labeled MADB106 tumor cells. When pulmonary tumor cell retention was measured, animals that underwent surgery showed 1.6% retention, compared with 0.2% in the control group—an 8-fold increase. Treatment in the immediate postoperative period with the β-blocker nadolol (0.6 mg/kg subcutaneously) did not affect the control group, but it reduced tumor cell retention by approximately one-third in the surgery group.[11] This suggests that mitigating the surgical stress response can limit the ability of cancer cells to spread.

Cyclooxygenase Inhibitors

Similar to β blockers, long-term use of cyclooxygenase inhibitors has been shown in epidemiologic studies to affect cancer; their use was associated with a decreased incidence of colon cancer. After prospective studies confirmed this benefit, the drugs are now indicated in patients considered to be at high risk for this disease. After short-term administration, more relevant to the perioperative setting, cyclooxygenase inhibitors also show benefit. In the study mentioned above in relation to β blockade,[11] the prostaglandin synthesis inhibitor indomethacin (4 mg/kg intraperitoneally) showed benefits similar to that of nadolol on lung tumor retention and metastatic load. When the 2 drugs were combined, lung tumor cell retention after surgery was decreased by two-thirds and the number of metastases was cut almost in half (see Figure 24–1).

Cyclooxygenase inhibitors may be of particular interest in mitigating the negative effects of opiates in the setting of cancer. In part, this is because of their opiate-sparing effect, but in addition, they may mitigate some of the negative effects of opiates. As discussed above, morphine provides a potent angiogenic stimulus to tumor cells, resulting in rapid vascular development in the tumor. Celecoxib was shown able to completely prevent the tumor vascular growth induced by 3 weeks of opiate treatment.[17] In agreement, tumor weight in experimental animals, which was significantly increased by opiate treatment, was reduced back to baseline if celecoxib was administered as well. Survival also was beneficially affected, and importantly, analgesia was not compromised.

Together, these findings suggest a significant benefit for the use of cyclooxygenase inhibitors in the setting of cancer surgery. This is particularly the case since use of these compounds perioperatively is already widespread because of their analgesic properties. One retrospective study has been published that compared breast cancer recurrence rates in patients who had received ketorolac 30 mg perioperatively (administered for analgesia) with those who had not received the drug. After 72 months, the recurrence rate in the group that had received ketorolac was approximately half of that in the control group (Figure 24–2).[2] This exciting finding needs to be confirmed by a prospective study (particularly since the same investigators could not show similar benefit of ketorolac in prostate cancer).[19]

Local Anesthetics

Local anesthetics have a special position in the list of anesthetic drugs implicated in affecting cancer recurrence. On the one hand, many of the studies claiming beneficial effects of specific anesthetic techniques on recurrence used them as part of a regional anesthesia approach.[1,3,4] On the other hand, the compounds themselves seem to have little action on cancer cells, unless very high concentrations are used, in which case they can induce cancer cell apoptosis and reduce motility. They do have several potential indirect actions that could be of importance: when used for neuraxial blockade, local anesthetics suppress the stress response to surgery, and when used systemically they have inflammation modulating properties. In addition, use of local anesthetics (either systemically or for nerve blockade) would be expected to result in opiate sparing and volatile anesthetic sparing, both of which would be beneficial during cancer surgery.

But all this is speculation. There are almost no mechanistic data available, leaving us in the uncomfortable position that the majority of retrospective clinical data suggests a role for local anesthetics, whereas they have not been specifically investigated to any significant degree in this setting.

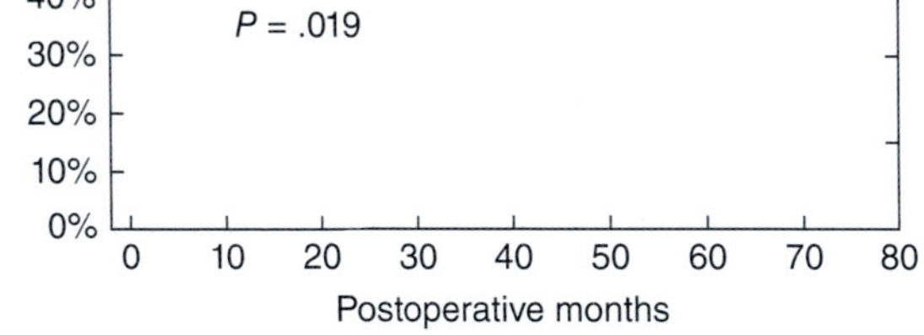

FIGURE 24–2 Kaplan-Meier recurrence-free survival estimated for 319 patients receiving (or not receiving) ketorolac. Univariate analysis by log-rank tests. Reproduced with permission from Forget P, Vandenhende J, Berliere M, Machiels JP, Nussbaum B, Legrand C, et al. Do intraoperative analgesics influence breast cancer recurrence after mastectomy? A retrospective analysis. *Anesth Analg*. 2010; un 1;110(6):1630-1635.

SELECTED PERIOPERATIVE EVENTS

Hypotension, Hypovolemia, Anemia, and Transfusion

Blood loss and the need for volume replacement are common in cancer surgery, and they may affect outcome. Hypovolemia has been shown to increase tumor growth in animals.[21] Human data are limited, but one study reviewing outcome after complete resection of colorectal liver metastases found the number of intraoperative hypotensive episodes to be "the most significant single factor that affected recurrence rates"[22]: patients with fewer than 3 episodes of intraoperative hypotension fared significantly better than those who suffered 3 or more episodes. This was independent of need for transfusion. Nonetheless, it is easy to see how other factors might have been causative to both intraoperative hypotension and poor outcome. Unfortunately, these older data (patient recruitment occurred from 1987 to 1989) have not been replicated. Avoidance of hypotension is a laudable goal for several reasons, and even if the data on its effect on cancer recurrence are not particularly solid, it seems worthwhile paying careful attention to blood pressure in tumor surgery cases.

A frequent result of intraoperative blood loss is anemia. Little data are available on the effect of brief periods of low hemoglobin levels on cancer outcome. Long-term anemia, however, is a dire predictor. A review of survival times in patients with or without anemia in a large number of cancer types showed anemia to be an independent predictor of shortened survival in every single type of cancer.[23] As with the data on intraoperative hypotension, it is difficult to determine if this is a causative effect or only a correlative relationship.

This question is particularly vexing as the treatment of anemia—transfusion—may similarly not be benign in the setting of cancer surgery. That blood transfusion has immune suppressant effects has been known for decades. Whether these effects are significant enough to affect cancer recurrence after perioperative transfusion is still being debated. Although more than 200 papers have been published on this topic, a consensus does not exist. Most convincing, maybe, is a meta-analysis of the effect of intraoperative transfusion in colon cancer, which found a modest correlation between transfusion and recurrence after resection of curable colon cancer (odds ratio, 1.42).[24] A causative relationship can, of course, not be determined from these data.

The age of red cells used for transfusion has recently been a focus of attention in several studies. Few data are available in the setting of cancer surgery, but although animal data suggested a critical role for aged red blood cells in cancer progression,[25] a recent clinical trial suggests that age of blood transfused does not predict recurrence. When biochemical recurrence (based on prostate-specific antigen measurements) was assessed in patients who underwent radical prostatectomy and were transfused during the procedure, no difference was found between those who received red blood cells older than 21 days compared with those who received blood 21 days or less old.[26]

Hypothermia

Intraoperative hypothermia, even to a modest degree, has been demonstrated in a number of prospective trials to have significant negative effects. It potentially would be detrimental in the setting of cancer surgery as well. The immune suppression associated with hypothermia could allow micrometastases to escape from "immune surveillance," and the increased blood loss and increased need for transfusion associated with hypothermia could lead to increased recurrence rates, as described above.

Animal studies support a negative effect of hypothermia in this setting. Rats, anesthetized for 2.5 hours with thiopental at either normothermia (38°C) or hypothermia (30–32°C) were compared as to their NK cell activity and the metastasis potential of injected tumor cells.[27] Thiopental anesthesia did not affect the number of metastases in normothermic animals (as compared with nonanesthetized normothermic controls), but hypothermia increased the number of metastases 4-fold. NK activity was decreased by thiopental even in normothermic animals (as would be expected from the known actions of the drug) but was reduced even further, to negligible levels, in the setting of hypothermia.

SUMMARY

We do not know if specifics of anesthetic management influence recurrence rates after cancer surgery. Some suggestive retrospective clinical data have been published, but just as many negative studies exist, prospective data are lacking altogether. The preclinical data, therefore, should be looked at as indications of potential mechanisms and suggestions for further research, not as prescriptions for practice.

We can, simplifying, roughly divide the various drugs and interventions into 2 groups: "good" versus "bad" (**Table 24–1**). If we survey this table, it will become clear that most of the things on the "good" side of the list we already do or should do: (1) we already tend to use propofol, administer cyclooxygenase inhibitors or use regional anesthesia for postoperative analgesia, (2) we administer β blockers for cardiovascular protection, and (3) we should be using systemic local anesthetic (at least in abdominal surgery) because of its documented benefits on surgical recovery.[28] Conversely, many items on the "bad" side of the list we already try to avoid for reasons separate from a postulated action

TABLE 24–1 The perioperative period and cancer recurrence: good versus bad.

Good
Propofol
Cyclooxygenase inhibitors
β blockers
Anything that reduces opiate requirements, volatile anesthetic requirements, and the surgical stress response:
Regional anesthesia
Intravenous local anesthetics
Adjuvants
Bad
Surgery
Volatile anesthetics
Opiates
Hypotension
Anemia
Blood transfusion
Hypothermia

on cancer recurrence: our surgical colleagues keep pushing the frontier on minimally invasive surgery, and we work hard to prevent hypotension, anemia, transfusion, and hypothermia. And we probably should be working even harder to minimize the use of opiates perioperatively, because of their side effect profile and particularly the risk of respiratory depression.

This leaves only one area where current practice does not match what is suggested to be optimal for the prevention of cancer recurrence: volatile anesthetics. Again, the data are far from conclusive, but it could be argued that in situations where one is particularly concerned about recurrence risk, the use of propofol total intravenous anesthesia could be an attractive alternative. Not only would it eliminate the need for volatile anesthetics, but, as discussed, the prolonged administration of propofol in laboratory studies resulted in cancer-suppressing effects.

But, once again, this is speculation. At the current level of evidence, there is nothing that would force the anesthesia provider to change customary anesthetic practice in the setting of cancer surgery. The data presented in this chapter are intriguing and interesting, but it will take prospective, randomized clinical trials to demonstrate that they matter in the clinical setting. As it turns out, however, and as Table 24–1 indicates, if one practices good anesthesia, one already does the right thing, even in the setting of cancer surgery.

REFERENCES

1. Exadaktylos AK, Buggy DJ, Moriarty DC, Mascha E, Sessler DI. Can anesthetic technique for primary breast cancer surgery affect recurrence or metastasis? *Anesthesiology*. 2006;105(4):660-664.
2. Forget P, Vandenhende J, Berliere M, et al. Do intraoperative analgesics influence breast cancer recurrence after mastectomy? A retrospective analysis. *Anesth Analg*. 2010;110(6):1630-1635.
3. Biki B, Mascha E, Moriarty DC, Fitzpatrick JM, Sessler DI, Buggy DJ. Anesthetic technique for radical prostatectomy surgery affects cancer recurrence: a retrospective analysis. *Anesthesiology*. 2008;109(2):180-187.
4. Christopherson R, James KE, Tableman M, Marshall P, Johnson FE. Long-term survival after colon cancer surgery: a variation associated with choice of anesthesia. *Anesth Analg*. 2008;107(1):325-332.
5. Gottschalk A, Ford JG, Regelin CC, et al. Association between epidural analgesia and cancer recurrence after colorectal cancer surgery. *Anesthesiology*. 2010;113(1):27-34.
6. Myles PS, Peyton P, Silbert B, Hunt J, Rigg JR, Sessler DI. Perioperative epidural analgesia for major abdominal surgery for cancer and recurrence-free survival: randomised trial. *BMJ*. 2011;342:d1491.
7. Yamashita JI, Kurusu Y, Fujino N, Saisyoji T, Ogawa M. Detection of circulating tumor cells in patients with non-small cell lung cancer undergoing lobectomy by video-assisted thoracic surgery: a potential hazard for intraoperative hematogenous tumor cell dissemination. *J Thorac Cardiovasc Surg*. 2000;119(5):899-905.
8. Brittenden J, Heys SD, Ross J, Eremin O. Natural killer cells and cancer. *Cancer*. 1996;77(7):1226-1243.
9. Kondo E, Koda K, Takiguchi N, et al. Preoperative natural killer cell activity as a prognostic factor for distant metastasis following surgery for colon cancer. *Dig Surg*. 2003;20(5):445-451.
10. Dunn GP, Old LJ, Schreiber RD. The immunobiology of cancer immunosurveillance and immunoediting. *Immunity*. 2004;21(2):137-148.
11. Melamed R, Rosenne E, Shakhar K, Schwartz Y, Abudarham N, Ben-Eliyahu S. Marginating pulmonary-NK activity and resistance to experimental tumor metastasis: suppression by surgery and the prophylactic use of a beta-adrenergic antagonist and a

prostaglandin synthesis inhibitor. *Brain Behav Immun.* 2005;19(2):114-126.

12. Melamed R, Bar-Yosef S, Shakhar G, Shakhar K, Ben-Eliyahu S. Suppression of natural killer cell activity and promotion of tumor metastasis by ketamine, thiopental, and halothane, but not by propofol: mediating mechanisms and prophylactic measures. *Anesth Analg.* 2003;97(5):1331-1339.
13. Kushida A, Inada T, Shingu K. Enhancement of antitumor immunity after propofol treatment in mice. *Immunopharmacol Immunotoxicol.* 2007;29(3-4): 477-486.
14. Mammoto T, Mukai M, Mammoto A, et al. Intravenous anesthetic, propofol inhibits invasion of cancer cells. *Cancer Lett.* 2002;184(2):165-170.
15. Moudgil GC, Singal DP. Halothane and isoflurane enhance melanoma tumour metastasis in mice. *Can J Anaesth.* 1997;44(1):90-94.
16. Gupta K, Kshirsagar S, Chang L, et al. Morphine stimulates angiogenesis by activating proangiogenic and survival-promoting signaling and promotes breast tumor growth. *Cancer Res.* 2002;62(15):4491-4498.
17. Farooqui M, Li Y, Rogers T, et al. COX-2 inhibitor celecoxib prevents chronic morphine-induced promotion of angiogenesis, tumour growth, metastasis and mortality, without compromising analgesia. *Br J Cancer.* 2007;97(11):1523-1531.
18. Singleton PA, Lingen MW, Fekete MJ, Garcia JG, Moss J. Methylnaltrexone inhibits opiate and VEGF-induced angiogenesis: role of receptor transactivation. *Microvasc Res.* 2006;72(1-2):3-11.
19. Forget P, Tombal B, Scholtes JL, et al. Do intraoperative analgesics influence oncological outcomes after radical prostatectomy for prostate cancer? *Eur J Anaesthesiol.* 2011;28(12):830-835.
20. Powe DG, Voss MJ, Zanker KS, et al. Beta-blocker drug therapy reduces secondary cancer formation in breast cancer and improves cancer specific survival. *Oncotarget.* 2010;1(7):628-638.
21. Younes RN, Rogatko A, Vydelingum NA, Brennan MF. Effects of hypovolemia and transfusion on tumor growth in MCA-tumor-bearing rats. *Surgery.* 1991;109(3 Pt 1):307-312.
22. Younes RN, Rogatko A, Brennan MF. The influence of intraoperative hypotension and perioperative blood transfusion on disease-free survival in patients with complete resection of colorectal liver metastases. *Ann Surg.* 1991;214(2):107-113.
23. Caro JJ, Salas M, Ward A, Goss G. Anemia as an independent prognostic factor for survival in patients with cancer: a systemic, quantitative review. *Cancer.* 2001;91(12):2214-2221.
24. Amato A, Pescatori M. Perioperative blood transfusions for the recurrence of colorectal cancer. *Cochrane Database Syst Rev.* 2006(1):CD005033.
25. Atzil S, Arad M, Glasner A, et al. Blood transfusion promotes cancer progression: a critical role for aged erythrocytes. *Anesthesiology.* 2008;109(6):989-997.
26. Cata JP, Klein EA, Hoeltge GA, et al. Blood storage duration and biochemical recurrence of cancer after radical prostatectomy. *Mayo Clin Proc.* 2011;86(2): 120-127.
27. Ben-Eliyahu S, Shakhar G, Rosenne E, Levinson Y, Beilin B. Hypothermia in barbiturate-anesthetized rats suppresses natural killer cell activity and compromises resistance to tumor metastasis: a role for adrenergic mechanisms. *Anesthesiology.* 1999;91(3):732-740.
28. Marret E, Rolin M, Beaussier M, Bonnet F. Meta-analysis of intravenous lidocaine and postoperative recovery after abdominal surgery. *Br J Surg.* 2008;95(11):1331-1338.

CHAPTER 25

The Pharmacology of Anesthetic Drugs in Elderly Patients

Philip N. Gnadinger, MD, MPH

In the past several decades, there has been a dramatic increase in the percentage of the world's population that is elderly, defined as people 65 years or older. This trend is projected to continue to increase in the future.[1] Understanding core principles of perioperative care of the elderly, particularly in the context of clinical pharmacology, will become increasingly more important for clinicians.

PHYSIOLOGIC CHANGES WITH AGING

As people age, there are important changes in physiology and response to pharmacologic interventions. Aging consists of the deterioration or loss of functional units (eg, neurons, nephrons, or alveoli) at the cellular, tissue, or organ level, as well as disruption of regulatory processes at the molecular level.[2] Basal organ function, in the otherwise healthy individual, is relatively preserved with aging,[3] but functional reserves and the ability to tolerate stress, such as occurs with anesthesia and surgery, declines significantly with age. However, with regard to organ function, wide intraindividual and interindividual variability does exist.[4] That is, biologic age does not linearly correlate with physiologic or medical age. The geriatric population is unique in its physical and medical heterogeneity, which only increases with advancing age. Acute or chronic disease states, genetics, environmental, socioeconomic and likely countless other factors play into the rate or degree of organ function decline. Advanced age, nevertheless, has been shown by many studies to be an independent predictor of perioperative outcome (Table 25–1).

Blood albumin concentration is decreased by approximately 10% in the elderly. This decrease has been associated with an increase in unbound fraction of many drugs. Acidic compounds (eg, salicylic acid, phenytoin, warfarin) bind primarily to albumin, while basic compounds (eg, lidocaine, propranolol) bind to α1-acid glycoprotein.[5] Drugs that are highly extracted by the liver or highly protein bound are more affected, including fentanyl, propofol, midazolam, and lidocaine.[6] Volume of distribution is affected by aging, related to age-related changes in body composition. Body fat increases by 20% to 40% and body water percentage decreases by 10% to 15%.[7] Polar drugs that are mainly water soluble will have higher serum levels in the elderly due to their smaller volume of distribution.[8] Nonpolar drugs, on the other hand, tend to be lipid soluble and therefore tend to have an increased volume of distribution and longer half-life in the elderly.

INFLUENCE OF AGE ON DRUG PHARMACOKINETICS AND PHARMACODYNAMICS

Altered drug absorption, distribution, metabolism, and excretion lead to different drug concentrations in the body for a given dose in the elderly compared with younger people (pharmacokinetics). Evidence also exists for a pharmacodynamic explanation for decreased anesthetic requirements in the elderly, with increased sensitivity for any given plasma concentration of certain drugs.

Propofol sensitivity is increased by about 30% to 50% in the elderly compared with younger patients,

TABLE 25–1 Physiologic changes with age and associated clinical consequences.

	Physiologic Changes With Age	Consequences of Changes
Cardiovascular	Increased: systolic blood pressure, pulse pressure, sinoatrial node conduction time[5] Decreased: LV compliance, β_1-receptor response, heart rate,[6] VO_2 max (10% per decade between age 20 and 80),[7] compliance of aorta and great arteries[8]	Increased: LV wall thickness, LV chamber size, LV mass, oxygen demand[9] Decreased: chronotropic responses to noxious stimulus or β agonist, ability to compensatorily increase cardiac output
Pulmonary	Increased: work of breathing, physiologic shunt, ventilation/perfusion mismatch, residual volume, closing capacity Decreased: FEV_1 (8%–10% per decade), chest wall compliance, vital capacity, respiratory muscle strength, maximal minute ventilation	Increased: propensity for hypoxemia, atelectasis Decreased: functional reserve to deal with stresses of anesthesia/surgery, gas exchange, arterial oxygenation, respiratory mechanics
Neurologic	Increased: enzymatic activity that leads to neuronal degradation Decreased: brain mass, neurotransmitter synthesis, hypoxic drive, hypercarbic ventilatory drive	Increased: propensity for postoperative delirium, cognitive dysfunction (41% and 13% at 3 months)[9] Additional risk factors include anticholinergics, opioids, preexisting cognitive impairment, blood urea nitrogen–to–creatine ration greater than 18, fever, blood loss, infections)
Renal	Maintained: acid–base balance Decreased: number of nephrons, renal mass, glomerular filtration rate and renal blood flow (30%–50% by age 70)	Decreased: clearance of certain drugs, urine concentrating ability during water deprivation[10]
Hepatic	Decreased: hepatic blood flow and volume, first-pass metabolism, mass (decreased 40% by age 80)	Increased: bioavailability of drugs that undergo significant first-pass metabolism (eg, labetalol, propranolol)[11] Decreased: onset/effectiveness of prodrugs (eg, ACE inhibitors)

ACE, angiotensin-converting enzyme; FEV_1, forced expiratory volume in 1 second; LV, left ventricular.

independently of the decrease in drug clearance. This is due to age-related changes of the central nervous system.[9] Studies have shown this increased sensitivity using electroencephalographic (EEG) measures, probability of responsiveness to verbal stimulus, and insertion of an endoscope. When 75-year-old volunteers were compared with 25-year-old subjects, effect-site concentrations of propofol needed to achieve a similar state of unconsciousness were about half in the older individuals.[10]

Age does not affect brain sensitivity to thiopental using EEG as a measure of effect, but there is slower intercompartment clearance in the elderly, leading to higher serum concentrations, for longer period of time, in the elderly versus young patients. This leads to a greater, longer lasting, clinical effect, following an intravenous bolus of thiopental in the elderly.[11]

One study examining etomidate, however, showed no significant increased brain sensitivity with aging, based on no observed age-related changes in the IC_{50} for etomidate, where the IC_{50} is the blood concentration (ng/mL) that produces 50% of the maximal median frequency depression on EEG. The administered dose needed to reach a uniform EEG end point, however, was decreased significantly in the elderly. This indicates pharmacokinetic differences, such as a decreased volume of distribution in the elderly; thus, higher initial blood concentrations for a given dose may be responsible for the observed clinical difference.

It is readily apparent in clinical practice that the elderly require smaller doses of opioids than younger adults. Data for fentanyl and alfentanil indicate that this seems to be a pharmacodynamic effect with increased brain sensitivity to opioids, using EEG slowing as the measured variable, rather than a pharmacokinetic explanation. Age-related changes in opioid receptors are suggested as a possible mechanism.[12] Other data suggest that there is a longer terminal elimination half-life with fentanyl in the elderly leading to a longer duration of action of an administered dose.[13] As is commonly observed clinically, a dose of fentanyl will have a more profound effect in the elderly and that effect tends to last longer.

Benzodiazepine pharmacodynamics are significantly different between young and older patients. Benzodiazepines use has been shown to be associated with falls and hip fractures in the elderly.[14,15] The EC_{50} (half maximal effective concentration) for intravenous infusion of midazolam is reduced by 50% in older people. One study examined the midazolam Cp_{50} for response to verbal command (Cp_{50} is defined as the steady-state plasma concentration at which 50% of patients would be expected to not respond to a specific stimulus). Cp_{50} was significantly reduced with increasing patient age; it is less than 25% in patients who are 80 years old compared with those who are 40 years old.[16] This observation is not accounted for by age-related pharmacokinetic differences, such as protein binding. Alprazolam, on the other hand, showed no age-related differences in pharmacodynamics.[17] In a number of studies on different benzodiazepines, the elderly have significant baseline differences in the tested response measures, such as postural sway or reaction time.[18] Interestingly, γ-aminobutyric acid receptors do not seem to be increased with aging. Although exact mechanisms for pharmacodynamic differences in the elderly have not been worked out, postulated mechanisms include increased drug distribution to the CNS in the elderly.

Minimum alveolar concentration (MAC) of a volatile anesthetic at one atmosphere that prevents movement in 50% of patients exposed to a surgical incision is deceased with aging. This decrease can be represented by the formula:

$$MAC_{age} = MAC_{40} \times 10^{-0.00269(age - 40)}$$

where MAC at a given age is related to MAC values at age 40.[19]

Iso-MAC tables for inhalational agents are clinically very useful in that they clearly reflect the effect of age on MAC for different end-expiratory concentrations of agents in 100% oxygen, as well as in different mixes of nitrous oxide in oxygen. The necessary reduction in end-expiratory concentration for agents is often underappreciated with the elderly, even more so if using nitrous oxide in oxygen. For example, at age 80, only 0.3% isoflurane in 67% $N_2O:O_2$ will achieve 1.2 MAC. If subsequently one were to switch to 100% oxygen, one would need to increase the end-expiratory concentration of isoflurane to ~1.0% to achieve 1.2 MAC, keeping in mind the different solubilities of agents and nitrous oxide will affect clinical onset and recovery times (ie, N_2O is relatively insoluble and has faster onset and recovery than isoflurane. Thus, despite a more than 3-fold increase in the isoflurane end-expiratory concentration during transition from 67% $N_2O:O_2$ to 100% O_2, there will be relative lightening of anesthesia, since the N_2O effect will dissipate faster than the concurrent increase in Isoflurane concentration).[20] **Figure 25–1** clearly shows a decreased volatile agent concentration requirement to achieve a given MAC with increasing age and a significant further reduction when using nitrous oxide in oxygen.

Age-related differences also exist with neuromuscular blocking drugs. Rocuronium, for example, has been shown to have prolonged onset times in the elderly versus younger subjects, thought to be due to overall lower cardiac output, prolonged circulation time, and decreased muscle blood flow with slower biophase equilibration.[22] Clinical duration was longer in the elderly and females, up to 3 times longer interval to recovery (train-of-four ratio, 0.9) in elderly females compared to young males.[23] Median clinical duration times (time to 25% recovery of first twitch height in train-of-four) for elderly females was 85 minutes (range, 70–90 min) after 0.6-mg/kg rocuronium, compared with 30 minutes (25–42 min) for young males.[23] Vecuronium's onset times for maximal neuromuscular blockade given at 70 mcg/kg was longer with increasing age. Infusion rates of vecuronium required to maintain 90% blockade were lower and recovery times were also slower in the elderly.[24]

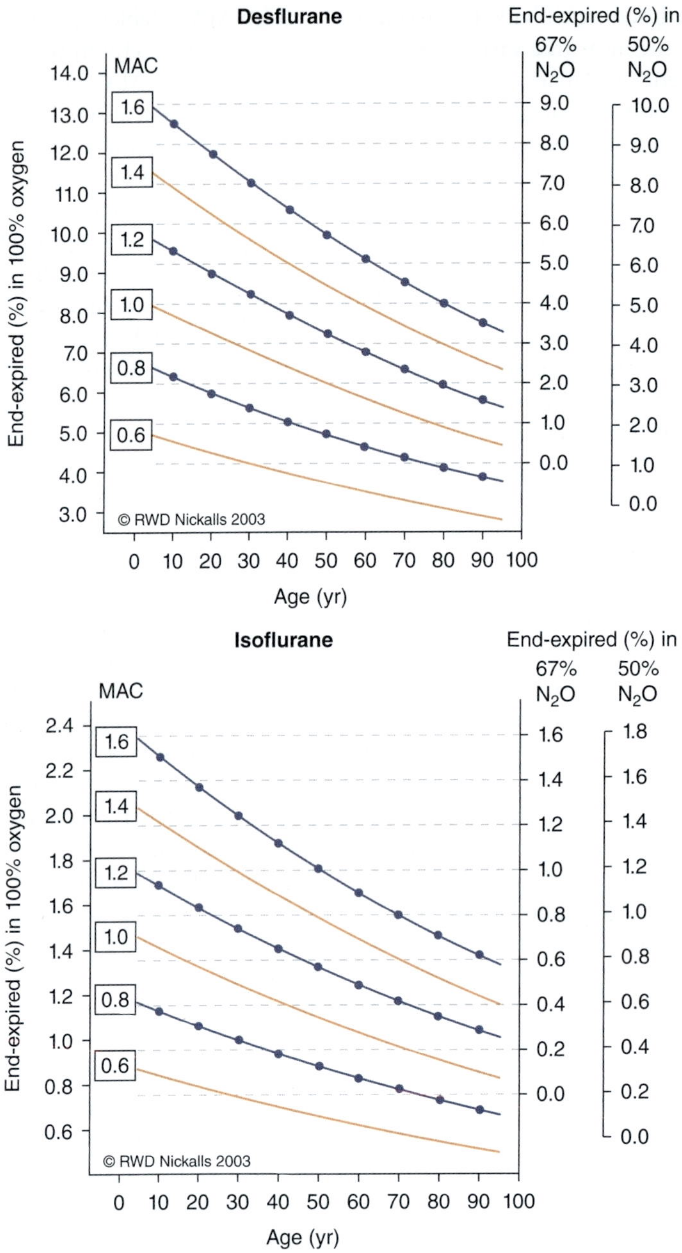

FIGURE 25–1 Iso-minimum alveolar concentration (MAC) charts for desflurane (top), isoflurane (middle), and sevoflurane (bottom) (age > 1 year). Curves are drawn for MAC (0.6–1.6). Dots on curves are present for help with alignment. The left scale indicates the end expiratory concentration of volatile agents using 100% oxygen. The right scales indicate end-expiratory volatile agent concentration in N_2O at 67% and 50% in oxygen. For a given age and MAC, the associated end-expiratory agent concentration is read from the appropriate ordinate scale. For example, a MAC of 1.2 in a 70-year-old patient, using 67% N_2O in oxygen, requires the end-expiratory concentration of sevoflurane to be ~0.6%.[20] (Reproduced with permission from Nickalls RWD, Mapleson WW. Age-related iso-MAC charts for isoflurane, sevoflurane and desflurance in man. *Br J Anaesth* 2003 Aug;91(2):170-174.)

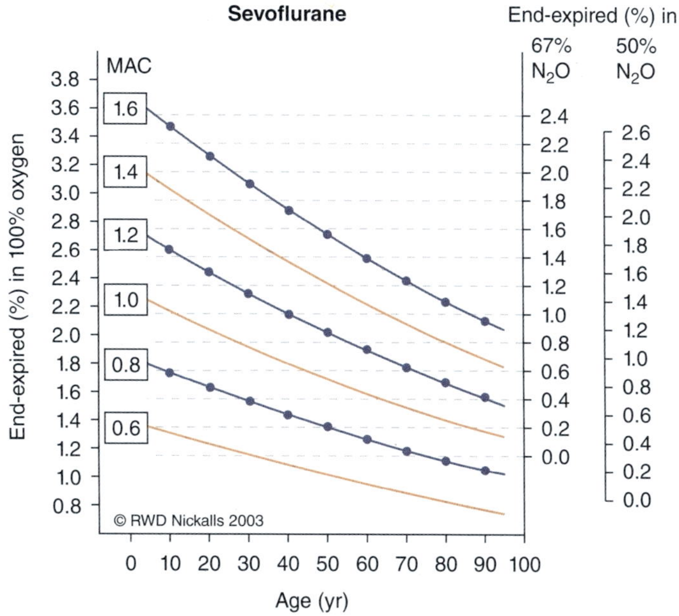

FIGURE 25–1 *(Continued)*

CASE DISCUSSION

An 80-year-old woman presents for surgery after sustaining an intertrochanteric femur fracture after tripping and falling. She has no other injuries and has had appropriate scans to rule out other fractures or pathology. She has a past medical history of compensated congestive heart failure, hypertension, hypothyroidism, and mild renal insufficiency. Medications include hydrochlorothiazide, a potassium supplement, metoprolol, levothyroxin, and multivitamins. She lives in an assisted living complex, and before the hip fracture had been ambulatory and able to achieve 4 metabolic equivalents of activity.

Spinal or General Anesthesia?

Consideration in choosing spinal versus general anesthesia requires a careful risk-benefit analysis. Often in orthopedic trauma surgery, spinal is not an option for a number of reasons. These include anticipated significant blood loss, making spinal and the subsequent sympathectomy relatively contraindicated, dangers of masking pain from compartment syndrome in lower extremity orthopedic surgery, iatrogenic or intrinsic anticoagulation issues, and length of surgery limitations. Positioning lateral for a total hip arthroplasty in an elderly person under spinal can also be challenging, as discomfort from positioning often ensues and there are safety limits to increasing the depth of sedation without a protected airway and in the lateral position. General anesthesia may also be preferable in that other monitors, such as transesophageal echocardiography, can be implemented to guide volume management. Benefits of a spinal, if not contraindicated for the above reasons and in a stable patient, include excellent pain control; avoidance of the cognitive disturbances from general anesthesia; and avoiding intubating the trachea and mechanically ventilating the lungs, both of which can add to overall perioperative risk.

Premedication

In elderly patients, cautious administration and decreased dosages are necessary. Anxiolysis can be beneficial in optimizing hemodynamics preoperatively (eg, reducing anxiety-related tachycardia or hypertension). These benefits, however, should be weighed against possible increased postoperative sedation, which can be more problematic in the elderly or those with preexisting cognitive deficits. Premedication with benzodiazepines has been shown to significantly reduce the dose requirements of propofol in both elderly and younger patients, and adjustment should be made accordingly.[21] In one randomized, placebo controlled trial, intravenous midazolam, in doses up to 2 mg, did not affect emergence, extubation ,or orientation times in geriatric patients undergoing brief surgical procedures. Postanesthesia care unit times, however, were significantly prolonged, and there was an increased incidence of oxygen saturations less than 94%, in a dose-dependent manner.

Induction

Induction of general anesthesia is typically achieved with a combination of intravenous agents, such as an opioid; a sedative–hypnotic agent, often given with lidocaine; and a neuromuscular blocking agent to facilitate tracheal intubation. Doses of opioids and sedative–hypnotics should be decreased up to 50% in the elderly, and agents should be titrated to effect. With a history of poor cardiac function, induction goals should be to attempt to maintain stable hemodynamics. This can be accomplished by achieving deep sedation with an opioid such as fentanyl prior to using a significantly decreased dose of an induction agent, such as etomidate, to achieve unconsciousness. It is important to remember there is no one best method or best agent to induce anesthesia, and a variety of patient and surgical characteristics play a role in clinical decision making regarding the induction of anesthesia. Obviously, any one patient can have multiple important considerations or comorbidities (eg, difficult airway, obesity, cardiovascular compromise, old age, chronic pain, hypovolemia).

A sample regimen might consist of the following:

- Opioid: fentanyl 1 to 3 mcg/kg, 3 to 5 minutes prior to induction
- Sedative–hypnotic: propofol, titrated to effect, often 1 mg/kg, or even less, sufficient to produce unconsciousness, when combined with an opioid. Alternatively, etomidate 0.1 to 0.3 mg/kg, depending on opioid dose and effect, can be used. This provides often better cardiovascular stability on induction versus alternative induction agents and is the induction drug of choice for many in unstable or high risks patients.
- Muscle relaxant: succinylcholine, 1.5 mg/kg after unconsciousness is achieved with the above agents, with an absence of known contraindications to succinylcholine. A nondepolarizing neuromuscular blocker as alternative, such as rocuronium 0.6 mg/kg, may be used, realizing it has a slower onset of action and longer duration in the elderly and females. Neuromuscular transmission (twitch) monitor should be used to guide neuromuscular blockade and timing of reversal.

Maintenance

Maintenance can be achieved with a balanced anesthetic of volatile agent and opioid. Again, increasing the end-tidal concentration of volatile anesthetic a bit more slowly and cautiously is prudent in elderly patients versus younger patients, watching closely for hemodynamic compromise. Elderly patients often require boluses of vasopressors, such as ephedrine or phenylephrine, immediately after induction to maintain a reasonable mean arterial pressure, especially in those patients with preexisting hypertension. One could also consider a total intravenous anesthesia (TIVA) technique, such as propofol and remifentanil infusions, to take advantage of the relatively short-acting effects of these agents and hopefully minimizing postoperative sedation and confusion. This technique is especially effective in surgical cases that do not generate high levels of postoperative pain, taking advantage of remifentanil's short context-sensitive half-time and where more precise titration of longer acting opioids is not as critical.

Sample regimens might consist of the following:

- Isoflurane 1/2 to 1 MAC with intermittent opioid boluses, such as fentanyl. One can consider using longer acting opioids with orthopedic surgery, such as hydromorphone or morphine, to avoid significant postoperative pain and accompanied adrenergic effects.

- TIVA single syringe: propofol 50 mL with remifentanil 1 mg added to make remifentanil concentration 20 mcg/mL of propofol. Start 80 to 100 mcg/kg/min as infusion. Again, maintenance doses may need to be titrated down in the elderly.

Emergence and Postoperative Care

Mental status and strength assessments are often more difficult in the elderly. Elderly patients may be hard of hearing and have cognitive decline, making communication and simple command assessments more challenging. As previously stated, they are more sensitive to anesthetics. If neuromuscular blockade is used during the case, full reversal and sustained tetanus with a twitch monitor should be ensured. If patients are obese, extubation in inclined or sitting position if appropriate should be recommended, to facilitate adequate ventilation (Chapter 20). It is necessary to observe for postoperative delirium or confusion. Frequent orientation to location and place is often necessary in the immediate postoperative period in the elderly. Sedating drugs, such as diphenhydramine or droperidol, should be avoided if possible. The elderly may require a very long time to recover postoperatively from a mental status standpoint due to residual effects of anesthetics. However, it is important to always first consider other causes of altered mental status in these patients. A differential diagnosis of postoperative altered mental status should include hypoxemia, hypercarbia, hypotension, or other cardiopulmonary compromise, metabolic disturbances, such as high or low sodium or glucose levels, or primary neurologic pathology, such as stroke or seizure. The elderly simply do not have the same functional reserve as younger patients and often require closer perioperative monitoring and care. A low threshold to escalate postoperative care to an intensive care unit or intermediate care unit is prudent in the elderly.

REFERENCES

1. United Nations. Implications of an Aging Society. Available at: www.un.org/esa/socdev/ageing/htm.
2. Fedarko NS. The biology of aging and frailty. *Clin Geriatr Med.* 2011;27(1):27-37.
3. Cook DJ, Rooke GA. Priorities in perioperative geriatrics. *Anesth Analg.* 2003;96(6):1823-1836.
4. Rivera R, Antognini JF. Perioperative drug therapy in elderly patients. *Anesthesiology.* 2009;110(5):1176-1181.
5. Fu A, Nair KS. Age effect on fibrinogen and albumin synthesis in humans. *Am J Physiol.* 1998;275:E1023-E1030.
6. Benet LZ, Hoener BA. Changes in plasma protein binding have little clinical relevance. *Clin Pharmacol Ther.* 2002;71:115-121.
7. Beaufrere B, Morio B. Fat and protein redistribution with aging: metabolic considerations. *Eur J Clin Nutr.* 2000;54:S48-S53.
8. McLean AJ, Le Couteur DG. Aging biology and geriatric clinical pharmacology. *Am Soc Pharmacol Exp Ther.* 2004;56:163-184.
9. Schnider TW, Minto CF, Shafer SL, et al. The influence of age on propofol pharmacodynamics. *Anesthesiology.* 1999;90(6):1502-1516.
10. Kazama T, Takeuchi K, Ikeda K, et al. Optimal propofol plasma concentration during upper gastrointestinal endoscopy in young, middle-aged, and elderly patients. *Anesthesiology.* 2000;93:662-669.
11. Homer TD, Stanski DR. The effect of increasing age on thiopental disposition and anesthetic requirement. *Anesthesiology.* 1985;62:714-724.
12. Scott JC, Stanski DR. Decreased fentanyl/alfentanil dose requirements with increasing age: a pharmacodynamic basis. *Anesthesiology.* 1985;63:159-166.
13. Bentley JB, Borel JD, Nenad RE Jr, Gillespie TJ. Age and fentanyl pharmacokinetics. *Anesth Analg.* 1982;61:968-971.
14. Ray W, Thap PB, Gideon P. Benzodiazepines and the risk of falls in nursing home residents. *J Am Geriatr Soc.* 2000;48(6):682-685.
15. Cumming RG, Le Couteur DG. Benzodiazepines and risk of hip fractures in older people: a review of the evidence. *CNS Drugs.* 2003;17(11):825-837.
16. Jacobs JR, Reves JG, Marty J, White WD, Bai SA, Smith LR. Aging increases pharmacodynamic sensitivity to the hypnotic effects of midazolam. *Anesth Analg.* 1995;80(1):143-148.
17. Pomara N, Tun H, DaSilva D, Hernando R, Deptula D, Greenblatt DJ. The acute and chronic performance effects of alprazolam and lorazepam in the elderly: relationship to duration of treatment and self-rated sedation. *Psychopharmacol Bull.* 1998; 34(2):139-153.

18. Bowie MW, Slattum PW. Pharmacodynamics in older adults: a review. *Am J Geriatr Pharmacother.* 2007;5(3):263-303.
19. Mapleson WW. Effect of age on MAC in humans. *Br J Anaesth.* 1996;76:179-185.
20. Nickalls RWD, Mapleson WW. Age-related iso-MAC charts for isoflurane, sevoflurane and desflurane in man, *Br J Anaesth.* 2003;91(2):170-174.
21. Cressey DM, Claydon P, Bhaskaran NC, Reilly CS. Effect of midazolam pretreatment on induction dose requirements of propofol in combination with fentanyl in younger and older adults. *Anaesthesia.* 2001;56(2):108-113.
22. Donati F. Onset of action of relaxants. *Can J Anaesth.* 1998;35:S52-S58.
23. Adamus M, Hrabalek L, Wanek T, Gabrhelik T, Zapletalova J. Influence of age and gender on the pharmacodynamic parameters of rocuronium during total intravenous anesthesia. *Biomed Pap Med Fac Univ Palacky Olomouc Czech Repub.* 2011; 115(4):347-354.
24. O'Hara DA, Fragen RJ, Shanks CA. The effects of age on the dose-response curves for vecuronium in adults. *Anesthesiology.* 1985;63:542-545.

CHAPTER 26

Premedicants

Dustin E. Coyle, MD

INTRODUCTION

Anesthesiologists recognize the expanding role of premedication in optimizing patient's condition prior to surgery. Important goals of premedication include reducing patient anxiety, providing analgesia as needed, facilitating induction of anesthesia, and optimizing patient comorbidities. This chapter will provide a brief overview of well-known premedication drugs, such as intravenous opioids and benzodiazepines, and explore how they interact with one another and how they may influence induction of anesthesia. This chapter will also review indications, controversies, and potential drawbacks of selected premedications used to manage common patient comorbidities.

MIDAZOLAM

Midazolam enjoys wide spread popularity among anesthesiologists because it has a rapid onset of anxiolysis with minimal side effects and provides anterograde amnesia. Midazolam is water-soluble, and unlike diazepam, does not cause irritation on injection. At relatively low doses (0.02 mg/kg), midazolam is an effective anxiolytic over a large age range (20–80 years), with minimal respiratory depression in healthy individuals of either gender.[1] Larger doses (0.05 mg/kg) increase the likelihood of sedation but are not more effective at reducing anxiety.[1] Elderly debilitated patients require up to 20% less midazolam (0.016 mg/kg) to achieve an equivalent anxiolytic effect.[2] For example, patients who have an American Society of Anesthesiologists (ASA) physical classification of 3 or greater and who are of age 55 or older should be dosed with caution.

An advantage of benzodiazepines is they attenuate catecholamine-induced stress response. For example, at doses of 0.025 mg/kg, midazolam attenuates stress responses; at 0.05 mg/kg it abolishes stress responses.[3] This may be especially useful in patients with severe coronary artery or cerebral vascular disease who are at significant risk for catecholamine-induced ischemia.

Midazolam has an interesting kinetic profile (Figure 26–1). It has a rapid rise in effect-site concentration with intravenous administration in comparison to other benzodiazepines. However, it requires a relatively long time to reach peak concentrations (6–9 minutes), and plasma concentrations dissipate more slowly in comparison to other intravenous sedatives (eg, propofol). An anxiolytic effect is typically observed within minutes; clinicians may be tempted to administer additional midazolam if an effect is not observed within 2 minutes. Given that peak concentrations are not achieved for up to 6 minutes, additional doses may lead to more pronounced effect. For example, Figure 26–1 presents the anticipated effects from 2 doses of midazolam (0.025 mg/kg or 2 mg to an 80-kg individual) separated by 2 minutes using the Ramsay Sedation Scale (RSS).[4] The RSS (range, 0–6) quantifies the effects of midazolam from anxiolysis (RSS = 2) to sedation (RSS = 3) to loss of responsiveness (RSS = 6). The additional midazolam dose prolongs reaching peak to 8 minutes and doubles the effect-site concentration, leading to an increased probability of sedation beyond just anxiolysis.

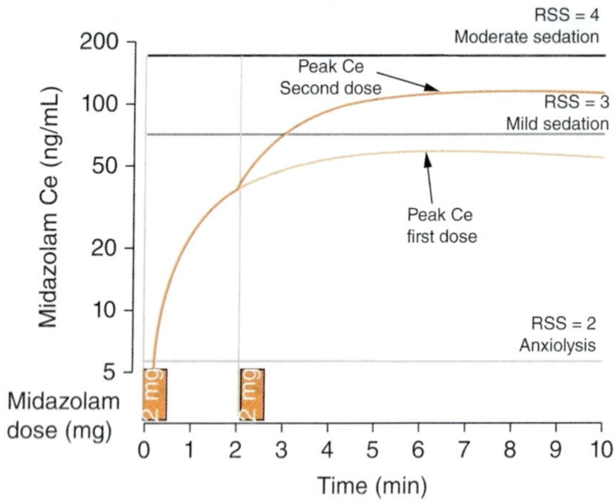

FIGURE 26–1 Simulations of midazolam effect-site concentrations (Ce levels) following 2 doses of midazolam (0.025 mg/kg each) separated by 2 minutes. The vertical axis is on the logarithmic scale. The gray horizontal lines represent midazolam C_{50} plasma concentrations for levels of sedation as defined by the Ramsay Sedation Scale (RSS).[4] C_{50} indicates the concentration where half of individuals exhibit a given effect and half do not. Of note, the peak concentration following a single dose occurs at approximately 6 minutes and after the second dose at 8 minutes. The single dose leads to primarily anxiolysis with little to no sedation, whereas the second dose leads to mild sedation.

MIDAZOLAM AND FENTANYL

Opioids can decrease anxiety by ameliorating pain, a common preoperative issue. Opioids are often given in combination with midazolam. Fentanyl is frequently used because it is has a fast onset (peak effect within 5 minutes), short duration of action, and produces intense analgesia.

Midazolam interacts synergistically with fentanyl and other opioids. The analgesic and respiratory effects of fentanyl are pronounced in the presence of midazolam, and the anxiolytic and sedative effects of midazolam are pronounced in the presence of fentanyl.[5] For example, in a study exploring the interaction between fentanyl and midazolam, fentanyl 2 mcg/kg by itself led to hypoxemia (SpO_2 < 90%) in half of recipients and midazolam 0.05 mg/kg caused no hypoxemia. When combined, however, essentially all study participants developed hypoxemia and half developed apnea.[6] Other researchers confirmed this finding[7] using similar dosing regimens for fentanyl (1.25 mcg/kg) combined with midazolam (0.05 mg/kg), emphasizing the importance of continuously monitoring patients when administering these drugs together.

Simulations of these dosing regimens visually illustrate the time course of effects presented in these reports (Figure 26–2) for a healthy male who stands 6 feet (183 cm)and weighs 176 pounds (80 kg). High-dose combinations (midazolam 0.05 mg/kg with fentanyl 2 mcg/kg) reach peak concentrations between 5 and 9 minutes. These doses in an 80-kg individual would be 4 mg of midazolam and 160 mcg of fentanyl and are perhaps higher than what anesthesiologists routinely administer. A high probability of analgesia is achieved within minutes and remains high for up to 1 hour. The probability of intolerable ventilatory depression (a respiratory rate less than 4 breaths/min) reaches a 40% probability within 5 minutes and then slowly diminishes over the next 30 minutes. As dosed, this combination of fentanyl and midazolam leads to a high probability of sedation for more than 40 minutes and a low probability of loss of responsiveness (< 20%) for 15 minutes. If using this dosing regimen for premedication, up to 30 minutes of continuous monitoring for apnea and hypoxemia would be prudent.

A more common dosing regimen is also presented in Figure 26–2. With midazolam 0.012 mg/kg and fentanyl 0.6 mcg/kg (approximately 1 mg of midazolam and 50 mcg of fentanyl in an 80-kg individual), the likelihood of analgesia is lower (25%–50%) for a much shorter period of time (< 15 minutes) compared to the high dose. The probability of intolerable ventilatory depression and loss of responsiveness is negligible. Some patients may develop sedation (15% probability) for 10 to 15 minutes.

INFLUENCE OF PREMEDICATION ON INDUCTION AGENTS

If administered in temporal proximity to induction, premedicants may enhance induction drug effect. Both midazolam and fentanyl interact with propofol.[5] One concern is that if during induction an unanticipated difficult airway is encountered, premedication may prolong emergence if it is necessary to wake up a patient rapidly.

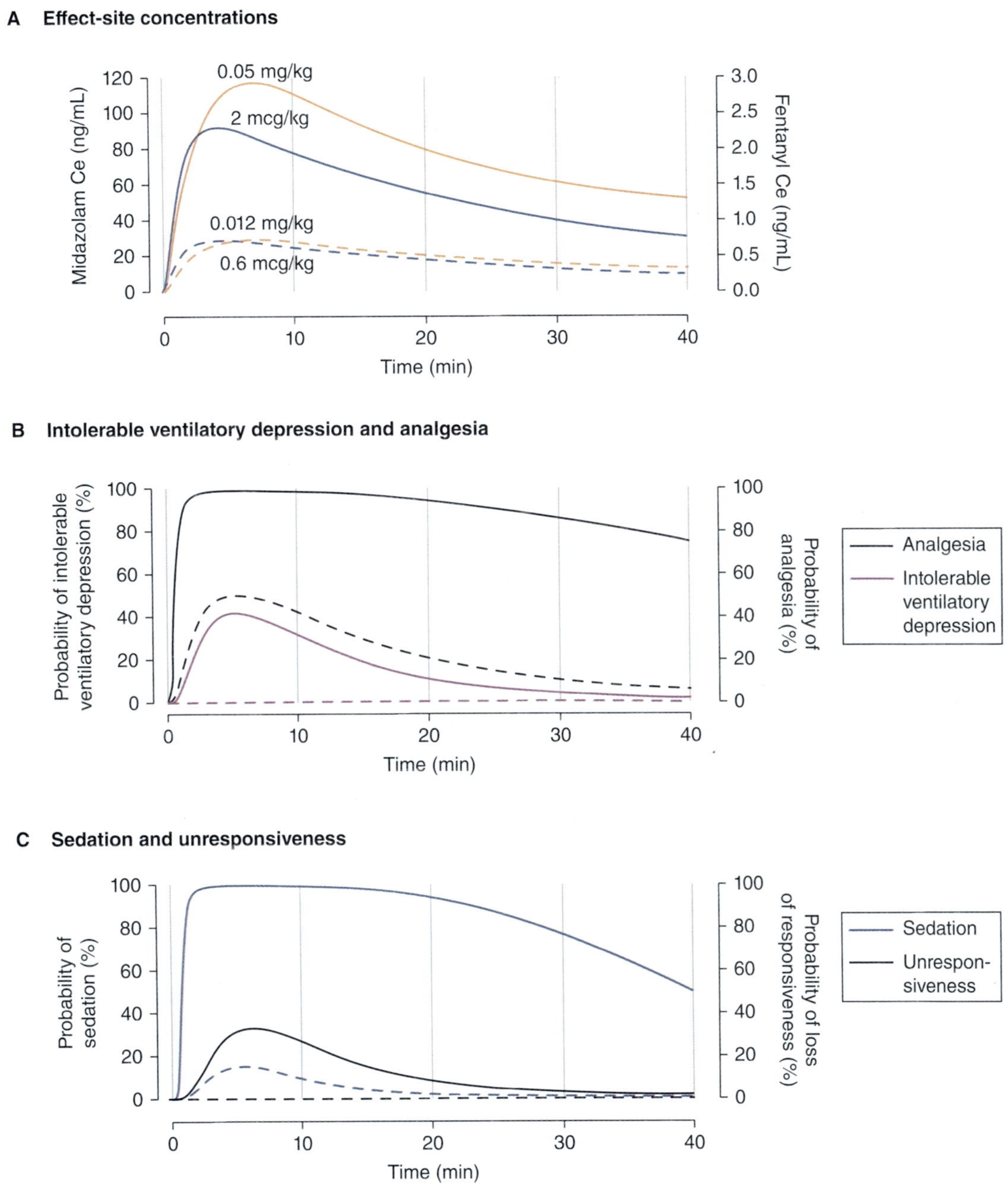

FIGURE 26–2 Simulations of effect-site concentrations (Ce levels) (A), intolerable ventilatory depression and analgesia (B), and sedation and unresponsiveness (C) for premedication with low- and high-dose fentanyl (0.6 and 2 mcg/kg) and midazolam (0.012 and 0.05 mg/kg). Intolerable ventilatory depression is defined as a respiratory rate of less than 4 breaths/min. Analgesia is defined as a loss of response to a moderately painful stimulus (30 pounds per square inch of tibial pressure). Sedation is defined as responsive only after loudly or repeatedly calling an individual's name. Unresponsiveness is defined as no response to tactile and verbal stimuli. Drug effects for high and low doses are represented as solid and dashed lines, respectively.

To explore this concern, a simulation of premedication followed by induction of anesthesia 10 minutes later is presented in Figure 26–3. In this simulation, midazolam 0.025 mg/kg is administered 5 minutes prior to induction of anesthesia as a premedication. Five minutes later, induction of anesthesia begins with fentanyl 2 mcg/kg, followed 5 minutes later by propofol 2 mg/kg. Simulations present the time course of unresponsiveness and sedation with and without the midazolam and fentanyl.

As dosed, propofol renders 50% and 95% of patients unresponsive for 6 and 3 minutes, respectively. With the addition of midazolam and fentanyl, the duration of unresponsiveness for 50% and 95% of patients is extended to 9 and 5 minutes, respectively. Midazolam or fentanyl added to the propofol prolongs the duration by 1 minute compared to propofol alone. Waiting an additional 3 minutes for a patient to emerge from induction in an unanticipated difficult airway may be unacceptable in a setting of "can't intubate and can't ventilate."

Midazolam and fentanyl substantially prolong sedation compared to propofol alone; their interaction is more pronounced than with loss of responsiveness. In these simulations, sedation is defined using the Observer's Assessment of Alertness and Sedation Scale.[8] Patients are considered sedated if they respond only after their name is called loudly or repeatedly. As dosed, propofol renders 50% and 95% of patients sedated for 7 and 4 minutes, respectively. With the addition of midazolam and fentanyl, the duration of sedation for 50% and 95% of patients is markedly extended to 44 and 24 minutes, respectively. Midazolam added to the propofol has minimal impact on the duration of sedation, but fentanyl added to the propofol prolongs the duration of sedation to 29 and 13 minutes for 50% and 95% of patients, respectively.

Another point of interest with premedicants is their impact on sedative–hypnotic dosing requirements for induction. Several researchers have explored how midazolam and/or fentanyl premedication, if administered near induction, decreases the amount of propofol needed to achieve loss of responsiveness.[9-12]

How midazolam (0.025 mg/kg) as a premedicant and fentanyl (2 mcg/kg) as part of the induction influences the propofol dose is illustrated in Figure 26–4. In the presence of midazolam and fentanyl, the time course of unresponsiveness from propofol 0.5, 1, 1.5, and 2 mg/kg is compared to propofol 2 mg/kg alone. With both midazolam and fentanyl, the amount of propofol required to achieve a near-equipotent effect to propofol 2 mg/kg in terms of unresponsiveness is 1 mg/kg (Table 26–1). With either midazolam or fentanyl, as dosed, the amount of propofol required to achieve a near-equipotent effect is 1.5 mg/kg.

These simulations are consistent with reports of the propofol-sparing effect by fentanyl and midazolam. For example, fentanyl dosed to achieve an effect-site concentration of 3 ng/mL (approximately 2.5 mcg/kg) decreases the propofol effect-site concentration required for loss of consciousness in 50% of patients by 40%.[9] Similarly, midazolam 0.05 mg/kg decreases the propofol required for loss of responsiveness in 50% of patients from 1.0 to 0.4 mg/kg.[10] As expected, smaller midazolam doses (0.025 mg/kg) require more propofol to achieve loss of responsiveness.[11]

Unlike propofol, not much data are available exploring the interactions of opioids and benzodiazepines with etomidate. With regard to opioids, in an animal model, etomidate was found to have a synergistic interaction with fentanyl in producing loss of the righting reflex (a measure of hypnosis) in rats.[13] In patients, increasing doses of fentanyl are more likely to produce apnea with an induction dose of etomidate, but apnea is fairly common with an induction dose of etomidate alone.[14] With regard to benzodiazepines, one study reported that there was no significant difference in sedation score or recovery time when patients were given either a small dose of midazolam (0.015 mg/kg) or placebo prior to a 0.3-mg/kg bolus of etomidate for cardioversion.[15] Given the small dose, it is difficult to ascertain any synergistic or additive effect between midazolam and etomidate with regard to producing hypnosis. In sum, there are very little data to determine how fentanyl and/or midazolam reduce etomidate requirements during induction.

Simulations

Simulations of drug effect-site concentrations were based on published pharmacokinetic models of midazolam,[16] fentanyl,[17] and propofol.[18] Simulations

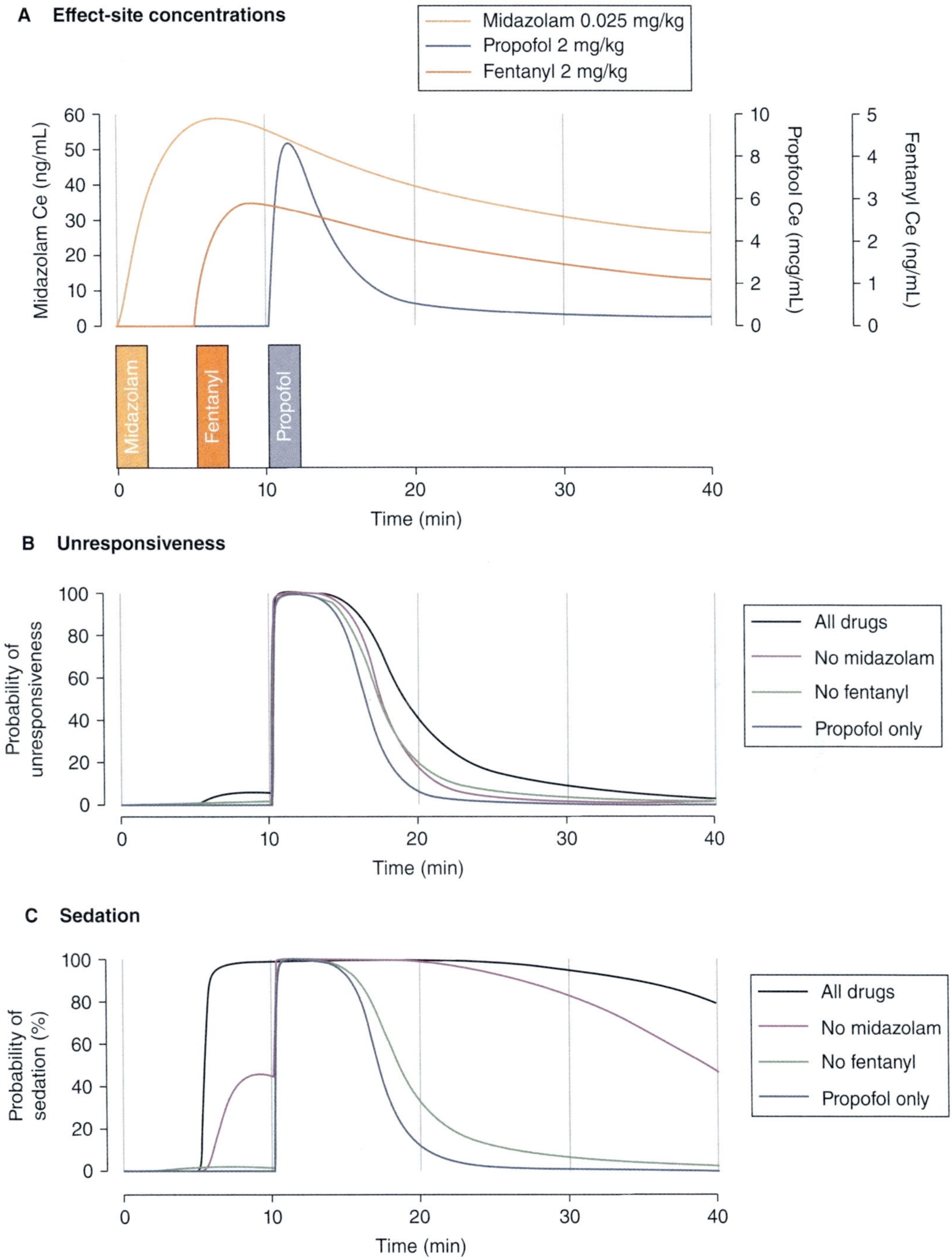

FIGURE 26–3 Simulations of effect-site concentrations (Ce levels) (A), unresponsiveness (B), and sedation (C) for premedication with midazolam followed by induction with fentanyl and propofol. Unresponsiveness is defined as no response to tactile and verbal stimuli. Sedation is defined as responsive only after loudly or repeatedly calling an individual's name.

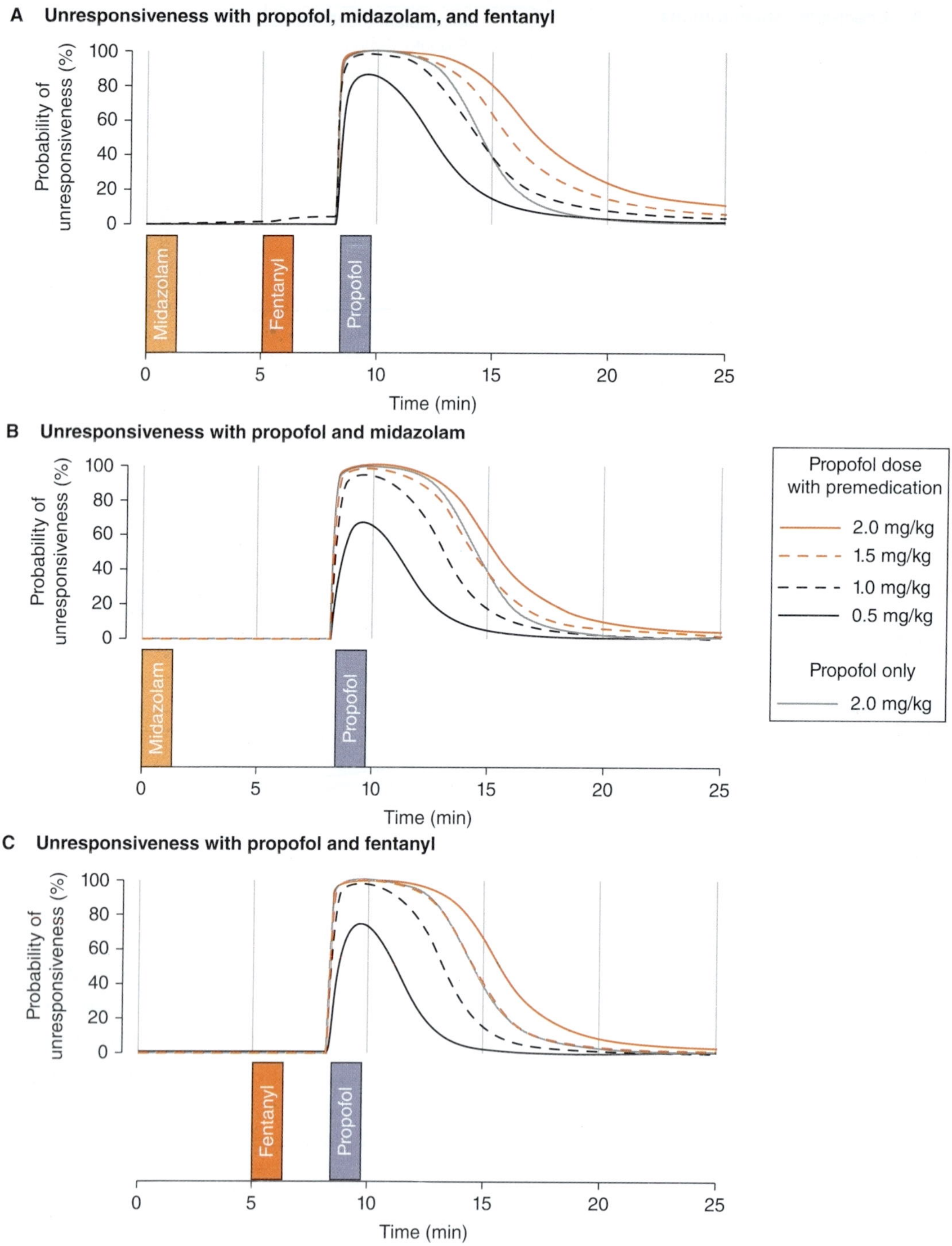

FIGURE 26–4 Simulations of unresponsiveness for various propofol doses (0.5, 1, 1.5, and 2 mg/kg). Ten minutes prior to induction with propofol, midazolam 0.025 mg/kg (time = 0) was administered followed 5 minutes later by fentanyl 2.5 mcg/mL). The probabilities of unresponsiveness with propofol, midazolam, and fentanyl are presented in A, with propofol and midazolam in B, and with propofol and fentanyl in C.

TABLE 26–1 Simulations of duration of unresponsiveness with and without premedication.

Propofol With Midazolam and Fentanyl				
Propofol dose (mg/kg)	**2**	**1.5**	**1**	**0.5**
Above 50% (min)	8	7	6	4
Above 95% (min)	5	4	3	0
Propofol With Midazolam (No Fentanyl)				
Propofol dose (mg/kg)	**2**	**1.5**	**1**	**0.5**
Above 50% (min)	7	6	4	2
Above 95% (min)	4	3	0	0
Propofol With Fentanyl (No Midazolam)				
Propofol dose (mg/kg)	**2**	**1.5**	**1**	**0.5**
Above 50% (min)	7	6	5	3
Above 95% (min)	4	3	1	0
Propofol Alone				
Propofol dose (mg/kg)	**2**			
Above 50% (min)	6			
Above 95% (min)	3			

Above 50% and 95% indicates the duration of time (in minutes) that the probability of unresponsiveness is above 50% and 95%, respectively. Midazolam 0.025 mg/kg was dosed 5 minutes prior to induction. Fentanyl 2 mcg/kg was administered at the time of induction, and propofol was administered 3 minutes after the fentanyl. The values in the gray cells represent times that are similar to a propofol bolus with no midazolam or fentanyl.

of drug effects used published work for sedation with midazolam,[4] and published models of sedation and loss of responsiveness[19] and models of analgesia and intolerable ventilatory depression[20-22] for propofol combined with remifentanil. Assumptions and limitations of these simulations are presented in Table 26–2.

TABLE 26–2 Simulation limitations and assumptions.

Limitations
Interaction models for sedation and unresponsiveness between propofol and midazolam are not available. Based on electroencephalographic changes,[21] equipotent effect-site concentrations for propofol and midazolam were used to convert midazolam to propofol equivalents. Interaction models for unresponsive and analgesia between fentanyl and midazolam also are not available. Prior work has indicated that interactions are synergistic.[6] For simulation purposes, the interaction was considered to be similar to that of propofol and fentanyl congeners.
Models that predict unresponsiveness have been created in the presence of a mild stimulus (i.e. shake and shout). More anesthetic is likely required to ensure unresponsiveness in the presence of moderate to severe stimuli (laryngoscopy, skin incision).
No model of *consciousness* or *awareness* exists; only models of *responsiveness*. Patients may be unresponsive but still be conscious or aware, although unlikely in the presence of a painful stimulus and no paralytic. By contrast, patients may be responsive but have no memory of an event. Although not identical, unresponsiveness is the best available surrogate of unconsciousness.
Assumptions
Cardiac output remains stable and intravascular volume is normal throughout the premedication period.
Patients are opioid and benzodiazepine naïve
Metabolic organ perfusion (the liver and kidney) remains constant

OTHER PREMEDICANTS

Antacids

Antacids are frequently given as premedication before induction of anesthesia, especially in patients at high risk for aspiration. The goal of giving an antacid preoperatively is to reduce stomach pH to a level above 2.5, because a pH below that level is considered a risk factor for acid aspiration syndrome.[23] Commonly used perioperative antacids include the histamine receptor-2 (H_2) antagonists ranitidine and famotidine, which can be given intravenously, and sodium citrate, a nonparticulate antacid, which is given orally.

Ranitidine and famotidine have both been shown to increase gastric pH and decrease gastric volume, although famotidine was superior at doing both.[24] Forty-five minutes after intravenous administration, famotidine increases gastric pH by 43% and decreases gastric volume by an average of 24%.[25]

Sodium citrate 30 mL given 5 minutes before induction raises gastric pH more than 2.5.[26,27] However, it significantly increases gastric volume[26] unless given concomitantly with an intravenous H_2 antagonist.[28]

Gastrokinetic Agents

Metoclopramide, a dopamine antagonist, increases gastrointestinal peristalsis and relaxes the pyloric sphincter to increase stomach emptying. It has been used in premedication regimens to prevent acid aspiration. A dose of 10 mg, given intravenously 15 to 30 minutes before induction, is effective at significantly reducing residual gastric volumes but does not reduce pH.[29] Other researchers have reported that doses of 0.15 mg/kg lower gastric volumes and increase gastric pH.[30]

Antiemetics

Postoperative nausea and vomiting (PONV) is a frequent complication of anesthesia, especially in high-risk patients. Many medications are now available for prevention and treatment of this problem. The timing of giving these drugs is somewhat important for optimal prevention of PONV. Only 2 of these drugs are more effective when given at the beginning of surgery: dexamethasone and scopolamine.

Dexamethasone in a dose of 2.5 to 5 mg, when administered before anesthesia induction, is effective at preventing PONV with a number needed to treat of about 4.[31] Transdermal scopolamine is most effective when applied the night prior to anesthesia, or at least 4 hours prior to the end of anesthesia.[31]

Other commonly used antiemetics such as $5HT_3$ antagonists, droperidol, and prochlorperazine are best given at the end of anesthesia.[31]

Beta Blockers

A recent debate in anesthesiology has been whether to start β-blocker therapy in certain patients prior to surgery. β Blockers are advocated for patients with coronary artery disease (CAD) undergoing vascular procedures.[32] Even though many studies have found a decrease in perioperative myocardial events in patients started on β-blocker therapy,[33,34] several recent large randomized trials,[35,36] as well as a large meta-analysis[37] have shown an increase in all-cause mortality and stroke.

Patients who are chronically on β blockers do not seem to show an increase in perioperative stroke when undergoing noncardiac surgery.[38] The incidence of postoperative stroke is lower in studies where β-blocker therapy is started at least a week prior to surgery.[39]

The dose and timing of initiating β blockers preoperatively to decrease myocardial morbidity but not increase stroke risk has not yet been determined by a large, randomized trial. Therefore, it is not recommended to start patients on β blockers prior to noncardiac surgery. However, patients on chronic β-blocker therapy should continue their medication in the perioperative period.[32,39]

Angiotensin-Converting Enzyme Inhibitors and Angiotensin Receptor Blockers

Continuing patients on their angiotensin-converting enzyme (ACE) inhibitors up to the morning of surgery is associated with significant intraoperative hypotension, which has led many to recommend withholding these anti-hypertensives the morning of surgery.[40-42] However, the decision about whether to continue ACE inhibitors the morning of surgery remains controversial, because despite the moderate hypotension, it appears that there is no increase in the incidence of severe hypotension or the use of vasopressors intraoperatively.[41] The hypotension appears to be transient and does not persist beyond the first 30 minutes after induction.[41] In conjunction with diuretic therapy, preoperative ACE inhibitors are associated with more need for intraoperative vasopressor use but no increase in the incidence of myocardial infarction or postoperative renal failure.[43] Patients taking ACE inhibitors who received spinal anesthesia did not experience hypotension any more severe than those not taking the medications.[44] There was no difference in the incidence of hypotension in patients with good left ventricular function continuing or omitting their ACE inhibitor the morning of coronary artery bypass graft surgery.[45]

Angiotensin receptor blockers (ARBs) appear to cause longer periods of more profound hypotension requiring vasopressor therapy than do ACE inhibitors.[46] The ARBs were also not associated with increased incidences of myocardial infarction or renal failure.[43]

There does not seem to be any convincing evidence that cancelling surgery because patients did not stop their ACE inhibitors or ARBs is necessary or beneficial. Furthermore, there is no convincing evidence that ACE inhibitors protect the kidneys from damage during surgery,[47] or offer any other benefit that would lead to a recommendation to start them on any particular patient population preoperatively.

Statins

Statins are another group of drugs that may be promising premedicants to give certain patient populations. Initially prescribed to treat cholesterol, these HMG-CoA reductase inhibitors have been shown to do the following: (1) reduce plasma inflammatory markers such as tumor necrosis factor-α and interleukin-6 [48] and (2) lower cardiovascular-related death in patients without hyperlipidemia but with elevated C-reactive protein.[49]

The 2007 American Heart Association/American College of Cardiology guidelines acknowledge that there is evidence supporting perioperative use of statins to prevent cardiac complications in noncardiac surgery, but that it is unclear how to identify which patients would benefit, when to initiate therapy, and for how long.[32] It appears that vascular surgery and cardiac surgery patients show varying degrees of benefit from decreased cardiovascular events[50,51] and mortality,[52] to decreased incidence of atrial fibrillation[53] and stroke.[54] The benefits of statins in noncardiac surgery have been suggested in retrospective studies but have not been established in prospective studies.

There is good evidence that continuing patients on their statins perioperatively is beneficial and that stopping them abruptly is associated with increased morbidity and mortality.[55] Statin withdrawal of over 4 days seems to be a risk factor for postoperative myocardial events.[56]

As with β blockers, it is unclear yet whether statins should be started preoperatively in patients not already on them. However, it is clear that patients already taking them chronically should be maintained on them throughout the perioperative period.[57]

REFERENCES

1. Sun GC, Hsu MC, Chia YY, et al. Effects of age and gender on intravenous midazolam premedication: a randomized double-blind study. *Br J Anaesth.* 2008;101:632-639.
2. Reeves JG, Fragen RJ, Vinik HR, et al. Midazolam: pharmacology and uses. *Anesthesiology.* 1985;62: 310-324.
3. Dorges V, Wenzel V, Dix S, et al. The effect of midazolam on stress levels during simulated emergency medical service transport: a placebo-controlled, dose-response study. *Anesth Analg.* 2002;95:417-422.
4. Somma J, Donner A, Zomorodi K, et al. Population pharmacodynamics of midazolam administered by target controlled infusion in SICU patients after CABG surgery. *Anesthesiology.* 1998;89(6):1430-1443.
5. Hendrickx JA, Eger EI, Sonner JM, et al. Is synergy the rule? A review of anesthetic interactions producing hypnosis and immobility. *Anesth Analg.* 2008;107:494-506.
6. Bailey PL, Pace NL, Ashburn MA, et al. Frequent hypoxemia and apnea after sedation with midazolam and fentanyl. *Anesthesiology.* 1990;73:826-830.
7. Deitch K, Chudnofsky CR, Domincini P. The utility of supplemental oxygen during emergency department procedural sedation and analgesia with midazolam and fentanyl: a randomized, controlled trial. *Ann Emerg Med.* 2007;49:1-8.
8. Chernik DA, Gillings D, Laine H, et al. Validity and reliability of the Observer's Assessment of Alertness/Sedation Scale: study with intravenous midazolam. *J Clin Psychopharmacol.* 1990;10:244–251.
9. Smith C, McEwan AI, Jhaveri R, et al. The interaction of fentanyl on the Cp50 of propofol for loss of consciousness and skin incision. *Anesthesiology.* 1994;81:820-828.
10. Short TG, Chui PT. Propofol and midazolam act synergistically in combination. *Br J Anaesth.* 1991;67: 539-545.
11. McClune S, McKay AC, Wright PMC, et al. Synergistic interactions between midazolam and propofol. *Br J Anaesth.* 1992;69:240-245.
12. Kazama T, Ikeda K, Morita K. Reduction by fentanyl of the Cp50 values of propofol and hemodynamic responses to various noxious stimuli. *Anesthesiology.* 1997;87:213-227.
13. Kissen I, Brown PT, Bradley EL. Morphine and fentanyl anesthetic interactions with etomidate. *Anesthesiology.* 1987;67:A383.
14. Stockham RJ, Stanley TH, Pace NL, et al. Fentanyl pretreatment modifies anaesthetic induction with etomidate. *Anaesth Intensive Care.* 1988;16:171-176.

15. Huter L, Schreiber T, Gugel M, et al. Low-dose intravenous midazolam reduces etomidate-induced myoclonus: a prospective, randomized study in patients undergoing elective cardioversion. *Anesth Analg.* 2007;105:1298-1302.
16. Albrecht S, Ihmsen H, Hering W, Geisslinger G, Dingemanse J, Schwilden H, Schüttler. The effect of age on the pharmacokinetics and pharmacodynamics of midazolam. *J Clin Pharmacol Ther.* 1999;65(6):630-639.
17. Shafer SL, Varvel JR, Aziz N, Scott JC. Pharmacokinetics of fentanyl administered by computer-controlled infusion pump. *Anesthesiology.* 1990;73(6):1091-1102.
18. Schnider TW, Minto CF, Gambus PL, et al. The influence of method of administration and covariates on the pharmacokinetics of propofol in adult volunteers. *Anesthesiology.* 1998;88(5):1170-1182.
19. Kern SE, Xie G, White JL, Egan TD. A response surface analysis of propofol-remifentanil pharmacodynamic interaction in volunteers. *Anesthesiology.* 2004;100(6): 1373-1381.
20. Johnson KB, Syroid ND, Gupta DK, et al. An evaluation of remifentanil propofol response surfaces for loss of responsiveness, loss of response to surrogates of painful stimuli and laryngoscopy in patients undergoing elective surgery. *Anesth Analg.* 2008;106(2):471-479.
21. LaPierre CD, Johnson KB, Randall BR, White JL, Egan TD. An exploration of remifentanil-propofol combinations that lead to a loss of response to esophageal instrumentation, a loss of responsiveness, and/or onset of intolerable ventilatory depression. *Anesth Analg.* 2011;113(3):490-499.
22. Egan TD Muir KT, Hermann DJ, Stanski DR, Shafer SL. The electroencephalogram (EEG) and clinical measures of opioid potency: defining the EEG-clinical potency relationship ('fingerprint') with application to remifentanil. *Int J Pharm Med.* 2001;15(1):1-8.
23. Brady M, Kinn S, Stuart P. Preoperative fasting for adults to prevent perioperative complications. *Cochrane Database Syst Rev.* 2003;4:CD004423.
24. Kulkarni PN, Batra YK, Wig J. Effect of different combinations of H2 receptor antagonists with gastrokinetic drugs on gastric fluid pH and volume in children—a comparative study. *Int J Clin Pharmacol Ther.* 1997;35:561-564.
25. Wagner, BK, Amory DW, Majcher CM, et al. Effects of intravenous famotidine on gastric acid secretion in patients undergoing cardiac surgery. *Ann Pharmacother.* 1995;29:349-353.
26. Jasson J, Lefevre G, Tallet F, et al. Oral administration of sodium citrate before general anesthesia in elective cesarean section. Effect on pH and gastric volume. *Ann Fr Anesth Reanim.* 1989;8:12-18.
27. Lim SK, Elegbe EO. The use of single dose of sodium citrate as a prophylaxis against acid aspiration syndrome in obstetric patients undergoing cesarean section. *Med J Malaysia.* 1991;46:349-355.
28. Lim SK, Elegbe EO. Ranitidine and sodium citrate as prophylaxis against acid aspiration syndrome in obstetric patient undergoing caesarean section. *Singapore Med J.* 1992;33:608-610.
29. Pandit SK, Kothary SP, Pandit UA, et al. Premedication with cimetidine and metoclopramide. Effect on the risk factors of acid aspiration. *Anaesthesia.* 1986;41:486-492.
30. Solanki DR, Suresh M, Ethridge HC. The effects of intravenous cimetidine and metoclopramide on gastric volume and pH. *Anesth Analg.* 1984;63:599-602.
31. Gan TJ, Meyer T, Apfel CC, et al. Consensus guidelines for managing postoperative nausea and vomiting. *Anesth Analg.* 2003;97:62-71.
32. Fleisher LA, Beckman JA, Brown KA, et al. ACC/AHA 2007 guidelines on perioperative cardiovascular evaluation and care for noncardiac surgery: executive summary. *J Am Coll Cardiol.* 2007;50:1707-32.
33. Mangano DT, Layug EL, Wallace A, et al. Effect of atenolol on mortality and cardiovascular morbidity after noncardiac surgery. *N Engl J Med.* 1996;335:1713-20.
34. Poldermans D, Boersma E, Bax JJ, et al. The effect of bisoprolol on perioperative mortality and myocardial infarction in high-risk patients undergoing vascular surgery (DECREASE). *N Engl J Med.* 1999;341: 1789-1794.
35. Devereaux PJ, Yang H, Yusuf S, et al. Effect of extended-release metoprolol succinate in patients undergoing non-cardiac surgery (POISE trial): a randomized, controlled trial. *Lancet.* 2008;371:1839-1847.
36. Dunkelgrun M, Boersma E, Schouten O, et al. Bisoprolol and fluvastatin for the reduction of preoperative cardiac mortality and myocardial infarction in intermediate-risk patients undergoing noncardiovascular surgery: a randomized, controlled trial (DECREASE-IV). *Ann Surg.* 2009;249:921-926.
37. Bangalore S, Wetterslev J, Pranesh S, et al. Perioperative beta blockers in patient having non-cardiac surgery: a meta-analysis. *Lancet.* 2008;372:1962-1976.
38. van Lier F, Schouten O, van Domburg RT, et al. Effect of chronic beta-blocker use on stroke after noncardiac surgery. *Am J Cardiol.* 2009;104:429-433.
39. Poldermans D, Schouten O, van Lier F, et al. Perioperative strokes and beta-blockade. *Anesthesiology.* 2009;111:940-945.
40. Coriat P, Richer C, Douraki T, et al. Influence of chronic angiotensin-converting enzyme inhibition on anesthetic induction. *Anesthesiology.* 1994;81:299-307.

41. Comfere T, Sprung J, Kumar MM, et al. Angiotensin system inhibitors in a general surgical population. *Anesth Analg.* 2005;100:636-644.
42. Schirmer U, Schurmann W. Preoperative administration of angiotensin-converting enzyme inhibitors. *Anaesthetist.* 2007;56:557-61.
43. Kheterpal S, Khodaparast O, Shanks A, et al. Chronic angiotensin-converting enzyme inhibitor or angiotensin receptor blocker therapy combined with diuretic therapy is associated with increased episodes of hypotension in noncardiac surgery. *J Cardiothorac Vasc Anesth.* 2008;22:180-186.
44. Hohne C. Meier L, Boemke W, et al. ACE inhibition does not exaggerate the blood pressure decrease in the early phase of spinal anaesthesia. *Acta Anaesthesiol Scand.* 2003;47:891-896.
45. Pigott DW, Nagle C, Allman K, et al. Effect of omitting regular ACE inhibitor medication before cardiac surgery on haemodynamic variables and vasoactive drug requirements. *Br J Anaesth.* 2000;83:715-720.
46. Brabant SM, Bertrand M, Eyaud D, et al. The hemodynamic effects of anesthetic induction in vascular surgical patients chronically treated with angiotensin II receptor antagonists. *Anesth Analg.* 1999;88:1388-1392.
47. Zacharias M, Conion NP, Herbison GP, et al. Interventions for protecting renal function in the perioperative period. *Cochrane Database Syst Rev.* 2008;4:CD003590.
48. Node K, Fujita M, Kitakaze M, et al. Short-term statin therapy improves cardiac function and symptoms in patients with idiopathic dilated cardiomyopathy. *Circulation.* 2003;108:839-843.
49. Ridker PM, Danielson E, Fonseca FA, et al. Rosuvastatin to prevent vascular events in men and women with elevated C-reactive protein. *N Engl J Med.* 2008;359:2195-2207.
50. Durazzo AES, Machado FS, Ikeoka DT, et al. Reduction in cardiovascular events after vascular surgery with atorvastatin: a randomized trial. *J Vasc Surg.* 2004;39:967-976.
51. Poldermans D, Schouten O, Bax J, et al. Reducing cardiac risk in non-cardiac surgery: evidence from the DECREASE studies. *Eur Heart J.* 2009;11:A9-A14.
52. Hindler K, Shaw AD, Samuels J, et al. Improved postoperative outcomes associated with preoperative statin therapy. *Anesthesiology.* 2006;105:1260-1272.
53. Patti G, Chello M, Candura D, et al. Randomized trial of atorvastatin for reduction of postoperative atrial fibrillation in patients undergoing cardiac surgery. *Circulation.* 2006;114:1455-1461.
54. Aboyans V, Labrousse L, Lacroix P, et al. Predictive factors of stroke in patients undergoing coronary bypass grafting: statins are protective. *Eur J Cardiothorac Surg.* 2006;30:300-304.
55. Schouten O, Hoeks SE, Welten GMJM, et al. Effect of statin withdrawal on frequency of cardiac events after vascular surgery. *Am J Cardiol.* 2007;100: 316-320.
56. Le Manach Y, Godet G, Coriat P, et al. The impact of postoperative discontinuation or continuation of chronic statin therapy on cardiac outcome after major vascular surgery. *Anesth Analg.* 2007;104: 1326-1333.
57. Brookes ZL, McGowan CC, Reilly CS. Statins for all: the new premed? *Br J Anaesth.* 2009;103:99-107.

CHAPTER 27

Key Concepts in Safe Sedation

Sean Runnels, MD, and Brian St. George, MD

INTRODUCTION

Although widely utilized in a variety of clinical venues and delivered by nurses and physicians with a broad range of clinical training and experience, core principles guiding safe sedation practice are not well established. Sedation practices (ie, drug choice and dose, patient preparation, procedure room equipment for safe sedation delivery, patient monitoring standards, practitioner training requirements, sedation goals) are often left to the discretion of the individual sedation practitioner and are not well regulated. The chapter will discuss core concepts of anesthetic pharmacology that apply to sedation practice (Table 27–1) that sedation practitioners should consider prior to administering sedatives and analgesics.

THE SEDATION CONTINUUM

No discussion of safe sedation techniques can begin without first asking "What is sedation?" In general, sedation is a drug-induced, depressed level of consciousness that allows a patient to safely tolerate a procedure or noxious stimuli, while maintaining innate cardiopulmonary functions. Defining sedation more specifically is a difficult task. Terms such as procedural sedation, conscious sedation, deep sedation, sedation and analgesia, monitored anesthetic care, moderate sedation, anxiolysis, and minimal sedation are often used interchangeably in the literature and in daily discussions between caregivers and medical specialists. This lack of standardized language and definitions concerning the practice of sedation has served to confuse communication as well inhibit the development of consistent sedation guidelines, standards, and techniques.[1,2]

Currently, the majority of position papers, practice guidelines, and medical literature use the definition and taxonomy put forth by the American Society of Anesthesiologist (ASA), called the sedation continuum.[3] This sedation continuum presents stages of central nervous system depression that eventually culminate in general anesthesia. Four sedation states are defined: minimal sedation, moderate sedation, deep sedation, and general anesthesia. Each of these states is differentiated by responsiveness to stimulation, ability to maintain a natural airway, adequacy of spontaneous airway, and impairment of cardiovascular functions. For purposes of clarity, the ASA sedation continuum will be used throughout this chapter (Table 27–2).[3]

An important consideration of the sedation continuum is the correlation of central nervous system depression and ability to maintain vital cardiopulmonary functions. As central nervous system depression increases, a patient's ability to maintain vital cardiopulmonary function decreases. Loss of responsiveness to verbal and tactile stimulation is an important transition increasing the likelihood of adverse cardiopulmonary events. Once the patient is unresponsive, mitigation of these risks is a function of the provider's skill in managing a patient under general anesthesia (Figure 27–1).

KEY POINT

Sedation is a drug-induced state of central nervous system depression that produces dose-related adverse cardiopulmonary effects along a continuum. As the dose increases, the patient moves along the continuum toward deeper sedation states, and the likelihood of intervention to counter adverse cardiopulmonary events increases.

TABLE 27–1 Core anesthetic pharmacology concepts in sedation practice.

The sedation continuum
The difference between moderate and deep sedation
The importance of recognizing deeper-than-intended sedation
The time to peak effect of common analgesics and sedatives used in sedation practice
The influence of sedative–analgesic interactions on responsiveness, respiratory depression, and analgesia

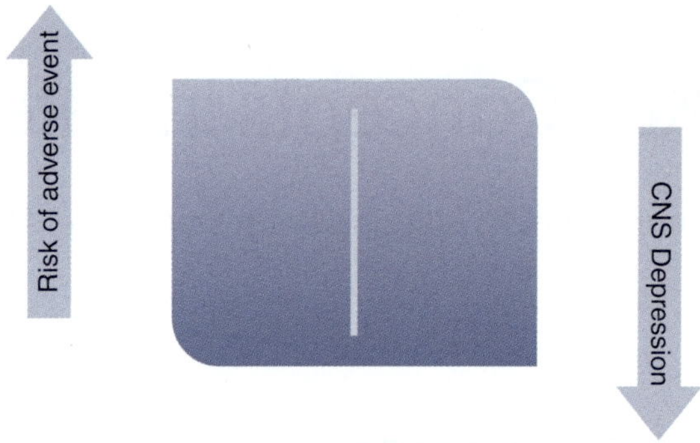

FIGURE 27–1 The relationship between central nervous system (CNS) depression and risk of adverse events and patient harm.

Limitations of the Sedation Continuum

Although the sedation continuum provides a conceptual and intellectual framework with which to understand sedation, its definitions and distinctions are artificial and imperfect. The continuum is a progression of central nervous system depression, which cannot always be rigidly categorized into distinct clinical states. A patient's physiologic features may overlap more than one sedation state, and the speed with which a patient moves through these states is unpredictable. Furthermore, a patient may clinically skip states all together.

Self-Rescue and Loss of Responsiveness

An important premise of the sedation continuum is that the loss of responsiveness to verbal and tactile stimulation is an important transition that correlates with the increasing likelihood of adverse cardiopulmonary events. The ability of a patient to respond

TABLE 27–2 The American Society of Anesthesiologist (ASA) sedation continuum.[a]

	Minimum Sedation ("Anxiolysis")	Moderate Sedation/ Analgesia ("Conscious Sedation")	Deep Sedation/ Analgesia	General Anesthesia
Responsiveness	Normal response to verbal stimulation	Purposeful response to verbal and tactile stimulation	Purposeful response following repeated painful stimulation	Unarousable, even with painful stimulus
Airway	Unaffected	No intervention required	Intervention may be required	Intervention often required
Spontaneous ventilation	Unaffected	Adequate	May be inadequate	Usually inadequate
Cardiovascular function	Unaffected	Usually maintained	Usually maintained	May be impaired

[a]Layered over the ASA's sedation continuum is shading that indicates sedation target by practitioner skill level required to rescue patients from adverse events such as bag-mask ventilation and placement of an oral or nasopharyngeal airway, and so on. Green indicates that the practitioner has basic airway management skills. Red indicates that the practitioner has advanced airway and cardiovascular management skills such as laryngoscopy to perform intubation, laryngeal mask airway placement, ventilator management, administration of vasoactive agents, and so on. The vertical blue line represents the transition from moderate to deep sedation, a transition associated with increased risk of adverse events, and skill level required to properly manage those adverse events.
From reference 3.

TABLE 27–3 Important considerations of provider rescue.

Call for help.
Stop administration of sedatives and analgesics.
Consider reversal agents if appropriate.
Notify proceduralist.
Return patient to intended sedation state.
Consider cancelling procedure if difficult to complete at intended sedation state.

purposefully to verbal commands is an important distinction between moderate and deep sedation. A patient who responds can self-rescue. This marks the increasing likelihood that a patient will lose the innate ability to maintain his or her cardiopulmonary function without provider rescue. Typically, if a patient remains responsive to voice and tactile stimulation (moderate sedation), with airway obstruction or hypoventilation, the situation can generally be resolved by stimulation and asking the patient to take a deep breath. If a patient is unresponsive, then the burden of rescue falls to the provider. Provider rescue may involve one or more simultaneous activities (Table 27–3).

KEY POINT

Preserving responsiveness is a critical safety feature in moderate sedation as it enables a patient to respond, with prompting, should airway obstruction or hypoventilation occur. If a patient becomes unresponsive, a feature of deep sedation and general anesthesia, then rescue is entirely dependent on the skills of the sedation practitioner.

PHARMACODYNAMIC MODELING FOR SEDATION

In this chapter, previously published pharmacodynamic models[4-11] are used to illustrate the profiles of anesthetic drugs used in sedation practice and illustrate key concepts vital to the practice of safe sedation. As with all models, their predictions are inherently wrong and are unlikely to consistently predict an individual patient's response. However, they are useful to visualize anesthetic behavior as it pertains to sedation. Model assumptions and limitations, presented in Table 27–4, should be considered when interpreting models predictions.

TABLE 27–4 Pharmacodynamic model assumptions and limitations.

Assumptions
All simulations assume the patient does not chronically consume opioids or other substances that may alter published concentration-effect relationships.
Simulations of sedation techniques will target moderate sedation (ie, maintain responsiveness).
Deeper-than-intended sedation state will include both deep sedation and general anesthesia without distinction.
Simulations will include a prediction of plasma concentrations, effect-site concentrations, drug effects, and the interaction of opioids and sedatives.
Limitations
Data used to construct pharmacodynamic models were primarily gathered in healthy volunteers. Not all patients presenting for sedation are young and healthy.
For selected effect measures (loss of responsiveness, sedation level, ventilatory depression), observed responses were measured in the absence of a persistent noxious stimulus. Hence, model predictions may overestimate the probability of a given effect.
Many patients consume substances that alter the concentration-effect relationship of opioids and benzodiazepines. This represents a substantial limitation in available pharmacodynamic models.

TITRATION: TIMING IS EVERYTHING!

Titration of small amounts of drug over time to achieve a desired effect using the least amount of drug possible is the safest method of drug delivery for targeting a sedation state. This involves use of a titration cycle: the delivery of small doses of medication punctuated by assessment of patient response and sedation state (Figure 27–2). Skilled titration requires an understanding of the time to peak effect of the drug and the concentration-effect relationship. Guiding principles to titration for sedation practice are presented in Table 27–5.

The time to peak effect for several anesthetic drugs used in sedation is presented in Table 27–6.

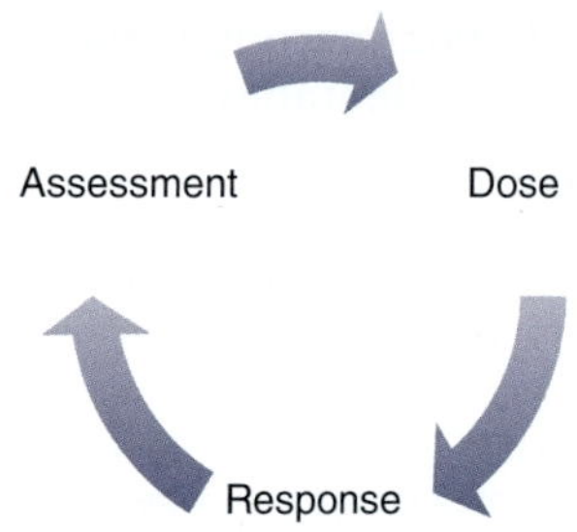

FIGURE 27–2 The sedation titration cycle.

Some drugs, such as propofol and remifentanil, have a rapid time to peak effect, whereas others, such as morphine, have a very slow time to peak effect. Figure 27–3 presents the time to peak effect for midazolam, fentanyl, and morphine. Of note, midazolam has a relatively slow time to peak concentration. This is an important consideration for sedation practitioners who may be tempted to administer additional midazolam before the prior dose reaches peak effect. Six to 9 minutes is a long time to wait during a brief procedure associated with noxious stimuli.

Next, consider dose amount for titration. Adverse effects from a deeper-than-intended sedation state are a function of the duration how long a patient remains in that state. Titration technique involves administering intermittent small doses as opposed to one single dose. The simulation presented in the Figure 27–4 illustrates two dosing schemes for the same amount of propofol (50 mg)

TABLE 27–5 Guiding principles to titration of sedative and analgesics for sedation.

The time to peak effect should be considered before administering additional doses of an anesthetic.
Initial bolus is tailored to a population; subsequent boluses are tailored to the individual's response.
The safest way to deliver sedation is titration of multiple small amounts of drugs with an adequate time for evaluation of effect. Due to individual variability in drug response, delivering a large dose of drug with the expectation of rapidly achieving a targeted sedation state will lead to an unacceptably high incidence of entry into as well as total time spent in a deeper-than-intended state-of-sedation, exposing the patient to needless risk.
Additional drug may be given if needed, but once a drug is given it may not be taken back.

TABLE 27–6 Time to peak effect for selected analgesics and sedatives used in sedation.

Drug	Time to Peak Effect (min)
Morphine	75–90
Fentanyl	3–5
Sufentanil	1–3
Alfentanil	1–1.5
Remifentanil	1–1.5
Propofol	1–1.5
Midazolam	6–9
Ketamine	2–10

Note: The times represent the time to peak effect when administered as a single agent. The times do not reflect the time to peak effect when used in combination with other analgesics or sedatives.

administered to a morbidly obese patient undergoing an endoscopy procedure. Simply administering the 50 mg in divided doses separated by 3 minutes produces a much different profile in the probability of unresponsiveness over time. This simulation clearly demonstrates the principle that the larger the bolus, the deeper the sedation and the greater the risk of spending more time in a deeper-than-intended state of sedation. If the goal is to target the state of moderate sedation, attempting to target a sedation state with a single standard bolus dose of propofol for every individual is unwise. For instance, if a 40-mg bolus of propofol is given as a standard dose to a population of patients, we can expect more than 10% of the patients to reach deep sedation or general anesthesia and remain in that state for about 3 minutes. In contrast, with a 15-mg propofol dose, the risk and duration of deeper-than-intended sedation is much less (Table 27–7).

One nuance to loss of responsiveness is that it is otherwise well tolerated as long as respiratory function is not compromised. Sedation practitioners may find it suitable to briefly render a patient unresponsive as long as the patient continues to breathe. Caution should be used with this practice, given that sedatives, especially propofol, relax airway structures, leading to an increased likelihood of partial (ie, snoring) or complete airway obstruction.

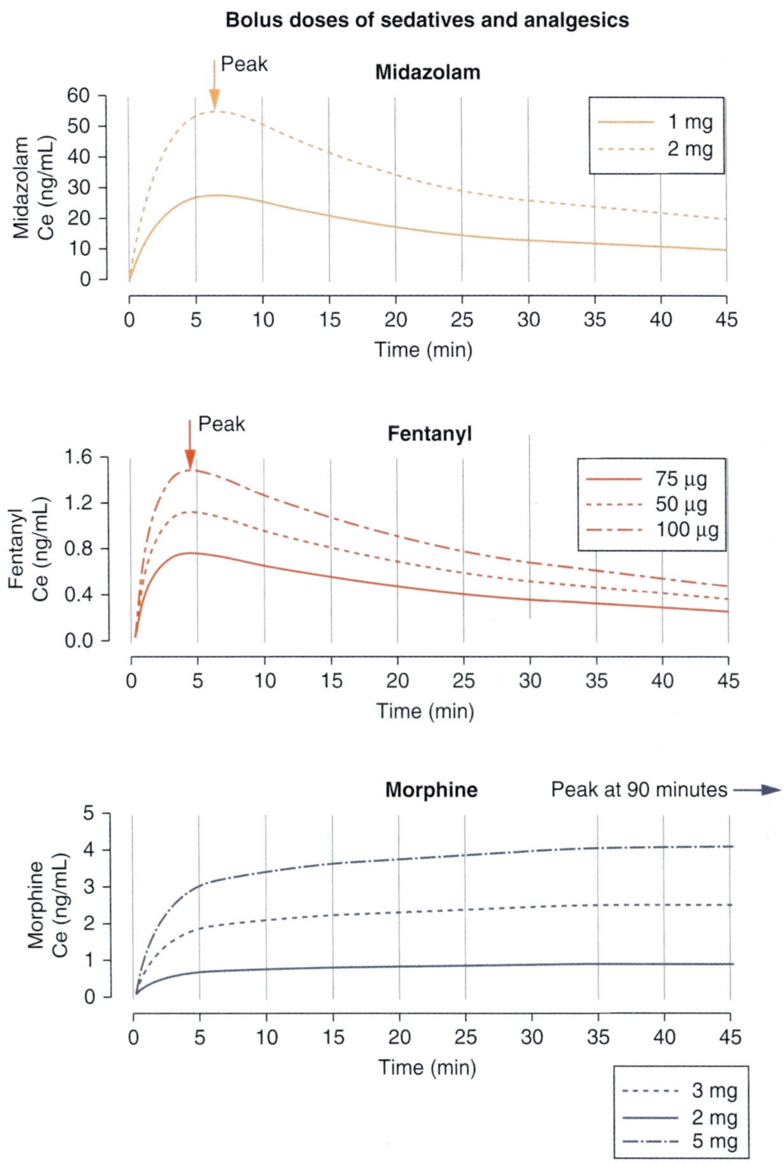

FIGURE 27–3 Simulation of predicted effect-site concentration (Ce) levels from bolus doses of midazolam, fentanyl, and morphine in a 30-year-old, 70-kg, 175-cm individual. The arrows indicate the peak Ce levels. Fentanyl has the fasted time to peak Ce, followed by midazolam and then morphine. These simulations assume that the pharmacokinetics are linear, meaning that the profile of drug concentration over time is independent of dose.

OPIOID–SEDATIVE INTERACTIONS

To illustrate opioid–sedative interactions, consider the interaction between the midazolam or propofol with fentanyl. Fentanyl is an opiate with analgesic properties that acts at primarily opioid receptors at the level of the spinal cord. When given alone, it produces little central nervous system depression. For example, substantially high doses are required to render a patient unresponsive. By contrast, midazolam and propofol are hypnotics that act primarily

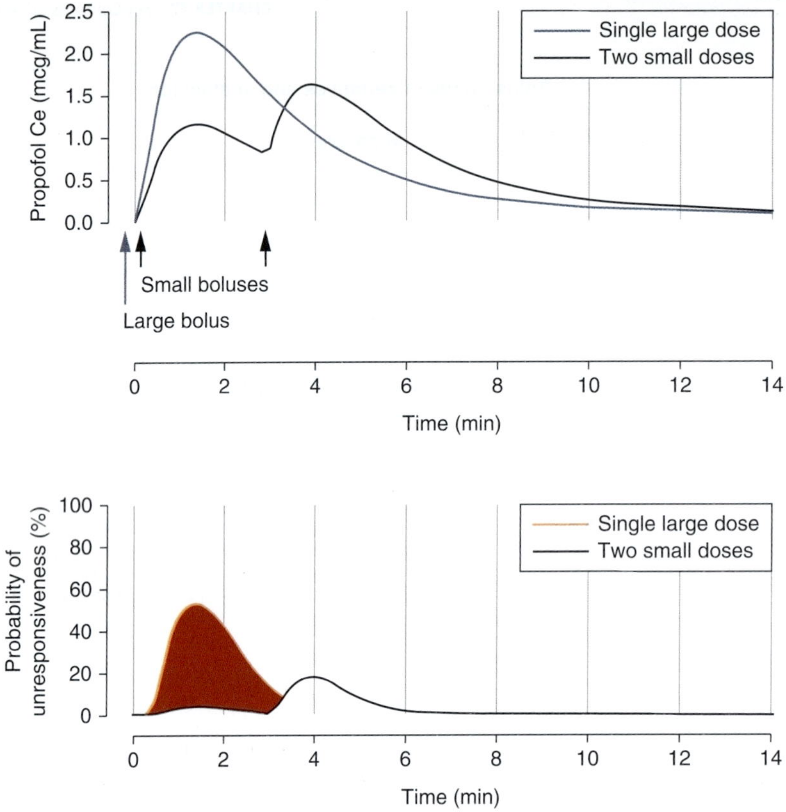

FIGURE 27–4 Simulation of a propofol bolus to a morbidly obese patient (100-kg, 155-cm patient with a body mass index of 46). This simulation presents two dosing schemes: (1) a single dose of 50 mg administered as a single bolus and (2) as more frequent smaller doses, in this case 2 smaller doses of 25 mg separated by 3 minutes. Both deliver the same amount of drug. The top plot presents the propofol effect-site concentration (Ce) levels, and the bottom plot presents the probability of unresponsiveness (an unwanted effect during moderate sedation) over time. Note that the single-dose technique leads to a higher probability of unresponsiveness over time for both dosing schemes.

TABLE 27–7 Simulations of loss of responsiveness for increasing propofol boluses.[a]

Propofol Bolus	Percent With Probability of Unresponsiveness (%)	Duration of Unresponsiveness
10 mg	0	0
20 mg	3	15–30 seconds
30 mg	20	1–1.5 minutes
40 mg	50	3 minutes
50 mg	75	4 minutes
60 mg	87	4.5 minutes

[a]Simulations assume an 80-kg patient.

via central nervous system depression. They have little analgesic effect. Toleration of painful procedures is accomplished via excessive central nervous system depression to the point where patients are likely to be unresponsive. When combined, advantages from both sedatives and analgesics help achieve sedation goals yet minimize the adverse effects from dosing them as a single agent.

Figure 27–5 presents a simulation of fentanyl coadministered with midazolam at the same time. The simulation predicts both the drug effect-site concentrations and selected drug effects to include predictions of analgesia, sedation, and ventilatory depression. It also presents the predicted effects from each drug individually. Of note, the predicted effects from each drug by itself are substantially less than when administered in combination. Midazolam is a

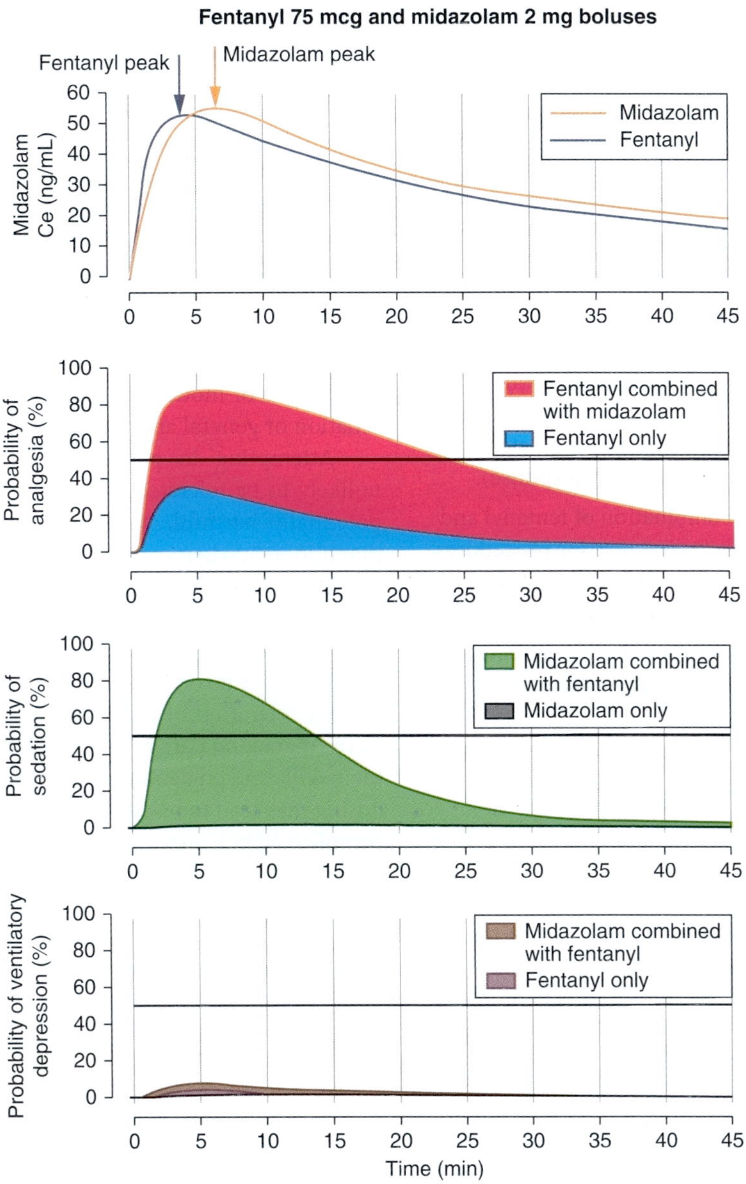

FIGURE 27–5 Simulations of a bolus dose of midazolam (2 mg) and fentanyl (75 mcg), assuming a 30-year-old, 70-kg, 175-cm person. Both are administered simultaneously. The top plot presents the predicted effect-site concentration (Ce) levels. The bottom three plots present the predicted probability of effect for analgesia, sedation, and ventilatory depression. For analgesia and ventilatory depression, predictions include the combination of both drugs combined and for fentanyl alone. For sedation predictions, include the combination of both drugs combined and for midazolam alone.

more effective sedative in the presence of fentanyl and fentanyl is a more effective analgesic in the presence of midazolam that if administered individually. Predictions of ventilatory depression form both drugs was low (< 6%) but not inconsequential. Ventilatory depression was defined as a respiratory rate less than 4 breath/min in an otherwise healthy individual in the absence of any painful stimuli.

Important key points and conclusions from this simulation include:

- The addition of opioids to hypnotics can increase the likelihood that a patient will tolerate a moderately stimulating procedure while remaining in the state of moderate sedation (retention of conscious response).
- This dose and the combination of fentanyl and midazolam is unlikely to suffice for procedures associated with prolonged painful stimulation while maintaining a state of moderate sedation.
- Patients are unlikely to tolerate a moderately stimulating procedure using midazolam alone.

INFUSIONS

It is the opinion of the authors that use of infusion for the sedatives requires expertise and experience not consistently available to nonanesthesia providers. Infusion techniques increase the risk of unrecognized entry into deeper-than-intended sedation states, as they break the dose-assessment cycle. Specific concerns are:

- Slow onset of infusions and impatience of the proceduralist, which may lead to combinations of bolus dosing on top of an infusion
- Increasing effect-site concentration creep over time, leading to unrecognized entry into deeper-than-intended states of sedation later in the sedation than expected
- Automatic continued drug delivery during a sedation crisis due to a distracted sedation team that does not turn off the infusion

Thus, sedation practitioners who consider using infusions should have the appropriate training to properly address the concerns listed above.

CHANGES IN THE APPROACH TO SEDATION PRACTICE

Recently, there has been an important shift in the end point of sedation practice. This shift is the notion of administration of sedation with the goal of targeting a defined sedation state on the sedation continuum versus targeting a sedation level so that a patient can tolerate a procedure. Targeting "toleration-of-the-procedure" can easily result in sedation states that exceed the skills and expertise of the sedation provider. In fact, some procedures cannot be tolerated in the state of moderate sedation and require deep sedation or general anesthesia.

Attempting to perform procedures that are unlikely to be tolerated in lighter sedation states is potentially harmful. Nonanesthesiologist sedation practitioners, when confronted with an uncomfortable patient and a proceduralist who would like to complete a procedure, lose track of targeting sedation states that are consistent with their level of training. They may go on to administer excessive doses to achieve toleration of the procedure, yet find themselves managing patient conditions that are beyond their skills and credentialing. For example, excessive dosing may lead to respiratory depression, partial or complete upper airway obstruction, or aspiration. All are avoidable if a patient can participate in his or her own rescue. Guiding principles to safe sedation practice with regard to practitioner training are presented in Table 27–8.

KEY POINT

Based on the sedation continuum, dosing to achieve moderate but not deep sedation is advised when non—anesthesia-trained practitioners administer sedatives and analgesics (green-shaded area in Table 27–2). This suggests that if patients cannot tolerate a procedure with moderate sedation, then an anesthesiologist may be required to provide deep sedation and/or general anesthesia. Practitioners providing sedation should practice within their scope of credentialing and clinical skills!

TABLE 27–8 Guiding principles in safe sedation practice.

Safe sedation always targets a sedation state appropriate to the rescue skill and credentialing of the sedation provider.
If the sedation provider is credentialed or trained to provide minimal and moderate sedation (green-shaded area on Table 27–2), targeting of those sedation states should always be the goal.
If the goal is toleration-of-the-procedure, without regard to sedation state, the provider should be trained and credentialed to deliver general anesthesia (red-shaded area in Table 27–2).
If the patient is unable to tolerate the procedure in the targeted sedation state (ie, moderate sedation), the procedure should be postponed until an anesthesia provider can be recruited to provide deep sedation and/or general anesthesia.

Computer-Assisted Personalized Sedation

Computer-assisted personalized sedation (CAPS) technology has been recently developed for the administration of propofol by a slow loading dose followed by an infusion to achieve and maintain moderate sedation for brief endoscopy procedures. CAPS uses patient response assessment technology, capnometry, pulse oximetry, and cardiovascular monitors to frequently assess patient responsiveness and cardiopulmonary status. When decreased responsiveness or decreased respiratory function is detected, CAPS decreases or stops propofol delivery. This automated patient assessment serves as a tool to avoid deeper-than-intended sedation. A pivotal trial evaluated this technology in 496 patients undergoing colonoscopy and upper endoscopy procedures. Endoscopist-sedation nurse teams successfully provided minimal to moderate sedation for these procedures using SEDASYS®, a CAPS system. SEDASYS® was recently approved for clinical use by the United States Food and Drug Administration; it is labeled only for use in ASA physical status I to II patients undergoing routine upper endoscopy and colonoscopy procedures.

SEDASYS takes advantage of the synergistic relationship between fentanyl and propofol, minimizing the amount of propofol required to achieve sedation during brief noxious stimuli. Figure 27–6 presents a simulation of the fentanyl–propofol-like dosing scheme used in a CAPS system. Fentanyl is administered 3 minutes before propofol. Propofol is administered as a slow loading dose over 3 minutes followed by an infusion for the remainder of a brief procedure. Key points from this simulation include:

- Fentanyl enhances the sedation effects of propofol, and propofol enhances the analgesic effects of propofol. This allows sedation practitioners to administer less of each drug, minimizing oversedation with propofol and respiratory depression with fentanyl.
- Fentanyl has a 3- to 5-minute latency to reach peak effect. Because fentanyl takes longer to reach peak effect, it is prudent to administer fentanyl early so that fentanyl and the propofol loading dose reach their peak effects at different times minimizing the risk of respiratory depression.
- The slow propofol loading dose is administered over 3 minutes. If an adverse effect (ie, respiratory depression) is detected, propofol administration is automatically decreased or terminated.
- Once propofol infusion is turned off, the rate of decline in concentration is rapid, offering an advantage over midazolam.

THE FUTURE OF SEDATION

Sedation delivered by nonanesthesiologists will continue to increase. Participation of the anesthesiologist in development of guidelines, training, and structuring of this discipline will be critical to the safety of these practices. The structure of sedation delivery models in the future will have to balance cost, scheduling flexibility, production pressure risk, and nurse–physician power imbalance, and availability of anesthesia expertise. Some possibilities include:

- Nurse-administered sedation under the supervision of a physician proceduralist

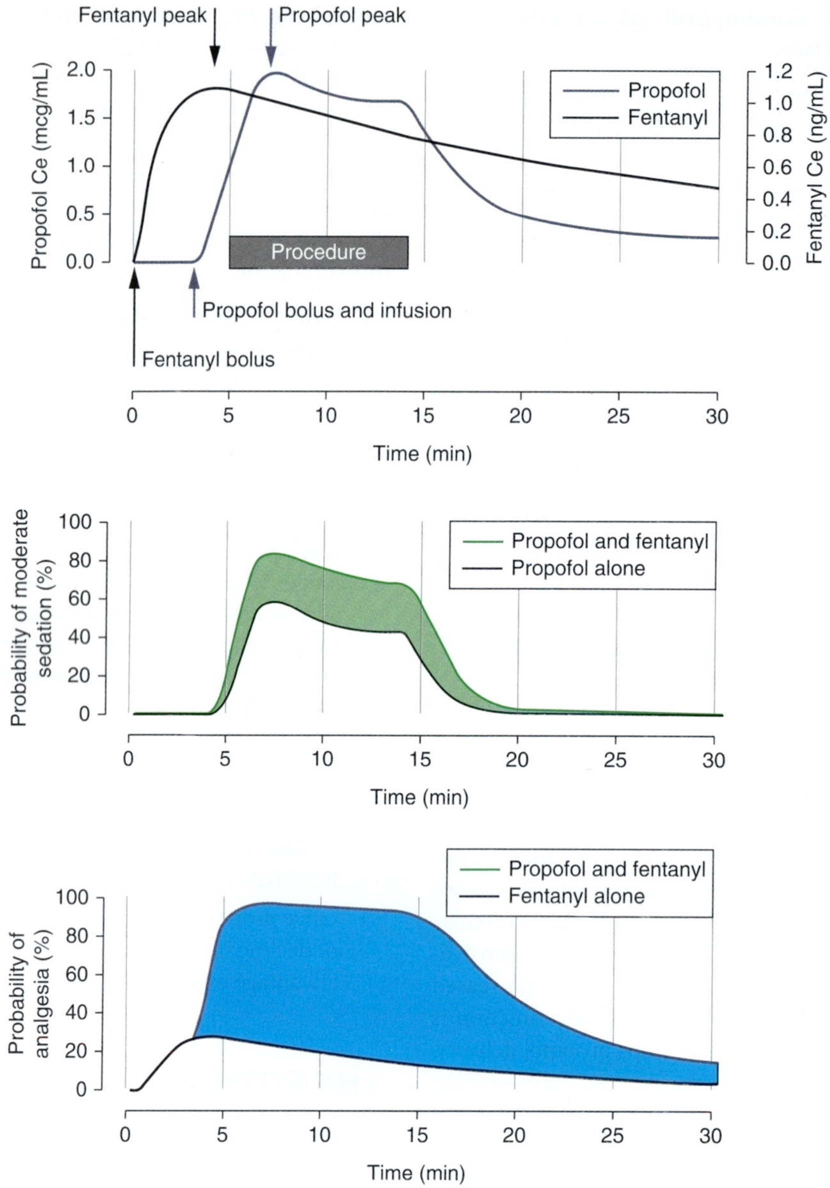

FIGURE 27–6 Simulations of effect-site concentration (Ce) levels (top plot) and the probability of selected effects (middle and bottom plots) for a fentanyl bolus (75 mcg) administered intravenously 3 minutes prior to the start of a slow propofol loading dose (0.5 mg/kg) over 3 minutes followed by a propofol infusion (75 mcg/kg/min) for 7 minutes. Simulations assume a 30-year-old, 80-kg, 183-cm male undergoing a colonoscopy where the propofol was turned off after reaching the cecum, the most uncomfortable part of the procedure. In the middle and bottom plots, the predictions of drug effect are based on a probability range of 1% to 100%. The green and blue areas represent the combined effects from propofol and fentanyl for moderate sedation and analgesia, respectively. In the presence of a noxious stimulus (eg, colonoscopy), these simulations likely overestimate the probability of effect.

TABLE 27–9 Sedation delivery models.

	Proceduralist-Directed, Nurse-Delivered Sedation	Anesthesiologist-Directed, Nurse-Delivered Sedation	Nurse-Delivered Sedation Under an Anesthesiology Umbrella
Availability of anesthesiology expertise	Low	High	High
Production pressure risk	High	Low	Low
Power balance risk	High	Low	Low
Cost	Low	High	Low

without involvement of an anesthesia care provider (most common in current medical practice). The major disadvantages are production pressure and inherent physician–nurse power imbalance. The sedation provider (nurse) often is employed directly by the proceduralist and may feel pressure to target toleration of the procedure without regard to sedation state or proper patient selection. An additional disadvantage is the lack of access to an anesthesiologist for backup or expert advice. Advantages include low cost and ease of scheduling.

- Sedation providers directly supervised by an anesthesiologist (less common in current medical practice). Disadvantages are cost and practicability. It is expensive and impractical to have an anesthesiologist directing every sedation case. Advantages are possible minimization of production pressure and lack of access to anesthesiology expertise.
- Sedation providers practicing under an anesthesiology umbrella (uncommon in clinical practice, but most promising sedation practice option). In this model, nurse sedation providers are part of a sedation team working under the umbrella of an anesthesiologist or anesthesia department. The training, credentialing, and scheduling of the nurse sedation providers is under the direction of an anesthesiology service. The nurses delivering sedation work under strict protocols and guidelines addressing patient selection, procedure selection, and drug delivery, without the direct supervision of an individual anesthesiologist unless needed. Sedation protocols and guidelines are developed by the anesthesiology service. If questions arise, an anesthesiologist is available to offer expertise and protect nurses from production pressure and the inherent power imbalance of the physician–nurse relationship. At our institution,we use PACU nurses with anesthesiology oversite, but not direction, to deliver moderate sedation in our operating rooms. We have found that the credible threat of an instant anesthesiology consultation on matters of patient selection, procedure selection, and targeting of sedation has greatly reduced inappropriate patient management.

A summary of the advantages and disadvantages of each sedation practice model is presented in Table 27–9.

REFERENCES

1. National Survey of Ambulatory Surgery. 2007. Available from: www.cdc.gov/nchs/nsas.htm. Accessed April, 2014.
2. Anghelescu D, Kaplan RF. Defining levels of sedation in pediatric patients. *AnesthAnalg*. 1998 Dec;87(6): 1454-1455.
3. Practice guidelines for sedation and analgesia by non-anesthesiologists. *Anesthesiology*. 2002;96(4): 1004-1017.
4. Kern SE, Xie G, White JL, Egan TD. A response surface analysis of propofol-remifentanil pharmacodynamic interaction in volunteers. *Anesthesiology*. 2004;100: 1373-1381.

5. Minto C, Vuyk J. Response surface modeling of drug interactions. *Adv Exp Med Biol.* 2003;523:35-43.
6. Bouillon TW, Bruhn J, Radulescu L, et al. Pharmacodynamic interaction between propofol and remifentanil regarding hypnosis, tolerance of laryngoscopy, bispectral index, and electroencephalographic approximate entropy. *Anesthesiology.* 2004;100:1353-1372.
7. Minto CF, Schnider TW, Egan TD, et al. Influence of age and gender on the pharmacokinetics and pharmacodynamics of remifentanil. *Anesthesiology.* 1997;86:10-23.
8. Schnider TW, Minto CF, Shafer SL, et al. The influence of age on propofol pharmacodynamics. *Anesthesiology.* 1999;90(6):1502-1516.
9. Minto CF, Schnider TW, Shafer SL. Pharmacokinetics and pharmacodynamics of remifentanil. II. Model application. *Anesthesiology.* 1997;86(1):24-33.
10. Minto CF, Schnider TW, Egan TD, et al. Influence of age and gender on the pharmacokinetics and pharmacodynamics of remifentanil. I. Model development. *Anesthesiology.* 1997;86(1):10-23.
11. Shafer SL, Varvel JR, Aziz N, Scott JC. Pharmacokinetics of fentanyl administered by computer. *Anesthesiology.* 1990;73(6):1091-1102.
12. Pambianco DJ1, Vargo JJ, Pruitt RE, Hardi R, Martin JF. Computer-assisted personalized sedation for upper endoscopy and colonoscopy: a comparative, multicenter randomized study, *Gastrointest Endosc.* 2011;73(4):765-772.

CHAPTER

28

Considerations for the Induction of Anesthesia

Ken B. Johnson, MD, Lara Brewer, PhD, and Cristen D. Lapierre, PhD

INTRODUCTION

Anesthesiologists often consider competing interests when formulating a plan for induction of anesthesia. Of particular concern is the onset and duration of various effects for combinations of anesthetic drugs used in induction. Some questions include:

- For a rapid-sequence induction, what is the optimal timing of drug administration so that peak effects occur at near the same time?
- If planning to induce anesthesia in patients with known or suspected difficult manual bag-mask ventilation, what is the duration of apnea and/or ventilatory depression for a given combination of induction agents should manual ventilation become inadequate?
- Following preoxygenation, what is the anticipated duration of maintaining reasonable oxygen saturations once a patient is rendered apneic?
- When using a high-dose opioid technique for induction, what dose of sedative–hypnotic provides a near-equivalent effect to a conventional induction technique?
- What is the role of sugammadex in a failed intubation when a nondepolarizing neuromuscular blocking agent is used?
- Is it necessary to completely block the response to laryngoscopy and tracheal intubation, or is it reasonable to simply blunt it?

The aim of this chapter is to briefly explore, through simulation, the clinical implications of these questions. The simulations present predictions based on available models of anesthetic drug behavior and human physiology. As with any model-based simulation, the predictions are as good as the models used to make them. When providing a clinical interpretation of the predictions, their assumptions and limitations will be discussed.

THE IMPORTANCE OF TIMING

A common combined anesthetic induction technique includes fentanyl, propofol, and either succinylcholine or a nondepolarizing neuromuscular blocker such as rocuronium. Given that laryngoscopy and tracheal intubation can be one of the most stimulating events during a surgical procedure, it is useful to maximize the combined analgesic effect of drugs used for induction. A basic understanding of induction drug kinetics can guide the timing of drug administration (Table 28–1). Fentanyl has a different kinetic profile from propofol and succinylcholine. In order for each induction drug to reach maximal effect at nearly the same time, fentanyl 2 to 3 mcg/kg is administered 3 to 4 minutes before propofol.

Fentanyl versus Remifentanil

A potentially attractive alternative to fentanyl during induction is remifentanil.[1,2] Authors have suggested that remifentanil not only can be used as an analgesic for induction but also that this analgesia can be so profound that no neuromuscular blocking agent is required.[2,3] A set of simulations comparing an induction sequence with propofol and remifentanil or fentanyl is presented in Figure 28–1.

In this simulation, fentanyl is administered 4 minutes before the propofol, such that both agents reach their peak concentrations at nearly the same

TABLE 28–1 Predicted time to onset and duration of effect for induction drugs.

Effect	Time (min)
Fentanyl 2 mcg/kg bolus	
Time to peak effect-site concentration	3.5
Time to probability of:	
No response to laryngoscopy > 95%	Never
Loss of responsiveness > 95%	Never
Propofol 2 mg/kg bolus	
Time to peak effect-site concentration	1.5
Time to probability of loss of responsiveness > 95%	0.5
Duration of probability of loss of responsiveness > 95%	4.5
Time to probability of no response to laryngoscopy > 95%	1
Duration of probability of no response to laryngoscopy > 95%	1.8
Combined technique	
Time to probability of loss of responsiveness > 95%[b]	0.5
Duration of probability of loss of responsiveness > 95%	5
Time to probability of no response to laryngoscopy > 95%[b]	0.5
Duration of probability of no response to laryngoscopy > 95%	3.5

[a]Combined technique consists of fentanyl followed by propofol 4 minutes later. Loss of responsiveness is defined as no response to verbal and vigorous tactile stimuli.
[b]From the time propofol was administered.

time (third plot from the top). Similarly, remifentanil is administered with the propofol. Propofol and remifentanil have a very similar kinetic profile when administered as a bolus, such that they reach their respective peak concentrations at nearly the same time (top plot). The simulations also present the predicted time course of no response to laryngoscopy. Of note, both opioids prolong the duration of this effect in a dose-dependent fashion. As dosed, they prolong the effect by 1 to 2 minutes. Although remifentanil has a rapid onset and offset, as dosed in these simulations, it does not appear to be any different from fentanyl in the duration of effect.

Remifentanil may lead to pronounced respiratory depression. In comparison to fentanyl, remifentanil's rapid onset does not allow for an accumulation of carbon dioxide as occurs with fentanyl. Elevated carbon dioxide levels can offset the respiratory depressant effects of opioids to some degree. Patients may not spontaneously breathe during the early phases of induction as they would with fentanyl. Another consideration with remifentanil is that when administered as a bolus, it can have a potent vagal effect, causing bradycardia. Caution should be used when administering large boluses. It may be prudent to administer boluses slowly in patients with known or suspected arrhythmias.

DRUG INTERACTIONS

An exploration of the duration of no response to laryngoscopy for a range of propofol and opioid combinations is presented in Figure 28–2. This figure presents a remifentanil-propofol pharmacodynamic interaction model for loss or response to laryngoscopy and tracheal intubation. For a range of propofol (0–2 mg/kg), fentanyl (0–2 mcg/kg), and remifentanil (0–1 mcg/kg) combinations, predictions of the duration of effect are made. Of interest, at higher opioid concentrations, much less propofol is required to achieve an equivalent effect. Note that 1 mg/kg of propofol combined with remifentanil 1 mcg/kg provides a similar duration of effect to 2 mg/kg of propofol in the absence of any opioid. This is an example of the isoeffect line (black line in the figure), where any combination of sedative and opioid effect-site concentrations yields a similar effect.

Two clinical implications of this set of simulations include:

- For patients with a known or suspected condition that will lead to a rapid oxygen desaturation following apnea during induction, it may be prudent to select an opioid-propofol combination that quickly dissipates.

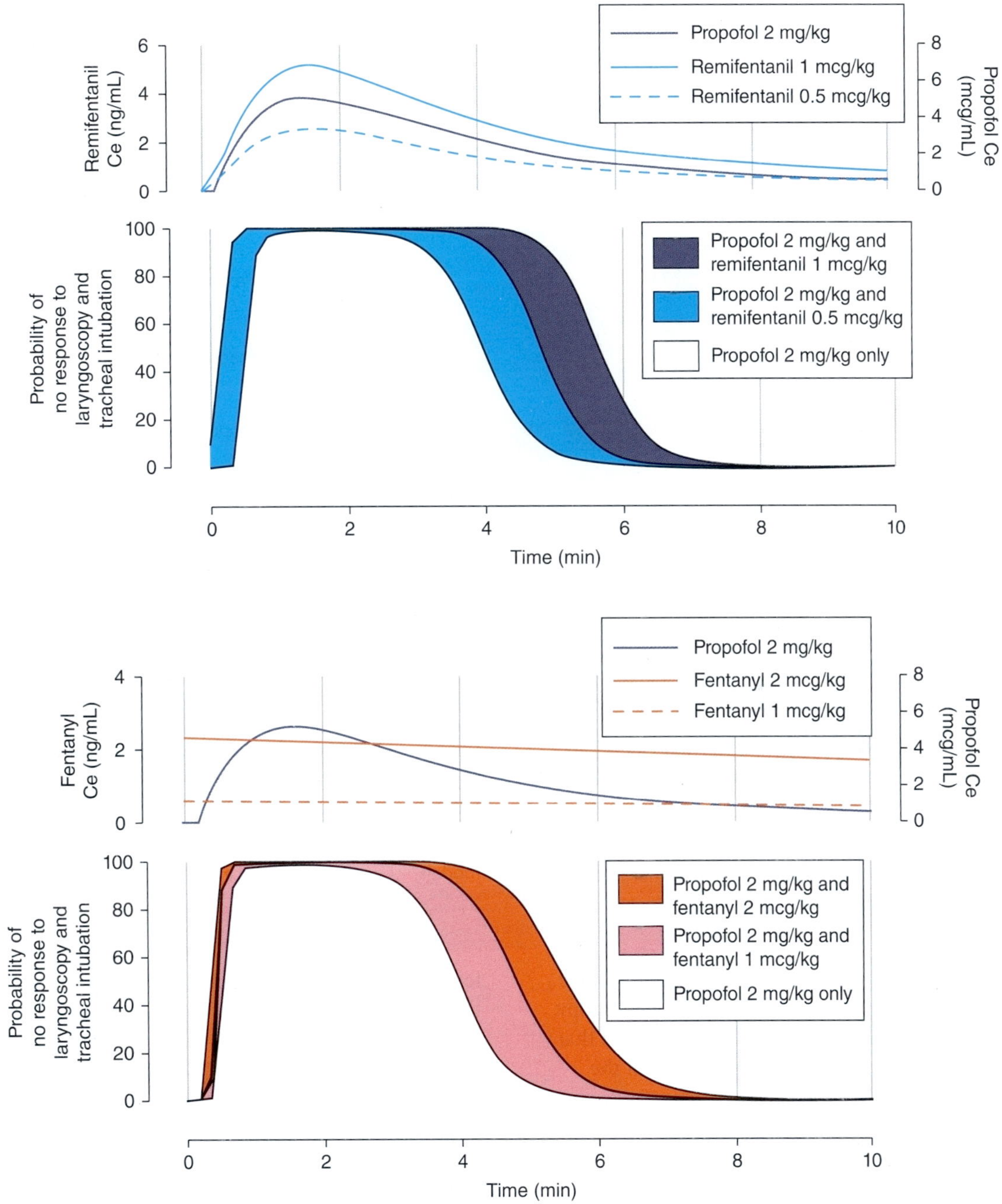

FIGURE 28–1 The importance of timing. Simulation of induction techniques using propofol in combination with either remifentanil (top plots) or fentanyl (bottom plots). Simulations include the predicted effect-site concentrations (Ce levels) and the probability of loss of response to laryngoscopy for the bolus doses presented in the graphs. The fentanyl was administered 4 minutes before the propofol, so that both agents would reach near-peak concentrations at the same time. With the addition of an opioid, the duration of effect for loss of response to laryngoscopy is prolonged (see Figure 28–2). This set of simulations assumes a 30-year-old, 100-kg, 183-cm male. Simulations were based on published pharmacokinetic and pharmacodynamic models.[4-9]

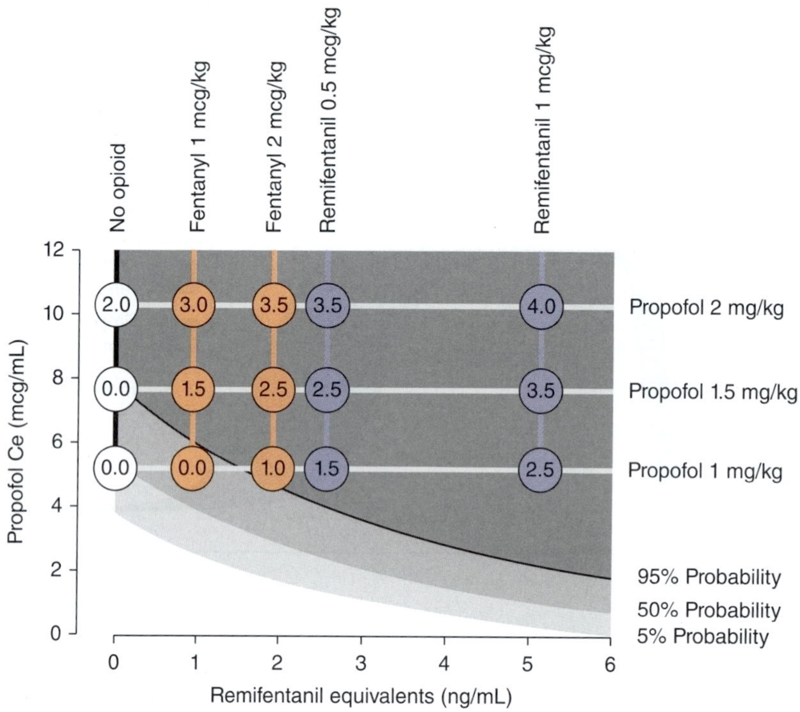

FIGURE 28–2 Propofol–opioid combinations for induction. Topographic representation of the propofol–remifentanil pharmacodynamic interaction model for loss of response to laryngoscopy. The gray shaded areas represent portions of the response surface associated with a 5% to 50% (light gray), 50% to 95% (gray), and greater than 95% (dark gray) probability of effect. Superimposed over the interaction model surface are the approximate maximal concentration pairs (large circles) for each of the dosing regimens presented in Figure 28–1. The time each concentration pair is above a 95% probability of no response to laryngoscopy is presented within each circle in minutes. Fentanyl concentrations are presented as remifentanil equivalents.[10] This set of simulations assumes a 30-year-old, 100-kg, 183-cm male. Simulations were based on published pharmacokinetic and pharmacodynamic models.[4-9] Ce, effect-site concentration.

- In patients where it is desirable to minimize the hemodynamic response to laryngoscopy, it may be useful to select a combination that best matches the duration of effect of the neuromuscular blocker.

When considering the clinical implications of an induction technique, it is useful to compare the duration of other effects such as loss of responsiveness and ventilatory depression. Figure 28–3 presents the time course of these effects for a conventional induction with fentanyl and propofol. These simulations illustrate the synergistic interaction between these 2 drugs. Propofol profoundly enhances and prolongs the analgesic effects of fentanyl, and fentanyl somewhat prolongs the sedative effects of propofol.

NEUROMUSCULAR BLOCKADE

With regard to neuromuscular blockade, the kinetic profile of propofol and succinylcholine are similar. Administering them in quick succession allows them to reach their peak effect-site concentrations at nearly the same time (Figure 28–4A). This figure presents the duration of effect for unresponsiveness, ventilatory depression, and loss of response to laryngoscopy. It also presents the duration of effect from succinylcholine. The duration of effect from succinylcholine is longer (6–7 minutes) than the

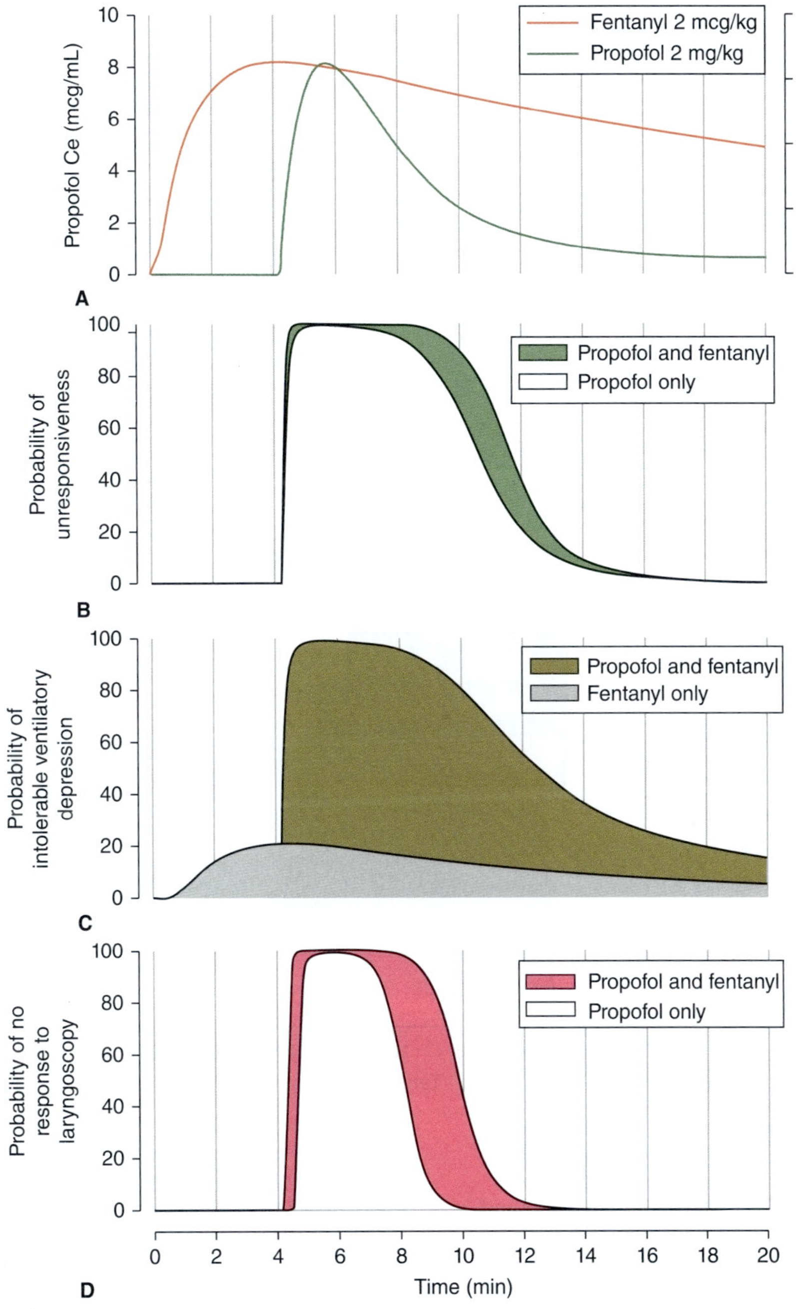

FIGURE 28–3 Predicted effects following induction with propofol 2 mg/kg and fentanyl 2 mcg/kg. The plot in A presents the time course of the effect-site concentrations (Ce levels). Fentanyl was administered 4 minutes before the propofol so that they would reach peak Ce levels at nearly the same time. The plots in B and C present the probability of unresponsiveness and intolerable ventilatory depression. For comparison, the plot in D presents the probability of loss of response to laryngoscopy from Figure 28-1. Unresponsiveness was defined as an observer's assessment of alertness and sedation less than 2.[11] Intolerable ventilatory depression was defined as respiratory rate less than 4 breaths/min.[12,13] Plots B, C, and D present the predicted effects resulting from the fentanyl and propofol in combination and the effects from just propofol or fentanyl by themselves. This set of simulations assumes a 30-year-old, 100-kg, 183-cm male. Simulations were based on published pharmacokinetic and pharmacodynamic models.[4-6,9,12-15]

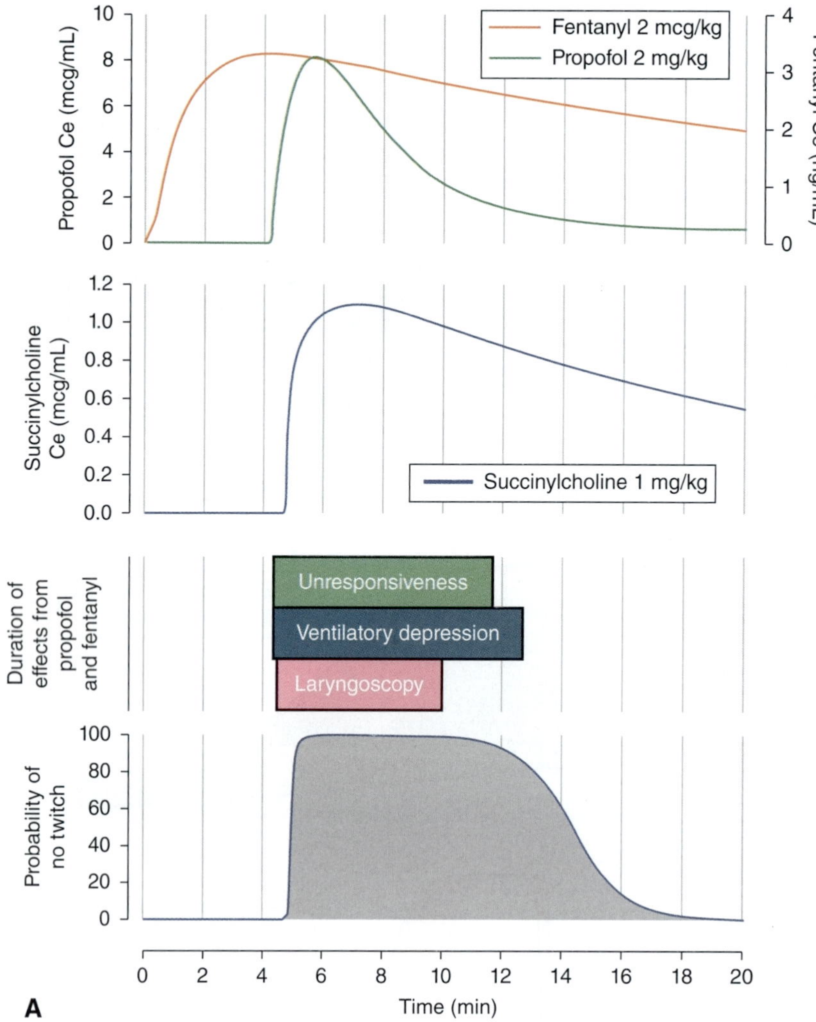

FIGURE 28–4 The time course of effect for selected approaches to neuromuscular blockade as part of an induction with fentanyl and propofol. Parts A, B, and C present the predicted effect-site concentration (Ce) and effects from succinylcholine, rocuronium, and rocuronium reversed 2.5 minutes later with sugammadex. The top and second-from-the-top plots in each part present the Ce levels over time for each drug. The third-from-the-bottom plot in each part presents the duration of loss of responsiveness, intolerable ventilatory depression, and loss of response to laryngoscopy (labeled laryngoscopy)—defined as the time the probability of effect is greater than 50%. The fourth-from-the-top plot presents the predicted duration of loss of train-of-four. Unresponsiveness was defined as an observer's assessment of alertness and sedation less than 2.[11] Intolerable ventilatory depression was defined as respiratory rate less than 4 breaths/min.[12,13] This set of simulations assumes a 30-year-old, 100-kg, 183-cm male. Simulations were based on published pharmacokinetic and pharmacodynamic models.[7,9,16-19]

other effects, especially loss of response to laryngoscopy (3.5 minutes). Similarly, the duration of effect from rocuronium is also much longer than the duration of unresponsiveness (Table 28–2 and Figure 28–4B).

This is important to consider when airway management is prolonged such as with an unanticipated difficult airway. This may explain why patients develop hypertension, tachycardia, and tearing following tracheal intubation. Although the patients

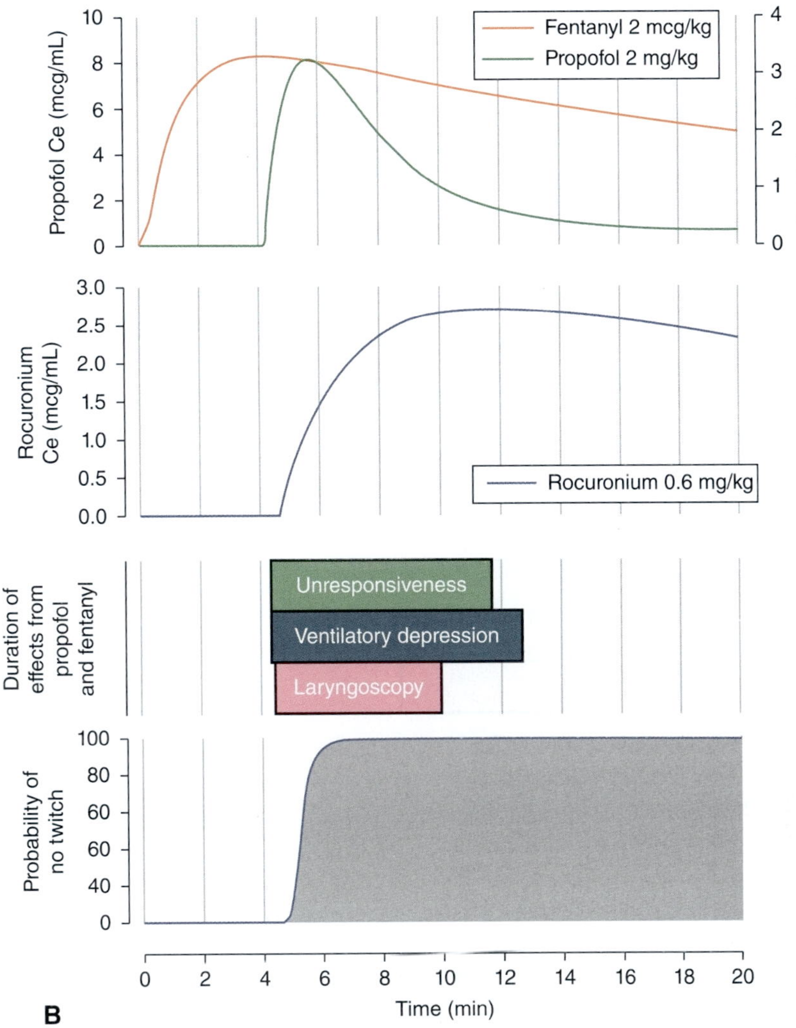

FIGURE 28–4 *(Continued)*

were immobile and apparently unresponsive, laryngoscopy was performed outside the time window of maximal drug effect.

Sugammadex has been introduced as a reversal agent for rocuronium and vecuronium. Figure 28–4C presents a simulation of a rocuronium 0.6 mg/kg followed 2.5 minutes later by sugammadex 4 mg/kg. Sugammadex rapidly reverses the paralytic effects. The reversal is so rapid that other effects, such ventilatory depression and unresponsiveness, are still present. This may be important to consider when rapidly attempting to resuscitate a hypoxic patient who is proving difficult to ventilate and intubate. Although the neuromuscular blockade has been reversed, the patient may remain unresponsive and in a state of intolerable ventilatory depression for several more minutes.

HEMOGLOBIN OXYGEN DESATURATION

An important element of induction is to consider the rate of hemoglobin oxygen desaturation once a patient has been rendered apneic (Figure 28–5).

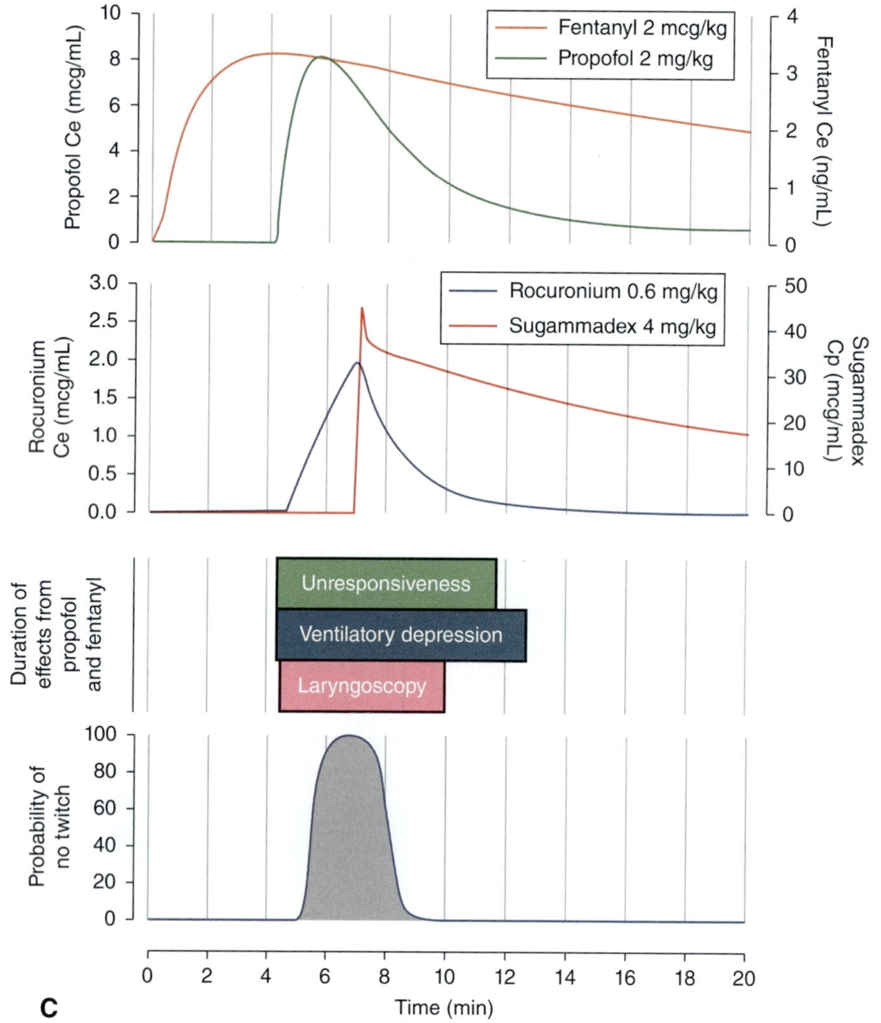

FIGURE 28–4 *(Continued)*

This simulation predicts the hemoglobin oxygen desaturation following 1 and 3 minutes of preoxygenation. Assumptions used in making this prediction are listed in Table 28–3.

The most important suggestion of this simulation is that in the rare instance that the patient can neither be intubated nor ventilated, the effects of succinylcholine may not dissipate before oxygen desaturation occurs. It is important to point out that these simulations assume normal pulmonary physiology. In patients with an increased metabolic rate (ie, sepsis) or decreased functional residual capacity (eg, obesity, pregnancy), the rate of hemoglobin oxygen desaturation will likely be faster (as depicted by the solid and dashed lines for 1 and 3 minutes of preoxygenation, respectively).

CLINICAL CONSIDERATION DURING INDUCTION

Opioids are known to produce less of a hemodynamic insult during induction. Patients with known or suspected cardiac instability may be better served using a high-dose opioid induction technique that minimizes the dose of sedative–hypnotics. Various combinations of opioid and a sedative can be used to

TABLE 28–2 Predicted time to onset and duration of effect for selected neuromuscular blocking agents.

Effect	Time (minutes)
Succinylcholine 1 mg/kg bolus	
Time to peak effect-site concentration	2.3
Time to probability of no twitches > 95%	< 1
Duration of probability of no twitches > 95%	6.5
Rocuronium 0.6 mg/kg bolus	
Time to peak effect-site concentration	7
Time to probability of no twitches > 95%	1.5
Duration of probability of no twitches > 95%	27
Rocuronium 0.6 mg/kg bolus followed 2.5 minutes later by sugammadex 4 mg/kg	
Time to peak effect-site concentration	2.5
Time to probability of no twitches > 95%	1.5 mi
Duration of probability of no twitches > 95%	1.5

achieve a near-equivalent loss of response to laryngoscopy. Figure 28–6 presents a set of simulated dosing regimens with propofol and fentanyl. In this simulation, 3 combinations are presented that are all near the isoeffect line for a 95% probability of no response to laryngoscopy. With higher doses of fentanyl, a very small dose of propofol can be used to achieve a similar effect.

Overall, propofol may not be a prudent choice. Even in small doses, it can cause severe cardiovascular depression in select patients. Propofol was used in these simulations because its interaction with opioids has been better characterized.

Similar to the patient with severe cardiovascular disease, other patient conditions merit scrutiny prior to administering induction agents. Some of these include:

- Preoperative nausea and vomiting presents an increased risk of aspiration on induction. If this issue is of primary concern, propofol followed immediately by succinylcholine in rapid sequence may be useful.
- Prolonged anorexia and frequent emesis may lead to severe intravascular volume depletion. Cardiovascular compensatory mechanisms may mask the true extent of dehydration (ie, peripheral vasoconstriction to maintain blood pressure). If this is of potential concern, intravenous etomidate 0.2 mg/kg followed immediately by succinylcholine in rapid sequence may be appropriate. Etomidate should be used with caution, especially in critically ill patients because of its associated adrenal suppression, evident even after a single induction dose. If this is of significant concern, consider ketamine (up to 1 mg/kg), ketamine with midazolam (up to 0.03 mg/kg), or etomidate (up to 0.2 mg/kg) in *incremental* doses until unresponsive. If the clinical setting allows, consider restoring intravascular volume and urine output to 0.5 to 1 mL/kg/h prior to induction.
- Assess the risk of aspiration risks versus intravascular volume depletion before induction of anesthesia. Consider rapid-sequence induction versus an incremental induction to minimize cardiovascular depression.

In summary, induction of anesthesia is the convergence of several potentially conflicting goals. Meeting those goals requires an in depth understanding of the drugs used for induction and how they synergistically interact with one another. Some key points include:

- Sedative effects: Opioids alone have a very low probability of generating unresponsiveness, but propofol alone does. When combined, opioids amplify the sedating effects of propofol but only by a small amount.
- Analgesic effects: Laryngoscopy is one of the most painful stimuli encountered in the operating room. The most pronounced synergism is with analgesic effects. Propofol or an opioid by itself will not consistently block the response to laryngoscopy. But when combined, they amplify the effects of one another and lead to a high probability of no response to laryngoscopy and tracheal intubation.

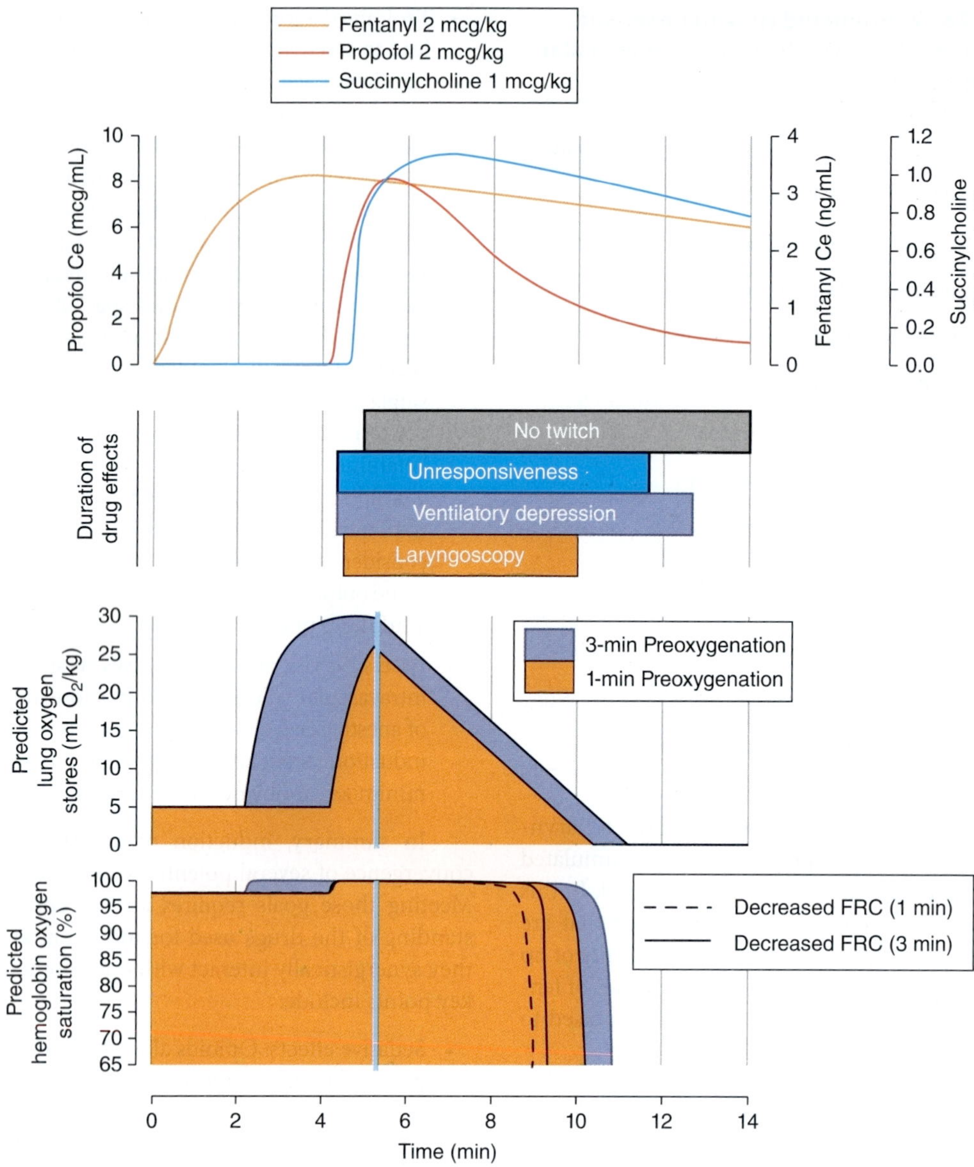

FIGURE 28–5 Simulations of the rate of oxygen desaturation following an induction with fentanyl, propofol, and succinylcholine. The top plot presents the effect-site concentration (Ce) levels for each drug. The second-from-the-top plot presents the duration of various effects for this combination of induction drugs. The duration of effect was defined as the time above a 50% probability of effect. The third-from-the-top plot presents the estimated amount of oxygen within the lungs as a function of preoxygenation (1 versus 3 minutes). The fourth-from-the-top plot presents the predicted rate of oxygen desaturation. The simulations of oxygen saturation assume that with the onset of neuromuscular blockade, delineated by the vertical green line, apnea is present with no gas exchange. A list of assumptions for this set of simulations is presented in Table 28–2. This set of simulations assumes a 40-year-old, 70-kg, 170-cm male. Simulations were based on published models of pulmonary physiology.[20-28] FRC, functional residual capacity.

TABLE 28–3 Assumptions and limitations of predicting oxygen saturation during apnea.

Assumptions
Preoxygenation with a well-sealed face mask on an anesthesia machine yields an inspired oxygen level (FiO_2) of 0.8.
Spontaneous respiratory rate is 10 breaths/min.
For each breath, the tidal volume is 7 mL/kg, anatomic dead space is 2.2 mL/kg, and alveolar tidal volume is 4.8 mL/kg.
Lung volumes are weight normalized to ideal body weight.
Cardiac output, hemoglobin concentration, arterial pH, arterial carbon dioxide, and temperature are within normal limits.
Exponential oxygen wash-in.[20,21]
Estimates of oxygen consumption assume the basal metabolic rate,[6] resting energy expenditure, and respiratory quotient are all within normal limits.[23]
The Harris Benedict formula estimates of basal metabolic are reasonable in morbidly obese individuals.[29]
The functional residual capacity in obese individuals is reduced.[24]
Increased alveolar–arterial oxygen gradient.[30]
Estimates of SpO_2 can be made from arterial oxygen tension levels.[25]
Limitations
Ventilatory response to elevated arterial carbon dioxide levels may be decreased in obese individuals.
Values for cardiac output and arterial carbon dioxide levels are likely to be abnormal in obese individuals.

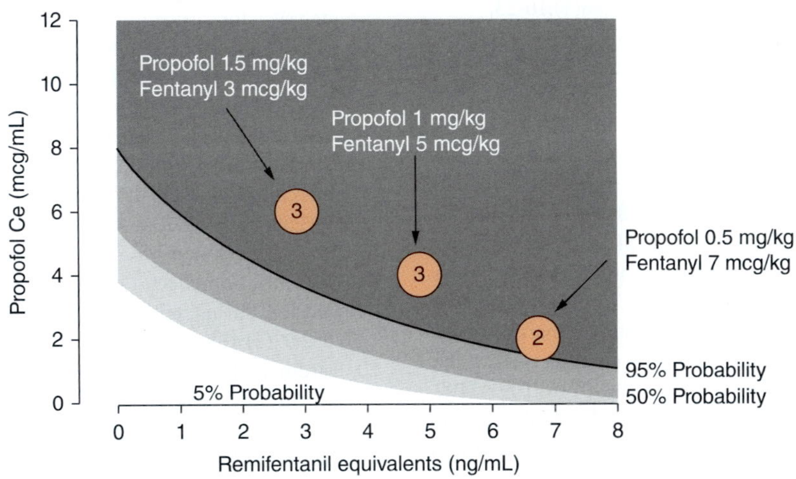

FIGURE 28–6 High-dose opioid induction techniques superimposed over a topographic representation of the propofol–remifentanil pharmacodynamic interaction model for loss of response to laryngoscopy. The gray shaded areas represent portions of the response surface associated with a 5% to 50% (light gray), 50% to 95% (gray), and greater than 95% (dark gray) probability of effect. The large red circles represent the approximate maximal concentration pairs for 3 different dosing regimens of fentanyl in combination with propofol. The time each concentration pair is above a 95% probability of no response to laryngoscopy is presented within each circle in minutes. Fentanyl concentrations are presented as remifentanil equivalents.[31] This set of simulations assumes a 50-year-old, 70-kg, 165-cm female. Simulations were based on published pharmacokinetic and pharmacodynamic models.[4-9] Ce, effect-site concentration.

REFERENCES

1. Alanoglu Z, Tolu S, Yalcin S, Batislam Y, Ozatamer O, Tuzuner F. Different remifentanil doses in rapid sequence anesthesia induction: BIS monitoring and intubation conditions. *Adv Clin Exp Med.* 2013;22(1):47-55.
2. Demirkaya M, Kelsaka E, Sarihasan B, Bek Y, Ustun E. The optimal dose of remifentanil for acceptable intubating conditions during propofol induction without neuromuscular blockade. *J Clin Anesth.* 2012;24(5):392-397.
3. Johnson KB, Swenson JD, Egan TD, Jarrett R, Johnson M. Midazolam and remifentanil by bolus injection for intensely stimulating procedures of brief duration: experience with awake laryngoscopy. *Anesth Analg.* 2002;94(5):1241-1243.
4. Bouillon TW, Bruhn J, Radulescu L, et al. Pharmacodynamic interaction between propofol and remifentanil regarding hypnosis, tolerance of laryngoscopy, bispectral index, and electroencephalographic approximate entropy. *Anesthesiology.* 2004;100(6):1353-1372.
5. Minto CF, Schnider TW, Egan TD, et al. Influence of age and gender on the pharmacokinetics and pharmacodynamics of remifentanil. I. Model development. *Anesthesiology.* 1997;86(1):10-23.
6. Minto CF, Schnider TW, Shafer SL. Pharmacokinetics and pharmacodynamics of remifentanil. II. Model application. *Anesthesiology.* 1997;86(1):24-33.
7. Schnider TW, Minto CF, Gambus PL, et al. The influence of method of administration and covariates on the pharmacokinetics of propofol in adult volunteers. *Anesthesiology.* 1998;88(5):1170-1182.
8. Schnider TW, Minto CF, Shafer SL, et al. The influence of age on propofol pharmacodynamics. *Anesthesiology.* 1999;90(6):1502-1516.
9. Shafer SL, Varvel JR, Aziz N, Scott JC. Pharmacokinetics of fentanyl administered by computer-controlled infusion pump. *Anesthesiology.* 1990;73(6):1091-1102.
10. Westmoreland CL, Sebel PS, Gropper A. Fentanyl or alfentanil decreases the minimum alveolar anesthetic concentration of isoflurane in surgical patients. *Anesth Analg.* 1994;78(1):23-28.
11. Chernick DA, Gillings D, Laine H, Hendler J, Silver JM, Davidson AB. Validity and reliability of the Observer's Assessment of Alertness/Sedation Scale: study with intravenous midazolam. *J Clin Psychopharmacol.* 1990;10(4):244-251.
12. LaPierre CD, Johnson KB, Randall BR, Egan TD. A simulation study of common propofol and propofol-opioid dosing regimens for upper endoscopy: implications on the time course of recovery. *Anesthesiology.* 2012;117(2):252-262.
13. LaPierre CD, Johnson KB, Randall BR, White JL, Egan TD. An exploration of remifentanil-propofol combinations that lead to a loss of response to esophageal instrumentation, a loss of responsiveness, and/or onset of intolerable ventilatory depression. *Anesth Analg.* 2011;113(3):490-499.
14. Johnson KB, Syroid ND, Gupta DK, et al. An evaluation of remifentanil propofol response surfaces for loss of responsiveness, loss of response to surrogates of painful stimuli and laryngoscopy in patients undergoing elective surgery. *Anesth Analg.* 2008;106(2):471-479.
15. Johnson KB, Syroid ND, Gupta DK, et al. An evaluation of remifentanil-sevoflurane response surface models in patients emerging from anesthesia: model improvement using effect-site sevoflurane concentrations. *Anesth Analg.* 2010;111(2):387-394.
16. Cooper RA, Maddineni VR, Mirakhur RK, Wierda JM, Brady M, Fitzpatrick KT. Time course of neuromuscular effects and pharmacokinetics of rocuronium bromide (Org 9426) during isoflurane anaesthesia in patients with and without renal failure. *Br J Anaesth.* 1993;71(2):222-226.
17. Kleijn HJ, Zollinger DP, van den Heuvel MW, Kerbusch T. Population pharmacokinetic-pharmacodynamic analysis for sugammadex-mediated reversal of rocuronium-induced neuromuscular blockade. *Br J Clin Pharmacol.* 2011;72(3):415-433.
18. Plaud B, Proost JH, Wierda JM, Barre J, Debaene B, Meistelman C. Pharmacokinetics and pharmacodynamics of rocuronium at the vocal cords and the adductor pollicis in humans. *Clin Pharmacol Ther.* 1995;58(2):185-191.
19. Roy JJ, Donati F, Boismenu D, Varin F. Concentration-effect relation of succinylcholine chloride during propofol anesthesia. *Anesthesiology.* 2002;97(5):1082-1092.
20. Hardman JG, Wills JS, Aitkenhead AR. Factors determining the onset and course of hypoxemia during apnea: an investigation using physiological modelling. *Anesth Analg.* 2000;90(3):619-624.
21. Hardman JG, Wills JS, Aitkenhead AR. Investigating hypoxemia during apnea: validation of a set of physiological models. *Anesth Analg.* 2000;90(3):614-618.
22. Harris JA, Benedict FG. A biometric study of human basal metabolism. *Proc Natl Acad Sci U S A.* 1918;4(12):370-373.
23. Weir JB. New methods for calculating metabolic rate with special reference to protein metabolism. *J Physiol.* 1949;109(1-2):1-9.

24. Jones RL, Nzekwu MM. The effects of body mass index on lung volumes. *Chest*. 2006;130(3):827-833.
25. Kelman GR. Digital computer subroutine for the conversion of oxygen tension into saturation. *J Appl Physiol*. 1966;21(4):1375-1376.
26. Greenbaum R, Kelman GR, Nunn JF, Prys-Roberts C. Arterial oxygen tensions. *Anesthesiology*. 1966;27(6):869-870.
27. Ibanez J, Raurich JM. Normal values of functional residual capacity in the sitting and supine positions. *Intensive Care Med*. 1982;8(4):173-177.
28. Kreymann G, Grosser S, Buggisch P, Gottschall C, Matthaei S, Greten H. Oxygen consumption and resting metabolic rate in sepsis, sepsis syndrome, and septic shock. *Crit Care Med*. 1993;21(7):1012-1019.
29. Muller B, Merk S, Burgi U, Diem P. [Calculating the basal metabolic rate and severe and morbid obesity]. *Praxis*. 2001;90(45):1955-1963.
30. Taylor RR, Kelly TM, Elliott CG, Jensen RL, Jones SB. Hypoxemia after gastric bypass surgery for morbid obesity. *Arch Surg*. 1985;120(11):1298-1302.
31. Syroid ND, Johnson KB, Pace NL, et al. Response surface model predictions of emergence and response to pain in the recovery room: an evaluation of patients emerging from an isoflurane and fentanyl anesthetic. *Anesth Analg*. 2010;111(2):380-386.

CHAPTER

29

Considerations for the Maintenance of Anesthesia

Ken B. Johnson, MD

INTRODUCTION

Anesthetic technique has expanded and improved with the advent of newer drugs, methods to deliver them, and drug displays that present real-time anesthetic drug interactions. This chapter will briefly explore the following:

- Use of pharmacodynamic interaction models to compare common anesthetic techniques
- How substantially different dosing regimens yield near-equivalent effects
- The pronounced opioid effect from common remifentanil dosing regimens
- How target-controlled infusion (TCI) and total intravenous anesthesia (TIVA) compare in terms of anesthetic effects

TOTAL INTRAVENOUS ANESTHESIA VERSUS COMBINED TECHNIQUE

Anesthesiologists have long used both TIVA and potent inhaled agents combined with opioids. Both techniques are effective. TIVA is better suited for patients with a known or suspected history of postoperative nausea and vomiting; procedures such as microlaryngoscopy and rigid bronchoscopy, where delivery of potent inhaled agents is not possible; and females of childbearing age. Potent inhaled agents are better suited for patients with known or suspected ischemic cardiovascular disease. Major advantages are that there is less postoperative nausea and vomiting; improved cognitive function, at least during the first few hours after surgery[1]; and smooth emergence; patients simply appear happier as well.

Potential disadvantages of TIVA are that it is more expensive; more complicated; and associated with a perception of more risk of awareness, although studies suggest a low risk of awareness.[2] Use of inhalation agents is popular because they are easier to use and less expensive, allow for the monitoring of end-tidal concentrations, and are associated with a perceived lower risk of awareness.

With regard to the ability of either technique to provide an adequate level of anesthesia, consider the simulations presented in Figure 29–1. They present predictions of unresponsiveness for a TIVA technique using infusion rates (ie, mcg/kg/min), an intravenous technique using TCIs, and a potent inhaled agent in combination with an opioid technique. The 3 techniques used common dosing regimens that led to a predicted high probability of unresponsiveness.

DIFFERENT DOSE, SAME EFFECT

Clinical pharmacologists have characterized anesthetic drug interactions for a variety of effects. This research has confirmed that various combinations of anesthetic drugs can have near-equivalent effects and that anesthetics with different mechanisms may enhance the effects of one another such that less overall anesthetic is required. Variations of the anesthetic techniques presented in Figure 29–1 illustrate this point (Table 29–1 and Figure 29–2). Low-dose opioid–high-dose sedative combinations versus high-dose opioid–low-dose sedative combinations have similar overall effects in terms of loss of responsiveness. This phenomenon persists across different types of sedatives (ie, propofol versus sevoflurane).

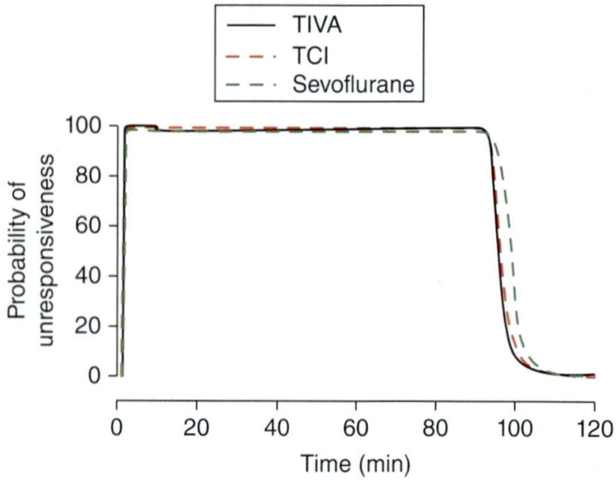

FIGURE 29–1 Total intravenous anesthesia (TIVA) versus target-controlled infusion (TCI) versus combined techniques: simulation of the probability of unresponsiveness for 3 anesthetic dosing regimens: TIVA, TCI, and a combined potent inhaled agent (sevoflurane) and opioid technique. Unresponsiveness was defined as an Observer's Assessment of Alertness and Sedation greater than 2. All simulations assumed a 50-year-old, 165-cm, 70-kg female undergoing a 90-minute procedure associated with minimal postoperative pain. All 3 techniques provide a high probability of unresponsiveness. The TIVA technique consisted of induction with fentanyl 1.5 mcg/kg and propofol 2 mg/kg followed by maintenance with propofol 100 mcg/kg/min and remifentanil 0.2 mcg/kg/min. A fentanyl bolus (1.5 mcg/kg) was administered as a transition opioid 15 minutes before the end of the procedure. The TCI technique consisted of a target propofol effect-site concentration of 3 mcg/mL and a target remifentanil effect-site concentration of 6 ng/mL. The combined potent inhaled agent–opioid technique consisted of induction as described for the TIVA followed by 2% sevoflurane in oxygen and remifentanil 0.2 mcg/kg/min. For both the TCI and sevoflurane techniques, a fentanyl bolus was administered as a transition opioid 15 minutes before the end of the procedure. Simulations were based on published pharmacokinetic and pharmacodynamic models.[3-17]

TABLE 29–1 Selected simulated dosing regimens for total intravenous anesthesia (TIVA), target-controlled anesthesia (TCI), and sevoflurane combined with fentanyl and remifentanil.

	Technique
TIVA	
Regimen 1	Propofol 100 mcg/kg/min Remifentanil 0.2 mcg/kg/min
Regimen 2	Propofol 130 mcg/kg/min Remifentanil 0.1 mcg/kg/min
Regimen 3	Propofol 200 mcg/kg/min No remifentanil
TCI	
Regimen 4	Propofol set to 3.5 mcg/mL Remifentanil set to 6 ng/mL
Regimen 5	Propofol set to 4.2 mcg/mL Remifentanil set to 3 ng/mL
Regimen 6	Propofol set to 6 mcg/mL No remifentanil
Inhaled Agent	
Regimen 7	Sevoflurane 1.6% Remifentanil 0.2 mcg/kg/min
Regimen 8	Sevoflurane 1.8% Remifentanil 0.1 mcg/kg/min
Regimen 9	Sevoflurane 2% No remifentanil

For all techniques, induction consisted of a 1.5-mcg/kg fentanyl bolus administered 4 minutes before a 2-mg/kg propofol bolus. Maintenance anesthetics were initiated just after the induction drugs. For postoperative analgesia, a 1.5-mcg/kg fentanyl bolus was administered 15 minutes before the end of procedure. All anesthetics were administered for 90 minutes.

REMIFENTANIL INFUSIONS

An advantage to using remifentanil as part of a combined technique with propofol, another sedative, or a potent inhaled agent is that it can be administered as a continuous infusion without much regard for residual effect. Recommended intraoperative infusion rates range from 0.1 to 0.25 mcg/kg/min. To put these infusion rates into more of a clinical context, it is interesting to estimate what dose of fentanyl would be required, either as a bolus or as a continuous infusion, to provide a near-equivalent opioid effect. Figure 29–3A and B present predicted remifentanil effect-site concentrations that result from common remifentanil infusion rates and the

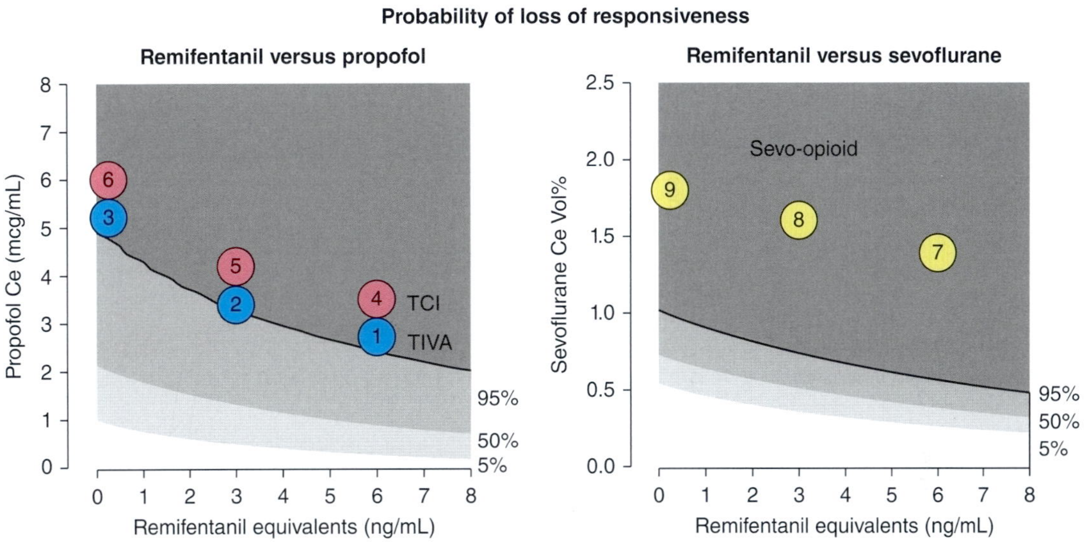

FIGURE 29–2 Different dose, same effect. Topographic representation of remifentanil–propofol (left) and remifentanil–sevoflurane (right) pharmacodynamic interaction models for loss of responsiveness. The gray shaded areas represent portions of the response surface associated with a 5% to 50% (light gray), 50% to 95% (gray), and greater than 95% (dark gray) probability of effect. Superimposed over the interaction model surface are approximate maximal concentration pairs for selected propofol and remifentanil infusion rates for various total intravenous dosing regimens (TIVA, blue circles), selected target propofol and remifentanil effect-site concentrations for various target-controlled infusion dosing regimens (TCI, pink circles), and selected sevoflurane (Sevo) vaporizer settings and remifentanil infusion rates for various potent inhaled agent–opioid dosing regimens (yellow circles). The numbers in the circles refer to dosing details presented in Table 29–1. Fentanyl concentrations are presented as remifentanil equivalents.[18] All simulations assumed a 50-year-old, 165-cm, 70-kg female undergoing a 90-minute procedure associated with minimal postoperative pain. Simulations were based on published pharmacokinetic and pharmacodynamic models.[3-5,11-16] *Many different dosing regimens yield a similar effect if dosed along isoeffect lines.* Ce, effect-site concentration.

predicted probability of no response to a painful stimulus and severe ventilatory depression. Both remifentanil infusion rates (0.1 and 0.2 mcg/kg/min) produce high probabilities of analgesia and the higher dose remifentanil infusion produces a high probability of intolerable ventilatory depression. In order to achieve a near-equivalent effect, a fentanyl infusion of 5 to 6 mcg/kg/h or a fentanyl bolus of 3 to 5 mcg/kg is required. Of note, the boluses only maintain similar drug effects for 20 to 30 minutes. The bolus fentanyl doses may be used, but the continuous infusion rates are excessive for routine use. These simulations illustrate the versatility of remifentanil to provide profound analgesia yet minimize prolonged opioid effects once administration is terminated. Remifentanil can be used to provide intense analgesia for procedures of short duration, even on an outpatient setting, whereas to do so with other opioids would be impractical.

COMPARISON OF TOTAL INTRAVENOUS ANESTHESIA VERSUS TARGET-CONTROLLED INFUSION

TCIs represent a method of delivering intravenous anesthetics. They use pharmacokinetic models to drive infusion pumps to quickly achieve and maintain a target plasma or effect-site concentration. TCI is available for several drugs but is primarily used for the delivery of propofol and remifentanil. TCI uses a more sophisticated approach to administering an anesthetic that is more akin to the delivery of potent

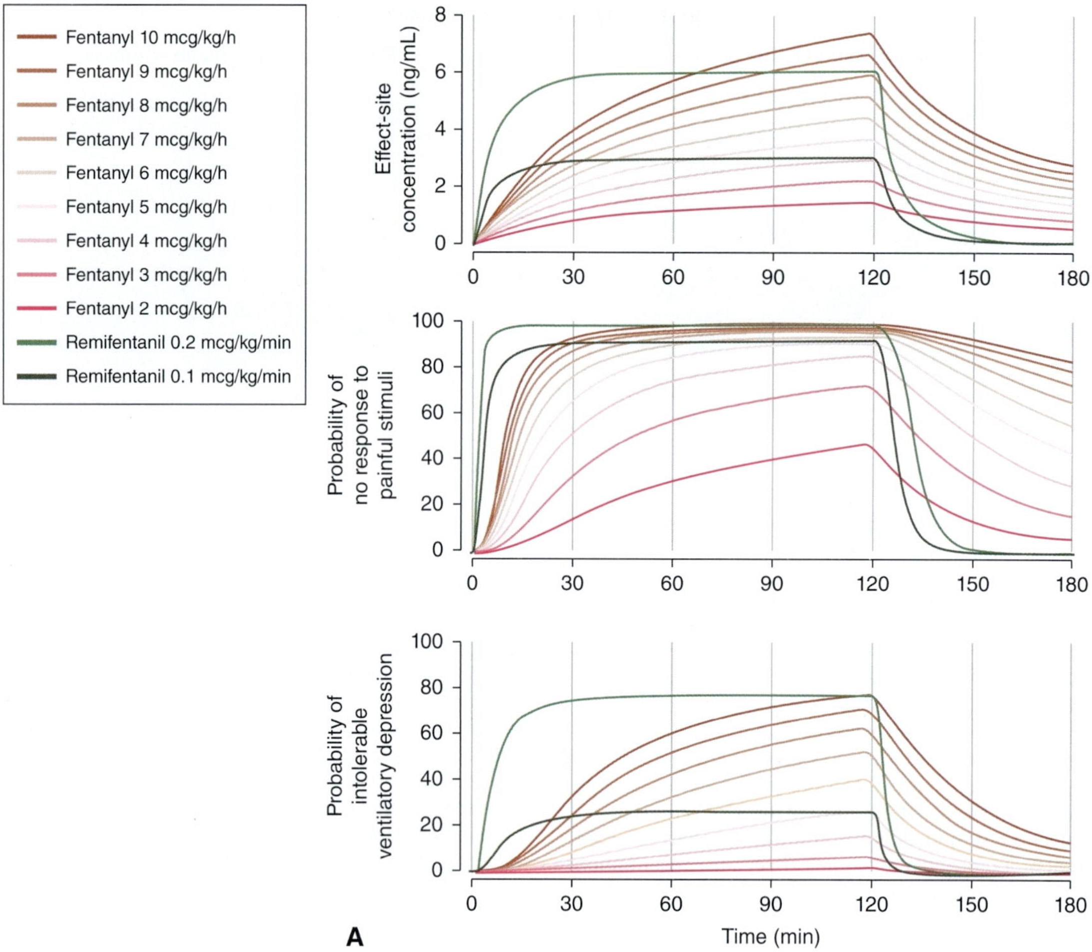

FIGURE 29–3 Remifentanil infusions: a high-dose opioid technique? Simulations of predicted effect-site concentrations from remifentanil continuous infusions (0.1 and 0.2 mcg/kg/min) and fentanyl infusions (2–7 mcg/kg/h, part A) and fentanyl boluses (2–8-mcg/kg bolus) and their associated effects (analgesia and intolerable ventilatory depression). Analgesia was defined as a loss of response to painful tibial pressure found to be consistent with pain experienced in the postanesthesia care unit, where patients requested analgesics.[4] Intolerable ventilatory depression was defined as a respiratory rate less than 4 breaths per min.[19,20] All simulations assumed a 50-year-old, 165-cm, 70-kg female. Simulations were based on published pharmacokinetic and pharmacodynamic models.[15,19,20] *A substantial amount of fentanyl (either bolus or infusion) is required to achieve a similar effect from a routine infusion rate of remifentanil.*

inhaled agents via a vaporizer. Anesthesiologists frequently consider their dosing of a potent inhaled agent in terms of estimated brain concentrations (volume %) or in terms of drug effect (ie, minimum alveolar concentration) but to a lesser extent with intravenous agents. Dosing intravenous agents is often thought of in terms of mcg/kg or mcg/kg/min. To bridge the gap between how anesthesiologists formulate doses of intravenous versus potent inhaled agents, TCI nudges anesthesiologists into thinking of their intravenous anesthetics in terms of target effect-site concentrations.

One advantage of TCI over conventional infusions is that computerized drug delivery can account

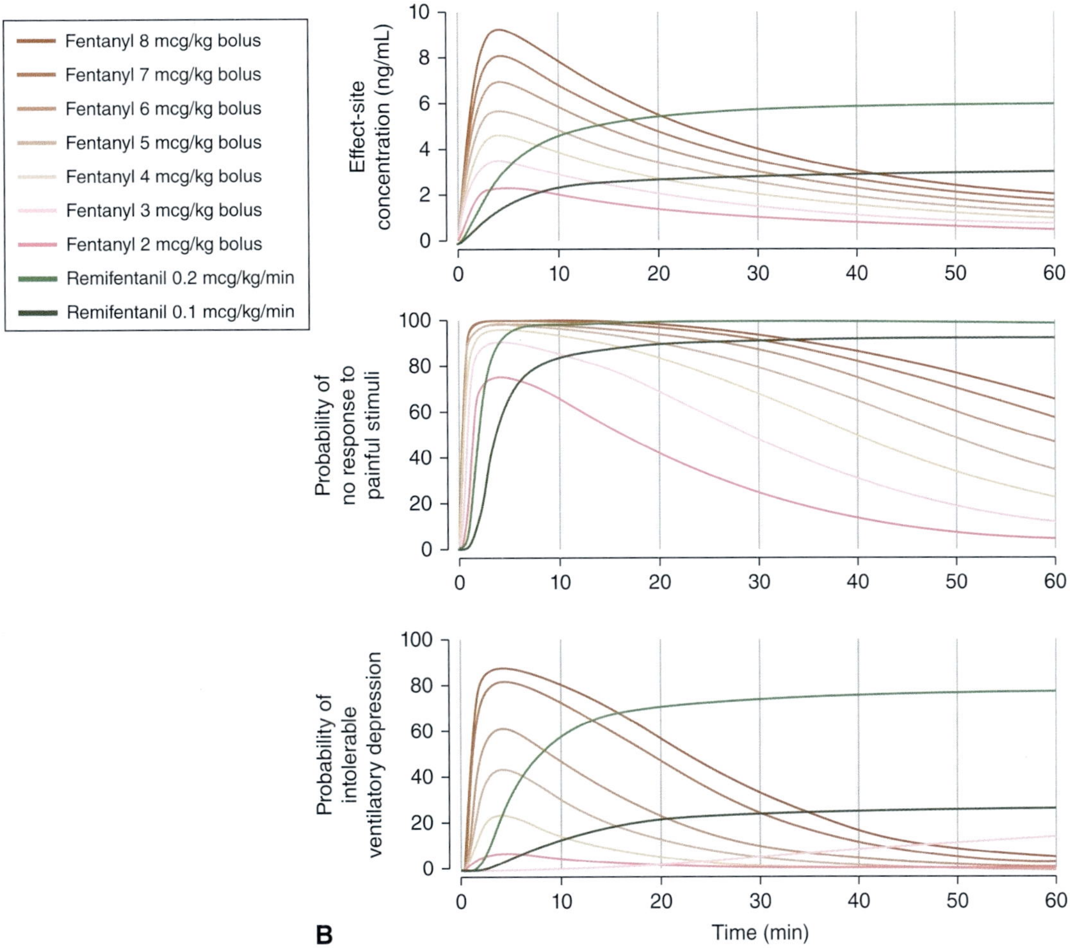

FIGURE 29–3 *(Continued)*

for nuances in drug kinetics that humans cannot perceive in real time without the aid of a computer that uses complex mathematical expressions. Thus, anesthesiologists use infusion rates and clinical judgment to "get by." With anesthetics that require substantial adjustment to meet dynamic changes in surgical stimuli, changes in infusion rates may require up to 15 to 20 minutes to reach a near steady state for either propofol or remifentanil. TCI can arrive at a new target concentration much faster.

Although there are clear advantages to TCI, drug administration using simple infusion rates can provide an adequate anesthetic. To explore this further, a sample TIVA and TCI technique is presented in Figure 29–4. It compares a TIVA technique of propofol 100 mcg/kg/min combined with remifentanil 0.2 mcg/kg/min with a TCI technique with the propofol and remifentanil set to 3 mcg/mL and 6 ng/mL, respectively, for 2 hours. One difference is how the drugs are administered. This is especially evident with propofol. The infusion rate starts out very high and decreases continuously until the infusion is terminated. This allows for a consistent predicted propofol effect-site concentration. The propofol continuous infusion, however, leads to concentrations that slowly climb until the infusion is terminated. Remifentanil is different. TCI boluses the remifentanil and then maintains an infusion rate identical

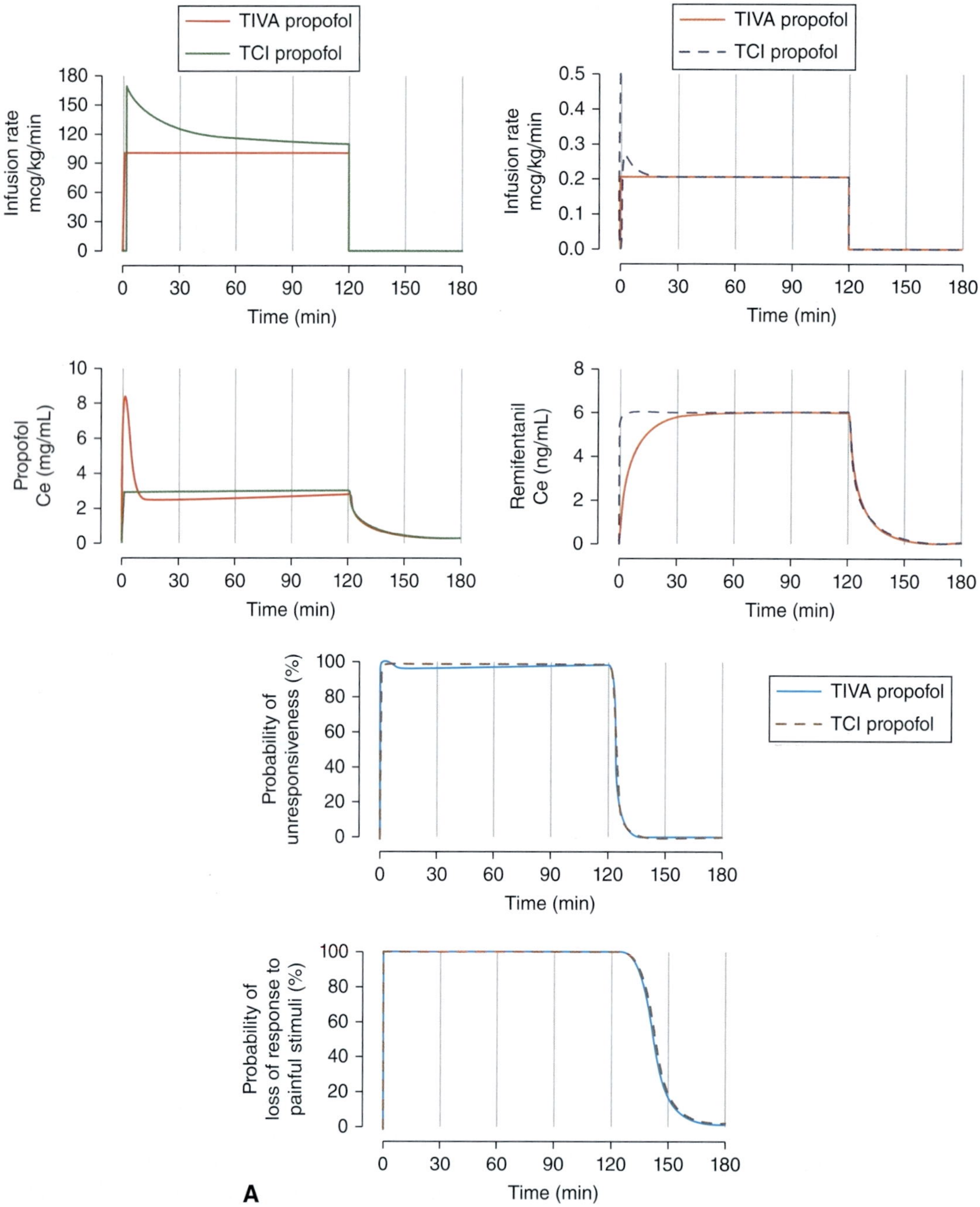

FIGURE 29–4 Comparison of total intravenous anesthesia (TIVA) to target-controlled infusion (TCI). A, Illustration of infusion rates (top plots), predicted effect-site concentrations (Ce, second row of plots), and selected predicted effects (bottom plots) comparing TIVA and TCI using propofol and remifentanil. The TIVA technique included an induction dose of 2-mg/kg propofol (not shown on the top left plot) followed by continuous infusions of propofol 100 mcg/kg/min and remifentanil 0.2 mcg/kg/min. The TCI technique consisted of a target propofol effect-site concentration (Ce) of 3 mcg/mL and a target remifentanil Ce of 6 ng/mL.

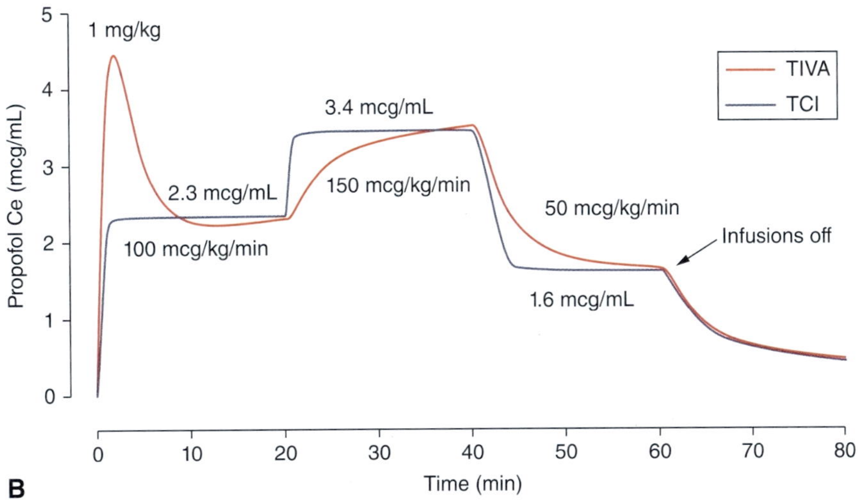

FIGURE 29–4 *(Continued)* B, Comparison of changes in infusion rate versus target Ce levels for a continuous 1-hour propofol infusion. In this simulation, there were 4 changes in drug administration. For the TIVA (pink line), there were (1) a 1-mg/kg bolus followed by an infusion of 100 mcg/kg/min, (2) a change in the infusion rate to 150 mcg/kg/min, (3) a change in the infusion rate to 50 mcg/kg/min, and (4) the infusion was turned off. For the TCI (blue line), there were (1) a change from a target Ce of 0 to 2.3 mcg/mL, (2) a change from 2.3 to 3.4 mcg/mL, (3) a change from 3.4 to 1.6 mcg/mL, and (4) a change from 1.6 to 0 mcg/mL. The target Ce levels were selected to be similar to the concentrations achieved with the continuous infusion rates after 20 minutes. This figure illustrates a key advantage of administering propofol via TCI. TCI can achieve and maintain a target concentration faster than a change in a continuous infusion. This advantage for propofol is more evident when increasing versus decreasing the infusion rates. All simulations assumed a 50-year-old, 165-cm, 70-kg female for a 2-hour anesthetic. Simulations were based on published pharmacokinetic and pharmacodynamic models.[3,5,12-14] *Both techniques yield very similar effects, yet TCI achieves and maintains target concentrations more effectively.*

to the TIVA approach (0.2 mcg/kg/min). With TCI, remifentanil quickly achieves its target concentration, whereas the remifentanil infusion requires up to 30 minutes to achieve its near–steady-state effect-site concentration.

Both techniques lead to similar profiles in anesthetic effects over time. Both quickly achieve and maintain a very high probability of unresponsiveness and analgesia. This simulation of a 2-hour anesthetic with no changes in infusion rates or target effect-site concentrations throughout the anesthetic indicate that both techniques can provide nearly equivalent results. These simulations, although interesting, do not, however, reflect clinical practice, where it is likely that several adjustments in either infusion rates or target effect-site concentrations would be required.

A limitation with TCI is that it uses pharmacokinetic models to drive the infusion pumps to reach and maintain target effect-site concentrations. Although available pharmacokinetic models capture much of the population, there are patient conditions (ie, morbid obesity, severe blood loss, elderly state) that render model predictions inaccurate to the point that adjustments are required to compensate for overdosing or underdosing. As with any anesthetic technique, constant vigilance is required to ensure optimal delivery.

REFERENCES

1. Larsen B, Seitz A, Larsen R. Recovery of cognitive function after remifentanil-propofol anesthesia: a comparison with desflurane and sevoflurane anesthesia. *Anesth Analg*. 2000;90(1):168-174.
2. Enlund M, Hassan HG. Intraoperative awareness: detected by the structured Brice interview? *Acta Anaesth Scand*. 2002;46(4):345-349.

3. Johnson KB, Syroid ND, Gupta DK, et al. An evaluation of remifentanil propofol response surfaces for loss of responsiveness, loss of response to surrogates of painful stimuli and laryngoscopy in patients undergoing elective surgery. *Anesth Analg*. 2008;106(2):471-479.
4. Johnson KB, Syroid ND, Gupta DK, et al. An evaluation of remifentanil-sevoflurane response surface models in patients emerging from anesthesia: model improvement using effect-site sevoflurane concentrations. *Anesth Analg*. 2010;111(2):387-394.
5. Kern SE, Xie G, White JL, Egan TD. A response surface analysis of propofol-remifentanil pharmacodynamic interaction in volunteers. *Anesthesiology*. 2004;100(6):1373-1381.
6. Lerou JG, Booij LH. Model-based administration of inhalation anaesthesia. 2. Exploring the system model. *Br J Anaesth*. 2001;86(1):29-37.
7. Lerou JG, Booij LH. Model-based administration of inhalation anaesthesia. 1. Developing a system model. *Br J Anaesth*. 2001;86(1):12-28.
8. Lerou JG, Booij LH. Model-based administration of inhalation anaesthesia. 3. Validating the system model. *Br J Anaesth*. 2002;88(1):24-37.
9. Lerou JG, Dirksen R, Beneken Kolmer HH, Booij LH. A system model for closed-circuit inhalation anesthesia. I. Computer study. *Anesthesiology*. 1991;75(2):345-355.
10. Lerou JG, Dirksen R, Beneken Kolmer HH, Booij LH, Borm GF. A system model for closed-circuit inhalation anesthesia. II. Clinical validation. *Anesthesiology*. 1991;75(2):230-237.
11. Lerou JG, Verheijen R, Booij LH. Model-based administration of inhalation anaesthesia. 4. Applying the system model. *Br J Anaesth*. 2002;88(2):175-183.
12. Minto CF, Schnider TW, Egan TD, et al. Influence of age and gender on the pharmacokinetics and pharmacodynamics of remifentanil. I. Model development. *Anesthesiology*. 1997;86(1):10-23.
13. Minto CF, Schnider TW, Shafer SL. Pharmacokinetics and pharmacodynamics of remifentanil. II. Model application. *Anesthesiology*. 1997;86(1):24-33.
14. Schnider TW, Minto CF, Shafer SL, et al. The influence of age on propofol pharmacodynamics. *Anesthesiology*. 1999;90(6):1502-1516.
15. Shafer SL, Varvel JR, Aziz N, Scott JC. Pharmacokinetics of fentanyl administered by computer-controlled infusion pump. *Anesthesiology*. 1990;73(6):1091-1102.
16. Syroid ND, Johnson KB, Pace NL, et al. Response surface model predictions of emergence and response to pain in the recovery room: An evaluation of patients emerging from an isoflurane and fentanyl anesthetic. *Anesth Analg*. 2010;111(2):380-386.
17. Wissing H, Kuhn I, Rietbrock S, Fuhr U. Pharmacokinetics of inhaled anaesthetics in a clinical setting: comparison of desflurane, isoflurane and sevoflurane. *Br J Anaesth*. 2000;84(4):443-9.
18. Westmoreland CL, Sebel PS, Gropper A. Fentanyl or alfentanil decreases the minimum alveolar anesthetic concentration of isoflurane in surgical patients. *Anesth Analg*. 1994;78(1):23-28.
19. LaPierre CD, Johnson KB, Randall BR, Egan TD. A simulation study of common propofol and propofol-opioid dosing regimens for upper endoscopy: implications on the time course of recovery. *Anesthesiology*. 2012;117(2):252-262.
20. LaPierre CD, Johnson KB, Randall BR, White JL, Egan TD. An exploration of remifentanil-propofol combinations that lead to a loss of response to esophageal instrumentation, a loss of responsiveness, and/or onset of intolerable ventilatory depression. *Anesth Analg*. 2011;113(3):490-499.

CHAPTER 30

Emergence from Anesthesia

Ken B. Johnson, MD, Jennifer J. Davis, MD, and Jeffrey Swenson, MD

INTRODUCTION

Emergence from anesthesia is complex period where, as with induction, several competing interests influence an anesthesiologist's course of action. Timely emergence from anesthesia, adequate ventilatory function, and pain control once emerged from anesthesia; prevention of postoperative nausea and vomiting; and proper management of other comorbidities are some of these interests. This chapter will briefly review the selected issues regarding emergence from anesthesia, including:

- Is there any advantage of target-controlled infusion (TCI) over total intravenous anesthesia (TIVA) when using conventional infusion rates in terms of a timely emergence from anesthesia?
- Are end-tidal potent inhaled agent levels under non–steady-state conditions, such as emergence, useful in predicting wake-up times?
- What is a rational approach to opioid administration for safe postoperative analgesia?
- What technique can be used to estimate intraoperative and postoperative opioid requirements in patients who chronically consume opioids?

TARGET-CONTROLLED INFUSION VERSUS TOTAL INTRAVENOUS ANESTHESIA

No definitive outcomes study has explored whether administering a total intravenous anesthetic via TCI or with conventional continuous infusion rates impacts emergence. One might hypothesize that if administering a lengthy anesthetic, TCI would provide a more economical anesthetic and avoid unnecessary drug delivery that would perhaps delay emergence. Figure 30–1 presents a simulation of 2 intravenous techniques: one using TCI and the other set infusion rates for 2, 4, 6, and 8 hours. Both approaches used a high-dose remifentanil and low dose propofol technique. In fact the TCI target effect-site concentrations were selected to be near the effect-site concentrations that resulted from propofol infusions of 100 mcg/kg/min and remifentanil 0.2 mcg/kg/min. In general, with increasing duration of the anesthetic, the simulation predicted the time to emergence would become longer. Time to emergence was defined as the time required for the model of loss of responsiveness to predict that only 1 out of 20 people would be unresponsive (5%). Either technique (TCI or TIVA) was within 1 or 2 minutes of the other. For shorter infusions (2 and 4 hours), the TIVA technique was 1 minute ahead of the TCI for emergence. For the long infusion (8 hours), that relationship was reversed; time for emergence from TCI occurred a few minutes before that for TIVA. A potential explanation for the negligible differences between TIVA and TCI is that a high-dose opioid technique was used reducing the amount of propofol used.

END-TIDAL INHALED AGENT CONCENTRATIONS

Gas monitors provide measurements of end-tidal inhaled agent concentrations that anesthesiologists may use to predict when patients will emerge from anesthesia. A key phenomenon illustrated in Figure 30–2 is that effect-site concentrations lag

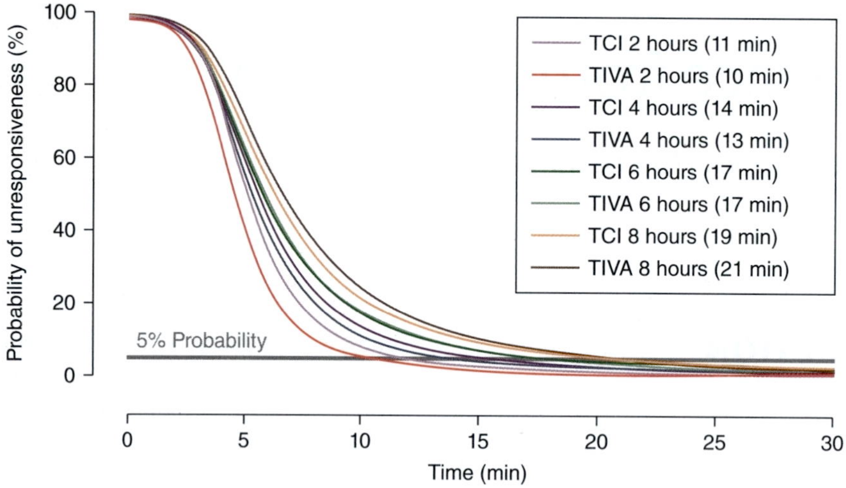

FIGURE 30–1 Emergence for anesthesia: is there a difference between total intravenous anesthesia (TIVA) and target-controlled infusion (TCI)? Here are simulations of the predicted probability of unresponsiveness once an anesthetic has been terminated for TCI and TIVA using propofol and remifentanil. TIVA consisted of propofol 100 mcg/kg/min and remifentanil 0.2 mcg/kg/min. TCI consisted of propofol and remifentanil target effect-site concentrations of 3 mcg/mL and 6 ng/mL, respectively. Each technique was administered for 2, 4, 6, and 8 hours. The end of emergence (gray horizontal line) was defined as a 5% probability of unresponsiveness (ie, 19 out of 20 people would be awake). The time from turning off all infusions until reaching a 5% probability of unresponsiveness is presented in parentheses. All simulations assumed a 50-year-old, 165-cm, 70-kg female. Simulations were based on published pharmacokinetic and pharmacodynamic models.[1-5] *The main point of these simulations is that for infusions up to 8 hours, technique (TIVA versus TCI) has minimal impact on the predicted time to emergence.*

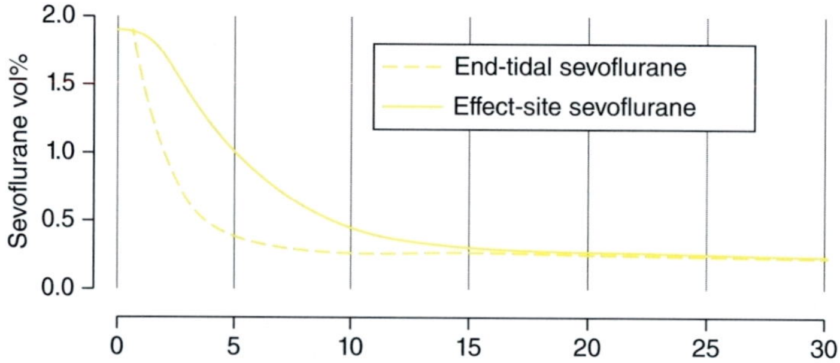

FIGURE 30–2 During emergence, are end-tidal agent levels useful in predicting time to wake-up? All simulations assumed a 30-year-old, 175-cm, 80-kg male undergoing a 4-hour anesthesia with sevoflurane combined with either hydromorphone or fentanyl. Simulations also assumed a minute volume of 6 L/min, normal pulmonary mechanics, and normal cardiopulmonary function. Hydromorphone or fentanyl was administered as a transition opioid near the end of the procedure. Hydromorphone, either 0.5 mg or 1 mg, was administered 1 hour before the end of the procedure. Fentanyl, either 2 or 3 mcg/kg, was administered 15 minutes before the end of the procedure. The top plot presents the predicted end-tidal and effect-site concentration (Ce) levels for sevoflurane. Of note, the effect concentration lags behind the end-tidal concentration by up to 15 minutes.

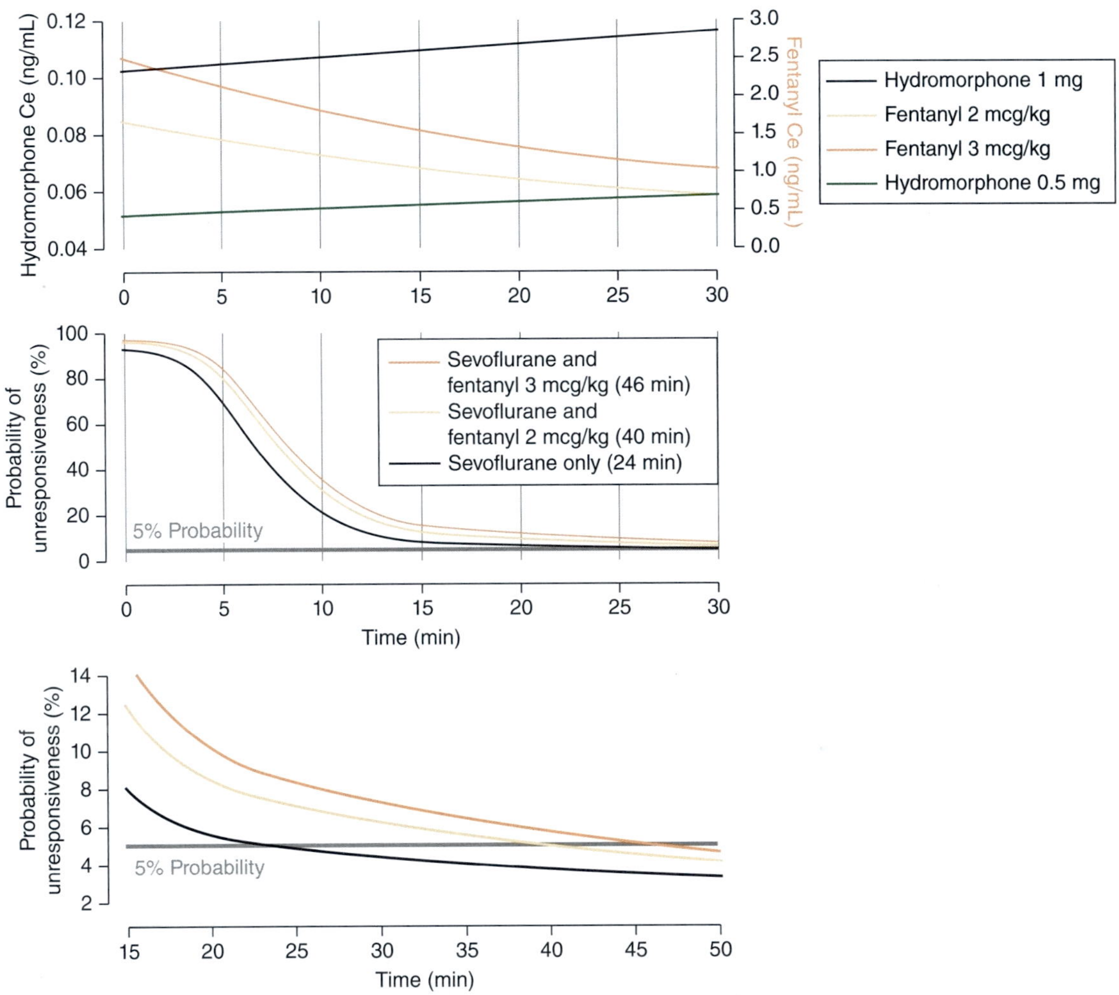

FIGURE 30–2 *(Continued)* The second plot presents the predicted Ce levels during the first 30 minutes following the 4-hour anesthetic use. Of note, although the hydromorphone was administered 1 hour before the end of the procedure, the Ce levels are still rising, whereas the fentanyl concentrations are on the decline. The third plot presents the predicted probability of unresponsiveness during the first 30 minutes after the anesthetic has been turned off. The end of emergence (gray horizontal line) was defined as a 5% probability of unresponsiveness (ie, 19 out of 20 people would be awake). The time from turning off the sevoflurane until reaching a 5% probability of unresponsiveness is presented in parentheses for sevoflurane alone and sevoflurane in combination with fentanyl (a simulation for sevoflurane in combination with hydromorphone is not available). The bottom plot presents an expanded view of the third plot to visualize where each sevoflurane–fentanyl combination crosses over the 5% probability of unresponsiveness. Simulations were based on published pharmacokinetic and pharmacodynamic models.[3-13] *The most important points from these simulations are that sevoflurane Ce levels lag behind end-tidal concentrations during non-steady-state conditions (such as emergence) and that the addition of a small amount of opioid can substantially prolong unresponsiveness.*

behind end-tidal concentrations under non–steady-state conditions (ie, emergence). In this example, sevoflurane has been maintained at 2% for 4 hours. Once administration is terminated, end-tidal concentrations quickly drop to below 0.5% in less than 5 minutes. In fact, effect-site concentrations do not catch up to end-tidal concentrations for up to 15 minutes. These times are somewhat arbitrary, given than anesthesiologists often manipulate ventilatory function to remove as much inhaled agent as quickly as possible, but the relationship stays the same. Thus, making prediction of emergence based on end-tidal concentrations is likely to be misleading.

The addition of even a small amount of opioid can substantially prolong emergence. In this simulation, an opioid was administered as a transition analgesic. Fentanyl was administered 15 minutes before the end of the procedure in either a 2- or 3-mcg/kg bolus. Hydromorphone was administered 1 hour before the end of the procedure in either a 0.5- or a 1-mg bolus. Although once the sevoflurane is discontinued, the time to emergence (again, time to reach a 5% probability of unresponsiveness) is markedly increased in the presence of fentanyl (from 24 to 40 minutes with 2 mcg/kg of fentanyl).

POSTOPERATIVE ANALGESIA

Figure 30–3 presents simulations of predicted effect-site concentrations following administration and effects for bolus doses of fentanyl, morphine, and hydromorphone. The aim of these simulations was to visualize the kinetic advantages and/or disadvantages of these opioids. The simulations demonstrate how effect-site concentrations of both hydromorphone and morphine persist for more than 8 hours in comparison to fentanyl, which lasts up to 1 hour. Both morphine and fentanyl provide analgesia and some probability of intolerable ventilatory depression, although these effects are short-lived for fentanyl but prolonged with morphine. Modeling parameters are not yet available to make similar predictions for hydromorphone.

These simulations suggest that if used in an outpatient surgery setting, morphine or hydromorphone will continue to exert an effect long after discharge. For patients who are discharged following procedures associated with moderate pain, it may be prudent to clarify pain control requirements and manage them with oral analgesics, as they would at home instead of administering long-acting opioids.

THE FENTANYL CHALLENGE

One of the vexing problems in the perioperative setting for patients, surgeons, anesthesiologists, and nursing staff is pain control for patients who chronically consume opioids. Conventional opioid dosing regimens are frequently inadequate. Health care professionals are uncomfortable administering opioid doses outside of recommended maximal dosing recommendations for fear of adverse events associated with ventilatory depression. By contrast, patients may experience poor pain control accompanied by debilitating anxiety and sleep disturbance. Although intending to provide better acute pain control, clinicians may inadvertently administer excessive opioid doses along with other sedating medications (eg, sleep aids, anxiolytics, antiemetics), provoking an adverse event.

A potential solution to managing pain for the patient who chronically consumes opioids is the fentanyl challenge. It is best suited for patients who undergo procedures associated with moderate to severe postoperative pain that require an inpatient stay for at least 36 to 48 hours. The fentanyl challenge consists of estimating an individual's opioid tolerance before surgery and then using that information to formulate a personalized fentanyl-dosing regimen for intraoperative and postoperative use (Table 30–1). In much the same way submarines use sonar to "ping" surrounding waters to estimate size and distance of objects in its path, the fentanyl challenge "pings" a patient's response to opioids. The aim of the "ping" is to identify a fentanyl effect-site concentration associated with ventilatory depression.[18,19]

Like other anesthetic drugs, opioids have several effects such as analgesia, ventilatory depression, and at higher doses, changes in the electroencephalogram. Prior work exploring the pharmacodynamics of these effects has proposed several key features of the concentration-effect relationships.[20] First, each effect has a unique C_{50} (effect-site concentration associated with a 50% probability of effect).

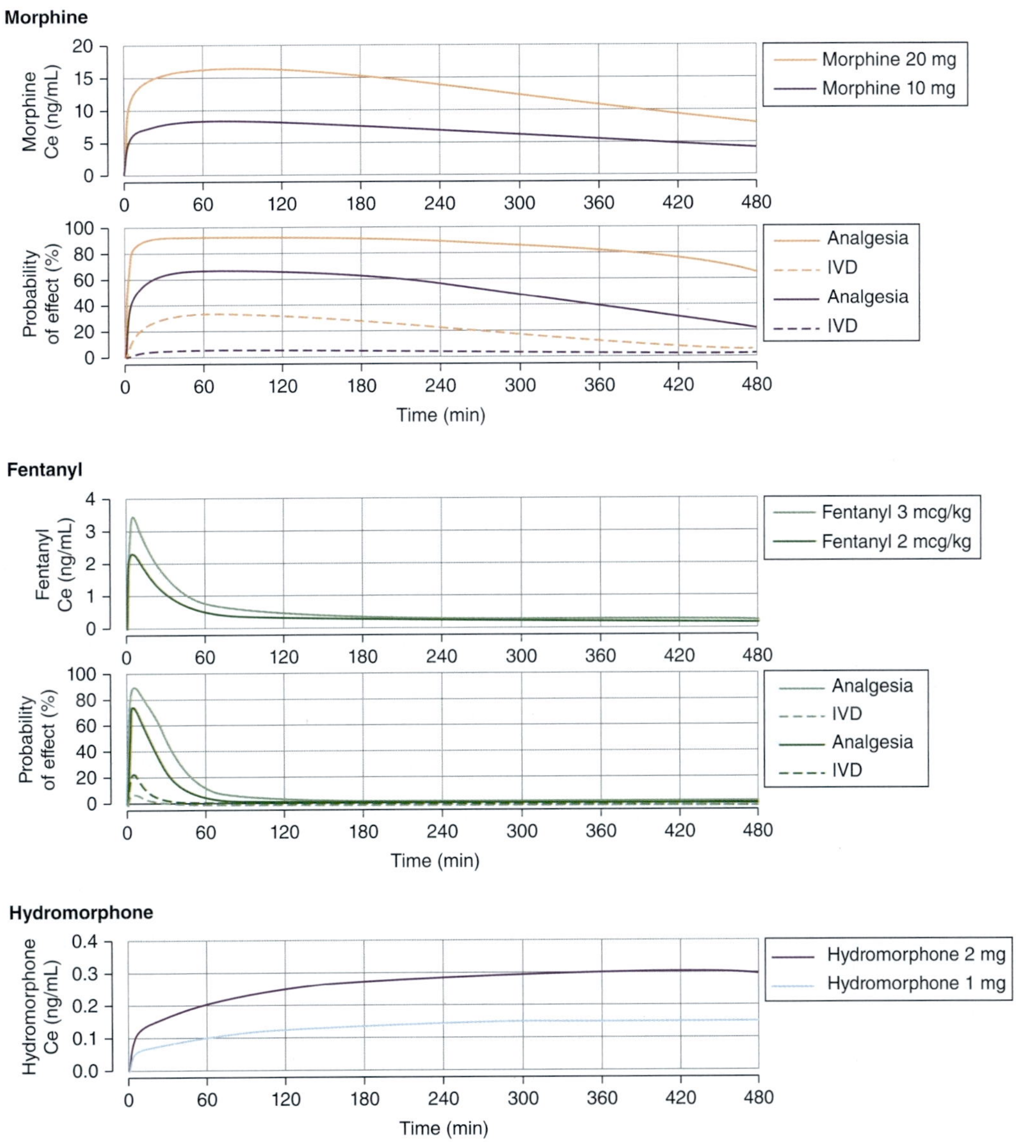

FIGURE 30–3 Which opioid is best for postoperative analgesia? Here are simulations of morphine, fentanyl, and hydromorphone boluses administered near the end of a surgical procedure for moderate postoperative pain. Simulations present predicted effect-site concentration (Ce) levels and drug effects including analgesia and intolerable ventilatory depression (IVD) for 8 hours after administration. Analgesia was defined as a loss of response to painful tibial pressure found to be consistent with pain experienced in the postanesthesia care unit where patients requested analgesics.[1,6] IVD was defined as respiratory rate less than 4 breaths/ min.[14,15] A simulation of analgesia and IVD for hydromorphone is not available. All simulations assumed a 30-year-old, 183-cm, 100-kg male. Simulations were based on published pharmacokinetic and pharmacodynamic models.[11-13,16,17] *The main points of this figure are that the kinetic profile of morphine and hydromorphone is substantially different than fentanyl. Both morphine and hydromorphone provide effect long after the fentanyl effect has dissipated. Higher dose morphine (20 mg) may lead to ventilatory depression for several hours after administration.*

TABLE 30–1 Important considerations of the fentanyl challenge.

Patient Safety

- Use of standard operating room patient monitoring to pulse oximetry, electrocardiogram, noninvasive blood pressure, and capnometry
- Readily available rescue equipment (eg, nasal and oral pharyngeal airways, bag-mask to delivery positive pressure ventilation, laryngoscopes, endotracheal tubes, supraglottic airways) and reversal medications (naloxone, induction drug to facilitate airway instrumentation)

Equipment

- Syringe pump that allows programming in mcg/kg/min and mcg/kg/h
- Timer with resolution to 1 second
- Pharmacokinetic simulation software that provides predicted fentanyl effect-site concentrations

Preparation

- Intravenous (IV) access with an infusion port near the IV insertion site. The fentanyl infusion line should be attached to the most proximal port to the IV insertion site. This is done to minimize IV line dead space that can increase the time between when the infusion is started and when fentanyl enters the circulatory system.
- No anxiolytics, sedatives, or other opioids should be administered before the fentanyl challenge. The interaction among these agents may lead to a predicted fentanyl effect-site concentration lower than what would be achieved without them.
- Patients may present to the preoperative area with recent (ie, same day) consumption of time-contingent opioids (ie, methadone, time-released oxycodone). A common practice, where appropriate, is to continue these opioids throughout the perioperative period. That may not be feasible in patients who will not be able to take medications by mouth after surgery for a few days. In those instances, it is best to ask patients to refrain from taking long-acting oral opioids on the day of surgery. Since oral medications will not be available in the immediate postoperative period, fentanyl will be used to replace them. The intent is to recreate the conditions for the fentanyl challenge that best mimic the patient condition in the postoperative period.

Detection of Ventilatory Depression

- Fentanyl is administered at a high rate to rapidly achieve the onset of ventilatory depression.
- The fentanyl challenge should be performed in an unstimulated state. Following placement of patient monitors and supplemental oxygen, tactile and verbal stimuli should be minimized and the ability to monitor respiratory function confirmed.
- Preoxygenation is strongly encouraged, especially in patients with known or suspected pulmonary disease or any reason to have a decrease in their function residual capacity (eg, obesity, pregnancy, ascites). The fentanyl challenge may not be suitable in patients with severe lung disease or acute pulmonary compromise.
- To optimally capture the onset of ventilatory depression, respiratory rate should be monitored via capnography. Common techniques include the addition of a side-stream capnography sensor to face mask or nasal cannula. The oxygen flow should be adjusted to allow detection of carbon dioxide with each breath. When used in this configuration, it is important to remember that end-tidal carbon dioxide values are not reliable estimates of alveolar carbon dioxide levels but rather simply evidence of a breath in the absence of airway obstruction.
- Airway obstruction may occur from an opioid infusion leading to respiratory effort without detection of carbon dioxide. Clinicians should carefully monitor patient chest excursion, potential recruitment of accessory muscles (suggestive of partial or complete airway obstruction), capnography waveforms, and pulse oximetry throughout the challenge. A chin lift/head tilt may be necessary to detect exhaled carbon dioxide.

Technique

- A high fentanyl infusion rate of 2 mcg/kg/min is administered using a syringe pump. Fentanyl is administered until the patient develops evidence of ventilatory depression (< 5 breaths/min).
- A timer is used to accurately measure the duration of the fentanyl infusion.
- Using pharmacokinetic simulations, the infusion duration is used to predict the fentanyl effect-site concentrations that correspond to the onset of ventilatory depression (see Figure 30–4).
- The target analgesic concentration is estimated as 0.30 times the predicted concentration at the onset of ventilatory depression.
- Using simulations of lower fentanyl infusion rates (1–6 mcg/kg/h), select the infusion rate that best approximates the target concentration (see Figure 30–5) for intraoperative administration.
- For postoperative administration, divide the intraoperative infusion rate by 2. One half is administered as a basal infusion and the other half is divided into interval doses and administered via patient-controlled analgesia.
- Basal infusion rates are adjusted based on the demand dose utilization every 4 hours. For patients who use less than 1 demand dose per hour, the basal infusion rate is decreased by 20%. For patients who use 3 or more demand doses per hour, the basal infusion is increased by 20%.

Second, the C_{50} levels for analgesia, ventilatory depression, and suppression of the electroencephalogram are at progressively higher concentrations such that analgesia typically occurs at concentrations lower than those that lead to ventilatory depression. Third, these various C_{50} levels are linearly proportioned, and the proportionality is consistent from one individual to the next. Thus, although an opioid-tolerant patient may have a higher C_{50} for analgesia, the ratio of the C_{50} for analgesia and the C_{50} for ventilatory depression is the same for an opioid-naive and opioid-tolerant patient: approximately 0.3.

To estimate the effect-site concentration for an individual, a high-dose fentanyl infusion (2 mcg/kg/min) is administered until the patient develops the onset of ventilatory depression (defined as a respiratory rate less than 5 breaths/min). Using published pharmacokinetic models of fentanyl,[16,21] the infusion duration is carefully recorded and based on Figure 30–4, an estimate of the fentanyl effect-site

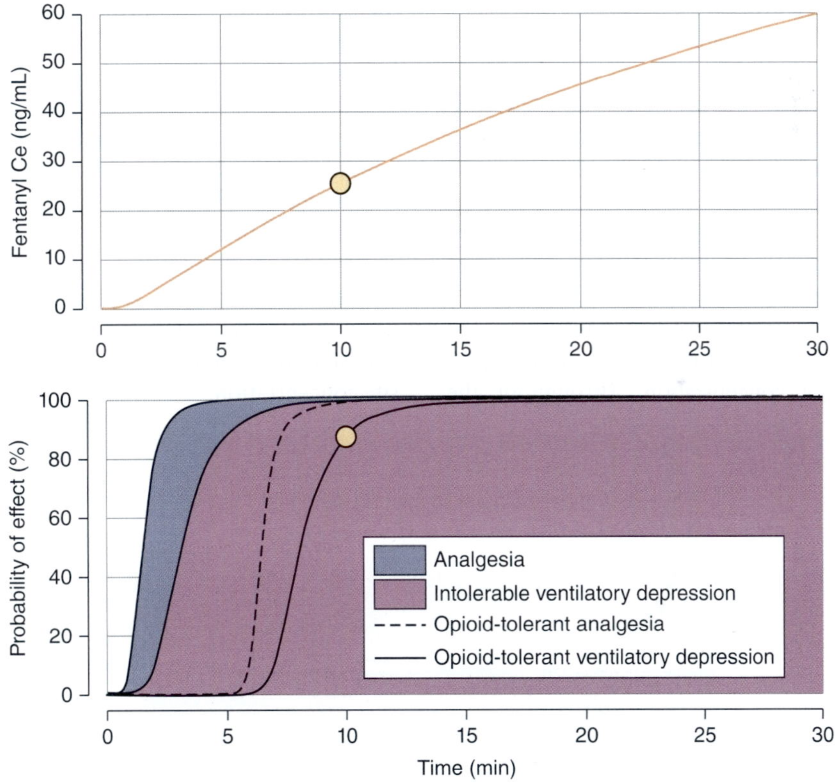

FIGURE 30–4 The fentanyl challenge. Simulation of predicted effect-site concentration (Ce) levels (top plot) and predicted effects (analgesia and intolerable ventilatory depression) that result from a 2-mcg/kg/min fentanyl infusion. Analgesia was defined as a loss of response to painful tibial pressure found to be consistent with pain experienced in the postanesthesia care unit where patients requested analgesics.[1,6] Intolerable ventilatory depression was defined as respiratory rate less than 4 breaths per min.[14,15] The bottom plot presents the predicted time course of analgesia and intolerable ventilatory depression in an opioid-naive person (solid blue and pink) and in an opioid-tolerant person (solid and dashed black line). The fentanyl challenge is administered preoperatively to predict a fentanyl Ce at which a patient develops ventilatory depression. In this example, the infusion is run for 10 minutes, and at that time, the patient develops ventilatory depression defined as a respiratory rate less than 6 breaths per min in an unstimulated state, signified by the large yellow circle. The time point corresponds to a predicted fentanyl Ce of 24 ng/mL (top plot). At 10 minutes, this patient is likely opioid tolerant. All simulations assumed a 30-year-old, 180-cm, 80-kg male. Simulations were based on published pharmacokinetic and pharmacodynamic models.[1,8,16]

concentration is made. In the example presented in this figure, the patient developed ventilatory depression after 10 minutes. This corresponded to a fentanyl effect-site concentration of 26 ng/mL. Using the analgesia to ventilatory depression ratio of 0.3, this individual's analgesic threshold is approximately 8 ng/mL. To achieve and maintain this analgesic threshold, an intraoperative and postoperative dosing regimen is developed.

Intraoperative Dosing

For intraoperative dosing, a continuous infusion is identified that approximates this target concentration for the anticipated duration of the procedure. Figure 30–5 presents the predicted effect-site concentrations for a series of fentanyl continuous infusion rates (1–6 mcg/kg/h) over 6 hours following the 10-minute fentanyl challenge. Based on this figure, an infusion rate of 5 mcg/kg/h provides a predicted fentanyl concentration near 8 ng/mL for a procedure that is anticipated to last 4 to 5 hours.

This figure illustrates two key points. First, the fentanyl infusion does not result in a constant predicted effect-site concentration. Throughout the infusion, fentanyl concentrations continue to climb. Thus, for procedures where the anticipated duration is longer than 5 hours, a slower rate (ie, 4 mcg/kg/min) is more appropriate. Second, for the first hour, the large dose of fentanyl delivered during the challenge maintains concentrations well above the target (8 ng/mL).

Postoperative Dosing

For postoperative dosing, the continuous infusion identified for intraoperative dosing is divided by 2. Half is administered as a basal infusion, and the other half is administered via a patient-controlled analgesia (PCA) pump. In this example, the basal infusion is 2.5 mcg/kg/h. The remainder of the fentanyl is administered in 50-mcg increments on a 15-minute lockout for a total possible 200 mcg/h (2.5 mcg/kg/h for an 80-kg patient) via the PCA pump. The aim of providing half the fentanyl by basal infusion and the remainder by PCA is to minimize respiratory depression by requiring that the patient administer part of the dose required to maintain the target effect-site concentration.

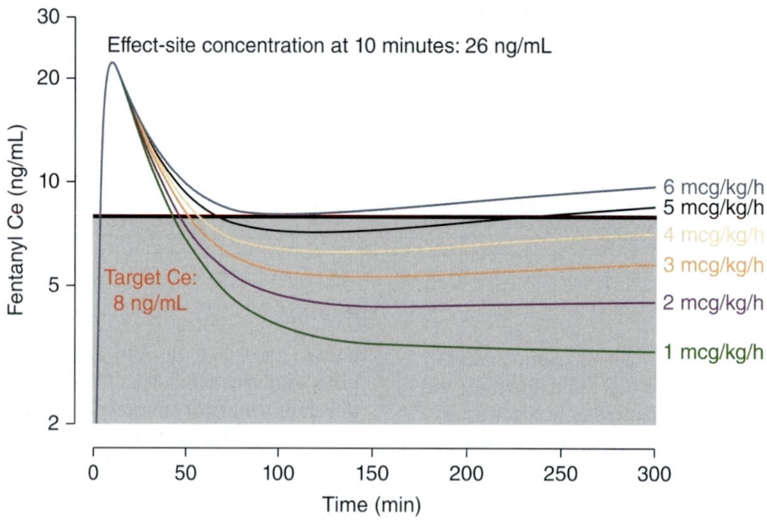

FIGURE 30–5 The fentanyl challenge—simulation of predicted effect-site concentration (Ce) levels for a range of intraoperative fentanyl infusion rates (1 to 6 mcg/kg/h) following a fentanyl challenge that was terminated after 10 minutes. The target effect-site concentration is estimated as 30% of the fentanyl Ce at the onset of respiratory depression (24 ng/mL). A continuous infusion of 5 mcg/kg/h achieves the target Ce the best. All simulations assumed a 30-year-old, 180-cm, 80-kg male. Simulations were based on published pharmacokinetic and pharmacodynamic models.[1,8,16]

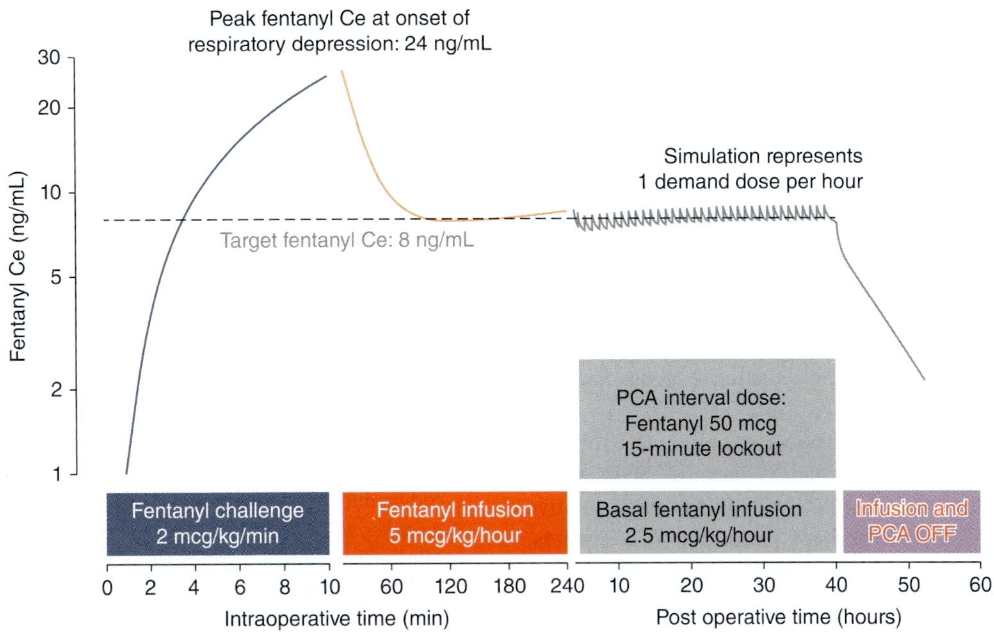

FIGURE 30–6 The fentanyl challenge—simulation of the intraoperative and postoperative course following a fentanyl challenge. As presented in Figures 30–4 and 3–5, after a 10-minute fentanyl challenge, the predicted fentanyl effect-site concentration (Ce) was 24 ng/mL. Subsequently, a fentanyl infusion was initiated at 5 mcg/kg/h (8 mL/h) for 4 hours with a target analgesic concentration of 8 ng/mL. Upon completion of the anesthetic, a basal infusion at 2.5 mcg/kg/h (4 mL/h) and a patient-controlled analgesia (PCA) pump with a 50-mcg bolus dose on a 15-minute lockout were started. The average PCA dose was 1 bolus/h. All simulations assumed a 30-year-old, 180-cm, 80-kg male. Simulations were based on published pharmacokinetic and pharmacodynamic models.[1,8,16]

Figure 30–6 presents a simulation of the fentanyl challenge followed by intraoperative and then postoperative dosing. Of note during the postoperative period is that 1 interval dose (50 mcg) per hour along with a basal infusion maintains the target concentration. During the postoperative period, the fentanyl concentrations continue to slowly climb over time with the basal infusion rate and interval bolus dosing.

Adjustments to the basal infusion rate in the postoperative period are based on the demand dose utilization. Adjustments are considered every 4 hours. For patients who use less than 1 demand dose per hour, the basal infusion rate is decreased by 20%. For patients who use 3 or more demand doses per hour, the basal infusion is increased by 20%. For patients who use 1 to 2 demand doses per hour, the basal infusion is maintained at its current settings.

Clinical Validation

In a clinical evaluation of the fentanyl challenge, arterial blood gas and fentanyl concentrations were measured in 20 chronic opioid consumers who were undergoing elective multilevel spine surgeries. Blood gas and fentanyl concentrations were measured once a PCA dosing reached a near steady state. Steady-state PCA dosing was defined as no changes in the basal infusion rate or bolus interval dosing for the past 8 hours and a minimum of at least 24 hours of postoperative PCA use. The arterial PCO_2 median level was 41 mm Hg with an interquartile range of 39-46 mm Hg. Measured plasma fentanyl concentrations correlated well with predicted levels over the range of concentrations measured. These results indicate that a preoperative fentanyl challenge may be a useful tool to personalize the administration of analgesics to patients who are chronic opioid consumers.

Limitations

A major limitation of the rapid fentanyl infusion rate is that patients typically develop ventilatory depression at a time point where the plasma (and effect-site concentrations) are rapidly changing and a difference of 1 minute in detecting the onset of ventilatory depression can lead to much different predicted fentanyl effect-site concentrations. For example, if the time point associated with ventilatory depression in Figure 30–4 was misidentified by 1 minute too soon or too late, the resultant fentanyl levels would range between 23 and 28 ng/mL. This discrepancy can mis-specify intraoperative and postoperative dosing regimens.

The fentanyl challenge uses fentanyl as opposed to other fentanyl congeners because of its ready availability and familiarity among perioperative clinicians. Other, perhaps better-suited congeners, from a kinetic standpoint, such as remifentanil, have less frequent use in the perioperative domain. Notwithstanding, remifentanil would be more appropriate because of its rapid kinetic profile.

A second limitation is associated with the limits of the fentanyl pharmacokinetic model used to predict effect-site concentrations. Like most pharmacokinetic models, it does not account for common comorbidities such as obesity, advanced age, and severe heart disease, all of which may influence fentanyl kinetic behavior.

A third limitation is that the fentanyl challenge calls for a large dose of fentanyl to be administered on induction. In the example shown in Figure 30–4, the patient received 20 mcg/kg (in this case, 32 mL of fentanyl at 50 mcg/mL in an 80-kg patient). High fentanyl doses may lead to muscle rigidity in select patients. As well, the large dose may have postoperative consequences should the surgical procedure be cancelled or end earlier than expected.

Summary

Opioid doses that cause ventilatory depression and analgesia may differ between chronically opioid-consuming and opioid-naive patients. A preoperative fentanyl challenge with pharmacokinetic simulation may be a useful tool for identifying concentrations that lead to respiratory depression and analgesia in an individual patient. With this information, a personalized dosing regime can be developed for the postoperative treatment of pain in patients who chronically consume opioids.

REFERENCES

1. Johnson KB, Syroid ND, Gupta DK, et al. An evaluation of remifentanil propofol response surfaces for loss of responsiveness, loss of response to surrogates of painful stimuli and laryngoscopy in patients undergoing elective surgery. *Anesth Analg*. 2008;106(2):471-479.
2. Kern SE, Xie G, White JL, Egan TD. A response surface analysis of propofol-remifentanil pharmacodynamic interaction in volunteers. *Anesthesiology*. 2004;100(6):1373-1381.
3. Minto CF, Schnider TW, Egan TD, et al. Influence of age and gender on the pharmacokinetics and pharmacodynamics of remifentanil. I. Model development. *Anesthesiology*. 1997;86(1):10-23.
4. Minto CF, Schnider TW, Shafer SL. Pharmacokinetics and pharmacodynamics of remifentanil. II. Model application. *Anesthesiology*. 1997;86(1):24-33.
5. Schnider TW, Minto CF, Shafer SL, et al. The influence of age on propofol pharmacodynamics. *Anesthesiology*. 1999;90(6):1502-16.
6. Johnson KB, Syroid ND, Gupta DK, et al. An evaluation of remifentanil-sevoflurane response surface models in patients emerging from anesthesia: model improvement using effect-site sevoflurane concentrations. *Anesth Analg*. 2010;111(2):387-394.
7. Lerou JG, Verheijen R, Booij LH. Model-based administration of inhalation anaesthesia. 4. Applying the system model. *Br J Anaesth*. 2002;88(2):175-183.
8. Syroid ND, Johnson KB, Pace NL, et al. Response surface model predictions of emergence and response to pain in the recovery room: An evaluation of patients emerging from an isoflurane and fentanyl anesthetic. *Anesth Analg*. 2010;111(2):380-386.
9. Westmoreland CL, Sebel PS, Gropper A. Fentanyl or alfentanil decreases the minimum alveolar anesthetic concentration of isoflurane in surgical patients. *Anesth Analg*. 1994;78(1):23-28.
10. Wissing H, Kuhn I, Rietbrock S, Fuhr U. Pharmacokinetics of inhaled anaesthetics in a clinical setting: comparison of desflurane, isoflurane and sevoflurane. *Br J Anaesth*. 2000;84(4):443-449.
11. Coda B, Tanaka A, Jacobson RC, Donaldson G, Chapman CR. Hydromorphone analgesia after intravenous bolus administration. *Pain*. 1997;71(1):41-48.
12. Coda BA, O'Sullivan B, Donaldson G, Bohl S, Chapman CR, Shen DD. Comparative efficacy of patient-controlled administration of morphine,

hydro- morphone, or sufentanil for the treatment of oral mucositis pain following bone marrow transplantation. *Pain*. 1997;72(3):333-346.

13. Drover DR, Angst MS, Valle M, et al. Input characteristics and bioavailability after administration of immediate and a new extended-release formulation of hydromorphone in healthy volunteers. *Anesthesiology*. 2002;97(4):827-836.
14. LaPierre CD, Johnson KB, Randall BR, Egan TD. A simulation study of common propofol and propofol-opioid dosing regimens for upper endoscopy: implications on the time course of recovery. *Anesthesiology*. 2012;117(2):252-262.
15. LaPierre CD, Johnson KB, Randall BR, White JL, Egan TD. An exploration of remifentanil-propofol combinations that lead to a loss of response to esophageal instrumentation, a loss of responsiveness, and/or onset of intolerable ventilatory depression. *Anesth Analg*. 2011;113(3):490-499.
16. Shafer SL, Varvel JR, Aziz N, Scott JC. Pharmacokinetics of fentanyl administered by computer-controlled infusion pump. *Anesthesiology*. 1990;73(6):1091-1102.
17. Dershwitz M, Walsh JL, Morishige RJ, et al. Pharmacokinetics and pharmacodynamics of inhaled versus intravenous morphine in healthy volunteers. *Anesthesiology*. 2000;93(3):619-628.
18. Davis JJ, Johnson KB, Egan TD, Vezina DP, Snell TE, Swenson JD. Preoperative fentanyl infusion with pharmacokinetic simulation for anesthetic and perioperative management of an opioid-tolerant patient. *Anesth Analg*. 2003;97(6):1661-1662.
19. Davis JJ, Swenson JD, Hall RH, et al. Preoperative "fentanyl challenge" as a tool to estimate postoperative opioid dosing in chronic opioid-consuming patients. *Anesth Analg*. 2005;101(2):389-395.
20. Egan TD, Muir KT, Hermann DJ, Stanski DR, Shafer SL. The electroencephalogram (EEG) and clinical measures of opioid potency: defining the EEG-clinical potency relationship ('fingerprint') with application to remifentanil. *Int J Pharm Med*. 2001;15(1):1-8.
21. Scott JC, Stanski DR. Decreased fentanyl and alfentanil dose requirements with age. A simultaneous pharmacokinetic and pharmacodynamic evaluation. *J Pharmacol Exp Ther*. 1987;240(1):159-166.

Anesthetic Considerations During Cardiopulmonary Bypass

CHAPTER 31

Ben Gmelch, MD

INTRODUCTION

Cardiothoracic surgery entails unique, often extreme, conditions in comparison to noncardiac surgery. Profound hemodynamic and physiologic perturbations associated with hypothermic cardiopulmonary bypass (CPB) and circulatory arrest lead to unique dosing considerations for anesthetic drugs, anticoagulants, vasoactives, inotropes, and antifibrinolytics. This chapter will review the pharmacologic considerations of cardiac anesthesia chronologically in stages, from premedication and induction to pre-CPB maintenance, initiation of CPB, separation from CPB, and the post-CPB period. A special discussion will review the unique pharmacologic approach to anticipated deep hypothermic circulatory arrest (DHCA).

PREMEDICATION

Anxiolysis/Amnesia

Benzodiazepine (eg, intravenous [IV] midazolam 0.02–0.04 mg/kg) may be given prior to arterial line and/or central line placement. Cardiac surgery has among the highest incidence of intraoperative awareness of any elective surgery (1%–2%). Benzodiazepine administration has been shown to decrease the risk of awareness.[1] Benzodiazepines also have a relatively slow offset time with respect to their hypnotic effects, particularly in elderly patients. Lorazepam (0.02 mg/kg IV) has a half-life of 12 to 14 hours in healthy young patients, with evidence of residual sedation and electroencephalographic (EEG) changes 8 hours after a single dose.[2] In comparison, the half-life of midazolam is 2.8 hours, with EEG returning to near baseline by 3 hours.[3] In the setting of cardiac surgery with CPB, delayed awakening attributed to the sedative effects of lorazepam may be more than 9 hours.[4] Residual postoperative sedation is of potential concern in patients where early extubation is desired (eg, "fast-track" anesthesia). Midazolam in anxiolytic doses administered preoperatively and pre-CPB is not typically associated with delayed awakening. However, caution should be exercised when considering even a single preoperative dose of lorazepam, or a post-CPB dose of any benzodiazepine, if early extubation is desired.

Analgesia

Beginning slow titration of IV fentanyl 0.5 to 1.0 mcg/kg or sufentanil 0.05 to 0.1 mcg/kg during placement of invasive lines may be considered.

INDUCTION

Analgesics

Similar blunting of the autonomic response to intubation and sternotomy has been demonstrated for fentanyl, sufentanil, alfentanil, and morphine at equianalgesic doses. Ideally, laryngoscopy should be performed adequate analgesia is in place to avoid or blunt an adverse hemodynamic effect. Although all these opioids are similar in pharmacologic action (ie, μ-receptor agonists), they each have quite different pharmacokinetics. One major difference is the time to peak effect. This difference is important to consider when dosing an opioid just prior to laryngoscopy. As is described in Chapter 5, Figure 5–1, the time to peak effect varies for each opioid: alfentanil, less than 2 minutes; fentanyl, 4 minutes; sufentanil, 6 minutes; and morphine, more than 80 minutes.

Sedative–Hypnotics

Induction drugs include propofol, etomidate, ketamine, high-dose midazolam, and the combination of ketamine and midazolam. Among the choices of induction agents, propofol leads to the greatest decrease in systemic vascular resistance (SVR) and may be associated with hypotension, even in modest doses. In comparison to ketamine (2 mg/kg), a propofol-based induction (0.5 mg/kg) produced a transient decrease in SVR, pulmonary vascular resistance (PVR), and mean arterial pressure (MAP). Although the cardiac index is decreased slightly (< 10%) with both induction drugs, no significant difference in cardiac index or heart rate was shown between the 2 strategies.[5] The decrease in SVR with propofol in this study was transient, with return to baseline after endotracheal intubation.

Etomidate, in comparison to propofol, is associated with significantly less decrease in SVR and MAP, without any difference in cardiac index in patients with coronary artery disease (CAD) or aortic valve disease.[6] This was also shown in patients with severe aortic stenosis, where propofol induction was associated with a greater incidence of hypotension than etomidate. However, etomidate is associated with transient adrenal suppression.[7] Even a routine induction dose can suppress adrenal function for more than 24 hours.[8] Etomidate may be dangerous in septic and critically ill patients who require steroids to maintain their immune function and metabolic homeostasis. Some authors have recommended abandoning etomidate in septic patients or providing supplemental corticosteroid therapy following etomidate administration.[9]

Midazolam as a sole sedative–hypnotic induction agent has been described, typically in higher doses (0.1–0.2 mg/kg) than used for anxiolysis. The time to peak effect of an induction dose of midazolam is significantly longer (6–8 minutes) than propofol, etomidate, or ketamine. Thus, it should be given earlier in the induction sequence. In patients with normal and decreased left ventricular function, midazolam has been shown to have minimal effect on heart rate, SVR, and cardiac index.[10]

Muscle Relaxants

The nondepolarizing muscle relaxants (NDMRs) such as rocuronium (0.6 mg/kg), vecuronium (0.05 mg/kg), or cisatracurium (0.1 mg/kg) will provide optimal conditions for direct laryngoscopy and endotracheal intubation without significant hemodynamic changes. Succinylcholine 1 mg/kg is used in the setting of a rapid-sequence induction or suspected difficult airway. Succinylcholine, although more rapid in onset than the NDMRs, has been associated with tachycardia and rarely dysrhythmias in certain patients.[11] One study in patients with CAD comparing succinylcholine and vecuronium demonstrated a transient increase in heart rate with succinylcholine (11% increase from baseline) and MAP (25% increase from baseline). These hemodynamic effects are short-lived and return to near baseline within 4 minutes of administration.[12] The benefits of succinylcholine should be balanced with its adverse effects in patients with ischemic coronary disease and valvular disease.

Special Consideration

The time required before peak plasma concentration of any IV medication is dependent upon both the diffusivity of the drug and the cardiac output. In patients with decreased cardiac output, the time of peak plasma concentration (and hence effect-site concentration) may be delayed by up to 60 seconds compared to individuals with normal cardiac output.[13] This applies to premedications, opioid and sedative induction agents, and muscle relaxants. Consideration should be given to this potential delay in peak effect to avoid "stacking" doses of medications prior to the peak of the initial dose.

MAINTENANCE OF ANESTHESIA (Pre-CPB)

Volatile Anesthetics

Of the 3 commonly used volatile anesthetics, isoflurane is the most studied in cardiac anesthesia and has been shown to play a role in ischemic preconditioning, helping to reduce infarct size and possibly improve morbidity and mortality in cardiac surgery. More recently, both desflurane and sevoflurane have been associated with decreased troponin release and shorter intensive care unit stay when compared to total IV anesthesia (TIVA).[14] The mechanisms of myocardial protection are multifactorial but appear to be unique to volatile anesthetics. The issue remains controversial, and a large retrospective analysis recently showed no difference in markers of ischemia or outcomes between sevoflurane-based and TIVA anesthetics. All volatile anesthetics decrease myocardial function to a modest degree. Isoflurane may preserve myocardial function better than sevoflurane at concentrations equivalent to 1 minimum alveolar concentration (MAC).[15]

It is well established that concomitant administration of opioids has a "MAC-reducing" effect, decreasing the concentration of volatile anesthetic required to maintain unresponsiveness and to blunt the adrenergic response to surgical stimulation.[16] When administering isoflurane to patients with substantial cardiac disease, dosing is reduced to avoid the cardiodepressant effects of isoflurane and opioids are used to make up unmet anesthetic requirements. One advantage of opioids is their minimal impact on cardiovascular function, even at high doses. This feature, although well characterized when administered alone, is not as distinct in the presence of other anesthetics, such as potent inhaled agents. Patients may have pronounced hemodynamic responses to opioids in the presence of other anesthetics.

The interaction between opioids and inhaled agents is often difficult to conceptualize in a clinical context. In general, the interactions are synergistic. As was described in Chapter 3, the extent of synergism varies for different effects. For example, the interactions are more pronounced for analgesia than for loss of responsiveness. Consider the simulations presented in **Figure 31–1**, which illustrate the synergy between isoflurane and intermittent boluses of fentanyl. This simulation assumes that the isoflurane vaporizer is set to 0.9% in a patient with normal cardiac function and normal ventilator settings. It also assumes that the isoflurane has been on for 20 minutes and has not yet reached near steady state. Three 1-mcg/kg fentanyl boluses were administered intermittently over a 1-hour period, each bolus separated by 15 minutes. Figure 31–1 presents the time course of predicted effect-site concentrations for each drug and 2 predicted effects: analgesia and loss of responsiveness. As with all simulations, this simulation makes several assumptions, which are described in **Table 31–1**.

A few points that are well visualized in this simulation merit discussion. First, under these conditions, predictions of isoflurane effect-site concentrations continue to climb despite no change in dosing. Isoflurane requires a long time to reach near steady state (Chapter 6). So in the context of a typical cardiac case, it is likely, if isoflurane dosing remains constant, that isoflurane effect-site concentrations will continue to slowly increase. Second, although the isoflurane vaporizer is set to 0.9%, the effect-site concentration is lower (over the 80-minute window, the isoflurane effect-site concentration starts at 0.5% and ends at 0.7%). Third, the 3 fentanyl doses, separated by 15 minutes, yield effect-site concentrations that continue stack up upon one another such that the peak fentanyl effect-site concentration of the third bolus is substantially higher than the first (ie, greater than a 2-fold increase). Fourth, the synergy between fentanyl and isoflurane is more pronounced for analgesia than it is for loss of responsiveness.

Four time points are labeled with letters to illustrate the synergistic interactions. They represent the time just prior to the first fentanyl bolus (A) and the peak fentanyl effect-site concentrations after each bolus (B–D) as presented in the top plot. The letters map out the fentanyl and isoflurane effect-site concentration pairs on a topographic rendering of fentanyl–isoflurane response surfaces for loss of responsiveness and analgesia (middle plots). The 5%, 50%, and 95% isoeffect lines (also known as isoboles) are superimposed on each plot.

Without fentanyl (point A), low dose isoflurane provides a moderate to high probability of loss of responsiveness (between the 50% and 95% isoboles) and moderate probability of analgesia (near the 50% isobole). However, with the first fentanyl bolus (point B), both probabilities of effect exceed the 95% isobole. The additional fentanyl boluses only drive the probabilities of effect closer to 100% (points C and D) and are likely unnecessary.

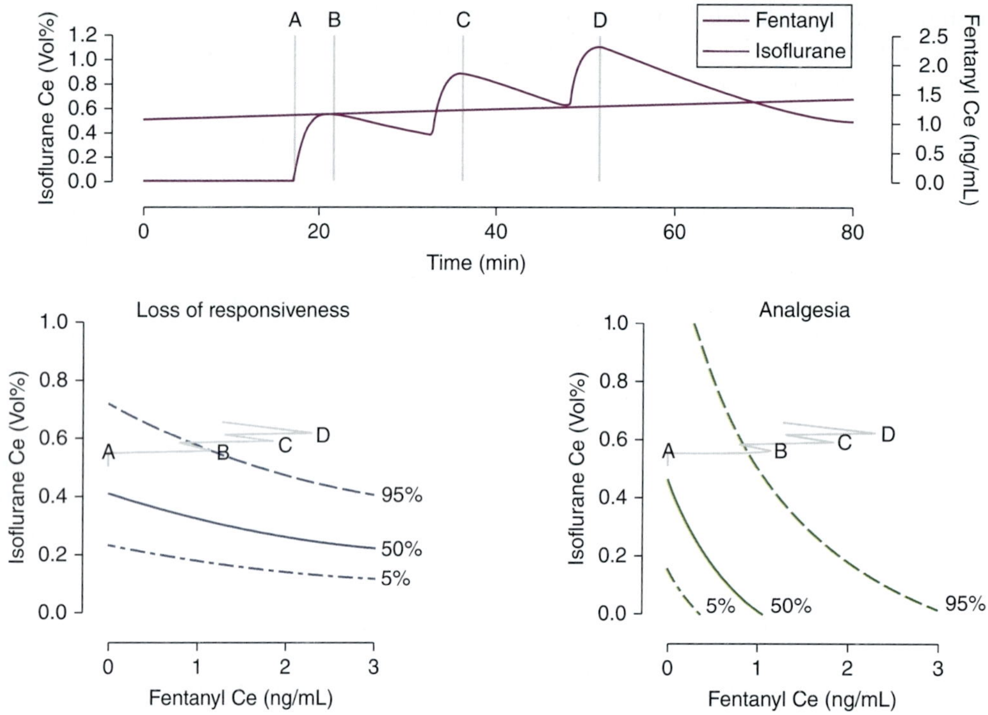

FIGURE 31–1 Simulations of isoflurane and fentanyl effect-site concentration (Ce) levels and predictions of drug effects (analgesia and loss of responsiveness) over time. Simulations used published pharmacokinetic parameters[17-24] for a 30-year-old, 100-kg, 183-cm male with normal cardiopulmonary physiology. Simulations assumed a mechanically ventilated patient with settings of 10 breaths per minute, tidal volume of 600 mL, and isoflurane vaporizer set to 0.9%. Interactions between fentanyl and isoflurane (analgesia and loss of responsiveness) were based on published interactions models for sevoflurane and remifentanil.[25-27] Isoflurane and fentanyl concentrations were modeled as sevoflurane and remifentanil equivalents.[28-30] The top plot presents the predicted Ce levels for isoflurane and fentanyl over an 80-minute time window. The fentanyl boluses are 1 mcg/kg and separated by 15 minutes. The letters represent a time point just prior to fentanyl administration (A) and at the peak fentanyl Ce levels for each fentanyl bolus (B–D). The middle plots present topographic representations of the interaction models for loss of responsiveness (left) and analgesia (right). The blue and green lines represent the isoeffect (isobole) lines. The dash-dot, solid, and dashed lines represent the 5%, 50%, and 95% probability of effect. The letters A through D mark the fentanyl–isoflurane concentration pairs at the time points described above.

The bottom two plots in Figure 31–1 present predictions of drug effect over time. The probability of loss of responsiveness over time is presented for isoflurane alone (gray area) and in combination with fentanyl (blue area). Fentanyl somewhat increases the sedative–hypnotic effect of isoflurane. The probability of analgesia over time is presented for fentanyl alone (gray area) and in combination with isoflurane (green area). Isoflurane substantially increases the analgesic effect of fentanyl.

Effects of Cardiac Output on Uptake and Distribution

As discussed in Chapter 22, patients with low cardiac output have decreased uptake of volatile anesthetic into the blood and will therefore more rapidly achieve equilibrium between alveolar concentration and effect-site concentration. Titration of volatile anesthetics will also be affected by cardiac output in a similar way. Changes in inspired concentration of volatile anesthetic will be reflected more rapidly in

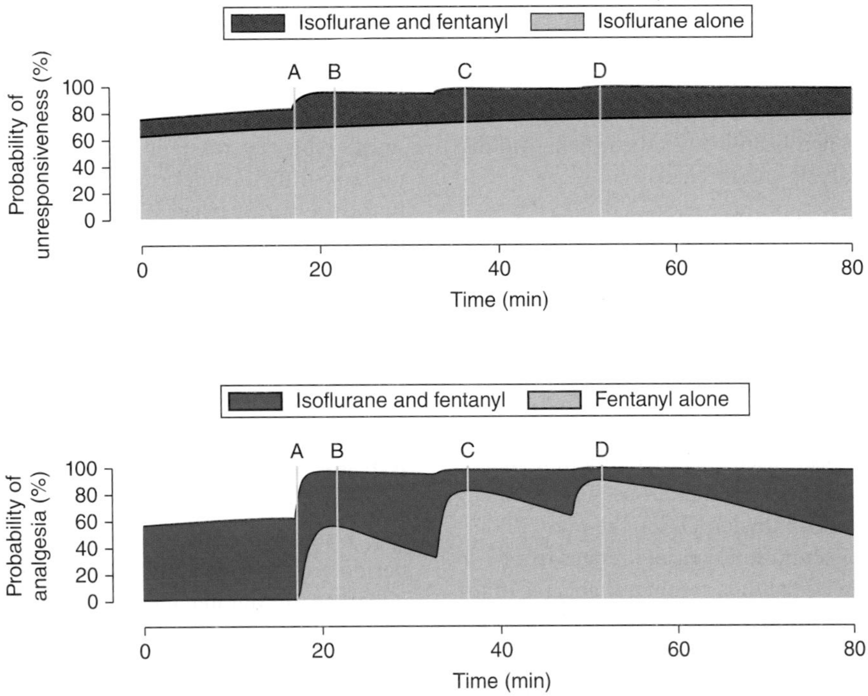

FIGURE 31–1 *(Continued)* The bottom two plots present the probability of effects over time. The probability of unresponsiveness is a blue area and the probability of analgesia is a green area for fentanyl combined with isoflurane. The probability of analgesia for fentanyl alone is a gray area, and the probability of loss of responsiveness for isoflurane alone is a gray area.

TABLE 31–1 Assumptions and limitations of simulations predicting fentanyl and isoflurane effect-site concentrations, analgesia, and loss of responsiveness.

Assumptions
Analgesia was defined as a loss of response to 30 pounds per square inch of pressure to the anterior tibia, a stimulus consistent with post-operative pain associated with laparoscopic surgery.[25,26]
Loss of responsiveness was defined as a loss to verbal and moderate prodding.[31]
Limitations
Interaction models for loss of responsiveness and analgesia were both based on observations in healthy volunteers. Responses in patients are likely to be different.
These models do not account for changes in cardiac output that are likely during heart surgery.

the brain in patients with low cardiac output. The more soluble the anesthetic, the more pronounced the effect of decreased cardiac output on the rate of equilibration. For example, simulations of isoflurane administration reveal that a change in cardiac output from 5 to 3 L/min is associated with a 15% to 20% increase in end-tidal concentration compared to target end-tidal concentration within 1 minute of the change in cardiac output.[32] The same change in cardiac output leads to an increase in the end-tidal concentration of desflurane, a less-soluble anesthetic, of less than 10%.

Like a high-cardiac output state, a significant left-to-right shunt (eg, uncorrected congenital defect such as an atrial septal defect, ventricular septal defect, patent ductus arteriosus, or large patent foramen ovale) leads to increased flow through the pulmonary circulation. This will slow the equilibration and titration of volatile anesthetics, with the most pronounced effects occurring in more soluble agents (ie, isoflurane). Predominantly right-to-left shunts do not significantly alter the uptake and distribution of volatile anesthetics.

Intravenous Anesthetic Infusion

Propofol may be used in conjunction with opioids (eg, TIVA) and/or volatile anesthetics to provide balanced anesthesia in the pre-CPB period. Although propofol-based anesthesia may be associated with decreased SVR and the potential for more hypotension compared to volatile anesthesia, the TIVA approach has been used to provide hemodynamically stable anesthesia in numerous studies. Using a target-controlled infusion (TCI), the pre-CPB target plasma concentration typically ranges from 1 to –3 mcg/mL. If TCI pumps are unavailable (as in the United States), this can be achieved with propofol infusion rates of 65 to 100 mcg/kg/min.[33]

An example of a propofol TCI set to 3 mcg/mL is compared to a continuous infusion set at 100 mcg/kg/min for 2 hours in Figure 31–2. In this simulation, both the TCI and the continuous infusion achieve a high probability of unresponsiveness, but the infusion may require a bolus to achieve unresponsiveness in a timely manner. If just using the infusion, it may take up to 20 minutes to reach a reasonable probability of unresponsiveness. Of note, both procedures have a similar recovery time.

Opioid Analgesics

Infusions of synthetic opioids are commonly used in cardiac anesthesia to maintain a steady-state level of analgesia during this period of intense stimulation. Fentanyl and sufentanil are frequent adjuncts to maintenance with volatile anesthesia, and their role in decreasing the volatile anesthetic requirement promotes preservation of myocardial function throughout the pre-CPB period. Prior studies of fentanyl have shown near-maximal analgesic effects at a plasma concentration of 7 ng/mL, whereas plasma concentrations less than 5 ng/mL are associated with an increased requirement for volatile anesthetic to control hemodynamic responses to the surgical stimuli of sternotomy, sternal lift, and sternal spreading.[16] Sample bolus and continuous infusion dosing regimens that achieve this range of fentanyl concentrations are presented in Figure 31–3. Underdosing the opioid may require higher concentrations of volatile anesthetic, which in turn can lead to an undesirable decrease in myocardial contractility, underscoring the importance of balanced anesthesia in the pre-CPB period. Where available, TCI may be used to maintain this target plasma concentration. Again, if TCI is unavailable, a sufentanil bolus of 1 mcg/kg followed by an infusion of 0.6 mcg/kg/h will maintain a predicted plasma concentration greater than 0.7 ng/mL, which is associated with adequate analgesia (Figure 31–4).

Muscle Relaxants

Dosing considerations for neuromuscular blockade in normothermic patients during the pre-CPB period are similar to those of noncardiac anesthesia (Chapter 9). Maintenance of neuromuscular blockade can be achieved with an infusion or intermittent boluses of rocuronium, vecuronium, or cisatracurium. Sample dosing regimens for a rocuronium are presented in Figure 31–5. In these simulations, the bolus dosing has been designed to achieve a near-equivalent effect of a continuous infusion.

Nonanesthetic Infusions During the Pre-CPB Period

Antifibrinolytics

CPB incites a significant inflammatory response involving a complex interaction of cytokines and coagulation factors. Among these, the fibrinolytic cascade, involving plasminogen, activated protein C, tissue plasminogen activator, and fibrin, is upregulated during and after CPB. This has been associated with increased postoperative bleeding risk, particularly in high-risk cardiac surgery (eg, reoperations, valve replacement, aortic surgery, combination coronary artery bypass grafting with valve replacement). Antifibrinolytic therapy, using either the synthetic lysine analogs, tranexamic acid (TXA) and epsilon-aminocaproic acid (EACA), or aprotinin (withdrawn by the Food and Drug Administration in 2008) has been shown to significantly decrease transfusion requirements and reoperation for bleeding.[39] There is also evidence that antifibrinolytic therapy may decrease the overall

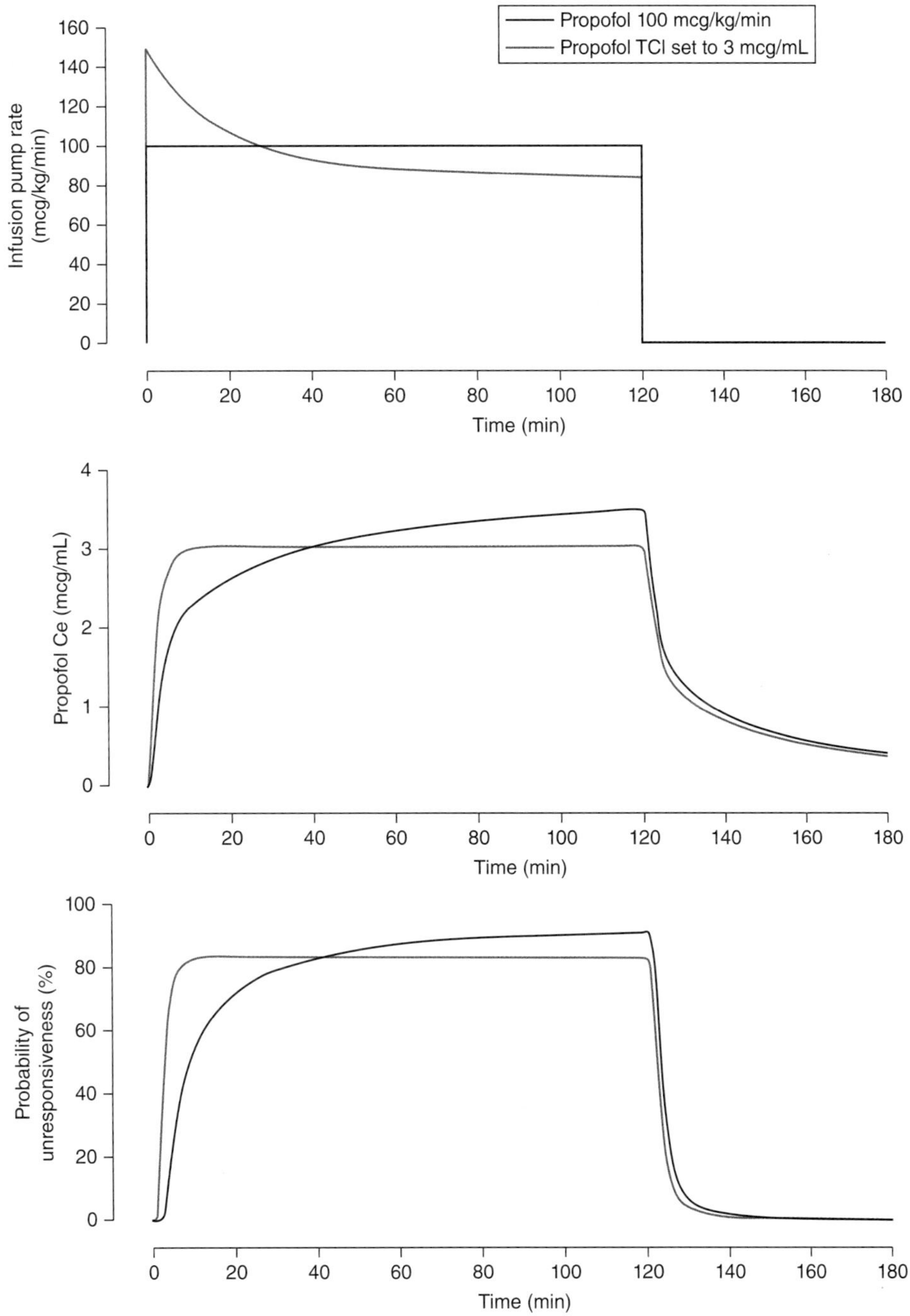

FIGURE 31–2 Simulation of a target-controlled propofol infusion set to 3 mcg/mL and a continuous propofol infusion set to a rate of 100 mcg/kg/min for 2 hours. The top plot presents the dosing regimen as infusion rates for the target-controlled infusion (blue line) and the continuous infusion (black line). The middle plot presents the propofol effect-site concentration (Ce) levels for each dosing regimen. The bottom plot presents the probability of unresponsiveness for each dosing regimen. Simulations used published pharmacokinetic parameters for propofol.[34,35]

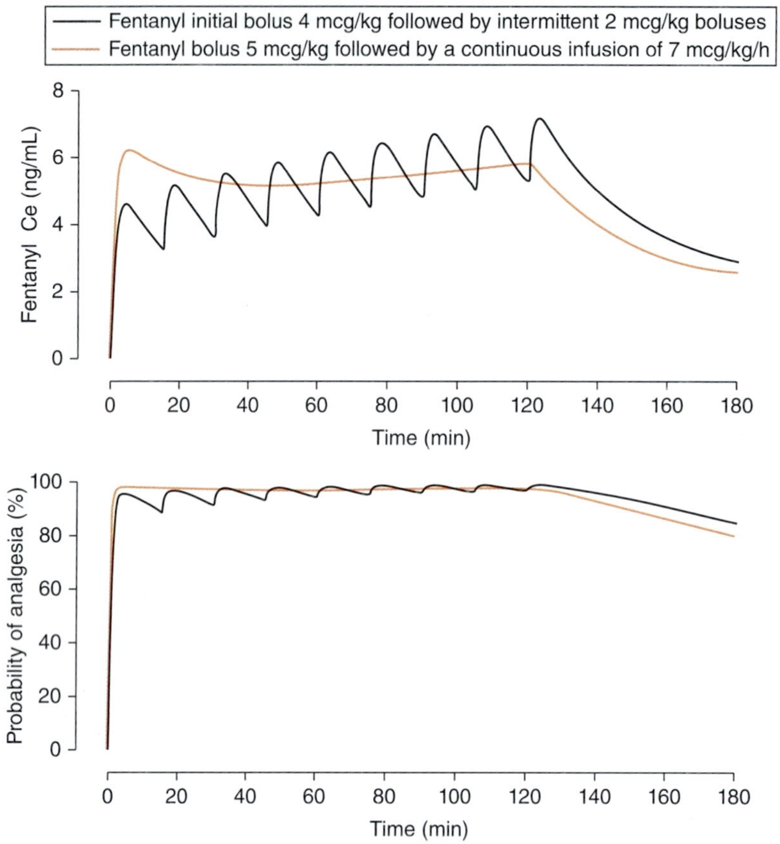

FIGURE 31–3 Simulations of 2 dosing regimens that achieve fentanyl effect-site concentration (Ce) levels between 5 and 7 ng/mL for 2 hours. The top plot presents the fentanyl Ce levels for each dosing regimen. The black line represents intermittent bolus dosing (4 mcg/kg followed by 2 mcg/kg every 15 minutes). The red line represents a bolus followed by continuous infusion technique (5 mcg/kg bolus followed by a continuous infusion at 7 mcg/kg/h). The bottom plot presents the probability of analgesia for each dosing regimen. Simulations used published pharmacokinetic parameters for fentanyl.[18]

systemic inflammatory response and the incidence of vasoplegic shock.[40] Because there is no firm consensus on the concentration threshold of efficacy for TXA and EACA, various dosing strategies have been proposed for these drugs. Pharmacokinetics are predicted by a 2-compartment model, with a plasma half-life of approximately 120 minutes for both drugs and a renal elimination that is independent of concentration.[41,42] Thus, a modest loading dose followed by a constant infusion is preferred to even a very large, single-bolus approach. Further, recent data have called into question the safety of high-dose tranexamic acid, due to an association with postoperative seizures.[43] The change in pharmacokinetic parameters upon initiation of CPB will be discussed in the next section.

Vasodilators

Pharmacologic management of hypertension (ie, afterload reduction) before initiation of CPB is sometimes necessary in order to decrease myocardial oxygen consumption and facilitate safe conditions for aortic cannulation. Nonanesthetic vasodilators are particularly useful in the setting of myocardial dysfunction, where increasing the anesthetic depth may lead to further depression in

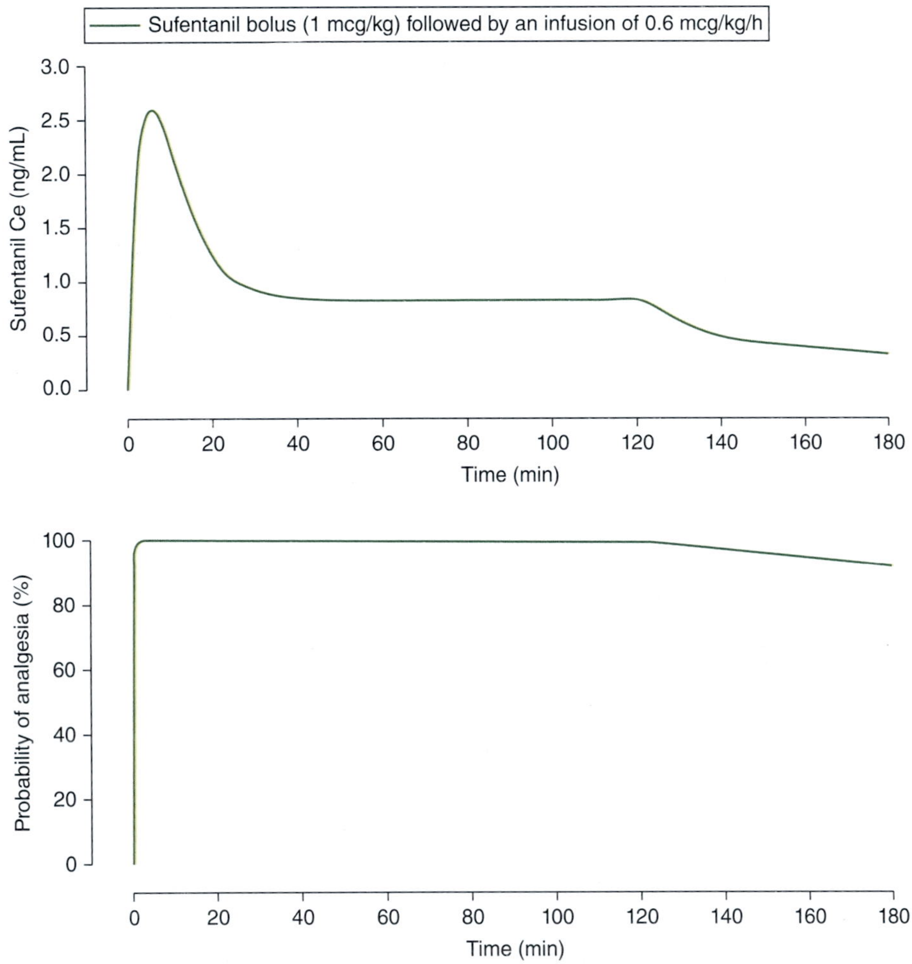

FIGURE 31–4 Simulation of a sufentanil bolus (1 mcg/kg) followed by continuous infusion (0.6 mcg/kg/h) that achieves sufentanil effect-site concentration (Ce) levels near 0.7 ng/mL for 2 hours. The top plot presents the sufentanil Ce levels. The bottom plot presents the probability of analgesia. This simulation used published pharmacokinetic parameters for sufentanil.[36]

cardiac output. Nitroglycerin, nitroprusside, and nicardipine are commonly used agents. The pharmacokinetics of these agents have been discussed previously (Chapter 14).

Heparinization

Heparin is administered several minutes prior to initiation of CPB for the purpose of anticoagulation. Heparin is a large, nonuniform mucopolysaccharoid; the molecular weights range from 10 to 30 kDa. Heparin quickly binds antithrombin III (AT-III) within 1 circulation time, potentiating its inhibitory effect on thrombin and several other coagulation factors. The peak effect of heparin occurs 2 to 3 minutes after IV administration. The anticoagulant response is variable and is dependent upon the type of heparin, existing AT-III levels, and levels of other coagulation factors. Most institutions, however, have standard heparin dosing in the range of 300 to 400 IU/kg. Heparinization is measured most readily by the activated clotting time (ACT), which measures the intrinsic cascade using either diatomaceous

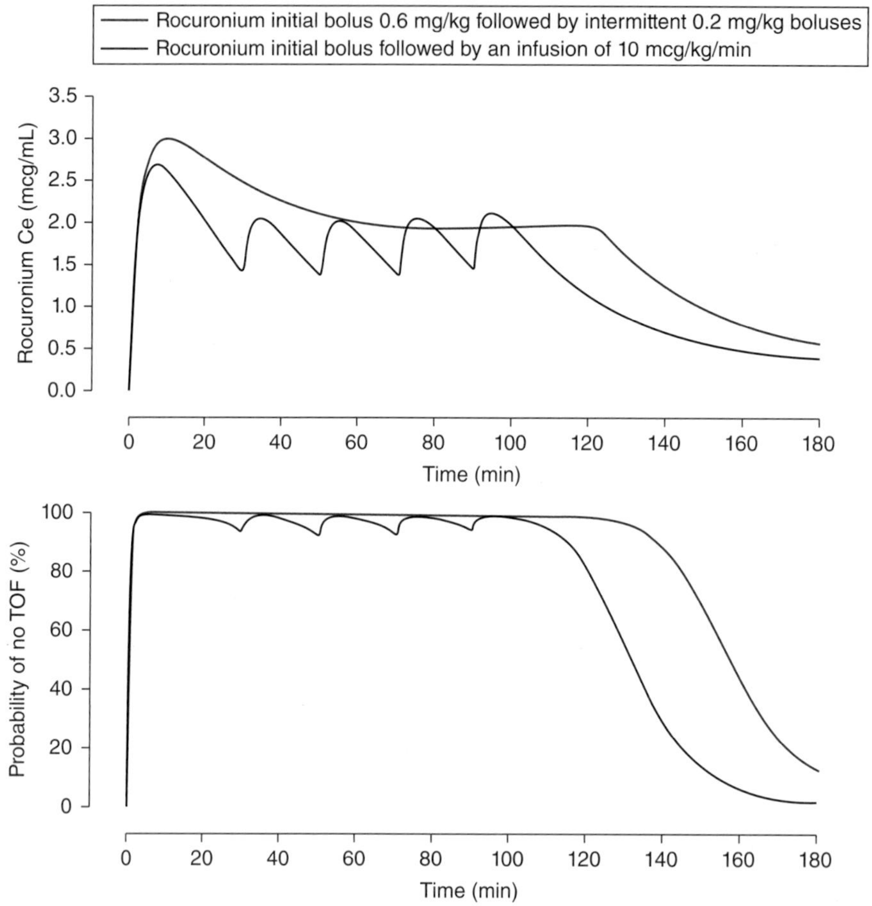

FIGURE 31–5 Simulations of 2 rocuronium dosing regimens that achieve a loss of train-of-four (TOF) for 2 hours. The top plot presents the rocuronium effect-site concentration (Ce) levels for each dosing regimen. The black line represents intermittent bolus dosing (0.6 mg/kg followed by 0.2 mg/kg every 20 minutes). The pink line represents a bolus followed by continuous infusion technique (0.6 mg/kg bolus followed by a continuous infusion at 20 mcg/kg/min). The bottom plot presents the probability of loss of TOF for each dosing regimen. Of note, in this simulation, a Ce of 2 mcg/mL provides adequate neuromuscular blockade. Simulations used published pharmacokinetic parameters for rocuronium.[37,38]

earth (Celite) or aluminum silicate (kaolin). Unlike measurements of partial thromboplastin time, there is a linear relationship between heparin dose and expected ACT. IV administration of 300 IU/kg of heparin, therefore, is expected to produce an ACT of approximately 480 seconds, which is considered adequate for initiation of CPB.

The pharmacokinetics of heparin are initially fairly simple. Because it is a large molecule that stays predominantly in the blood, it has a predictable volume of distribution. Its elimination (renal and reticuloendothelial) is dose-dependent, with a half-life of 120 minutes after a 300-IU/kg dose. However, there is evidence that, over time, heparin binds not only to the CPB circuit (minimal effect since most are heparin-bonded already) but to reticuloendothelial cells and vascular smooth muscle cells. This may explain to some degree explain "heparin rebound," an unexplained increase in ACT after protamine reversal (see Protamine Reversal of Anticoagulation, below).

INITIATION OF CARDIOPULMONARY BYPASS

Pharmacokinetic Changes During Cardiopulmonary Bypass

Upon initiation of CPB, several changes take place. The added volume of pump prime, typically ranging from 1.5 to 2 L, causes significant hemodilution and increases the volume of distribution of many drugs, particularly those confined to the plasma volume. Sequestration of drugs in the pulmonary circulation and the lungs at the onset of full CPB contributes to this dilutional effect by functionally decreasing the amount of active drug in the body. Drugs may also bind to the CPB circuit or membrane oxygenator, decreasing their plasma concentration.

Offsetting these dilutional effects to some degree is the effect of decreased plasma protein binding, predicted by the law of mass action, which may lead to an increased free fraction of some drugs. Notably, the administration of heparin releases free fatty acids, which displace some protein-bound drugs (eg, propofol, propranolol), further increasing their unbound fraction in plasma.

The onset of nonpulsatile flow and lower perfusion pressures may alter drug delivery to effect sites, lowering their expected effect-site concentration. Decreased drug delivery to the liver and kidneys may occur as a result of the change in organ perfusion, slowing the clearance of some drugs. Finally, pH changes and hypothermia during CPB can have variable effects on protein binding, organ blood flow (eg, increased cerebral blood flow with pH stat analysis), and enzymatic metabolism.

Pharmacodynamic Changes of Cardiopulmonary Bypass

Hypothermia significantly decreases anesthetic requirements of the central nervous system (CNS) and affects the affinity of receptors and metabolic enzymes for certain drugs. Tissue acidosis may occur despite optimization of blood pH management. This can also affect drug–receptor interactions. Electrolyte concentrations (principally calcium, magnesium, and potassium) are frequently altered during CPB, affecting the activity of drugs such as neuromuscular blockers (NMBs) and inotropic agents. Also, there are a number of changes at the molecular level related to the systemic inflammatory response during CPB, which may influence drug–receptor interaction, as well as up-regulation or down-regulation of plasma-binding proteins.

Specific Agents

Volatile Anesthetics

During CPB, volatile anesthetic is delivered by vaporizer via the membrane oxygenator (Figure 31–6). Because the wash-in with an oxygenator is significantly slower than via the lungs, there may be a delay in attainment of the target partial pressure by up to 50 minutes with isoflurane.[44] With the lack of a feedback mechanism (end-tidal measurement) by which to titrate levels of volatile anesthetic, such a subtherapeutic partial pressure may go undetected for some time. However, hypothermia decreases the anesthetic requirement of the CNS, and lipid-rich tissues typically store a significant amount of equilibrated volatile anesthetic from the pre-CPB period. Therefore, this delay in equilibration is unlikely to lead to awareness or light anesthesia. Hemodilution with the CPB prime and hypothermia produce two opposing effects on the blood–gas partition coefficient of volatile anesthetics. First, the addition of crystalloid prime decreases the blood solubility of isoflurane by approximately 30%. However, upon institution of hypothermia, the blood solubility of isoflurane is increased by approximately 5% (per degree Celsius), so that the net change in solubility is clinically insignificant.[41] If albumin or plasma prime is used, or if more profound hypothermia is achieved (< 30°C), volatile anesthetic solubility may increase significantly, exacerbating the delayed equilibration inherent to delivery via a membrane oxygenator. If this is a concern, a higher concentration of volatile anesthetic, supplemental benzodiazepine, or propofol bolus/infusion may be administered at the onset of CPB until equilibration is achieved.

Propofol

Conflicting data exist regarding the pharmacokinetics of propofol infusions after initiation of CPB. Some studies show decreased plasma concentration and some show no change. Two recent studies[45,46]

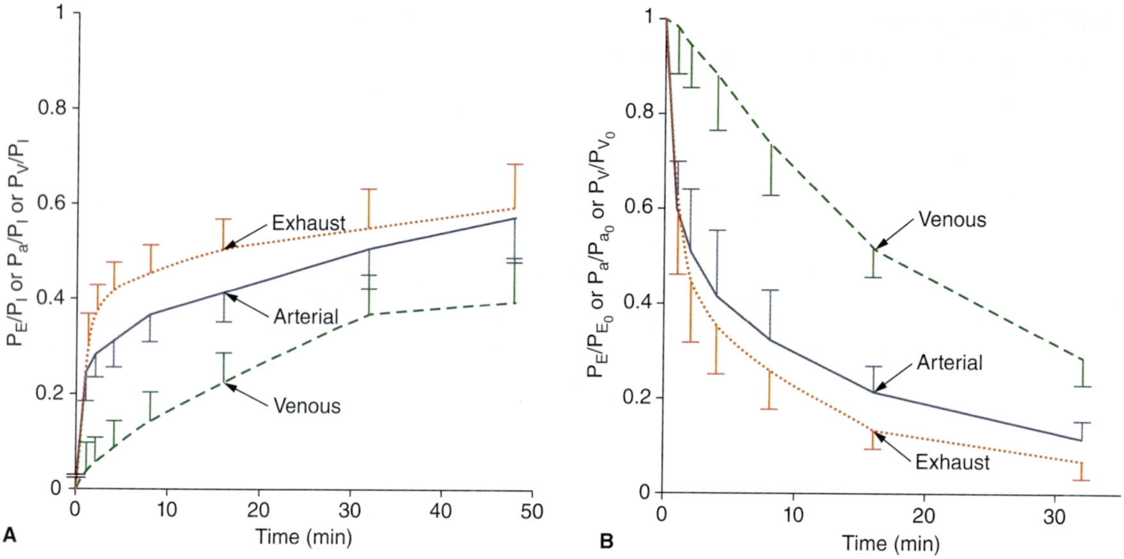

FIGURE 31–6 Ratio of partial pressure of isoflurane in exhaust gas (P_E) and arterial (P_A) and venous (P_V) blood to partial pressure of inlet gas (P_I) during washin (top plot) and washout (bottom plot). For washin, P_E, P_A, and P_V progressively rise with increasing duration of anesthetic administration. There is an initial rise in the arterial and exhaust curves to a "knee" at 1 to 2 minutes, and then the curve continues to slowly rise over the next 30 minutes. For washout, P_E and P_A decrease rapidly, but P_V drops more slowly. (Reproduced with permission from Nussmeier, N.A., M.L. Lambert, G.J. Moskowitz, N.H. Cohen, R.B. Weiskopf, D.M. Fisher, and E.I. Eger, 2nd, Washin and washout of isoflurane administered via bubble oxygenators during hypothermic cardiopulmonary bypass. *Anesthesiology*, 1989; Oct;71(4):519-525.)

demonstrated evidence of increased anesthetic effect (decreased Bispectral Index Scale [BIS] values) during CPB for propofol/narcotic-based anesthetics. This was in part due to a 2-fold increase in the free fraction of propofol during CPB, which is attributed to both administration of heparin (which competes with propofol for binding sites) and hemodilution of plasma proteins. CPB is also associated with an increase in CNS sensitivity to propofol. BIS values are decreased in patients during CPB compared to off-pump cardiac surgery with equivalent plasma concentrations.[46] No consensus exists on adjustment of propofol infusions during CPB, but these data would suggest that a slight decrease in infusion rate may be appropriate.

Opioids

Fentanyl and sufentanil are highly lipophilic and distribute rapidly to lipid-rich tissues in the pre-CPB period. Because of this large volume of distribution, the hemodilutional effect of the pump prime is very brief. If a bolus followed by an infusion of opioid is initiated during the pre-CPB period, the plasma concentration of fentanyl or sufentanil decreases by approximately 25% during the 5 minutes immediately after initiation of CPB. This is primarily due to hemodilution, with binding to the membrane oxygenator and CPB circuit as minor contributing factors. This initial decrease in plasma concentration is offset to some degree by increased fraction of free drug. The synthetic opioids stored in tissue then follow their concentration gradient back into the plasma, eventually restoring the plasma concentration to near pre-CPB levels by 30 minutes. Clearance of fentanyl and sufentanil is decreased during CPB, and the intensity of surgical stimulation during CPB and opioid requirements during hypothermia are decreased. Therefore, the 3-compartment, CPB-adjusted pharmacokinetic models for fentanyl and sufentanil suggest that infusion rates be decreased significantly during CPB.[47,48] However, if a large, single-bolus approach is used (eg, fentanyl 60-75 mcg/kg at the start of anesthesia), the initial decrease in plasma concentration with CPB may be up to 60%, with a slower return to baseline.[49] This highlights an advantage of opioid infusions over bolus approaches in the setting of CPB.

Muscle Relaxants

The nondepolarizing NMBs vecuronium, rocuronium, and cisatracurium have all been extensively studied in the setting of CPB. As polar, hydrophilic, highly protein-bound compounds, their volume of distribution is initially increased by the hemodilution effect of the CPB prime, although less than with synthetic opioids. This is slightly offset by an increase in free fraction of the drugs. The net effect is a transient increase in muscle relaxant requirement upon initiation of CPB. However, the onset of hypothermia has profound pharmacodynamic effects which increase the sensitivity of muscles to the effects of NMBs. Hypothermia alone decreases neuromuscular transmission; below 35°C, twitch tension decreases by 15% per degree Celsius in the absence of muscle relaxants.[50] Hypothermia also decreases clearance of NMBs, prolonging their elimination half-lives during CPB. For rocuronium and vecuronium, this is due to decreased hepatic and renal blood flow. Cisatracurium clearance (enzymatic Hofmann degradation) may be even more profoundly affected by hypothermia and tissue acidosis.[51] Decreasing the infusion dose of cisatracurium and vecuronium by 50% to 60% is recommended during hypothermic CPB.

Heparin

Heparin's therapeutic effect on the ACT during CPB is difficult to quantify accurately, because hypothermia and hemodilution of coagulation factors have significant effects on the coagulation cascade and prolong the ACT independent of heparin. Like many other drugs, the clearance of heparin is reduced during CPB and its volume of distribution is increased. The increase in volume of distribution is transient, however, due to routine addition of heparin to the CPB priming solution. Adsorption of heparin to the CPB circuit and membrane oxygenator is minimal with modern, heparin-bonded equipment. Traditionally, management of heparinization is performed via serial ACT measurements, but the ACT is not specific to the presence of heparin. Even with a "therapeutic" ACT, low heparin levels may lead to the undesirable effects of platelet activation, thrombin activity, and fibrin formation. Newer heparin assays such as the HepCon HMS have been adopted by many centers. The advantage of such systems is to provide accurate, timely information at the point of care, with the intent of reducing thrombin activation, neutrophil activation, and fibrinolysis.[52] More advanced systems may also help to detect depleted levels of AT-III during long CPB runs, guiding not only repeated heparin administration but supplementation of AT-III.

Antifibrinolytics

The pharmacokinetics of TXA and EACA are similar.[41,42] With the initiation of CPB, the volume of distribution of TXA and EACA increases by 15% and 50%, respectively, and the clearance decreases by 30% and 10-fold, respectively. As discussed previously, dosing regimens of TXA and EACA vary widely, without firm agreement upon the plasma concentration (Cp) at which fibrinolysis is maximally inhibited. Threshold efficacy values range from 200 to 800 μm for TXA and from 70 to 200 mcg/mL for EACA. The true value is likely dependent upon the patient's inherent bleeding risk and the intensity of the systemic inflammatory response, but recent studies have focused on maintaining a plasma concentration of greater than 330 μm for TXA and greater than 130 mcg/mL for EACA. This target value can be maintained for the duration of surgery by an initial bolus, followed by constant infusion until separation from CPB, with or without a supplemental dose added to the pump prime. A large bolus dose alone is inadequate to maintain plasma concentration above these targets until separation from CPB. Recent data associating tranexamic acid administration with postoperative seizures have triggered further investigation into the optimal safe dose of this drug.

SEPARATION FROM CARDIOPULMONARY BYPASS

The physiologic and pharmacologic changes associated with discontinuation of CPB have less dramatic implications on pharmacokinetics than the initiation of CPB. Rewarming and return of pulsatile pulmonary circulation leads to improved blood flow to peripheral tissues and elution of sequestered drugs from the lungs and pulmonary circulation. This recirculation of nonmetabolized drug leads to a transient increase in plasma concentration of opioids, propofol, and, to a lesser extent, neuromuscular blockers. Sufentanil concentration, for example, increases by 20% immediately upon separation from CPB but returns to baseline in less than 5 minutes due to its redistribution from the blood into lipid-rich tissues.[48]

Because of increased organ perfusion and normal enzymatic function at normothermia, improved elimination of most drugs is also restored, although full return to baseline elimination is contingent upon normal organ function. The clearance of benzodiazepines, in particular midazolam, is decreased throughout the post-CPB period. This may significantly delay emergence and extubation in the setting of midazolam infusions or boluses of midazolam given just prior to separation from CPB.[52]

Neuromuscular transmission returns very quickly to pre-CPB levels upon return to normothermia, so infusion adjustment back to pre-CPB rates or rebolusing of NMBs is often necessary. (NMB infusions can be decreased by 50%–60% just prior to bypass.)

In theory, sensitivity of the CNS to volatile anesthetics and sedative–hypnotics should return to baseline after normothermia is achieved, although BIS values are consistently lower after CPB compared to off-pump cardiac surgery patients at equivalent propofol concentrations.[46] This suggests a persistent pharmacodynamic change in the CNS response to anesthetics after termination of CPB.

Inotropic Regimen

Inotropic support is frequently required after CPB, even in patients with normal preoperative myocardial function. Myocardial stunning or low cardiac output syndrome, with transient left ventricular and right ventricular dysfunction, is often related to CPB duration. Etiologies include metabolic effects, ischemia–reperfusion injury, and suboptimal cardioplegia and myocardial preservation techniques.

Milrinone

This inotropic agent is the most studied with respect to pharmacokinetics in the setting of CPB. An advantage of milrinone, a phosphodiesterase inhibitor, in the setting of separation from CPB is that it is less dysrhythmogenic than the commonly used β agonists epinephrine and dobutamine. However, milrinone is an "inodilator" which is associated with significant decreases in SVR, particularly in bolus doses. The pharmacokinetics of milrinone is not significantly altered by administration prior to separation from CPB. Two studies[53,54] elegantly describe milrinone's pharmacokinetics with a 3-compartment model in patients with initial cardiac index initially less than 2.5. A dose of 50 mcg/kg while on CPB, followed by an infusion of 0.5 mcg/kg/min, was found to maintain milrinone plasma concentrations above the target threshold for therapeutic effects (ie, increase in cardiac index) of 100 ng/mL for the duration of the post-CPB anesthetic, with minimal effect on SVR, heart rate, or dysrhythmias. Single-dose administration of milrinone prior to separation from CPB was also associated with improved inotropy, but milrinone levels decreased below the target threshold after 30 to 40 minutes.[53] Of note, supplemental vasopressors (phenylephrine or norepinephrine) were required in approximately half of patients from both studies to maintain SVR. An added advantage to milrinone in patients with pulmonary hypertension is its effectiveness in lowering pulmonary vascular resistance (standard infusion range is as effective as 20 ppm of inspired nitric oxide).[55]

Epinephrine

There are limited data on the pharmacokinetics of epinephrine infusion during and after CPB. In patients with septic shock receiving epinephrine infusions to maintain hemodynamic parameters, epinephrine plasma concentration was accurately described by a 1-compartment model with linear pharmacokinetics, with mean elimination half-life of 3.5 minutes in this study.[56] Epinephrine has a wide range of variability in dose-response relationships, dependent upon disease severity, neurohormonal status, and preoperative use of β blockers. Clearance is also highly dependent upon disease severity in trauma and sepsis patients. Future studies may elucidate the pharmacokinetics particular to cardiac surgery patients. Epinephrine appears to result in less decrease in SVR than milrinone at equally therapeutic doses and slightly more tachycardia, and it is associated with increased postoperative lactate in cardiac patients.[57]

Dobutamine

Like epinephrine, dobutamine is a short-acting adrenergic inotrope. Because it is β-receptor specific, it is associated with more tachycardia than either epinephrine or milrinone, and decreased SVR.[55] At therapeutic doses, dobutamine increases heart rate by up to 35%, compared to 10% for milrinone. As with epinephrine, dose-response relationships are difficult to quantify, with significant interpatient variability based upon β-receptor density, disease severity, and preoperative β blockade.

Vasopressors

Vasodilatory shock, or "vasoplegia," post-CPB, is associated with significant morbidity. The etiology is multifactorial, with a reported incidence of 10%.[58] Two agents commonly used to increase SVR in these patients are norepinephrine and vasopressin.

Norepinephrine

As an endogenous catecholamine with predominantly α-adrenergic activity, norepinephrine reliably increases SVR with minimal effect on inotropy compared to epinephrine. As with epinephrine, there is considerable interpatient variability in hemodynamic response to norepinephrine infusions. A 2-compartment, linear pharmacokinetic model has been established in trauma and septic shock patients, with a half-life of 2 to 2.5 minutes.[59] As with epinephrine, the clearance of norepinephrine is decreased in patients with higher disease severity. Although norepinephrine is used frequently post-CPB, the pharmacokinetics have not been well described in cardiac patients.

Vasopressin

Vasopressin is an endogenous peptide hormone; in synthetic form, it may be given IV as a bolus or infusion. The half-life ranges from 10 to 35 minutes. The benefits of vasopressin have been clearly established in septic shock, where many patients have a functional vasopressin deficiency. After CPB, many patients also have inappropriately low endogenous vasopressin concentrations; this is the clinical basis for vasopressin use. Several studies have demonstrated a sustained improvement in hemodynamic parameters and a decrease in norepinephrine requirements in patients with vasodilatory shock after CPB.[58] Vasopressin has also been shown to decrease the incidence of vasodilatory shock when the infusion is started prior to initiation of CPB.[60] The therapeutic dose range used in the setting of post-CPB (0.01–0.1 U/min) is slightly wider than in patients with sepsis (0.02–0.04 U/min). Higher doses (0.06 U/min) have been shown to be more efficacious in maintaining SVR and decreasing lactate levels than doses of 0.03 U/min in certain patients.

Protamine Reversal of Anticoagulation

Protamine is a polycationic molecule derived from salmon roe. The only drug approved to reverse heparin anticoagulation, it is typically administered slowly after separation from CPB during removal of the arterial and venous cannulae. Protamine forms ionic bonds with circulating heparin, neutralizing the heparin. Protamine is rapidly eliminated, with a 2-compartment pharmacokinetic model predicting an elimination half-life of 12 minutes.[61] A slow infusion of protamine, therefore, may be necessary to maintain protamine levels long enough to neutralize all the remaining heparin. Slow administration is also prudent given the risk of a type 1 protamine reaction (histamine release and hypotension) associated with rapid administration. In large doses, protamine can cause significant platelet dysfunction and paradoxically increase the risk of bleeding, so that more accurate methods of heparin/protamine titration systems (such as Hepcon) are preferred over empiric dosing. "Heparin rebound" may still occur after protamine administration due to elution of heparin from vascular and reticuloendothelial cells, and this is usually corrected by small additional doses of protamine.

In addition to a type 1 reaction, protamine can rarely trigger an anaphylactic or anaphylactoid reaction (type 2), as well as an increase in PVR (type 3). Contrary to the practice of "protamine prophylaxis" in all patients with prior exposure to protamine (eg, redo operations), there are only 3 statistically significant risk factors for a protamine reaction: (1) NPH insulin exposure, (2) nonprotamine drug allergy, and (3) true allergy to fish.[62] In patients at risk, a commonly accepted prophylactic strategy consists of a dose of corticosteroids (hydrocortisone 100 mg IV), H_1 blocker (diphenhydramine 25 mg IV), and H_2 blocker (famotidine 20 mg IV), all administered within 24 hours of anticipated protamine exposure.[63]

The effect of protamine administration on the pharmacokinetics of anesthetic drugs is primarily mediated by its reversal of heparin's effect on protein binding. The unbound fraction of circulating propofol, for example, has been shown to decrease after administration of protamine.[60] However, since CNS sensitivity to propofol tends to be greater after weaning from CPB, dosing changes of propofol infusions are probably unnecessary.

SPECIAL CONSIDERATION: DEEP HYPOTHERMIC CIRCULATORY ARREST

DHCA is performed during repair of the aortic root, arch, or great vessels, where blood flow to the brain must be temporarily stopped to facilitate the surgical repair or exposure. Neurophysiologic and pharmacologic considerations are used to optimize cerebral protection. The hallmark of cerebral protection is hypothermia. Prior to circulatory arrest, nasopharyngeal temperature range should be 16 to 18°C. This active cooling may be augmented by the use of pH stat acid-base management, which promotes higher CO_2 and increased cerebral blood flow for more effective cooling and subsequent rewarming. The duration of "safe" time for duration circulatory arrest is typically considered to be 45 to 50 minutes, but methods of anterograde or retrograde cerebral perfusion, which maintain brain cooling and oxygenation, have lengthened this time considerably for complex operations.[57]

Pharmacologic adjuncts used for improved cerebral protection are empirical and have not shown improved outcome in human studies. Thiopental or propofol in burst-suppression doses has been used, although near-maximal burst-suppression is already achieved at brain temperatures less than 20°C. High-dose steroids (eg, methylprednisolone 500 mg IV) and ketamine have also been used, based on evidence of benefit in animal studies.[64] If pharmacologic adjuncts are administered, they should be given long enough before onset of circulatory arrest to ensure adequate effect-site concentrations. If pharmacologic adjuncts are given, consideration should be given to implications such as hyperglycemia, immune suppression, or delayed emergence.

REFERENCES

1. Phillips AA, McLean RF, Devitt JH, Harrington EM. Recall of intraoperative events after general anaesthesia and cardiopulmonary bypass. *Can J Anaesth.* 1993; 40(10):922-926.
2. Greenblatt DJ, Ehrenberg BL, Gunderman J, et al. Kinetic and dynamic study of intravenous lorazepam: comparison with intravenous diazepam. *J Pharmacol Exp Ther.* 1989;250(1):134-140.
3. Greenblatt DJ, Ehrenberg BL, Gunderman J, et al. Pharmacokinetic and electroencephalographic study of intravenous diazepam, midazolam, and placebo. *Clin Pharmacol Ther.* 1989;45(4):356-365.
4. McNulty SE, Gratch D, Costello D, Heropoulos M, Kim JY. The effect of midazolam and lorazepam on postoperative recovery after cardiac surgery. *Anesth Analg.* 1995; 81(2):404-407.
5. Basagan-Mogol E, Goren S, Korfali G, Turker G, Kaya FN. Induction of anesthesia in coronary artery bypass graft surgery: the hemodynamic and analgesic effects of ketamine. *Clinics (Sao Paulo).* 2010;65(2):133-138.
6. Haessler R, Madler C, Klasing S, Schwender D, Peter K. Propofol/fentanyl versus etomidate/fentanyl for the induction of anesthesia in patients with aortic insufficiency and coronary artery disease. *J Cardiothorac Vasc Anesth.* 1992;6(2):173-180.
7. Lundy JB, Slane ML, Frizzi JD. Acute adrenal insufficiency after a single dose of etomidate. *J Intensive Care Med.* 2007;22(2):111-117.
8. Bloomfield R, Noble DW. Etomidate and fatal outcome—even a single bolus dose may be detrimental for some patients. *Br J Anaesth.* 2006;97(1):116-117.
9. Jackson WL Jr. Should we use etomidate as an induction agent for endotracheal intubation in patients with septic shock? A critical appraisal. *Chest.* 2005;127(3):1031-1038.
10. Schulte-Sasse U, Hess W, Tarnow J. Haemodynamic responses to induction of anaesthesia using midazolam in cardiac surgical patients. *Br J Anaesth.* 1982;54(10): 1053-1058.
11. Naguib M, Magboul MM. Adverse effects of neuromuscular blockers and their antagonists. *Drug Saf.* 1998;18(2):99-116.
12. Delboy NJ, Tomichek RC, Shields JA. The hemodynamic effects of rapacuronium in patients with coronary

artery disease: succinylcholine and vecuronium compared. *Anesth Analg.* 2002;94(5):1100-1106.

13. Weiss M, Krejcie TC, Avram MJ. Transit time dispersion in pulmonary and systemic circulation: effects of cardiac output and solute diffusivity. *Am J Physiol Heart Circ Physiol.* 2006;291(2):H861-H870.
14. Landoni G, Bignami E, Oliviero F, Zangrillo A. Halogenated anaesthetics and cardiac protection in cardiac and non-cardiac anaesthesia. *Ann Card Anaesth.* 2009;12(1):4-9.
15. Gentry-Smetana S, Redford D, Moore D, Larson DF. Direct effects of volatile anesthetics on cardiac function. *Perfusion.* 2008;23(1):43-47.
16. Thomson IR, Henderson BT, Singh K, Hudson RJ. Concentration-response relationships for fentanyl and sufentanil in patients undergoing coronary artery bypass grafting. *Anesthesiology.* 1998;89(4):852-861.
17. Wissing H, Kuhn I, Rietbrock S, Fuhr U. Pharmacokinetics of inhaled anaesthetics in a clinical setting: comparison of desflurane, isoflurane and sevoflurane. *Br J Anaesth.* 2000;84(4):443-449.
18. Shafer SL, Varvel JR, Aziz N, Scott JC. Pharmacokinetics of fentanyl administered by computer-controlled infusion pump. *Anesthesiology.* 1990;73(6):1091-1102.
19. Lerou JG, Verheijen R, Booij LH. Model-based administration of inhalation anaesthesia. 4. Applying the system model. *Br J Anaesth.* 2002;88(2):175-183.
20. Lerou JG, Dirksen R, Beneken Kolmer HH, Booij LH, Borm GF. A system model for closed-circuit inhalation anesthesia. II. Clinical validation. *Anesthesiology.* 1991;75(2):230-237.
21. Lerou JG, Dirksen R, Beneken Kolmer HH, Booij LH. A system model for closed-circuit inhalation anesthesia. I. Computer study. *Anesthesiology.* 1991;75(2):345-355.
22. Lerou JG, Booij LH. Model-based administration of inhalation anaesthesia. 3. Validating the system model. *Br J Anaesth.* 2002;88(1):24-37.
23. Lerou JG, Booij LH. Model-based administration of inhalation anaesthesia. 2. Exploring the system model. *Br J Anaesth.* 2001;86(1):29-37.
24. Lerou JG, Booij LH. Model-based administration of inhalation anaesthesia. 1. Developing a system model. *Br J Anaesth.* 2001;86(1):12-28.
25. Syroid ND, Johnson KB, Pace NL, et al. Response surface model predictions of emergence and response to pain in the recovery room: An evaluation of patients emerging from an isoflurane and fentanyl anesthetic. *Anesth Analg.* 2010;111(2):380-386.
26. Johnson KB, Syroid ND, Gupta DK, et al. An evaluation of remifentanil-sevoflurane response surface models in patients emerging from anesthesia: model improvement using effect-site sevoflurane concentrations. *Anesth Analg.* 2010;111(2):387-394.
27. Manyam SC, Gupta DK, Johnson KB, et al. Opioid-volatile anesthetic synergy: a response surface model with remifentanil and sevoflurane as prototypes. *Anesthesiology.* 2006;105(2):267-278.
28. Westmoreland CL, Sebel PS, Gropper A. Fentanyl or alfentanil decreases the minimum alveolar anesthetic concentration of isoflurane in surgical patients. *Anesth Analg.* 1994;78(1):23-28.
29. Lang E, Kapila A, Shlugman D, Hoke JF, Sebel PS, Glass PS. Reduction of isoflurane minimal alveolar concentration by remifentanil. *Anesthesiology.* 1996;85(4):721-728.
30. Eger EI II. Age, minimum alveolar anesthetic concentration, and minimum alveolar anesthetic concentration-awake. *Anesth Analg.* 2001;93(4):947-953.
31. Chernik D, Gillings D, Harriet L, et al. Validity and reliability of the Observer's Assessment of Alertness/Sedation Scale: study with intravenous midazolam. *J Clin Psychopharmacol.* 1990;10:244-251.
32. Kennedy RR, Baker AB. The effect of cardiac output changes on end-expired volatile anaesthetic concentrations—a theoretical study. *Anaesthesia.* 2001;56(11):1034-1040.
33. Massey NJ, Sherry KM, Oldroyd S, Peacock JE. Pharmacokinetics of an infusion of propofol during cardiac surgery. *Br J Anaesth.* 1990;65(4):475-479.
34. Schnider TW, Minto CF, Shafer SL, et al. The influence of age on propofol pharmacodynamics. *Anesthesiology.* 1999;90(6): 1502-1516.
35. Schnider TW, Minto CF, Gambus PL, et al. The influence of method of administration and covariates on the pharmacokinetics of propofol in adult volunteers. *Anesthesiology.* 1998;88(5):1170-1182.
36. Gepts E, Shafer SL, Camu F, et al. Linearity of pharmacokinetics and model estimation of sufentanil. *Anesthesiology.* 1995;83(6):1194-1204.
37. Cooper RA, Maddineni VR, Mirakhur RK, Wierda JM, Brady M, Fitzpatrick KT. Time course of neuromuscular effects and pharmacokinetics of rocuronium bromide (Org 9426) during isoflurane anaesthesia in patients with and without renal failure. *Br J Anaesth.* 1993;71(2):222-226.
38. Plaud B, Proost JH, Wierda JM, Barre J, Debaene B, Meistelman C. Pharmacokinetics and pharmacodynamics of rocuronium at the vocal cords and the adductor pollicis in humans. *Clin Pharmacol Ther.* 1995;58(2):185-191.
39. Fergusson DA, Hebert PC, Mazer CD, et al. A comparison of aprotinin and lysine analogues in high-risk cardiac surgery. *N Engl J Med.* 2008;358(22):2319-2331.
40. Jimenez JJ, Iribarren JL, Lorente L, et al. Tranexamic acid attenuates inflammatory response in cardiopulmonary bypass surgery through blockade of fibrinolysis: a case control study followed by a

randomized double-blind controlled trial. *Crit Care.* 2007;11(6):R117.

41. Dowd NP, Karski JM, Cheng DC, et al. Pharmacokinetics of tranexamic acid during cardiopulmonary bypass. *Anesthesiology.* 2002;97(2):390-399.
42. Butterworth J, James RL, Lin Y, Prielipp RC, Hudspeth AS. Pharmacokinetics of epsilon-aminocaproic acid in patients undergoing aortocoronary bypass surgery. *Anesthesiology.* 1999;90(6):1624-1635.
43. Martin K, Wiesner G, Breuer T, Lange R, Tassani P. The risks of aprotinin and tranexamic acid in cardiac surgery: a one-year follow-up of 1188 consecutive patients. *Anesth Analg.* 2008;107(6):1783-1790.
44. Nussmeier NA, Lambert ML, Moskowitz GJ. Washin and washout of isoflurane administered via bubble oxygenators during hypothermic cardiopulmonary bypass. *Anesthesiology.* 1989;71(4):519-525.
45. Takizawa E, Hiraoka H, Takizawa D, Goto F. Changes in the effect of propofol in response to altered plasma protein binding during normothermic cardiopulmonary bypass. *Br J Anaesth.* 2006;96(2):179-185.
46. Barbosa RA, Santos SR, White P.F, et al. Effects of cardiopulmonary bypass on propofol pharmacokinetics and bispectral index during coronary surgery. *Clinics (Sao Paulo).* 2009;64(3):215-221.
47. Hudson RJ, Thomson IR, Jassal R, Peterson DJ, Brown AD, Freedman JI. Cardiopulmonary bypass has minimal effects on the pharmacokinetics of fentanyl in adults. *Anesthesiology.* 2003;99(4):847-854.
48. Hudson RJ, Thomson IR, Jassal R. Effects of cardiopulmonary bypass on sufentanil pharmacokinetics in patients undergoing coronary artery bypass surgery. *Anesthesiology.* 2004;101(4):862-871.
49. Gedney JA, Ghosh S. Pharmacokinetics of analgesics, sedatives and anaesthetic agents during cardiopulmonary bypass. *Br J Anaesth.* 1995;75(3):344-351.
50. Heier T, Caldwell JE, Sessler DI, Miller RD. The effect of local surface and central cooling on adductor pollicis twitch tension during nitrous oxide/isoflurane and nitrous oxide/fentanyl anesthesia in humans. *Anesthesiology.* 1990;72(5):807-811.
51. Cammu G, Coddens J, Hendrickx J, Deloof T. Dose requirements of infusions of cisatracurium or rocuronium during hypothermic cardiopulmonary bypass. *Br J Anaesth.* 2000;84(5):587-590.
52. Koster A, Fischer T, Praus M, et al. Hemostatic activation and inflammatory response during cardiopulmonary bypass: impact of heparin management. *Anesthesiology.* 2002;97(4):837-841.
53. Butterworth JFT, Hines RL, Royster RL, James RL. A pharmacokinetic and pharmacodynamic evaluation of milrinone in adults undergoing cardiac surgery. *Anesth Analg.* 1995;81(4):783-792.
54. Bailey JM, Mora CT, Shafer SL. Pharmacokinetics of propofol in adult patients undergoing coronary revascularization. The Multicenter Study of Perioperative Ischemia Research Group. *Anesthesiology.* 1996;84(6):1288-1297.
55. Gillies M, Bellomo R, Doolan L, Buxton B. Bench-to-bedside review: inotropic drug therapy after adult cardiac surgery—a systematic literature review. *Crit Care.* 2005;9(3):266-279.
56. Abboud I, Lerolle N, Urien S, et al. Pharmacokinetics of epinephrine in patients with septic shock: modelization and interaction with endogenous neurohormonal status. *Crit Care.* 2009;13(4):R120.
57. Maillet JM, Le Besnerais P, Cantoni M, et al. Frequency, risk factors, and outcome of hyperlactatemia after cardiac surgery. *Chest.* 2003;123(5):1361-1366.
58. Albright TN, Zimmerman MA, Selzman CH. Vasopressin in the cardiac surgery intensive care unit. *Am J Crit Care.* 2002;11(4):326-330; quiz 331-332.
59. Beloeil H, Mazoit JX, Benhamou D, Duranteau J. Norepinephrine kinetics and dynamics in septic shock and trauma patients. *Br J Anaesth.* 2005;95(6):782-788.
60. Papadopoulos G, Sintou E, Siminelakis S, Koletsis E, Baikoussis NG, Apostolakis E. Perioperative infusion of low- dose of vasopressin for prevention and management of vasodilatory vasoplegic syndrome in patients undergoing coronary artery bypass grafting—a double-blind randomized study. *J Cardiothorac Surg.* 2010;5:17.
61. Butterworth J, Lin YA, Prielipp RC, Bennett J, Hammon JW, James RL. Rapid disappearance of protamine in adults undergoing cardiac operation with cardiopulmonary bypass. *Ann Thorac Surg.* 2002;74(5):1589-1595.
62. Levy JH, Adkinson NF Jr. Anaphylaxis during cardiac surgery: implications for clinicians. *Anesth Analg.* 2008;106(2):392-403.
63. Kimmel SE, Sekeres MA, Berlin JA, Ellison N, DiSesa VJ, Strom BL. Risk factors for clinically important adverse events after protamine administration following cardiopulmonary bypass. *J Am Coll Cardiol.* 1998;32(7):1916-1922.
64. Dewhurst AT, Moore SJ, Liban JB. Pharmacological agents as cerebral protectants during deep hypothermic circulatory arrest in adult thoracic aortic surgery. A survey of current practice. *Anaesthesia.* 2002;57(10):1016-1021.

CHAPTER

32 Anesthetic Management for Abdominal Aortic Aneurysm Repair

Warner Smith, MD

CASE DISCUSSION

A 72-year-old, 96-kg, 179-cm male is scheduled for a transperineal repair of a 6-cm suprarenal abdominal aortic aneurysm repair. His past medical history is significant for coronary artery disease, hypertension, gastroesophageal reflux, smoking, and chronic obstructive pulmonary disease. His current medical management includes metoprolol, losartan, atorvastatin, and omeprazole. He has not taken any medications this morning. His current vital signs are: pulse 95/min, blood pressure 165/96 mm Hg, oxygen saturation 92%, and respiratory rate 19/min.

PREMEDICATION

- **Anxiolytic:** Intravenous midazolam
- **β blocker:** Intravenous metoprolol, esmolol infusion, or propranolol
- **Antihypertensive:** Intravenous labetalol, hydralazine, or nicardipine
- **Statin:** Oral atorvastatin, simvastatin, pravastatin, or fluvastatin
- **Thoracic epidural:** Preoperative placement

Sample Dosing Regimen

- **Anxiolytic:** Intravenous midazolam 1 to 2 mg, 15 to 30 minutes prior to induction
- **β blocker:** Consider slowly titrating intravenous metoprolol 1 to 10 mg (0.1 mg/kg) to a heart rate of < 65 beats/min, 30 minutes prior to induction.
- **Antihypertensive:** Consider intravenous labetalol 5 to 50 mg titrated to blood pressure within 20% above baseline blood pressure if not achieved with anxiolysis 10 minutes prior to induction.
- **Statin:** Oral atorvastatin 20 to 40 mg, 30 minutes prior to induction
- **Thoracic epidural:** Placement of an epidural catheter in the T10–11 interspace 30 minutes preoperatively, with administration of 3 mL of 1.5% lidocaine with 1:200,000 epinephrine as a test dose

Clinical Pharmacology

Anxiolysis prior to major vascular surgery can have the additional benefit of reducing adrenergic tone. Anxiolysis may be sufficient to return this patient's heart rate and blood pressure to baseline. Midazolam is frequently chosen due to its rapid onset, but the slower offset of midazolam can be a source of sedation into the postoperative period. Prolonged sedation is of more concern in the elderly and those with preexisting cognitive dysfunction.

β Blockers should not be acutely discontinued, because this can result in rebound tachycardia, hypertension, and angina. Evidence supports the continuation of chronic β-blocker therapy.[1] Initiation of perioperative β blockade has been questioned based on the PeriOperative Ischemic Evaluation (POISE) trial. The POISE trial demonstrated that perioperative β blockade decreased the incidence

TABLE 32–1 Revised cardiac risk index (RCRI) predictors of perioperative cardiac risk.[3]

Ischemic heart disease	High-risk surgery (aortic aneurysm repair)
Diabetes requiring insulin therapy	Congestive heart failure
Chronic renal insufficiency	Cerebrovascular disease

Each predictor has the value of 1, for a score of 0 to 6.
Adapted with permission from Lee, T.H., et al., Derivation and prospective validation of a simple index for prediction of cardiac risk of major noncardiac surgery. *Circulation* 1999,Sep 7;100(10):1043-1049.

of myocardial infarction but increased overall mortality and stroke.[2] There are several limitations to the POISE trial; the 2 major limitations are (1) the fixed high dose of metoprolol (100 mg) and (2) the revised cardiac risk index (RCRI) of 1 or 2 in most of the patients (Table 32–1). Therefore, there may still be overall benefit in patients with high cardiac risk (RCRI ≥ 3).

The Dutch Echocardiographic Cardiac Risk Evaluation Applying Stress Echocardiography (DECREASE) IV trial demonstrated significant reduction in cardiac mortality and myocardial infarction using bisoprolol 2.5 mg.[4] In contrast to the POISE trial, β blockade was initiated a month prior to the procedure, and β blockade was titrated to a heart rate of 50 to 70 beats/min in the DECREASE IV trial. Comparing the results of the DECREASE IV and POISE trials, β blockade is likely still of benefit in most patients presenting for abdominal aortic repair when initiated at least 1 month in advance, titrated to heart rate of 60 to 70 beats/min; hypotension is avoided. Table 32–2 summarizes the recommendations for perioperative β blockade.

TABLE 32–2 Recommendations for perioperative β blockade.

Initiate > 30 days preoperatively	Avoid initiation immediately prior to surgery
Use β_1-selective agent (bisoprolol, metoprolol, atenolol)	Avoid perioperative discontinuation
Titrate to 60–70 beats/min	Avoid hypotension
Use long-acting agent (bisoprolol)	Continue > 30 days postoperatively

It is extremely important that statins are continued in the perioperative period. Observational data suggest a significant increase in the risk of adverse cardiac events with acute perioperative cessation of statins. Unfortunately, there is no intravenous statin, and most patients are not fed for several days after open abdominal aortic aneurysm repair. Administration via nasogastric tube during this fasting period to avoid discontinuation of statins in the perioperative period has been shown to prevent the increase in cardiac events.[5] Statins have benefit in excess of their lipid-lowering effect, including plaque stabilization, anti-inflammation, and reduction of thrombogenesis. There is good evidence supporting initiation of statin therapy in patients undergoing major vascular surgery.[6] Ideally, statin therapy should be initiated at least 30 days prior to the operation and continued for at least 30 days afterward. When initiating therapy, the extended-release formulation of fluvastatin is the best choice. The increase in adverse cardiac events is less after the cessation of extended release fluvastatin when compared to shorter acting statins.[7] In urgent cases, there may still be benefit in acute initiation of therapy, and there is unlikely to be any harm. Table 32–3 summarizes the recommendations for perioperative statin therapy.

Thoracic epidural analgesia using a combination of local anesthetics and opiates is the standard practice for aortic aneurysm repairs at many institutions. A Cochrane systematic review demonstrated a reduction in pain, postoperative intubation, cardiac complications, gastric complications, and renal complications when comparing thoracic epidural analgesia with systemic opioid analgesia.[8]

TABLE 32–3 Recommendations for perioperative statin therapy.

Avoid perioperative discontinuation	Initiation in immediate preoperative period acceptable
Ideally initiated > 30 days preoperatively	Use long-acting agent (fluvastatin ER)
Continue > 30 days postoperatively	Can be administered via nasogastric tube

ER, extended release.

No overall reduction in postoperative mortality has been demonstrated. Epidural placement appears to be safe in the setting of intraoperative heparinization, especially if heparinization occurs at least 1 hour after placement. In the event of a bloody tap, it is typical to proceed with surgery, but this should be communicated to the surgical team. There is no evidence to support cancellation of surgery based on a bloody or traumatic neuraxial procedure.[9] Patients presenting for vascular surgery are often on chronic anticoagulants and antiplatelet medications. Some of these therapies significantly increase the risk of epidural hematoma and contraindicate epidural placement, as discussed in Chapter 16.

INDUCTION

- **Analgesic:** intravenous fentanyl, sufentanil, morphine, or hydromorphone
- **Local anesthetic:** Intravenous lidocaine
- **Sedative–hypnotic:** Intravenous propofol, etomidate, or ketamine
- **Muscle relaxant:** Intravenous succinylcholine, rocuronium, vecuronium, or cisatracurium
- **Hemodynamic agent:** Consider intravenous esmolol, intravenous nitroglycerin, or intravenous labetalol.

Sample Dosing Regimen

- **Analgesic:** Intravenous fentanyl 2 to 3 mcg/kg 5 minutes prior to induction
- **Local anesthetic:** Intravenous lidocaine 1 mg/kg 15 seconds prior to propofol
- **Sedative–hypnotic:** Intravenous propofol titrated to loss of consciousness, approximately 1 mg/kg at induction
- **Muscle relaxant:** Intravenous succinylcholine 1.5 mg/kg administered immediately after propofol
- **Hemodynamic agent:** Consider intravenous esmolol 1 to 2 mg/kg 2 minutes prior to intubation if blood pressure and heart rate remain poorly controlled.

Clinical Pharmacology

Propofol is an ideal induction agent for the patient in this case. Propofol minimizes airway responses to intubation to a greater extent than other induction agents,[10] which is beneficial in this smoker. Elderly patients require lower doses of propofol, especially when paired with opioids.[11] Propofol can cause excessive decreases in blood pressure and cardiac output, especially in patients with decreased intravascular volume or reduced cardiac function. Lidocaine is often given just prior to propofol administration to reduce the risk of pain with injection. Mixing lidocaine with propofol in a single syringe should be avoided based on experimental data that demonstrates droplet formation, which theoretically could lead to pulmonary embolism.[12]

There is a large gap in the anesthetic requirements to ensure unconsciousness and the requirements to prevent a significant adrenergic surge. Dosing induction agents to achieve the latter goal can result in persistently elevated drug levels and prolonged hypotension, especially once an inhaled anesthetic is added. The addition of esmolol can be used to bridge this gap in anesthetic requirements, and esmolol's effects dissipate very rapidly, minimizing the risk of prolonged hypotension. Esmolol is a extremely short-acting β_1-selective adrenergic antagonist with rapid onset within 60 seconds and a short duration of action of 10 to 20 minutes.[13] Nitroglycerin and lidocaine are also advocated to help decrease the adrenergic response to laryngoscopy, but when compared with esmolol, neither of these is very effective.[14,15] Esmolol has been shown to reduce propofol requirements by as much as 20%.[16] If prolonged airway manipulation or awake intubation is anticipated, a bolus of 0.5 mg/kg followed by an infusion of 50 to 300 mcg/kg/min can be used.

Labetalol has also been shown to be useful in preventing hypertension and tachycardia associated with laryngoscopy. Labetalol is a selective α_1- and nonselective β-adrenergic antagonist with a 1:7 α/β ratio in the intravenous formulation.[17] Labetalol 0.5 mg/kg was shown to be superior to low-dose esmolol (0.25 mg/kg) in controlling heart rate, blood pressure, and rate pressure product during laryngoscopy and intubation.[18] Labetalol should be administered 5 minutes prior to laryngoscopy in order to utilize peak drug effect. Labetalol's 2- to 4-hour duration of action may be beneficial in reducing postoperative hypertension but may also be detrimental during cross-clamp release or significant blood loss.

MAINTENANCE OF ANESTHESIA

- **Sedative–hypnotics:** Sevoflurane, desflurane, isoflurane, nitrous oxide, or propofol infusion
- **Analgesics:** Fentanyl, sufentanil, alfentanil, remifentanil, morphine sulfate, or hydromorphone
- **Muscle relaxants:** Rocuronium, vecuronium, or cisatracurium
- **Antiemetics:** Ondansetron, dolasetron, metoclopramide, dexamethasone, or droperidol as needed

Sample Dosing Regimen

- **Sedative–hypnotic:** Inhaled isoflurane 0.5 to 1.5 vol% can be titrated to prevent awareness and patient movement as well as to attenuate adrenergic response to surgical stimulus. The minimum alveolar concentration (MAC) value for adults is 1.15, but MAC values are greatly reduced with a balanced anesthetic technique that includes opioids.
- **Analgesic:** Intravenous fentanyl in incremental doses of 0.5 to 1 mcg/kg with an epidural for postoperative analgesia or sufentanil infusion 0.5 to 1 mcg/kg/h without an epidural
- **Muscle relaxant:** Vecuronium infusion of 0.03 to 0.06 mcg/kg/min titrated to a train-of-four of 1/4 to 2/4
- **Antiemetic:** Intravenous dexamethasone 8 mg, administered early in the procedure

Clinical Pharmacology

Isoflurane paired with low-dose fentanyl is a good choice for maintenance of anesthesia. MAC and MACbar are significantly lowered by the addition of low-dose fentanyl. Higher doses of fentanyl are not necessary when an epidural is present for postoperative pain relief, and no additional reduction of isoflurane requirements is seen with higher doses.[19] Isoflurane also has the benefit of ischemic preconditioning.[20]

Comparing isoflurane, desflurane, and sevoflurane, there is significant cost savings with isoflurane. All of the inhaled anesthetics are greenhouse gases but differ significantly in their impact. Sevoflurane has the lowest 20-year global warming potential (GWP), with isoflurane having twice the 20-year GWP and desflurane having 27 times the 20-year GWP. Nitrous oxide is similar to desflurane in impact but persists for a much longer time in the atmosphere.[21] Although there are many factors that influence the choice of inhaled anesthetic, isoflurane appears to represent a good balance between cost and environmental impact.

The thoracic epidural is typically not used for intraoperative analgesia. Epidural local anesthetic causes a sympathetic block that can exacerbate hypotension during the large fluid shifts that are common in abdominal aortic aneurysm repair. Researchers have hypothesized that running an epidural intraoperatively with a light general anesthetic may have benefit over just using the epidural for postoperative analgesia, but a double-blind randomized control trial failed to demonstrate any difference.[22]

Dexamethasone, a corticosteroid, is a very effective antiemetic[23] and has been shown to have analgesic benefits.[24] Dose finding studies have shown a dose-dependent antiemetic response, with 8 mg being much more effective than 4 mg.[25] Dexamethasone has a very favorable side-effect profile, but there is evidence that a single preoperative dose causes significant adrenal suppression.[26] Whether this represents a clinical risk to patients is unclear, and 2 recent studies looking at the risk of postoperative infection yielded conflicting results[27,28]. It appears that a randomized control trial is needed to clarify this issue, but at this time the benefits of dexamethasone as an antiemetic outweigh its risks.[29]

ANTICIPATED INTRAOPERATIVE EVENTS

Hemodynamic Management of Aortic Cross-Clamping

The repair of abdominal aortic aneurysms requires cross-clamping of the aorta proximal to the area of repair. This clamping causes a rapid and dramatic challenge for the cardiovascular system (as well as for the anesthesiologist). The most direct change is a large increase in afterload by excluding low resistance vascular beds from aortic outflow. In addition to the increase in afterload, there is a surge in catecholamine release as well as variable changes in preload.[30] The magnitude of the change is proportional to the level of aortic cross-clamping: the higher the cross-clamp, the more dramatic the changes. Many patients can tolerate these perturbations without significant hemodynamic compromise, especially with infrarenal clamping. However, some patients require pharmacologic intervention, particularly those with underlying coronary artery disease or heart failure. It is important to consider reduced collateral perfusion below the clamp when pharmacologic agents are used to decrease pressures above the clamp. Traditionally, above cross-clamp pressures are kept below 120% of baseline pressures. Transesophageal echocardiography is a more clinically useful guide in that myocardial performance and volume status can be monitored continuously. Distal perfusion can be maximized by reserving vasodilators for patients who demonstrate inadequate myocardial reserve. In addition to changes with initiation of aortic cross-clamping, release of the cross-clamp causes significant changes in the opposing direction. Potential vasodilators are presented in Table 32–4. Ideal pharmacologic agents for this purpose would have rapid onset, short half-life, result in optimal myocardial oxygen supply/demand, and have minimal side effects.

Intravenous Nitroglycerin

A dose of 0.5 to 5 mcg/kg/min is initiated 10 minutes prior to cross-clamping. Nitroglycerin is an ideal agent due to its very rapid onset and short duration of action. The mechanism is primarily venodilation, increasing venous capacitance with a resultant reduction in preload and cardiac output. This venodilation also helps minimize myocardial oxygen demand by reducing wall tension and helps improve supply through the reduction of left ventricular end-diastolic pressure. In some patients with significant blood pressure elevation during cross-clamping, nitroglycerin may not provide adequate reduction in blood pressure because of its minimal arterial dilation. Other disadvantages include cerebral vasodilation, inhibition of hypoxic pulmonary vasoconstriction and, rarely, methemoglobinemia.

Sodium Nitroprusside

The dose is 0.5 to 3 mcg/kg/min. This agent has a very rapid onset and offset and much more potent arterial dilation. However, sodium nitroprusside does not have favorable effects on myocardial oxygen supply/demand and can result in hyperperfusion above the clamp. The risks of cyanide toxicity and methemoglobinemia also make this agent less ideal. It can be useful at low doses as an adjunct to nitroglycerin in patients whose blood pressure is not adequately controlled by nitroglycerin alone.

Inhaled Anesthetics

The potent inhaled anesthetics are a viable option to control blood pressure elevations during cross-clamping and have the obvious advantage of providing surgical anesthesia. The reduction in blood pressure is almost exclusively due to vasodilation. The inhaled anesthetics do depress myocardial contractility, but usually there is no reduction in cardiac index. In many patients with infrarenal cross-clamping, increasing the depth of anesthesia with an inhaled anesthetic is sufficient to control blood pressure within 120% of baseline. The additional myocardial depression may not be tolerated in patients with preexisting heart failure or coronary disease, which limits the use of inhaled anesthetics for blood pressure management.

TABLE 32–4 Agents for hemodynamic management of aortic cross-clamping.

Agent	Mechanism	Advantages	Disadvantages
Nitroglycerin	Venous dilation	Improves myocardial supply/demand	Limited reductions in blood pressure
Sodium nitroprusside	Arterial dilation	Profound reductions in blood pressure	Cyanide toxicity, methemoglobinemia
Inhaled anesthetics	arterial dilation	Provides anesthesia	Myocardial depression

Renal Protection During Aortic Cross-Clamping

Renal failure following abdominal aortic aneurysm repair is a somewhat common and devastating complication. In repairs involving suprarenal clamping, the mechanism is primarily ischemia from the direct interruption of blood flow. In the more common infrarenal cross-clamping, the decrease in renal blood flow is due to an increase in renal vascular resistance and a redistribution of blood flow. This reduction of renal blood flow persists after the cross-clamp has been removed. Many pharmacologic agents have been utilized to offer some degree of protection. There is little evidence to suggest that they offer any significant protection, other than fenoldopam, which does show some promise in renal protection. These agents are summarized in Table 32–5.

Fenoldopam

Fenoldopam should be initiated at the beginning of surgery and continued for at least 24 hours. The dose is 0.1 mcg/kg/min for this period. There is demonstrated benefit with a wide range of dosages from 0.03 to 0.3 mcg/kg/min, but 0.1 mcg/kg/min appears to be the ideal dose to reduce acute kidney injury.[31] At this dose there is a significant increase in renal blood flow without any significant effect on systemic blood pressure.[32,33] Fenoldopam is a selective dopamine 1 receptor agonist that dilates renal and splanchnic vasculature. Improvement of blood flow to the renal cortex and outer medulla is thought to provide renal protection. There is evidence that fenoldopam reduces the risk of acute renal failure in abdominal aortic aneurysm repair.[34-36] Fenoldopam is an effective antihypertensive at higher doses[37] and could be used to control excessive hypertension during aortic cross-clamping.

Mannitol

There is no evidence that the osmotic diuretic mannitol given prior to cross-clamping offers any renal protection.[38] The amount of 12.5 g/70 kg is appropriate. The proposed mechanisms include free-radical scavenging and redistribution of blood flow to the renal cortex. Despite lack of evidence, mannitol is commonly requested by surgeons prior to cross-clamping. Mannitol is unlikely to be harmful but can cause electrolyte and fluid derangement, primarily hyponatremia and hypovolemia. The initial, transient increase in intravascular volume can exacerbate pulmonary edema in patients with poor left ventricular function.

Furosemide

Furosemide is a loop diuretic that inhibits sodium pumps in the loop of Henle. The dose is 20 to 40 mg. This agent is thought to be protective by reducing renal oxygen consumption. There is no evidence that furosemide provides any protection.[39] In fact, some studies demonstrate that furosemide actually increases the risk of acute kidney injury.[40] Furosemide causes a hypokalemic, hyperchloremic metabolic alkalosis and can cause hyponatremia.

Renal-Dose Dopamine

The use of dopamine at low doses for renal protection has been disproved in multiple studies and many different clinical situations.[40-42] The dose is 1 to 3 mcg/kg/min. There appears to be no justification

TABLE 32–5 Agents for renal protection during aortic cross-clamping.

Agent	Mechanism	Beneficial	Side Effects
Fenoldopam	Selective dopamine$_1$ agonist	Yes	Minimal at doses ≤ 0.1 mcg/kg/min
Mannitol	Osmotic diuretic	No	Hypovolemia, hyponatremia and rarely pulmonary edema
Furosemide	Loop diuretic	No	Increased risk of acute kidney injury, hypokalemia, hyponatremia
Dopamine	Nonselective dopamine, α and β agonist	No	Dysrhythmias, increased cardiac work, hypertension

to use dopamine for renal protection in vascular surgery. The α- and β-adrenergic properties of dopamine pose the risk of dysrhythmias, increased cardiac workload, hypertension, and decreased renal perfusion. In addition, dopamine pharmacokinetics are extremely variable and weight based infusions result in vastly different plasma concentrations.[43] Based on lack of efficacy, potential harm, and unpredictable dosing, renal-dose dopamine should be avoided.

Anticoagulation for Aortic Aneurysm Repair

Unfractionated heparin is typically administered shortly before aortic cross-clamp placement in communication with the surgeon. Dosing suggestions are 60 to 70 units/kg, but 5000 units is the typical dose irrespective of patient weight. It is common practice to administer another 1000 units of heparin for each additional hour of cross-clamp time. No monitoring of this low-dose anticoagulation with heparin is usually undertaken. Some surgeons ask for reversal with protamine, but evidence suggests that this is unnecessary and that protamine is associated with significant adverse reactions.[44] There is some reluctance to administer heparin during ruptured abdominal aortic aneurysms, but a recent study demonstrated that systemic heparinization in leaking aneurysms is safe and possible beneficial.[45]

EMERGENCE

- **Thoracic epidural:** Bupivacaine, in combination with fentanyl, morphine, or hydromorphone
- **Analgesia:** Fentanyl, hydromorphone, morphine, or sufentanil
- **Blood pressure management:** Labetalol, hydralazine, metoprolol, nicardipine, esmolol, or fenoldopam
- **Reversal of muscle relaxation:** Neostigmine or glycopyrrolate
- **Antiemetic:** Ondansetron, droperidol, or metoclopramide

Sample Dosing Regimen

- **Thoracic epidural:** Once the risk of significant hemorrhage is over, the epidural catheter is dosed with 75 mcg of fentanyl and 6 mL of 0.25% bupivacaine. The epidural infusion is then initiated using 0.125% bupivacaine with 2-mcg/mL fentanyl at 8 mL/h.
- **Analgesia:** With a working thoracic epidural, a transitional opioid for postoperative pain relief is not necessary. If a sufentanil infusion was used intraoperatively, it is discontinued approximately 30 minutes prior to emergence. If there is evidence of inadequate analgesia just prior to emergence based on respiratory rate, 0.5 mg of hydromorphone is administered.
- **Blood pressure management:** A nicardipine infusion of 2.5 to 15 mg/h is administered for a systolic blood pressure greater than 20% baseline once there is adequate analgesia.
- **Reversal of muscle relaxation:** Neostigmine 4 mg and glycopyrrolate 0.6 mg are administered intravenously as soon as the fascial closure is complete.
- **Antiemetics:** Intravenous ondansetron 4 mg is given around the time of abdominal closure.

Clinical Pharmacology

Despite the advantages of a thoracic epidural for postoperative analgesia, there are many circumstances when it is not an option. Some surgeons are adamantly against such use, and many patients presenting for vascular procedures are on chronic anticoagulants that are a contraindication for thoracic epidural placement. A sufentanil infusion is a very attractive alternative in these situations. When administered as an infusion, sufentanil frequently provides stable hemodynamics.[46] Sufentanil is very lipophilic and undergoes extensive tissue distribution, but it is more protein bound than alfentanil and fentanyl. This partially explains sufentanil's shorter context-sensitive half-time.[47] Sufentanil's context-sensitive half-time makes it attractive for maintenance of analgesia in longer cases with a need for postoperative analgesia. The question that still arises is when to discontinue sufentanil infusions to retain postoperative analgesia without causing delayed awakening or extubation. Pharmacokinetic modeling demonstrates greater than 50% chance of postoperative analgesia for up to 3 hours after a 0.5-mcg/kg/h sufentanil infusion is discontinued and a less than 50% probability of unconsciousness after 30 minutes, as shown in Figure 32–1. Therefore, discontinuing the sufentanil infusion 30 minutes prior to emergence balances the goals of postoperative analgesia and rapid emergence. This

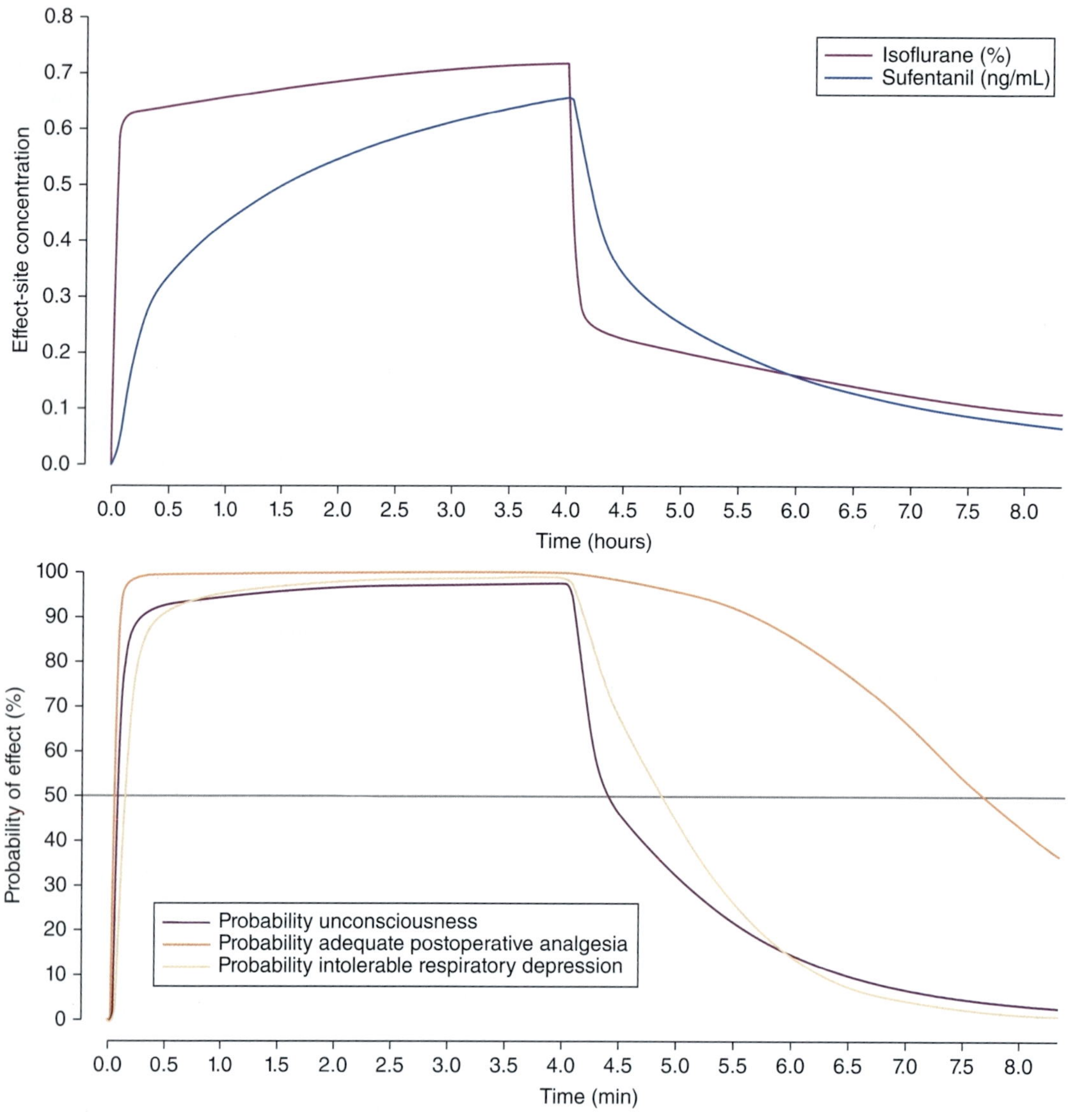

FIGURE 32–1 Simulation of an isoflurane–sufentanil 4-hour general anesthetic in a 100-kg, 185-cm male. The isoflurane vaporizer is set to 1%, and the sufentanil infusion is set to 0.5 mcg/kg/h for the entire anesthetic. Resultant effect-site concentrations for these dosing schemes are presented in the top plot. This simulation assumes normal cardiac output and normal ventilatory function. Predictions of unresponsiveness, intolerable ventilatory depression, and postoperative analgesia are presented in the bottom plot. As defined in previous chapters, intolerable ventilatory depression is defined as a respiratory rate less than 4 breaths per minute and postoperative analgesia is defined as a loss of response to pressure (30 pounds per square inch) on the anterior tibia.

pharmacokinetic modeling is based on opioid-naive volunteers. In patients with significant opioid tolerance, the sufentanil infusion can be continued until the time of emergence. A prolonged elimination has been demonstrated in those with higher percentages of adipose tissue (obese, elderly) as would be expected with sufentanil's lipophilic properties.[48,49]

Hypertension is common occurrence during emergence and the early postoperative period, occurring in 25% of hypertensive patients. Hypertension increases myocardial workload and creates significant stress on the vascular anastomoses. Nicardipine is very effective in controlling perioperative hypertension. Nicardipine is a dihydropyridine calcium channel blocker with an onset of 5 to 15 minutes and duration of action of 4 to 6 hours. Bolus administration of 2.5 mg can be used to speed the onset of the antihypertensive effect. Typical infusion doses are 2.5 to 15 mg/h, but it is often administered at doses as high as 45 mg/h. It is particularly useful in patients at risk of myocardial ischemia in that it provides selective coronary vasodilation.[37]

REFERENCES

1. van Klei WA, Bryson GL, Yang H, Forster AJ. Effect of beta-blocker prescription on the incidence of postoperative myocardial infarction after hip and knee arthroplasty. *Anesthesiology*. 2009;111(4):717-724.
2. POISE Study Group,Devereaux PJ, Yang H, et al. Effects of extended-release metoprolol succinate in patients undergoing non-cardiac surgery (POISE trial): a randomised controlled trial. *Lancet*. 2008; 371(9627):1839-1847.
3. Lee TH, Marcantonio ER, Mangione CM, et al. Derivation and prospective validation of a simple index for prediction of cardiac risk of major noncardiac surgery. *Circulation*. 1999;00(10):1043-1049.
4. Dunkelgrun M, Boersma E, Schouten O, et al. Bisoprolol and fluvastatin for the reduction of perioperative cardiac mortality and myocardial infarction in intermediate-risk patients undergoing noncardiovascular surgery: a randomized controlled trial (DECREASE-IV). *Ann Surg*. 2009;249(6):921-926.
5. Le Manach Y, Godet G, Coriat P, et al. The impact of postoperative discontinuation or continuation of chronic statin therapy on cardiac outcome after major vascular surgery. *Anesth Analg*. 2007;104(6):1326-1333.
6. Kertai MD, Boersma E, Westerhout CM. A combination of statins and beta-blockers is independently associated with a reduction in the incidence of perioperative mortality and nonfatal myocardial infarction in patients undergoing abdominal aortic aneurysm surgery. *J Vasc Surg*. 2005;41(2):370.
7. Schouten O, Hoeks SE, Welten GM, et al. Effect of statin withdrawal on frequency of cardiac events after vascular surgery. *Am J Cardiol*. 2007;100(2):316-320.
8. Nishimori M, Ballantyne JC, Low JH. Epidural pain relief versus systemic opioid-based pain relief for abdominal aortic surgery. *Cochrane Database Syst Rev*. 2006;3:CD005059.
9. Horlocker TT, Wedel DJ, Rowlingson JC, et al. Regional anesthesia in the patient receiving antithrombotic or thrombolytic therapy: American Society of Regional Anesthesia and Pain Medicine Evidence-Based Guidelines (3rd Edition). *Reg Anesth Pain Med*. 2010;35(1):64-101.
10. Eames WO, Rooke GA, Wu RS, Bishop MJ. Comparison of the effects of etomidate, propofol, and thiopental on respiratory resistance after tracheal intubation. *Anesthesiology*. 1996;84(6):1307-1311.
11. Smith I, White PF, Nathanson M, Gouldson R. Propofol. An update on its clinical use. *Anesthesiology*. 1994;81(4):1005-1043.
12. Masaki Y, Tanaka M, Nishikawa T. Physicochemical compatibility of propofol-lidocaine mixture. *Anesth Analg*. 2003;97(6):1646-1651.
13. Lowenthal DT, Porter RS, Saris SD, Bies CM, Slegowski MB, Staudacher A. Clinical pharmacology, pharmacodynamics and interactions with esmolol. *Am J Cardiol*. 1985;56(11):14F-18F.
14. Singh H, Vichitvejpaisal P, Gaines GY, White PF. Comparative effects of lidocaine, esmolol, and nitroglycerin in modifying the hemodynamic response to laryngoscopy and intubation. *J Clin Anesth*. 19957(1): 5-8.
15. Feng CK, Chan KH, Liu KN, Or CH, Lee TY. A comparison of lidocaine, fentanyl, and esmolol for attenuation of cardiovascular response to laryngoscopy and tracheal intubation. *Acta Anaesthesiol Sin*. 1996;34(2):61-67.
16. Johansen JW, Flaishon R, Sebel PS., Esmolol reduces anesthetic requirement for skin incision during propofol/nitrous oxide/morphine anesthesia. *Anesthesiology*. 1997;86(2):364-371.
17. Lund-Johansen P. Pharmacology of combined alpha-beta-blockade. II. Haemodynamic effects of labetalol. Drugs. 1984;28 (suppl 2):35-50.
18. Singh SP, Quadir A, Malhotra P. Comparison of esmolol and labetalol, in low doses, for attenuation of sympathomimetic response to laryngoscopy and intubation. *Saudi J Anaesth*. 2010;4(3):163-168.

19. Daniel M, Weiskopf RB, Noorani M, Eger EI II. Fentanyl augments the blockade of the sympathetic response to incision (MAC-BAR) produced by desflurane and isoflurane: desflurane and isoflurane MAC-BAR without and with fentanyl. *Anesthesiology.* 1998;88(1):43-49.
20. Kehl F, Krolikowski JG, Mraovic B, Pagel PS, Warltier DC, Kersten JR. Is isoflurane-induced preconditioning dose related? *Anesthesiology.* 2002;96(3):675-680.
21. Ryan SM, Nielsen CJ. Global warming potential of inhaled anesthetics: application to clinical use. *Anesth Analg.* 2010;111(1):92-98.
22. Norris EJ, Beattie C, Perler BA, et al. Double-masked randomized trial comparing alternate combinations of intraoperative anesthesia and postoperative analgesia in abdominal aortic surgery. *Anesthesiology.* 2001;95(5):1054-1067.
23. Carlisle JB, Stevenson CA. Drugs for preventing postoperative nausea and vomiting. *Cochrane Database Syst Rev.* 2006;3:CD004125.
24. Wu JI, Lu SF, Chia YY, Yang LC, Fong WP, Tan PH. Sevoflurane with or without antiemetic prophylaxis of dexamethasone in spontaneously breathing patients undergoing outpatient anorectal surgery. *J Clin Anesth.* 2009;21(7):469-473.
25. Fujii Y, Itakura M. Reduction of postoperative nausea, vomiting, and analgesic requirement with dexamethasone for patients undergoing laparoscopic cholecystectomy. *Surg Endosc.* 2010;24(3):692-696.
26. Cowie BS, Allen KJ, Said SA, Inder WJ. Anti-emetic doses of dexamethasone suppress cortisol response in laparoscopic cholecystectomy. *Anaesth Intensive Care.* 2010;38(4):667-670.
27. Corcoran TB, Truyens EB, Ng A, Moseley N, Doyle AC, Margetts L. Anti-emetic dexamethasone and postoperative infection risk: a retrospective cohort study. *Anaesth Intensive Care.* 2010;38(4):654-660.
28. Percival VG, Riddell J, Corcoran TB. Single dose dexamethasone for postoperative nausea and vomiting–a matched case-control study of postoperative infection risk. *Anaesth Intensive Care.* 2010;38(4):661-666.
29. Jakobsson J. Preoperative single-dose intravenous dexamethasone during ambulatory surgery: update around the benefit versus risk. *Curr Opin Anaesthesiol.* 2010;23(6):682-686.
30. Gelman S. The pathophysiology of aortic cross-clamping and unclamping. *Anesthesiology.* 1995;82(4): 1026-1060.
31. Landoni G, Biondi-Zoccai GG, Marino G, et al. Fenoldopam reduces the need for renal replacement therapy and in-hospital death in cardiovascular surgery: a meta-analysis. *J Cardiothorac Vasc Anesth.* 2008;22(1):27-33.
32. Mathur VS, Swan SK, Lambrecht LJ, et al. The effects of fenoldopam, a selective dopamine receptor agonist, on systemic and renal hemodynamics in normotensive subjects. *Crit Care Med.* 1999;27(9):1832-1837.
33. Meco M, Cirri S. The effect of various fenoldopam doses on renal perfusion in patients undergoing cardiac surgery. *Ann Thorac Surg.* 2010;89(2):497-503.
34. Gilbert TB, Hasnain JU, Flinn WR, Lilly MP, Benjamin ME. Fenoldopam infusion associated with preserving renal function after aortic cross-clamping for aneurysm repair. *J Cardiovasc Pharmacol Ther.* 2001;6(1):31-36.
35. Halpenny M, Rushe C, Breen P, Cunningham AJ, Boucher-Hayes D, Shorten GD. The effects of fenoldopam on renal function in patients undergoing elective aortic surgery. *Eur J Anaesth.* 2002;19(1):32-39.
36. Landoni G, Biondi-Zoccai GG, Tumlin JA, et al. Beneficial impact of fenoldopam in critically ill patients with or at risk for acute renal failure: a meta-analysis of randomized clinical trials. *Am J Kidney Dis.* 2007;49(1):56-68.
37. Varon J, Marik PE. Perioperative hypertension management. *Vasc Health Risk Manag.* 2008;4(3): 615-627.
38. Hersey P, Poullis M. Does the administration of mannitol prevent renal failure in open abdominal aortic aneurysm surgery? *Interact Cardiovasc Thorac Surg.* 2008;7(5):906-909.
39. Kellum JA. The use of diuretics and dopamine in acute renal failure: a systematic review of the evidence. *Crit Care.* 1997;1(2):53-59.
40. Lassnigg A, Donner E, Grubhofer G, Presterl E, Druml W, Hiesmayr M. Lack of renoprotective effects of dopamine and furosemide during cardiac surgery. *J Am Soc Nephrol.* 2000;11(1):97-104.
41. Kellum JA, M Decker J. Use of dopamine in acute renal failure: a meta-analysis. *Crit Care Med.* 2001; 29(8):1526-1531.
42. Marik PE, Iglesias J. Low-dose dopamine does not prevent acute renal failure in patients with septic shock and oliguria. NORASEPT II Study Investigators. *Am J Med.* 1999;107(4):387-390.
43. MacGregor DA, Smith TE, Prielipp RC, Butterworth JF, James RL, Scuderi PE. Pharmacokinetics of dopamine in healthy male subjects. *Anesthesiology.* 2000;92(2):338-346.
44. Dorman BH, Elliott BM, Spinale FG, et al. Protamine use during peripheral vascular surgery: a prospective randomized trial. *J Vasc Surg.* 1995;22(3): 248-256.
45. Chinien G, Waltham M, Abisi S, Smith A, Taylor P, Burnand KG. Systemic administration of heparin

intraoperatively in patients undergoing open repair of leaking abdominal aortic aneurysm may be beneficial and does not cause problems. *Vascular*. 2008;16(4): 189-193.

46. Flacke JW, Bloor BC, Kripke BJ, et al. Comparison of morphine, meperidine, fentanyl, and sufentanil in balanced anesthesia: a double-blind study. *Anesth Analg*. 1985;64(9):897-910.
47. Egan TD, Lemmens HJ, Fiset P, et al. The pharmacokinetics of the new short-acting opioid remifentanil (GI87084B) in healthy adult male volunteers. *Anesthesiology*. 1993;79(5):881-892.
48. Hudson RJ, Bergstrom RG, Thomson IR, Sabourin MA, Rosenbloom M, Strunin L. Pharmacokinetics of sufentanil in patients undergoing abdominal aortic surgery. *Anesthesiology*. 1989;70(3):426-431.
49. Schwartz AE, Matteo RS, Ornstein E, Young WL, Myers KJ. Pharmacokinetics of sufentanil in obese patients. *Anesth Analg*. 1991;73(6):790-793.

CHAPTER

33

Anesthetic Considerations for Liver Transplant

Charles Galaviz, MD

OVERVIEW OF LIVER FUNCTION

The liver plays a wide variety of roles in the overall scheme of the normal physiology of the body. The liver is involved in many aspects of metabolism, such as (1) lipid metabolism through fatty acid synthesis and lipoprotein conversion and (2) carbohydrate metabolism via glycogen storage, release. It is also the site of gluconeogenesis and amino acid metabolism. The liver is involved in synthesis of important proteins such as albumin and some of the coagulation factors. It also plays a role in immune system response, filtering out toxins and bacteria from the gastrointestinal tract, as well as amplifying the immune response via immune cells present in the liver. In addition, the liver is involved in endocrine control, via synthesis and secretion of hormones such as insulin-like growth factor 1 and angiotensinogen, as well as through inactivation of hormones such as insulin and corticosteroids. The liver also plays a major role in the coagulation system via synthesis of proclotting and anticlotting factors. Finally, it functions in modulating blood volume, acting as a reservoir for blood volume that can then be released into the bloodstream when stimulated by the sympathetic nervous system.[1]

CIRRHOSIS OF THE LIVER

Because of the liver's central role in normal physiology, when the liver fails, there are wide-ranging effects on other organ systems. The degree of secondary involvement can alter dosing strategies and also influences the approach to certain parts of anesthetic use. Notable organs or organ systems at risk for secondary impairment due to liver failure are the cardiovascular system, brain, lungs, kidneys, gastrointestinal system, endocrine, immune system, and bone marrow. Liver transplant is the only definitive treatment for end-stage liver disease.[2,3]

The cardiovascular manifestations are arteriolar vasodilation and increased cardiac output, characterized as a hyperdynamic state due to decreased metabolism of vasoactive substances. Brain manifestations are the result of accumulation of toxic metabolites and can lead to hepatic encephalopathy and increased intracranial pressure. Possible pulmonary manifestations are restrictive lung disease, intrapulmonary shunts, pulmonary hypertension, and ventilation–perfusion mismatch, and hypoxemia in the absence of ascites or intrinsic lung disease (hepatopulmonary syndrome). The kidneys can fail in patients with end-stage renal disease without a primary cause of renal disease, known as hepatorenal syndrome. Common gastrointestinal manifestations are ascites, esophageal varices, portal hypertension, and delayed gastric emptying. Hematologic effects are anemia due to malnutrition, chronic disease, or bleeding, and coagulopathy due to platelet defects (number of platelets, function of platelets, or both), decreased number of clotting factors, decreased clearance of activated factors, and hyperfibrinolysis.[3]

The Child-Turcotte-Pugh (CTP) scoring system is commonly used to grade the severity of liver disease and life expectancy at 1 and 2 years. The CTP classification includes 5 factors: ascites, level of encephalopathy, prothrombin time, plasma bilirubin level, and serum albumin level (Pugh's modification of the original scoring system replaced nutritional status with prothrombin time). The severity of each variable is assessed, and based on the total score patients are placed into class A (minimal), B (moderate), or C (advanced) disease.[2,4] Although the CTP class offers an assessment of severity of liver disease, it offers only minimal guidance on how to adjust drug dosing in liver disease because it does not address the specific ability of the liver to metabolize individual drugs.[5]

CTP was initially used in allocation of organs for transplant but has been supplanted by the model for end-stage liver disease (MELD) score. The MELD score offers an estimate of 3-month mortality, making it more useful in identifying liver transplant recipients. The MELD score is calculated from serum creatinine and bilirubin concentrations and the international normalized ratio (INR). The higher the MELD score, the more severe the underlying liver disease.[4] MELD scores less than 20 indicate a low 30-day mortality (less than 6%). MELD scores above 20, 30, and 40 indicate approximately a 20%, 50%, and 70% 30-day mortality, respectively. Like the CTP score, the MELD score offers minimal guidance on how to adjust an anesthetic for patients with liver disease.

HEPATIC DRUG CLEARANCE

Decreased liver function can substantially alter the behavior of several anesthetic drugs. Changes may be due to alteration in drug pharmacokinetics, drug pharmacodynamics, or both. How these changes affect the onset and duration of effect for anesthetic drugs is not well defined but worth considering when formulating a dosing regimen in patients undergoing a liver transplant.[6] In general, anesthetics metabolized by the liver can have a prolonged effect, especially if administered as a continuous infusion, and will require lower infusion rates. For bolus-dose administration, careful titration is recommended to achieve anesthetic goals of unresponsiveness, analgesia, and muscle relaxation. In otherwise healthy individuals, conventional dosing schemes are often adequate. Unfortunately, guidelines that indicate how doses should be adjusted in the setting of liver failure based on liver function scores do not exist.

For drugs that are metabolized by the liver, *clearance is a function of liver blood flow and intrinsic clearance.* These processes are quantified using the *hepatic extraction ratio,* defined as the rate of drug removal divided by the rate of drug delivery to the liver.

Intrinsic clearance refers to the ability of the liver to extract a drug independent of blood flow or protein binding. Each drug has its own intrinsic clearance; it can be low, intermediate, or high. Drugs with a low intrinsic clearance typically have a low extraction ratio (ie, the rate of drug's entering and exiting the liver are nearly the same). Drugs with a high intrinsic clearance typically have a high extraction ratio (ie, the rate of drug's leaving the liver is much lower than the rate of drug's entering the liver). Doubling the intrinsic clearance of a drug with a low intrinsic clearance will lead to an almost proportional change in extraction and thus clearance. However, if a drug has a high intrinsic clearance, doubling the intrinsic clearance will have little effect on drug clearance or extraction ratio.[6]

The effect of hepatic blood flow changes on the extraction ratio is also dependent on intrinsic clearance. In general, the extraction ratio is inversely proportional to hepatic blood flow. Decreasing hepatic blood flow leads to a relatively small increase in the extraction ratio for drugs with a high intrinsic clearance and a larger increase in the extraction ratio for drugs with a low intrinsic clearance. The effects of changes in flow on hepatic clearance are compensated by an opposing trend in extraction for drugs with small intrinsic clearance values, and their clearance is essentially independent of blood flow. If a drug has a high intrinsic clearance and extraction, hepatic clearance is essentially determined by the delivery of drug to the liver, and changes in the hepatic blood flow will lead to proportional changes in clearance.[6]

THE EFFECT OF LIVER FAILURE ON PHARMACOKINETICS AND PHARMACODYNAMICS

The liver plays a central role in drug metabolism. Hepatic dysfunction affects drug pharmacokinetics by a variety of possible mechanisms. One mechanism is reduced oxidation and reduction of anesthetic drugs via hepatocyte microsomal enzymes in damaged liver tissue. A second mechanism is reduced biliary excretion. Conjugated drugs are delivered via biliary excretion back to the gastrointestinal tract for reabsorption, eventually leading

TABLE 33–1 Drugs of interest that are substrates for selected hepatocyte microsomal enzymes of the cytochrome P450 (CYP) system.

1A2	2B6	2C19	2D6	2E1	3A4 3A5 3A7
Ondansetron	Methadone	Lansoprazole	Lidocaine	Enflurane	Alprazolam
Ropivacaine		Omeprazole	Ondansetron	Halothane	Diazepam
Cyclobenzaprine		Pantoprazole	Promethazine	Isoflurane	Midazolam
		Rabeprazole		Methoxyflurane	Triazolam
		Diazepam		Sevoflurane	Alfentanil
		Phenytoin			Fentanyl
					Cocaine

Microsomal enzymes CYP2C8 and 2C9 do not have substrates that are significant from an anesthetic standpoint.

Data from Lockhart DA: Drug Interactions: Cytochrome P450 Drug Interaction table. Indiana University; 2007.

to reduced renal excretion. A third mechanism is a function of liver production of plasma proteins. A reduction in plasma proteins can increase the free fraction of drug, allowing more of it to be eliminated (ie, some drugs may pass through the glomerular apparatus when unbound to protein but remain in the blood when bound). Portosystemic shunting, which occurs in varying degrees depending on the blood pressure required to perfuse a diseased liver, will decrease the presystemic elimination of orally administered drugs (ie, the first-pass effect), leading to an increase in bioavailability.[1,5]

Metabolic pathways are differentially affected in liver dysfunction. In early cirrhosis, drug glucuronidation is spared relative to oxidative metabolism. In advanced cirrhosis, drug glucuronidation may also be substantially impaired. Liver dysfunction can also affect the clearance of drugs or active metabolites that are normally cleared by the kidney. Even moderate degrees of hepatic impairment lead to a decrease in clearance of drugs normally cleared by the kidney.[7] Table 33–1 lists common drugs in anesthesia that undergo oxidative metabolism via the cytochrome enzyme system; as liver function worsens, it may be necessary to consider lowering the dose of these drugs.[8]

There are a couple of potentially important pharmacodynamic alterations in patients with cirrhosis. One, with rising plasma ammonia levels and brain swelling, there can be an increased sensitivity to sedative drugs. Two, there may also be a decrease in sensitivity to catecholamines and other vasoconstrictors.[1]

LIVER TRANSPLANTATION SURGERY

The goal of a liver transplant surgery is to remove the diseased native organ and replace it with a functioning liver. There are many factors that affect graft function, such as the ischemia time (warm and cold), steatosis of the donor liver, and age of the donor. Assuming an uneventful transplant, the donor liver should begin functioning prior to the end of the surgery. Signs of liver graft function are bile production, correction of coagulopathy without transfusion directed at correcting it, decreasing lactate level, and a rise in core temperature.[3,9]

There are 3 main phases to a liver transplant surgery: preanhepatic, anhepatic, and reperfusion. Each phase has unique challenges. Communication between surgical and anesthesia teams is critical because the surgical technique, particularly during the preanhepatic phase, will influence anesthetic management.

Preanhepatic Phase

The preanhepatic phase starts at the time of surgical incision and ends with the clamping of the liver blood supply. The surgical goals of this phase are to devascularize the liver by ligating and dividing the hepatic artery and portal vein and to mobilize the suprahepatic and infrahepatic inferior vena cava to enable hepatectomy.[9] Major challenges during this phase are hemorrhage, coagulopathy, citrate toxicity, hypothermia, acidosis, and electrolyte abnormalities. The amount of bleeding is influenced by the magnitude of preexisting coagulopathy, severity of portal hypertension, and whether the patient has had previous abdominal surgeries. Coagulopathy is usually due to deficiencies of plasma clotting factors manufactured by the liver. Citrate is used as an anticoagulant when storing red blood cells. When transfused, the liver quickly metabolizes the citrate. Citrate toxicity occurs when large volumes of stored red blood cell units are rapidly transfused or when the liver is unable to metabolize the citrate. Unmetabolized citrate causes hypocalcemia and hypomagnesemia, leading to a coagulopathy or myocardial depression. Hypothermia is common during liver transplant surgery due to prolonged large abdominal exposure. Strategies for rewarming are necessary. Hyponatremia and hypokalemia are common but do not require aggressive treatment. Plasma sodium levels may rise later in the procedure when normal saline and sodium bicarbonate are used. Plasma potassium levels may rise during liver reperfusion. Thus, treating hypokalemia during the preanhepatic phase is usually not advisable.[3,9]

Anhepatic Phase

The anhepatic phase begins with the clamping of the blood vessels to the native liver and ends when the newly anastomosed blood vessels of the graft liver to the recipient's native vasculature are reperfused. The surgical technique is important, because the hemodynamic response to the clamps is influenced by the technique. In the classical technique, both the suprahepatic and infrahepatic vena cava are clamped, leading to a drop in venous return of up to 50%. In the piggyback technique, inferior vena cava flow is preserved, leading to a smaller drop of venous return. If the classical technique is chosen, fluid management is guided by volume loading in preparation for the drop in venous return, whereas in the piggyback technique, volume loading is not performed and is undesirable. Massive bleeding is uncommon during the anhepatic phase due to isolation of the blood supply to the liver; however, fibrinolysis will occur during this phase due to a lack of liver produced inhibitor of plasminogen activation. Lactate levels will also rise during the anhepatic phase, as the liver is no longer metabolizing any lactate.[3,9]

Reperfusion Phase

The reperfusion phase begins with restoration of blood flow through the portal vein to the new liver. It is associated with abrupt decrease in systemic vascular resistance, increase in preload, increase in hydrogen ion concentration, and increase in potassium level. As such, major challenges during the reperfusion phase are hyperkalemia, dysrhythmias, hemodynamic instability with or without bleeding, and acidosis. Hyperkalemia can be life threatening, and careful observation of the electrocardiogram for changes consistent with hyperkalemia is important. Treatment includes calcium chloride, sodium bicarbonate, insulin, and albuterol. Reperfusion syndrome is defined as systemic hypotension and pulmonary hypertension in the period immediately following reperfusion (within the first 5 minutes). Many factors may influence this, including hyperkalemia, acidosis, hypothermia, or thrombi. Assuming no problems during the initial reperfusion or the successful treatment of any problems that arise, the surgery is completed with the arterial anastomoses and reconstructing the biliary tree.[3,9] A summary of clinical considerations during liver transplant surgery is presented in Table 33–2.

DRUG DISPOSITION DURING LIVER TRANSPLANT SURGERY

Anticipated liver function during each phase of a liver transplant provides an approximate guide for dosing adjustments. During the preanhepatic phase the liver is diseased, and anesthetic drugs metabolized by the liver may need to have their doses reduced to minimize prolonged effect, but conventional doses are often well tolerated. During the

TABLE 33–2 Clinical considerations during liver transplant surgery.

Preanhepatic phase	
Bleeding[a]	Risk increased if coagulopathy severe or patient technically difficult from surgical perspective Treated with transfusion
Coagulopathy[a]	Severity depends on degree of underlying liver dysfunction Treated with transfusion of blood components targeted at the area of deficiency Fresh-frozen plasma most common, followed by platelets and cryoprecipitate
Citrate toxicity[a]	Citrate in PRBC units metabolized by liver Extent of toxicity based on degree of underlying liver dysfunction and amount and rate of PRBC units transfused Treated with calcium May minimize by use of red cell salvage suction (minimizes need for units stored in citrate).
Hypothermia	Large surgical exposure facilitates heat loss
Hypokalemia	Aggressive treatment not necessary Transfusion of PRBC and donor liver reperfusion will raise potassium levels
Hyponatremia	Aggressive treatment not necessary
Anhepatic phase	
Lactic acidosis	Liver metabolizes lactate Lactate levels will rise during anhepatic phase
Fibrinolysis	Liver makes fibrinolysis inhibitor Anticipate fibrinolysis during anhepatic phase
Hypothermia	Large surgical exposure Donor organ is commonly stored on ice and not rewarmed prior to transplantation
Reperfusion phase	
Dysrhythmias[a]	Anticipate during immediate reperfusion period
Reperfusion syndrome[a]	During first 5 minutes of reperfusion, anticipate Pulmonary hypertension Cardiovascular instability
Hyperkalemia[a]	Donor liver is stored in potassium-rich solution Much of this solution flushed from the liver prior to reperfusion Some potassium may still remain
Hypothermia	Cold preservative in donor liver joins central circulation upon reperfusion
Acidosis	Accumulated acid metabolites join central circulation

[a]May require prompt treatment.
PRBC, packed red blood cells.

anhepatic phase, there is no liver function, so dosing adjustments may be required, especially for continuous infusions. A lower infusion rate is sufficient to achieve the desired drug effect. During reperfusion, assuming normal liver function, the donor liver will begin to metabolize drugs, and continuous infusions may need to be increased to achieve desired drug effects. A prolonged duration of action of vecuronium or rocuronium is an indicator of an abnormally functioning graft.[10-12] Suggested dosing adjustments are summarized in Table 33–3.

TABLE 33–3 Suggested anesthetic dosing adjustments for liver transplant surgery.

Premedicants	
Benzodiazepines	Reduced or none at all for severe disease or presence of encephalopathy
Opioids	Reduced; may have exaggerated respiratory depression
Induction medications	
Propofol	No reduction
Etomidate	No reduction
Opioids	No reduction; risk of respiratory depression is less concerning given imminent endotracheal intubation
Succinylcholine	No reduction
Rocuronium	No reduction
Maintenance medications	
Inhalational anesthetics	Consider reduced dose for MELD score > 20[13]
Opioids	No reduction
Neuromuscular blockers	Consider reduced dose prior to reperfusion

MELD, model for end-stage liver disease.

CASE DISCUSSION

A 51-year-old, 95-kg, 179-cm male with cirrhosis of the liver secondary to hepatitis C is scheduled to undergo an orthotopic liver transplant. His MELD score is 25, which indicates severe disease.

PREMEDICANTS

Consider the following as needed

- **Nonparticulate antacid:** Sodium citrate by mouth
- **Antacid:** Intravenous famotidine
- **Anxiolytic:** None

Sample Dosing Regimen: Famotidine and Sodium Citrate

- **Antacids:** Intravenous famotidine 20 mg 30 minutes prior to induction. Oral sodium citrate 30 mL should be given 5 to 15 minutes prior to induction.

Clinical Pharmacology

- **Antacids:** Famotidine undergoes minimal metabolism by the liver. Similarly, sodium citrate does not have a mechanism of action or properties that are affected by liver dysfunction.
- **Anxiolytic:** It is recommended to avoid midazolam, a common anxiolytic, because it has a prolonged duration of action in patients with diseased livers.[14] A benzodiazepine-like ligand not present in normal brain has been suggested as a factor in development of hepatic encephalopathy.[15]

INDUCTION

A rapid-sequence technique using one of the following sedative–hypnotics and muscle relaxants is appropriate.

- **Sedation and hypnosis:** Propofol or etomidate
- **Muscle relaxation:** Succinylcholine, rocuronium, or vecuronium

Sample Dosing Regimen: Propofol and Succinylcholine

- **Induction agent:** Propofol 1.5 to 2 mg/kg
- **Muscle relaxant:** Succinylcholine 1 mg/kg immediately following the propofol. Rocuronium 0.6 mg/kg can be used as an alternative to succinylcholine in these cases,[12] and some experienced centers will use vecuronium 0.1 mg/kg.[16]

Dosing Considerations

- A rapid-sequence induction is the most common induction technique. There are multiple reasons to assume a full stomach;

patients do not have advance warning of when an organ will be available and may not be nothing by mouth (NPO), and ascites can lead to abnormal gastric emptying.

- The choice of propofol or etomidate will be guided by clinician judgment based on the patient's preoperative status. Etomidate 0.2 mg/kg can be substituted for propofol in patients who are cardiovascularly unstable.

MAINTENANCE OF ANESTHESIA

Consider using a combined inhalation/intravenous agent or total intravenous anesthesia technique with the following drugs. Also listed below are other intravenous therapies that are commonly used during maintenance of general anesthesia.

- **Sedation and hypnosis:** Isoflurane, sevoflurane, desflurane, or propofol infusion
- **Analgesia:** Fentanyl, sufentanil, remifentanil, morphine, or hydromorphone
- **Muscle relaxation:** Cisatracurium, rocuronium, or vecuronium
- **Vasopressor support:** Epinephrine, norepinephrine, or vasopressin
- **Acid–base management:** Sodium bicarbonate
- **Electrolyte correction:** Calcium chloride, insulin, or dextrose

Sample Dosing Regimen: Isoflurane, Fentanyl, Vecuronium

- **Sedative–Hypnotic:** Following induction, isoflurane 0.6 to 1.4 vol% mixed with oxygen is titrated to maintain unconsciousness. Under steady-state conditions, end-tidal isoflurane concentrations can estimate effect-site concentrations. Desflurane and sevoflurane can be substituted for isoflurane; however, isoflurane is often chosen because it has the least detrimental effect on liver blood flow.
- **Analgesic:** Additional fentanyl boluses of 1 to 2 mcg/kg, or an infusion of 1 to 3 mcg/kg/h, are used to deepen anesthetic level in response to changes in intraoperative stimuli.
- **Muscle relaxant:** Vecuronium 0.1 mg/kg is administered at periodic intervals to maintain a train-of-four twitch response of 1/4. Alternatively, rocuronium or cisatracurium can be used, with dosing titrated to the same twitch response. Neuromuscular blocker infusions are another alternate choice (eg, vecuronium with a starting dose of 0.1 mg/kg/h, titrated to desired effect).[17]
- **Vasopressor support:** Norepinephrine infusion 0.05 mcg/kg/min starting dose, titrated to effect (mean blood pressure > 60 mm Hg). An intravenous vasopressin bolus of 1 to 5 U or an infusion can be added to supplement norepinephrine to keep the mean blood pressure greater than 60 mm Hg. Epinephrine infusion, starting dose 0.02 mcg/kg/min, titrated to effect (maintain cardiac output > 5 L/min).[18]
- **Acid–base management:** Sodium bicarbonate infusion or boluses are used to correct base deficit; the dose is selected based on magnitude of correction needed.[18] When administering sodium bica rbonate, caution should be used as it is a hypertonic solution (high sodium content) and may lead to paradoxical intracellular acidosis if ventilation is inadequate.
- **Electrolyte correction:** Calcium chloride is used to maintain normocalcemia, with the dose being chosen based on magnitude of correction needed.[18] Severe hyperkalemia, if encountered on reperfusion, is treated with insulin 5 to 10 U, dextrose, and calcium chloride.[19]

Clinical Pharmacology

- Liver failure has a minimal effect on termination of effect of inhaled anesthetics. Cardiac output, alveolar ventilation, and fresh gas flow have a much greater effect on termination of effect than liver function. Dose may need to be modified based on severity of underlying liver disease.[13]

- If intravenous infusions are being used to maintain portions of the anesthetic, they will likely need to be titrated carefully to clinical effect. Multiple studies have shown that during the anhepatic phase concentrations of drugs that have liver involvement in metabolism and clearance increase.[17,20] If infusions are turned down during this phase, they will likely need to be titrated up to maintain the same clinical effect during the reperfusion phase as the new liver begins to function.
- Prolonged response to standard dosing of vecuronium or rocuronium during the reperfusion phase strongly correlates to primary graft dysfunction.[11,12]

EMERGENCE

Goals for emergence hinge on the following question: is the patient going to be extubated? Guidelines exist for assisting in this decision; the safe operating room extubation after liver transplant (SORELT) score is one such guideline.[21] If the decision is made to extubate the patient, the anesthetic plan will include a timely return to consciousness, adequate analgesia, avoidance of respiratory depression, and avoidance of nausea. If the patient is unable to be extubated, the plan will include adequate sedation during transport to the intensive care unit.

- **Analgesia:** Fentanyl, morphine, or hydromorphone
- **Rescue antiemetics:** Ondansetron or dolasetron

Sample Dosing Regimen (Assuming Planned Extubation): Fentanyl, Ondansetron

- **Transition opioid:** As the patient regains respiratory function, additional fentanyl boluses of 0.5 to 1 mcg/kg can be given and titrated to effect.
- **Rescue antiemetic:** Ondansetron 0.1 mg/kg, up to 4 mg can be administered if nausea is present.

REFERENCES

1. Kaufman BS, Roccaforte JD. Hepatic anatomy, function, and physiology. In: Barash PG, et al, eds. *Clinical Anesthesia*. 6th ed. Philadelphia: Lippincott Williams & Wilkins; 2009:1247-1278.
2. Wiklund RA. Preoperative preparation of patients with advanced liver disease. *Crit Care Med*. 2004;32(4 suppl):S106-S115.
3. Steadman RH. Anesthesia for liver transplant surgery. *Anesthesiol Clin North Am*. 2004;22(4):687-711.
4. Wiesner RH, McDiarmid SV, Kamath PS, et al. MELD and PELD: application of survival models to liver allocation. *Liver Transpl*. 2001;7(7):567-580.
5. Verbeeck RK. Pharmacokinetics and dosage adjustment in patients with hepatic dysfunction. *Eur J Clin Pharmacol*. 2008;64(12):1147-1161.
6. Wilkinson GR, Shand DG. Commentary: a physiological approach to hepatic drug clearance. *Clin Pharmacol Ther*. 1975;18(4):377-390.
7. Morgan, DJ, McLean AJ. Clinical pharmacokinetic and pharmacodynamic considerations in patients with liver disease. An update. *Clin Pharmacokinet*. 1995;29(5):370-391.
8. Flockhart DA. Drug interactions: cytochrome P450 drug interaction table. 2007; http://medicine.iupui.edu/clinpharm/ddis/table.asp. Accessed January 16, 2011.
9. Saggi BH, Farmer DG, Yersiz H, Busuttil RW. Surgical advances in liver and bowel transplantation. *Anesthesiol Clin North Am*. 2004;22(4):713-740.
10. Kelley SD, Cauldwell CB, Fisher DM, Lau M, Sharma ML, Weisiger RA. Recovery of hepatic drug extraction after hypothermic preservation. *Anesthesiology*. 1995;82(1):251-258.
11. Lukin CL, Hein HA, Swygert TH, et al. Duration of vecuronium-induced neuromuscular block as a predictor of liver allograft dysfunction. *Anesth Analg*. 1995;80(3):526-533.
12. Marcel RJ, Ramsay MA, Hein HA, et al. Duration of rocuronium-induced neuromuscular block during liver transplantation: a predictor of primary allograft function. *Anesth Analg*. 1997;84(4):870-874.
13. Kang JG, Ko JS, Kim GS, Gwak MS, Kim YR, Lee SK. The relationship between inhalational anesthetic requirements and the severity of liver disease in liver transplant recipients according to three phases of liver transplantation. *Transplant Proc*. 2010;42(3):854-857.
14. MacGilchrist AJ, Birnie GG, Cook A, et al. Pharmacokinetics and pharmacodynamics of intravenous midazolam in patients with severe alcoholic cirrhosis. *Gut*. 1986;27(2):190-195.

15. Riordan SM, Williams R. Treatment of hepatic encephalopathy. *N Engl J Med.* 1997;337(7):473-479.
16. Mandell MS, Stoner TJ, Barnett R, et al. A multicenter evaluation of safety of early extubation in liver transplant recipients. *Liver Transpl.* 2007;13(11):1557-1563.
17. O'Kelly B, Jayais P, Veroli P, Lhuissier C, Ecoffey C. Dose requirements of vecuronium, pancuronium, and atracurium during orthotopic liver transplantation. *Anesth Analg.* 1991;73(6):794-798.
18. Hannaman MJ, Hevesi ZG. Anesthesia care for liver transplantation. *Transplant Rev (Orlando).* 2011;25(1):36-43.
19. Prough DS, Funston JS, Svensen CH, Wolf SW. Fluids, electrolytes, and acid-base physiology. In: Barash PG, et al, eds. *Clinical Anesthesia.* 6th ed. Philadelphia: Lippincott Williams & Wilkins; 2009:290-325.
20. Takizawa D, Sato E, Hiraoka H, et al. Changes in apparent systemic clearance of propofol during transplantation of living related donor liver. *Br J Anaesth.* 2005;95(5):643-647.
21. Skurzak S, Stratta C, Schellino MM, et al. Extubation score in the operating room after liver transplantation. *Acta Anaesthesiol Scand.* 2010;54(8):970-978.

CHAPTER 34

Application of Pharmacokinetic and Pharmacodynamic Modeling to Guide Propofol Administration for Endoscopy Procedures

Jeff E. Mandel, MD, MS

INTRODUCTION

Sedation for endoscopy is a rapidly emerging endeavor in anesthesia. Growth in this area has been steady, and anesthesiologists are increasingly becoming involved in endoscopic sedation. Endoscopy is distinguished from other anesthetic challenges by 2 factors. First, these procedures are performed with natural airways, and excessive sedation may induce obstruction and respiratory depression. Second, the procedure time is short, and there is insufficient time to tune the anesthetic. These factors affect the anesthetic strategy. Anesthesiologists assume that the skills learned in the operating room transfer to the endoscopy suite, but a bolus of propofol sufficient for a 99% probability of obtunding response to intubation may exceed the total propofol requirement for a diagnostic esophagogastroduodenoscopy (EGD) several times and result in a prolonged period of jaw thrust to overcome obstruction. Conversely, starting a propofol infusion at the infusion rate for maintenance of loss of consciousness will take a considerable period of time to achieve this outcome. Target-controlled infusion (TCI) may achieve a specified effect-site concentration reliably, but the variability of patient response complicates the selection of the target.[1] Thus, in a relatively short encounter, anesthesiologists must pick the appropriate induction dose for deep sedation and from this infer the proper maintenance dose.

Experienced clinicians use a number of strategies, but these can be divided into 2 broad camps based on whether an infusion pump or a handheld syringe is employed in titration. This chapter will present 2 strategies that use a pharmacokinetic model of propofol with little more than a few bits of information, a watch, and a calculator. This model enables anesthesiologists to optimize sedation and analgesia for EGD procedures that rivals the performance of real-time optimal control algorithms. It is important to recognize that these techniques are not a substitute for years of experience or sophisticated monitoring technology. Rather, they represent an application of drug simulation at the point of care that permits a novice to consistently "hit the dartboard."

Simulations will be used to illustrate the 2 dosing strategies. These simulations will utilize a propofol 3-compartment pharmacokinetic model introduced by Cortinez et al.[2] This model permits consideration of increasing weight without the problems associated with the high body mass indices encountered in earlier models of propofol pharmacokinetics. The model parameters are included in Table 34–1.

Compartment volumes are scaled by weight/70 kg, and clearances by weight/70 kg raised to the

TABLE 34–1 Propofol pharmacokinetic parameters.

Volumes (L/70 kg)	$V1_{std}$	4.48
	$V2_{std}$	21.2
	$V3_{std}$	237
Clearances (L/min/70 kg)	$CL1_{std}$	1.92
	$Q2_{std}$	1.45
	$Q3_{std}$	0.86
Age correction	SL_{V2}	-0.0164
	SL_{Q2}	-0.0153

0.75 power (referred to as allometric scaling). Age corrections are applied to model parameters V2 and Q2, as indicated in Equations 34–1 and 34–2.

$$V2 = V2_{std} \times \frac{TBW}{70} \times e^{SL_{V2} \times (AGE - 50)} \quad (34\text{–}1)$$

$$CL2 = CL2_{std} \times \left(\frac{TBW}{70}\right)^{3/4} \times e^{SL_{CL2} \times (AGE - 50)} \quad (34\text{–}2)$$

where TBW is total body weight. An effect-site is adjoined, with ke_0 calculated to yield a time to peak effect of 1.6 minutes. Simulations will also use a pharmacodynamic model of loss of consciousness based on estimated propofol effect-site concentrations.[3] Unless otherwise stated, simulations throughout this chapter are for a 50-year-old, 70-kg patient undergoing an EGD.

In developing strategies to rapidly determine the appropriate depth of anesthesia for a given patient, several assumptions will be used:

1. A loading sequence (ie, a slow bolus or rapid propofol infusion) can be determined that will cause a smooth increment in the probability of achieving loss of consciousness that is similar across all patients.
2. If the rate of change in probability of loss of consciousness is low, it is possible to infer the patient's sensitivity from the time to loss of consciousness.
3. Given this estimate of sensitivity, a maintenance sequence (ie, either intermittent boluses or a continuous infusion) will be identified that will maintain the effect-site concentration associated with loss of consciousness for the short duration of the procedure.

For the purposes of this effort, we will define loss of consciousness as lack of response to verbal stimulus.

For each strategy, a control system is used to find the optimum solution to the titration sequence. This is done by defining a desired trajectory for the effect-site, as described in Technique One. The infusion sequence is then adjusted so that the predicted trajectory is as close to the specified trajectory as possible. This is done by repeatedly running the simulation with adjustments in the infusion sequence until the difference between the desired and predicted trajectories (termed the error) is as low as possible, perhaps even zero. This process requires seconds on a modern computer running specialized software, such as MATLAB. Although this is no obstacle to the author, to make the examples workable by the reader, the strategies have been restated as recipes that can be "scaled to the size of the dinner party."

TECHNIQUE ONE

The first strategy is a bolus technique suitable for a handheld syringe or a pump used in bolus mode (a patient-controlled anesthesia [PCA] pump such as the Graseby 3300 works well for this). It begins with an initial loading dose of propofol, typically 20 to 80 mg, followed by small fixed doses (one-fifth the loading dose) until adequate sedation is obtained, which is then repeated periodically to maintain adequate sedation. The advantage of this technique is that it can be performed with a schedule for boluses. A combined pharmacokinetic–pharmacodynamic model can be used to advise clinicians when to administer the boluses, as was previously reported.[4] Model predictions of effect-site concentrations, drug effect (in this case unresponsiveness), and suggested bolus dosing regimen are illustrated in Figure 34–1.

An initial bolus of 30 mg is administered over 10 seconds; subsequent 6-mg boluses are administered over 2 seconds. The interval between boluses

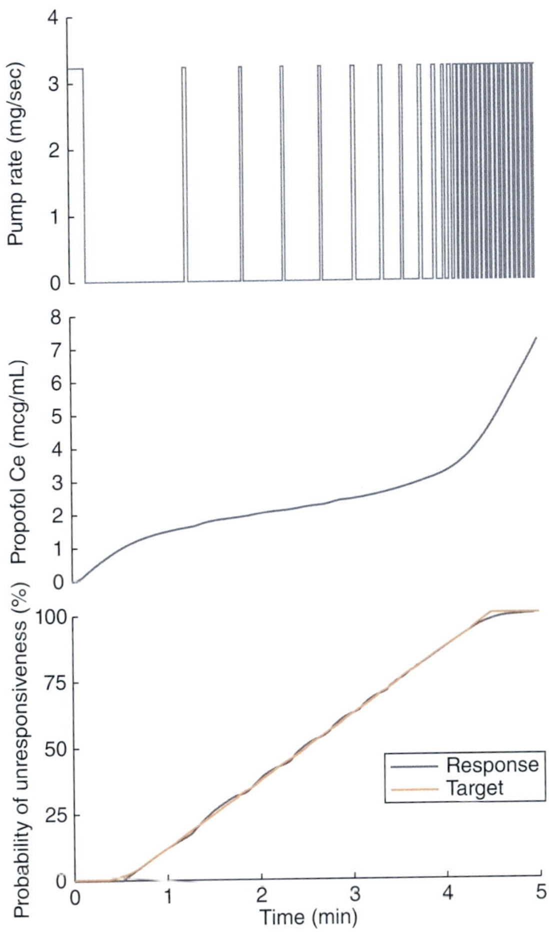

FIGURE 34–1 Propofol bolus dosing regimen (top plot), resultant predictions of propofol effect-site concentration (Ce) levels (middle plot), and probability of unresponsiveness (bottom plot) using intermittent small propofol boluses. The intermittent boluses are presented as burst from an infusion pump that delivers propofol at a rate of 3 mg/sec (1 mL every 3 seconds). The first bolus is for 10 seconds and subsequent boluses are for 2 seconds. The duration of time between boluses is progressively shorter (top plot).

decreases as a function of time, and the depth of anesthesia can be controlled by the period between boluses. To implement this strategy, all that is needed is a value for the loading dose and the schedule for bolusing. This dosing regimen can be implemented by following these steps:

1. Administer the loading dose.
2. Wait 72 seconds.
3. Administer the first incremental dose.
4. Wait 36 seconds.
5. For every subsequent incremental dose, decrease the waiting time by 5 seconds (to a minimum of 2 seconds).
6. Repeat until the patient loses consciousness up to a total of 20 incremental doses.

For the loading dose and 20 incremental doses, a total of 161 mg (2.3 mg/kg) is required for a 99% probability of loss of responsiveness within 5 minutes. There will be a few patients for whom this will be inadequate, but most patients will require less, and the average patient should be unresponsive by 3 minutes and 50 mg.

Once the dosing sequence to achieve loss of unconsciousness is identified, the bolus sequence that will maintain that effect-site concentration can be determined, as shown in Figure 34–2. With this technique, there is a slight overshoot because there was no way of knowing when a patient will lose consciousness—in this example, shortly after the third bolus. The bolus rate, however, rapidly stabilizes at a constant interval for the duration of the brief anesthetic, and is well approximated by a linear function of the time to loss of consciousness (T).

For maintenance, 3 more steps are added to the previous list.

7. When the patient loses consciousness, note the elapsed time T (in seconds) from start of the loading dose.
8. The bolus interval I is $78 - 0.1825 \times T$ (seconds).
9. After loss of consciousness, give the next bolus $1.25 \times I$ seconds after the preceding bolus.

To use this technique in clinical practice, a PCA pump can be programmed to deliver the appropriate bolus, and a computer can be programmed to beep every time a button press is needed. Although this method was not easy, it was successfully used to manage 25 patients undergoing colonoscopy.[4] It provides an appreciation of what can be accomplished using application of propofol pharmacokinetics to automatic control.

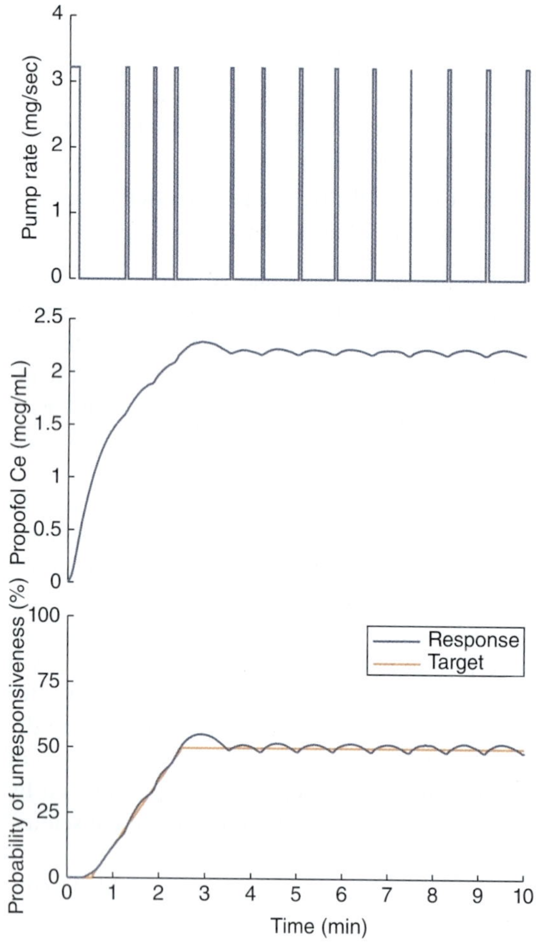

FIGURE 34–2 Propofol bolus dosing regimen to achieve and maintain unresponsiveness in a patient of average sensitivity. The top plot presents the bolus dosing regimen, the middle plot presents the predicted propofol effect-site concentration (Ce), and the bottom plot presents the predicted probability of unresponsiveness. In this example, the patient looses responsiveness at a 50% probability of unresponsiveness (ie, in a group of 100 patients, with this exact dosing regimen, 50 would be unresponsive and 50 would be responsive).

TECHNIQUE TWO

The second strategy uses a small propofol bolus followed by a large infusion to render a patient unconscious. Using a combined pharmacokinetic–pharmacodynamic model, the bolus dose and infusion rate are calculated with the goal of achieving a 50% probability of loss of consciousness in 140 seconds and a 90% probability of loss of consciousness at 360 seconds. For a 50-year-old, 70-kg patient, a bolus of 299 mcg/kg and infusion rate of 210 mcg/kg/min will achieve these target probabilities (50% and 90%) at the target times (140 and 360 seconds), as depicted in Figure 34–3.

Although this approach does not track a straight line as well as the bolus technique did, it does so with significantly less effort, and the algorithm is

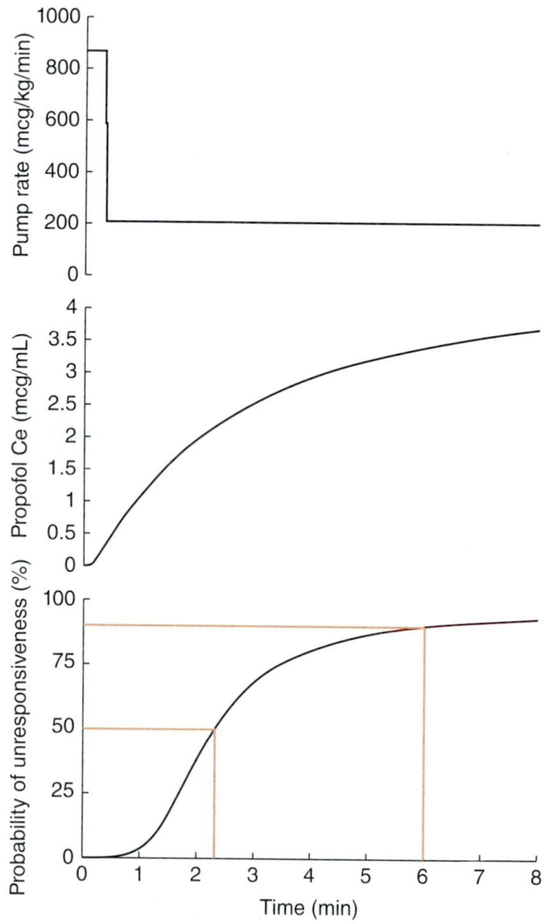

FIGURE 34–3 Propofol bolus and continuous infusion regimen to render a patient unresponsive. The top plot presents the bolus and continuous infusion dosing regimen, the middle plot presents the predicted propofol effect-site concentration (Ce), and the bottom plot presents the predicted probability of unresponsiveness. The gray lines represent the time at which a 50% and 90% probability of unresponsiveness will be attained in a 50-year-old, 70-kg patient.

much simpler. This second technique only specifies a bolus and an infusion rate rather than determining at what instant to administer 1 of 20 boluses as was described with the first technique, but the probability is constantly increasing and can be used to estimate patient sensitivity based on the duration of the infusion needed to lose consciousness. The author has used this approach to titrate propofol to an end point of moderate obstruction for diagnosis of sleep apnea.[5]

As with Technique One, by increasing the effect-site concentration smoothly, the infusion rate that maintains the effect-site concentration associated with loss of consciousness can be identified. The longer the infusion must run to achieve loss of consciousness, the higher the dose required to maintain this effect-site concentration. This relationship is closely approximated over a range of patient sensitivities by the following polynomial:

$$\textit{Maintenance rate} = -8.845 + 1.195 \cdot T_{Loc} - 0.003 \cdot T_{Loc}^{2} + 0.00000287 \cdot T_{Loc}^{3} \quad (34\text{–}3)$$

Where T_{LOC} is the time (in seconds) required for the patient to lose consciousness, and maintenance is given in mcg/kg/min for the 70-kg patient (Figure 34–4).

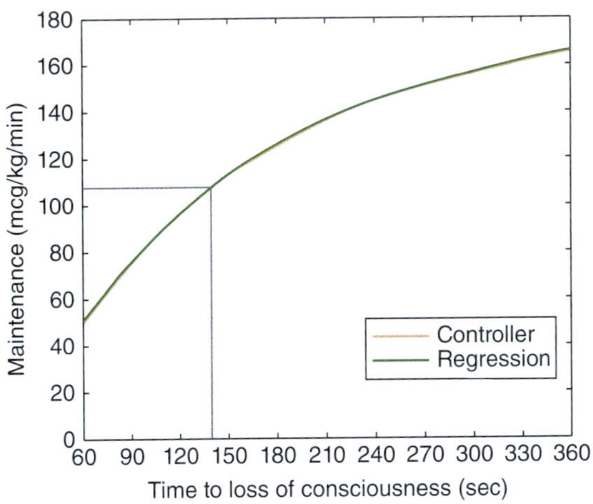

FIGURE 34–4 Predicted maintenance infusion rates (mcg/kg/min) based on the time (in seconds) required for loss of consciousness. The gray lines present a sample patient where the time to loss of consciousness was 140 seconds, indicating a maintenance infusion rate of 108 mcg/kg/min.

To implement this algorithm, the bolus and infusion values are programmed into the pump, and when loss of consciousness is observed, the time is used to determine the maintenance infusion, either graphically from Figure 34–4 or computationally from Equation 34–3. For a patient with average sensitivity (ie, the patient becomes unconscious at a propofol effect-site concentration associated with a 50% probability of loss of consciousness), the maintenance infusion of 108 mcg/kg/min starts when the patient loses consciousness at 140 seconds (Figure 34–5).

As with Technique One, there is some overshoot because the infusion rate cannot be lowered until the onset of loss of consciousness. However, the target probability of loss of consciousness (in this case 50%) is achieved within a few minutes. This approach works fairly reliably and is easily implemented in clinical practice.

ADJUSTING FOR AGE AND WEIGHT

For the first technique, the loading doses are presented in Table 34–2; the intermittent boluses are one-fifth of the loading dose. For example, a 45-year-old, 115-kg patient will have a propofol loading dose of 405 mcg/kg and intermittent boluses of 81 mcg/kg. These doses are given with the timing indicated in the recipe.

For the second technique, the initial propofol bolus and subsequent infusion (based on Equation 34–3) for a range of ages and weights is presented in Table 34–3. For a 75-year-old, 55-kg patient, the bolus is 251 mcg/kg and the infusion is 200 mcg/kg/min, while for a 25-year-old, 175-kg patient, the bolus is 431 mcg/kg and the infusion is 189 mcg/kg/min. The relationship between time to loss of consciousness and maintenance infusion rate varies with age and weight. This is depicted in Figure 34–6 for a range of ages (left part) and weights (right part)

All of these curves have similar shapes, and can be transformed from the standard 70-kg 50-year-old patient by a first order equation:

$$\textit{Maintenance}_{age,weight} = a_0 + a_1 \cdot \textit{Maintenance}_{50,70} \quad (34\text{–}4)$$

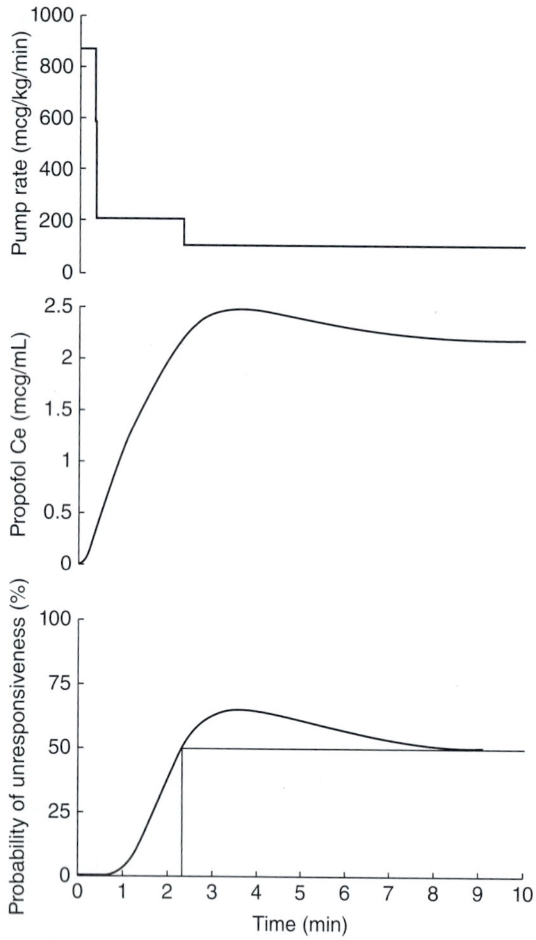

FIGURE 34–5 Application of Equation 34–3 (plotted in Figure 34–6) to identify the appropriate propofol infusion rate to maintain unresponsiveness for a patient with average sensitivity (ie, the patient actually loses consciousness at a model predicted probability of 50%). The top plot presents the bolus and infusion rate dosing regimen, the middle plot presents the predicted propofol effect-site concentration (Ce), and the bottom plot presents the probability of unresponsiveness. In this example, a propofol bolus of 300 mcg/kg followed by an infusion of 108 mcg/kg/min maintains the probability of unresponsiveness near 50% in a 70-kg patient.

The values for a_0/a_1 are given in Table 34–4.

As noted above, the 50-year-old, 70-kg patient losing consciousness at 140 seconds will require a maintenance infusion of 108 mcg/kg/min. For a 25-year-old, 65-kg patient losing consciousness at 140 seconds, the infusion will be $-2.82 + 1.11 \times 108 =$ 123 mcg/kg/min.

COMBINED TECHNIQUES WITH PROPOFOL AND OPIOIDS

A common practice in endoscopic anesthesia is to combine an opioid such as remifentanil with propofol. This allows us to attenuate the swings in response associated with varying levels of stimulus that occur in endoscopy. Although the dose-sparing effect of remifentanil for propofol is not as great for loss of consciousness as for response to noxious stimuli such as pain or intubation,[3] it cannot be ignored. In the dose ranges typically used in endoscopy, the effect of remifentanil on the pharmacokinetics of propofol will be negligible, and only the pharmacodynamic response will be noticeably altered.[6] For the 50-year-old, 70-kg patient undergoing the first strategy, this is depicted in Figure 34–7. Similarly, for the second strategy, the doses will be reduced (Figure 34–8).

These principles will apply equally to fentanyl and other opioids coadministered with propofol.[7] The reader is cautioned that the respiratory effects of opioid doses associated with significant propofol dose-sparing effects can be breath-taking; the longest breath interval noted in the previously mentioned study[4] was 18 minutes.

LIMITATIONS

These techniques are designed to identify an individualized propofol effect-site concentration associated with loss of consciousness and then use that information to maintain propofol levels at that concentration—with limited information about the patient and simple drug delivery systems. There are several important limitations to consider. First, loss of responsiveness to verbal stimulation may not be adequate for tolerance of endoscopy, and different end points such as tolerance of jaw thrust may be employed. Second, propofol can cause airway obstruction and respiratory depression that may require intervention to maintain adequate ventilation, and these effects may be seen at different

TABLE 34–2 Loading dose (mcg/kg) for bolus control for age and weight ranges.

	Age (years)					
Weight (kg)	**20–29**	**30–39**	**40–49**	**50–59**	**60–69**	**70–79**
50–59	629	569	522	485	455	430
60–69	588	534	491	457	430	407
70–79	557	507	467	436	410	389
80–89	531	484	447	418	394	375
90–99	509	466	431	403	381	362
100–109	491	450	417	391	369	352
110–119	476	436	405	380	360	343
120–129	462	425	395	370	351	335
130–139	450	414	385	362	343	328
140–149	439	405	377	355	337	322
150–159	430	396	370	348	330	316
160–169	421	389	363	342	325	311
170–179	413	382	357	336	320	306

TABLE 34–3 Bolus (mcg/kg)/infusion (mcg/kg/min) for pump control for age and weight ranges.

	Age (years)					
Weight (kg)	**20–29**	**30–39**	**40–49**	**50–59**	**60–69**	**70–79**
50–59	457/262	391/245	341/230	303/219	273/209	251/200
60–69	433/250	370/234	323/220	288/209	261/199	239/191
70–79	417/240	356/225	312/212	278/201	252/192	232/184
80–89	406/232	347/217	304/205	271/194	246/186	227/179
90–99	399/225	341/210	299/199	267/189	242/180	223/174
100–109	395/218	337/205	295/193	264/184	240/176	221/169
110–119	394/213	336/200	294/189	262/180	239/172	220/165
120–129	395/208	336/195	294/185	262/176	239/168	220/162
130–139	397/204	337/191	295/181	263/172	239/165	221/159
140–149	403/200	341/188	297/178	265/169	241/162	222/156
150–159	410/196	346/184	300/175	268/166	243/159	224/153
160–169	420/192	352/181	305/172	271/164	246/157	227/151
170–179	431/189	359/178	310/169	275/161	249/154	230/149

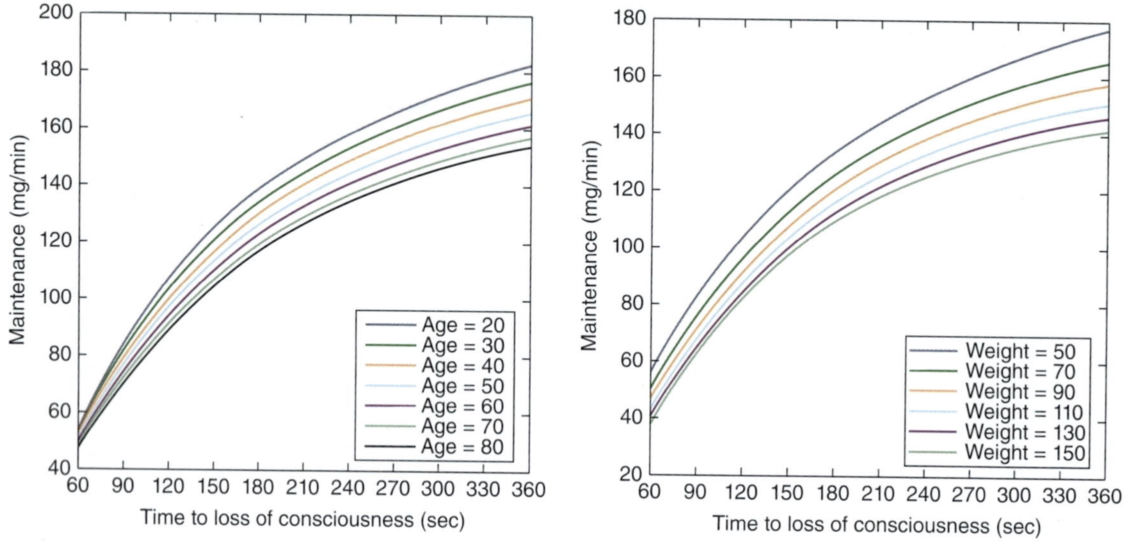

FIGURE 34–6 Propofol maintenance infusion rates versus time to loss of consciousness for a 70-kg patient over a range of ages (left) and a 50-year-old patient over a range of weights (right).

TABLE 34–4 Coefficients a_0/a_1 for Equation 34–4 across a range of ages and weights.

	Age (years)					
Weight (kg)	**20–29**	**30–39**	**40–49**	**50–59**	**60–69**	**70–79**
50–59	3.89/1.13	3.11/1.10	2.18/1.08	1.23/1.05	0.32/1.04	−0.50/1.02
60–69	2.82/1.11	2.20/1.08	1.40/1.05	0.57/1.02	−0.23/1.00	−0.96/0.99
70–79	1.81/1.09	1.38/1.05	0.72/1.03	−0.00/1.00	−0.70/0.98	−1.35/0.96
80–89	0.85/1.07	0.62/1.04	0.10/1.01	−0.51/0.98	−1.12/0.96	−1.69/0.94
90–99	−0.10/1.06	−0.13/1.02	−0.48/0.99	−0.98/0.96	−1.50/0.94	−2.00/0.92
100–109	−1.05/1.05	−0.83/1.01	−1.04/0.97	−1.43/0.94	−1.86/0.92	−2.29/0.90
110–119	−2.03/1.04	−1.53/1.00	−1.58/0.96	−1.85/0.93	−2.21/0.91	−2.57/0.88
120–129	−3.05/1.03	−2.26/0.99	−2.13/0.95	−2.28/0.92	−2.54/0.89	−2.84/0.87
130–139	−4.17/1.03	−3.01/0.98	−2.67/0.94	−2.70/0.91	−2.87/0.88	−3.11/0.86
140–149	−5.40/1.02	−3.79/0.97	−3.24/0.93	−3.14/0.90	−3.22/0.87	−3.38/0.85
150–159	−6.77/1.02	−4.67/0.97	−3.85/0.92	−3.58/0.89	−3.57/0.86	−3.67/0.84
160–169	−8.43/1.02	−5.61/0.96	−4.49/0.92	−4.07/0.88	−3.94/0.85	−3.96/0.83
170–179	−10.43/1.03	−6.69/0.96	−5.19/0.91	−4.58/0.88	−4.33/0.85	−4.27/0.82

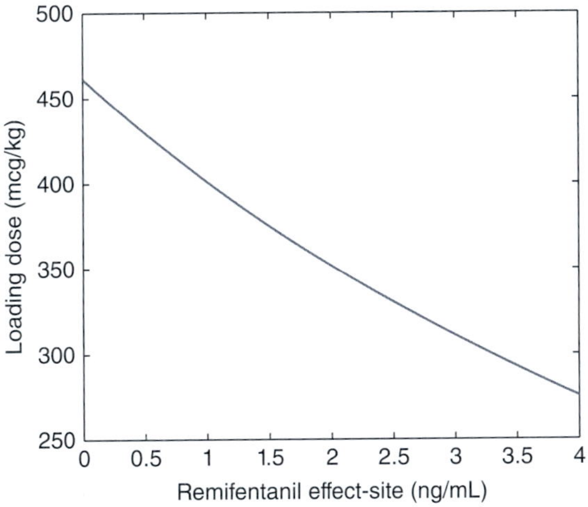

FIGURE 34–7 Suggested propofol loading bolus doses as a function of predicted remifentanil effect-site concentrations.

effect-site concentrations than loss of consciousness (both higher and lower).[8] Third, the model incorporates only patient age and weight. The pharmacokinetics of propofol are known to vary by gender,[9] ethnicity,[10] and genetic polymorphisms,[11] but a grand unifying model of propofol pharmacokinetics that incorporates all these factors has yet to emerge. Finally, use of commercially available TCI pumps may permit a more direct approach to the problem.

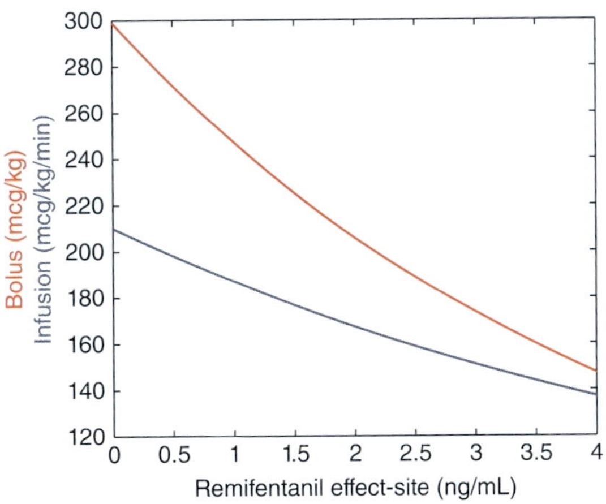

FIGURE 34–8 Suggested propofol bolus and infusion doses as a function of predicted remifentanil effect-site concentrations.

With this technology, the pump can be programmed for a target in excess of that typically required for endoscopy (4 mcg/mL), and the infusion suspended when adequate depth is observed and restarted at this effect-site concentration, as described by Rabelo.[12]

CONCLUSIONS

The intent of this chapter is to illustrate how pharmacokinetic and pharmacodynamic models of propofol can be used to guide dosing during brief procedures that require deep sedation and/or general anesthesia. By utilizing these models, dosing regimens can be refined to avoid excessive overdosing or underdosing and quickly achieve conditions that allow patients to tolerate endoscopy. Although technology that brings this capability to the point of care is under development, it not yet readily available. It is not the intent to have the reader laminate this chapter and go forth to the endoscopy suite but to understand how to adjust doses in a systematic fashion. The technology will eventually follow.

REFERENCES

1. Mandel JE, Sarraf E. The variability of response to propofol is reduced when a clinical observation is incorporated in the control: a simulation study. *Anesth Analg*. 2012;114:1221-1229.
2. Cortínez LI, Anderson BJ, Penna A, et al. Influence of obesity on propofol pharmacokinetics: derivation of a pharmacokinetic model. *Br J Anaesth*. 2010;105: 448-456.
3. Johnson KB, Syroid ND, Gupta DK, et al. An evaluation of remifentanil propofol response surfaces for loss of responsiveness, loss of response to surrogates of painful stimuli and laryngoscopy in patients undergoing elective surgery. *Anesth Analg*. 2008;106:471-479.
4. Mandel JE, Lichtenstein GR, Metz DC, Ginsberg GG, Kochman ML. A prospective, randomized, comparative trial evaluating respiratory depression during patient-controlled versus anesthesiologist-administered propofol-remifentanil sedation for elective colonoscopy. *Gastrointest Endosc*. 2010;72:112-117.
5. Atkins, JH, Mandel, JE, Rosanova, G. Safety and efficacy of drug induced sleep endoscopy employing a probability ramp propofol infusion system in patients with severe obstructive sleep apnea. *Anesth Analg*, in press.

6. Vuyk J. Clinical interpretation of pharmacokinetic and pharmacodynamic propofol-opioid interactions. *Acta Anaesthesiol Belg*. 2001;52:445-451.
7. Lysakowski C, Dumont L, Pellegrini M, Clergue F, Tassonyi E. Effects of fentanyl, alfentanil, remifentanil and sufentanil on loss of consciousness and bispectral index during propofol induction of anaesthesia. *Br J Anaesth*. 2001;86:523-527.
8. Noffsinger WJ, Eastwood PR, Hillman DR, et al. Evolution of changes in upper airway collapsibility during slow induction of anesthesia with propofol. *Anesthesiology*. 2009;111:63.
9. Hoymork SC, Raeder J. Why do women wake up faster than men from propofol anaesthesia? *Br J Anaesth*. 2005;95:627-633.
10. Ortolani O, Conti A, Ngumi ZW, et al. Ethnic differences in propofol and fentanyl response: a comparison among Caucasians, Kenyan Africans and Brazilians. *Eur J Anaesthesiol*. 2004;21:314-319.
11. Iohom G, Ni Chonghaile M, O'Brien JK, Cunningham AJ, Fitzgerald DF, Shields DC. An investigation of potential genetic determinants of propofol requirements and recovery from anaesthesia. *Eur J Anaesthesiol*. 2007;24:912-919.
12. Rabelo FA, Braga A, Küpper DS, et al. Propofol-induced sleep: polysomnographic evaluation of patients with obstructive sleep apnea and controls. *Otolaryngol Head Neck Surg*. 2010;142:218-224.

CHAPTER

35

Anesthesia for Craniotomy

John Hille, MD

INTRODUCTION

Providing an anesthetic for neurosurgical procedures that include a craniotomy can involve unique anesthetic goals otherwise not encountered in routine practice. For example, tight hemodynamic control and cerebral protection techniques during aneurysm clipping or providing moderate sedation during intracranial tumor resection allow patients to cooperate during speech mapping. Anesthesiologists have suggested numerous dosing regimens to meet these goals. This chapter will briefly summarize a few of those designed for aneurysm clipping and awake procedures for tumor resection.

CRANIOTOMY FOR ANEURYSM CLIPPING

The incidence of unruptured intracranial aneurysms is thought to be near 2%. Approximately 10 in 100,000 people suffer a brain aneurysm rupture, making it frequently encountered problem in the operating room. The prognosis is poor; 40% of ruptured brain aneurysms are fatal and of those that survive, about two thirds have permanent neurologic deficits.[1,2]

Perioperative management of these patients focuses on 5 potentially conflicting goals:

1. Maintain adequate cerebral perfusion pressure (CPP) to prevent cerebral ischemia and cerebral vasospasm.
2. Maintain a low transmural pressure (TMP) gradient to prevent rupture of the aneurysm.[3]
3. Minimize brain swelling.
4. Minimize large swings in intracranial pressure (ICP).
5. Provide an anesthetic that allows for a rapid emergence.

To accomplish this goal, a basic understanding of the aneurysm's TMP is useful. TMP (the equivalent of the CPP) is defined by Equation 35–1.

$$\text{TMP} = \text{CPP} = \text{MAP} - \text{ICP or CVP} \qquad (35\text{–}1)$$

where MAP is the mean arterial pressure and CVP is the central venous pressure. Normal values for MAP, ICP, CVP, and CPP are presented in Table 35–1. The higher value between ICP and CVP is used. TMP describes the relationship between the pressure within the aneurysm (arterial blood pressure) and the pressure surrounding the aneurysm. Abrupt increases in the transmural pressure gradient may lead to aneurysmal rupture and poor outcomes.

Subarachnoid hemorrhage (SAH) associated with aneurysmal rupture can be linked with numerous physiologic derangements (Table 35–2) that should be considered when formulating an appropriate anesthetic as well as drugs that may be used in the perioperative period to manage these derangements.

Premedication

With this hemodynamic goal in mind, premedication to treat anxiety and pain should be considered for each patient, keeping in mind that no specific agent or combination of agents is applicable for all patients. It may be useful to consider the clinical grade of SAH, patient comorbidities, cardiac and pulmonary status, and ICP when formulating the premedication plan to put into perspective the

TABLE 35–1 Normal values for pressures that influence aneurysm transmural pressures.

Hemodynamic Parameter	Normal Values (mm Hg)
Mean arterial blood pressure (MAP)	80–100
Central venous pressure (CVP)	3–8
Intracranial pressure (ICP)	7–15
Cerebral perfusion pressure (CPP)	70–90

amount of drug if any that will be required. Tables 35–3 and 35–4 present two grading systems used to classify SAHs (ie, the Hunt and Hess grading scale for SAH and the World Federation of Neurological Surgeons Grading Scale for aneurysmal SAH)[5,6]; these events can be associated with significant cardiac and pulmonary morbidity.

Although anxiety can lead to worrisome hypertension, possibly resulting in aneurysmal rupture, oversedation may cause respiratory depression and unwanted increase in ICP and increased cerebral blood flow with rising arterial PCO_2 levels. Careful titration of benzodiazepines and/or opioids is warranted given that many patients present in the preoperative period already on medications such as calcium channel blockers (ie, nimodipine to minimize cerebral vessel vasospasms), anticonvulsants, steroids, and possible analgesics (to treat severe headaches). These medications should be continued throughout the perioperative period. Special care should be taken when administering a benzodiazepine in the presence of an opioid, as each drug can enhance the effects of one another in a synergistic fashion.

Induction

As with premedication, a major goal of induction is to properly manage blood pressure. A primary focus is to limit the hypertensive response to laryngoscopy while at the same time maintaining appropriate CPP to minimize changes in the TMP gradient across the aneurysm. The depth of anesthesia should match the stimulation associated with laryngoscopy, tracheal intubation, and subsequent 3-point rigid cranial fixation. This can

TABLE 35–2 Physiologic derangements associated with subarachnoid hemorrhage.

Adverse Physiologic Problem	Management
Central nervous system	
Cerebral vasospasm	Triple H therapy (contraindicated prior to aneurysm clipping) Nimodipine[a] Oral dosing: 60 mg orally every 4 hours, with a maximal daily dose of 360 mg, continued for 21 days Intravenous dosing: 1 mg/h. Consider escalating after 6 hours if blood pressure remains stable up to 2 mg/h by 0.5 mg/h increments. Intravenous dosing may cause more pronounced hypotension.
Increased ICP and volume	Mannitol 0.25–1 g/kg Furosemide 0.25–1 mg/kg Consider draining CSF (maximal volume, 20–30 mL)[b] Consider temporary hyperventilation titrated to a $PaCO_2$ of 30–33 mm Hg until the dura is opened (prolonged hypocapnia may lead to unwanted cerebral ischemia).[c]
Seizures	Levetiracetam 500–1000 mg twice daily
Cardiopulmonary system	
Systemic and pulmonary hypertension	Induced systemic hypotension is no longer recommended for aneurysm clipping[4]
Electrolytes	
Hyponatremia for SIADH	Normal saline Consider hypertonic saline Consider steroids
Hypokalemia	
Hypocalcemia	
Hypomagnesemia	

[a]Nimodipine may cause hypotension; maintaining blood pressure (systolic pressures of 130-150 mm Hg) is the priority. Nimodipine administration may need to be reduced or terminated.
[b]The entire cerebrospinal fluid volume is 150 mL.
[c]Hyperventilation to decrease in ICP is time limited and acutely used to decrease ICP until more definitive treatments have an effect. Its effect is attenuated as the pH of the CSF equilibrates to the new $PaCO_2$ and cerebral arterioles redilate.
Triple H therapy includes hypertension, hypervolemia, and hemodilution.
CSF, cerebrospinal fluid; ICP, intracranial pressure; SIADH, syndrome of inappropriate antidiuretic hormone.
From reference 3.

TABLE 35–3 Hunt and Hess grading scale for subarachnoid hemorrhage.[5]

Grade	Clinical Description
I	Asymptomatic or minimal headache and slight nuchal rigidity
II	Moderate to severe headache, nuchal rigidity, and no neurologic deficit other than cranial nerve palsy
III	Drowsiness, confusion, or mild focal deficit
IV	Stupor, moderate to severe hemiparesis, and possibly early decerebrate rigidity and vegetative disturbances
V	Deep coma, decerebrate rigidity, and moribund appearance

be accomplished using multiple techniques, and achieving these goals is more imperative than the actual drugs used. Amnesia can be induced by thiopental 2 to 5 mg/kg (where available), propofol 1 to 2 mg/kg, or etomidate 0.1 to 0.3 mg/kg. Adrenal suppression with etomidate should be considered when selecting an induction agent in critically ill patients.[7,8] These induction agents all decrease cerebral blood flow and subsequently ICP. An opioid is necessary to blunt the sympathetic stimulation and hypertensive response to laryngoscopy and intubation. Fentanyl 3 to 5 mcg/kg or remifentanil 0.25 to 1 mcg/kg will achieve this goal.

TABLE 35–4 World federation of neurological surgeons grading scale for aneurysmal subarachnoid hemorrhage.[6]

Grade	Glasgow Coma Scale Score	Motor Deficit
I	15	Absent
II	13–14	Absent
III	13–14	Present
IV	7–12	Present or absent
V	3–6	Present or absent

Fentanyl and remifentanil should be administered 3 to 5 minutes and 1 minute, respectively, before laryngoscopy and tracheal intubation to allow effect-site concentrations to reach their maximal level (Figure 35–1). Caution should be exercised when administering remifentanil in large bolus doses, as it is vagotonic and may cause bradycardia. Muscle relaxation for intubation and patient positioning is typically accomplished with a nondepolarizing muscle relaxant. Succinylcholine causes an undesirable increase in ICP, while nondepolarizing muscle relaxants do not. Rocuronium 0.7 to 1.2 mg/kg or vecuronium 0.15 mg/kg is typically used to achieve adequate muscle relaxation. Additionally, lidocaine 1.5 to 2 mg/kg or esmolol 0.5 mg/kg can be administered to further blunt the hemodynamic response to laryngoscopy and intubation.

As is common with induction, hypotension may occur and should be treated promptly to maintain the TMP. A reasonable goal is to maintain the mean arterial blood pressure within 10% to 20% of baseline pressures.

Maintenance

Maintenance of anesthesia is most often achieved through a balanced technique using volatile agents or sedative–hypnotics in combination with opioids. Opioids are used to reduce volatile agent or sedative–hypnotic requirements. All volatile agents have been used effectively. Although they all decrease the cerebral metabolic rate (with the exception of nitrous oxide, which increases the cerebral metabolic rate), all volatile anesthetics increase cerebral blood flow and thus have the potential to increase ICP. As a result, if a volatile agent is used, it is typically done so at less than 1 minimum alveolar concentration (MAC).

Unlike volatile anesthetics, propofol and benzodiazepines not only decrease the cerebral metabolic rate but also decrease cerebral blood flow. Hence, propofol is often used as the sole anesthetic if brain relaxation is inadequate with a volatile agent. Propofol is typically administered as a continuous infusion at a rate of 75 to 150 mcg/kg/min, resulting in predicted effect-site concentrations of 3 to 6 mcg/mL when used as the primary anesthetic (Figure 35–2). It is then titrated according to the patient's hemodynamics.

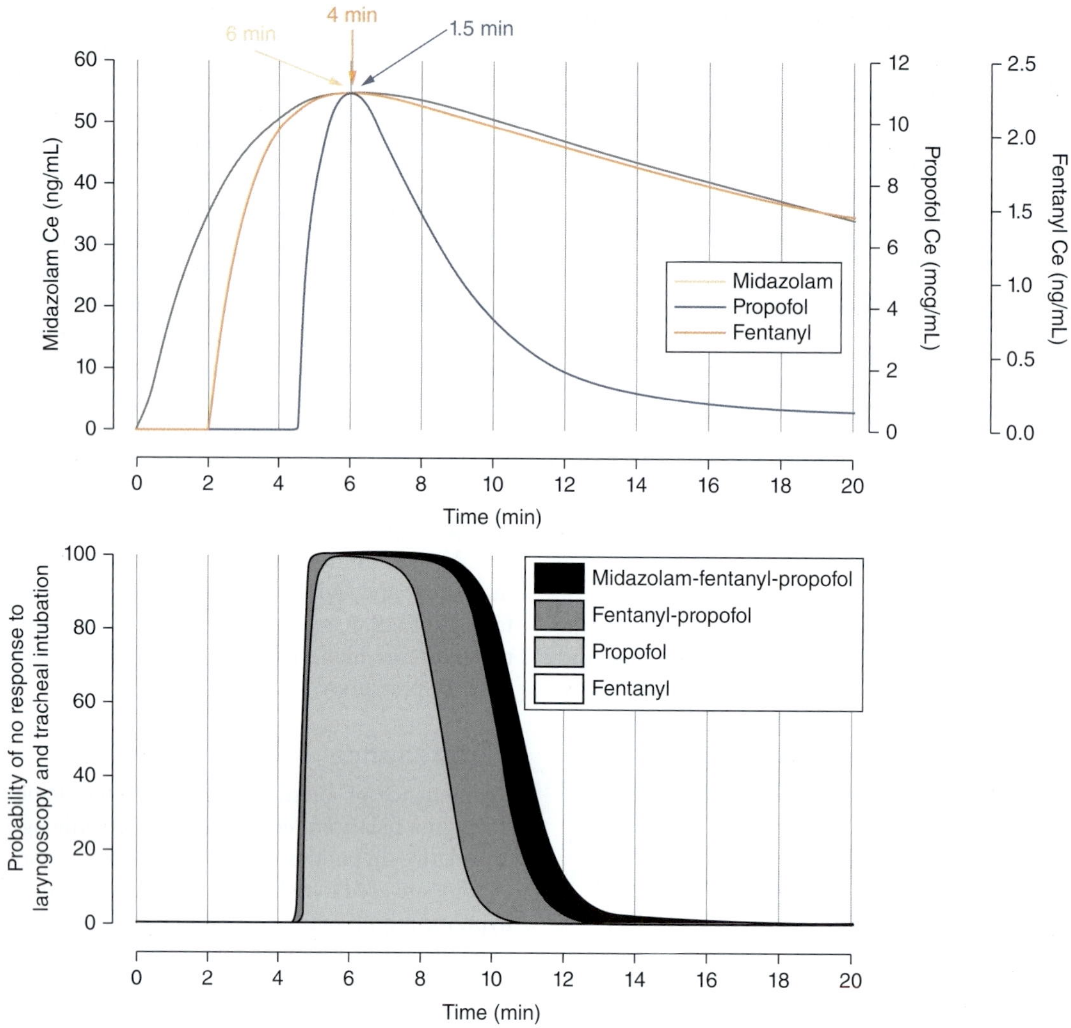

FIGURE 35–1 Simulation of an induction with midazolam (2 mg), fentanyl (2 mcg/kg), and propofol (2 mg/kg). The top plot presents the predicted effect-site concentration (Ce) levels, and the bottom plot presents the predicted loss of response to laryngoscopy and tracheal intubation. Simulations used published pharmacokinetic and pharmacodynamic models to predict effect site concentrations and effects.[9-14] The top plot illustrates the differences between drugs in the time required to reach the peak Ce (approximately 6 minutes for midazolam, 4 minutes for fentanyl, and 1.5 minutes for propofol). The timing of each bolus was such that each drug reached a peak concentration at nearly the same time to provide maximal effect during laryngoscopy (midazolam, followed 2 minutes later by fentanyl, followed 2.5 minutes later by propofol). The bottom plot presents the difference in the duration of effect for all 3 drugs combined, for propofol and fentanyl, for propofol alone, and for fentanyl alone. Of note, the midazolam prolonged the duration of effect (no response to laryngoscopy and tracheal intubation) for approximately 1 minute. Propofol administered without an opioid provided a shorter window of no response to laryngoscopy (4–5 versus 2–3 minutes above a 95% probability of no response for propofol alone and propofol combined with fentanyl and midazolam).

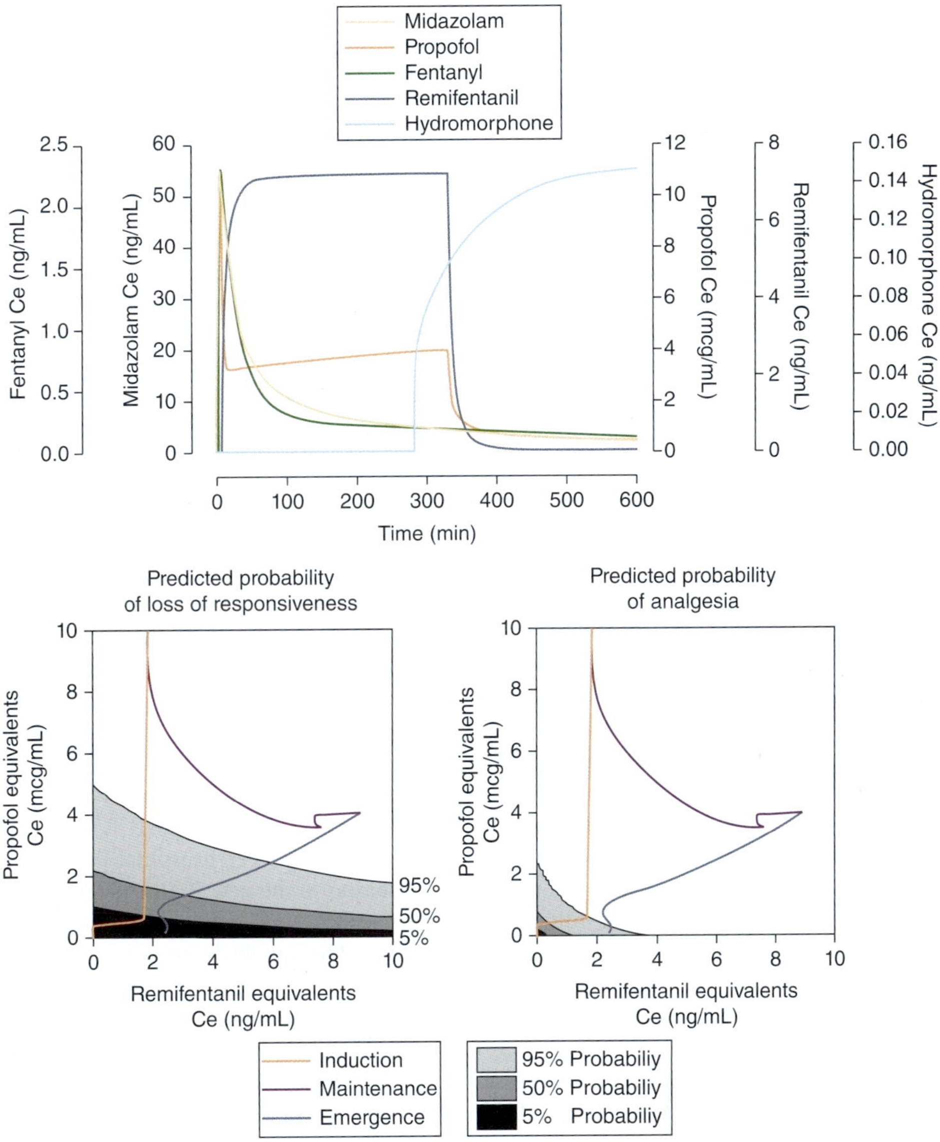

FIGURE 35–2 Infusion rates and simulation of predicted midazolam (2 mg), fentanyl (2 mcg/kg), propofol 2 mg/kg bolus followed by a 100 mcg/kg/min infusion), remifentanil (0.2 mcg/kg/min infusion), and hydromorphone (1 mg 30 minutes prior to the end of the procedure) effect-site concentration (Ce) levels and selected drug effects for a 6.5-hour craniotomy procedure. Predictions of drug Ce levels and drug effects were based on published pharmacokinetic and pharmacodynamic models.[9,11-19] The top plot presents the predicted Ce levels, and the bottom plots present the propofol and remifentanil equivalents of all drugs plotted over topographic representations of the pharmacodynamic interaction models of loss of responsiveness (left) and analgesia (right). Loss of responsiveness is defined as no response to verbal and vigorous tactile stimuli and analgesia is defined as a loss of response to a moderately painful pressure on the anterior tibia.[18] As dosed, the technique is more than adequate for maintaining a patient in an unresponsive state. During induction (red line) and maintenance (pink line), the resultant Ce levels are well above the 95% probability of response in both plots. Important assumptions made with these simulations are that (1) the patient is otherwise healthy and does not chronically consume opioids, (2) opioid equivalencies (Chapter 6) were used to estimate the remifentanil equivalent, and (3) the interaction between propofol and midazolam was considered additive (Chapter 3).

The avoidance of volatile agents may also be necessary when evoked potential monitoring is used. Volatile agents interfere with these types of monitoring, particularly motor-evoked potentials. Ketamine should also be avoided because it can increase ICP.

Opioid infusions with fentanyl 1 to 2 mcg/kg/kg, remifentanil 0.05 to 1 mcg/kg/min, or sufentanil 0.2 to 0.5 mcg/kg/h have been successfully used. Selection of the opioid may depend on the postoperative management of the patient. If extubation is desired, a short-acting opioid such as remifentanil is preferable. This will allow for extubation and early neurologic assessment of the patient. Neuromuscular blockage is not necessary but may be added if movement is a concern. A nondepolarizing agent such as rocuronium or vecuronium is most often chosen. These have to be avoided if motor-evoked potentials are being monitored.

Emergence

The anesthetic should be titrated to allow for a rapid emergence where appropriate (ie, Hunt and Hess grading scale of I to III). Techniques should also be used that prevent coughing, straining, and hypertension to reduce intracranial bleeding and edema formation. A common practice is for early discontinuation of the volatile agent with supplementation of anesthesia using propofol boluses or infusion. Hypertension is managed with labetalol and esmolol. Administration of lidocaine 1.5 mg/kg is another technique to reduce airway responsiveness during the extubation process.

Vasospasm is one of the most significant causes of morbidity and mortality in patients with SAH following aneurysmal rupture. The exact etiology remains unclear, but it appears to be related to the blood from the ruptured aneurysm irritating the nearby vessels. The vasospasm leads to decreased cerebral blood flow and ischemia. Treatment is aimed at prevention of vasospasm. Nimodipine, a cerebral selective calcium channel blocker, is used prophylactically to prevent vasospasm. The typical dose of nimodipine is 30 to 60 mg orally every 4 hours and is continued for 21 days. If vasospasm does occur, "triple H" therapy is initiated; this therapy consists of hypertension, hypervolemia, and hemodilution. Intravascular volume expansion with crystalloid or colloid is began with the goal of a CVP of 10 to 12 mm Hg and pulmonary capillary wedge pressure of 15 to 18 mm Hg. Hematocrit should be lowered to 30% to 35%. Systolic blood pressure should be raised to 120 to 150 mm Hg prior to aneurysm clipping. Once the aneurysm is clipped, higher blood pressures may be warranted but must be balanced with the potential risk of recurrent hemorrhage. This elevation of blood pressure can be achieved with phenylephrine or vasopressin.

Pharmacologic Approaches to Minimize Brain Swelling

Elevated ICP is a commonly encountered problem in neuroanesthesia. Increased ICP should be aggressively treated as it leads to decreases cerebral blood flow, possibly producing neuronal damage or infarction leading to permanent injury. Intraoperatively, there are a variety of methods to rapidly reduce ICP (Table 35–2). Hyperventilation is commonly employed to decrease the $PaCO_2$. This will acutely decrease ICP by causing vasoconstriction of the cerebral arteries leading to decreased cerebral blood volume. Hyperventilation to a $PaCO_2$ between 25 and 30 mm Hg will decrease ICP. Its effect is limited as the pH of the cerebrospinal fluid (CSF) rapidly equilibrates to the new $PaCO_2$ level and the cerebral arterioles will soon redilate. Hyperventilation is typically used to acutely decrease ICP to allow for more definitive treatments.

All intravenous anesthetics, analgesics and sedatives will decrease cerebral blood flow and cerebral metabolic rate, resulting in lowered ICP. On the other hand, all volatile agents result in a dose-dependent increase in cerebral blood flow through cerebral dilation.

Osmotherapy is also commonly used to quickly decrease ICP. Mannitol, glycerol, and hypertonic saline have all been used for this purpose. Mannitol is often used intraoperatively. It increases serum tonicity, drawing edema fluid from the cerebral parenchyma and lowering ICP. It is given as a bolus dose of 0.25 to 1 g/kg, and its effects last from 1.5 to 6 hours. It causes massive osmotic diuresis, resulting fluid and electrolyte imbalances, and these must be monitored. Hypertonic saline also creates the osmotic force to draw water from the interstitial space of the brain parenchyma to the intravascular compartment. Concentrations ranging from 3% to 23.4% have been used. Hypertonic saline may be advantageous over mannitol in patients who are hypovolemic or hypotensive because it lacks the diuretic effects of mannitol.

Other options to reduce ICP are primarily surgical in nature. A ventricular drain may be placed to reduce CSF volume. Surgical resection of damaged tissue or intracranial masses may be the only effective intervention to reduce ICP.

Burst Suppression

A common practice by neurosurgeons is to request burst suppression during neurosurgical procedures, particularly for aneurysm clipping. The goal of burst suppression is to achieve cortical electrical suppression. Burst suppression on the electroencephalogram (EEG) is characterized by 5 to 10 activity bursts/min but an otherwise flat line. Multiple anesthetic drugs, including volatile anesthetics, propofol, barbiturates, and etomidate, can be used to obtain burst suppression. Opioids, ketamine, and benzodiazepines are incapable of producing burst suppression. Volatile anesthetics typically produce burst suppression at concentrations greater than 1.5 MAC. The 2 most commonly used medications to achieve burst suppression are propofol and thiopental. Burst suppression is typically initially achieved with a bolus dose ranging from 1 to 2.5 mg/kg. A propofol infusion is then started ranging from 50 to 300 mcg/kg/min and titrated to obtain the desired EEG pattern of burst suppression. Thiopental is administered as a 5-mg/kg bolus dose and infusion ranging from 0.3 to 9 mg/kg/h. The infusion is titrated to achieve burst suppression on the EEG. Because these medications are used in high doses to obtain burst suppression, hemodynamic depression can ensue. Phenylephrine or epinephrine infusions should be available to counteract the hemodynamic effects of the propofol and thiopental.

Seizure Prevention

Intraoperative seizure is a potential complication in neuroanesthesia, particularly in the awake craniotomy for epilepsy. The incidence in craniotomies, awake or asleep, ranges from 0% to 24%, with an average of 9.5%. Seizures are often related to cortical electrostimulation and may be short and focal. Generalized seizures, such as tonic-clonic seizures, are less common. Most seizures self-terminate or can be controlled by irrigation of the surgical field with cold saline. Administration of an intravenous benzodiazepine (midazolam 2–5 mg or diazepam 5–10 mg) can also be used to treat intraoperative seizures. Propofol also possesses antiepileptic properties and can be used to manage seizures. Administration of propofol, benzodiazepines, and barbiturates may interfere with monitoring.

AWAKE CRANIOTOMY

The awake craniotomy is used for surgical treatment of epilepsy, deep-brain stimulation for the treatment of Parkinson disease, and supratentorial tumors involving critical areas of the brain. Critical areas include language areas of the brain, Broca and Wernicke areas, and motor and somatosensory portions of the brain. The awake craniotomy is used in conjunction with functional magnetic resonance imaging to excise lesions while preventing functional disabilities. At critical points during the tumor resection, intraoperative patient participation in neuropsychiatry testing can be performed to identify critical motor and speech centers near tissue marked for excision.

This technique is challenging in that anesthesiologists are called upon to provide adequate sedation and analgesia without impairing patient participation.[20] Sufficient anesthesia for bone flap removal followed by an appropriate level of mild sedation for cortical speech or seizure focus mapping while keeping the patient comfortable yet immobile throughout a long procedure can be difficult to achieve.[21] A list of important considerations for an awake craniotomy is presented in Table 35–5.

Two major anesthetic techniques have been successfully used for awake craniotomies.

1. Induction of general anesthesia for surgical exposure followed emergence from anesthesia for patient participation, followed by reinduction of anesthesia for closure. To facilitate

TABLE 35–5 Important patient considerations for an awake craniotomy.[20]

Patient selection
Willing to participate and cooperate during intraoperative testing
Understand and be comfortable with the procedure and anesthetic plan (moderate sedation)
Absence of extreme anxiety, claustrophobia or other psychiatric disorders
Anesthetic goals
Maintain adequate oxygenation and ventilation.
Maintain a patent airway.
Optimize systemic and cerebral hemodynamics.
Maintain normal intracranial pressure.
Provide sedation and analgesia.
Prepare to manage oversedation and unwanted respiratory depression, airway obstruction, or poor patient cooperation.
Prepare to manage undersedation and unstable hemodynamics and patient agitation or discomfort.

airway management, a laryngeal mask airway may be used.

2. Monitored anesthesia care (most common), where the patient maintains spontaneous ventilation and remains responsive yet comfortable throughout the procedure. This discussion will primarily focus on the monitored anesthesia care approach.

Premedication

As with all patients presenting for a neurosurgical procedure, choice and dose of premedicant should be determined by patient condition and comorbidities. A common choice is intravenous midazolam 1 to 2 mg just prior to going to the operating room. Caution should be used in patients who have depressed cognitive function from their disease process as premedication may lead to oversedation and subsequent respiratory depression and/or poor patient cooperation.

Maintenance

Drug selection for an awake craniotomy should include those anesthetics that are short-acting and rapidly titratable to allow the anesthesiologist to respond to varying degrees of surgical stimuli throughout the procedure. Common drugs include propofol and remifentanil in that they allow a rapid modulation of analgesia and sedation to meet the needs of a long awake craniotomy. An example illustrating their use in combination is presented in Figure 35–3.

Features of propofol that make it ideal include (1) a rapid onset and offset of effect, (2) ability to decrease cerebral metabolic rate and ICP allowing for better surgical operating conditions, and (3) anticonvulsant and antiemetic properties. It is administered by intravenous bolus or continuous infusion. Common infusion rates range from 20 to 75 mcg/kg/min titrated to the desired level of sedation, and bolus doses of 10 to 20 mg can be administered to rapidly achieve a desired level sedation. Other sedatives, such as thiopental (where available) and etomidate, can be used as intermittent bolus doses for sedation throughout awake craniotomies.

Remifentanil is administered as a continuous infusion at rates of 0.05 to 0.1 mcg/kg/min. Intravenous boluses of 0.25 to 0.5 mcg/kg can be administered for more stimulating segments of the procedure such as pinning. Fentanyl can also be administered in small intermittent intravenous boluses of 25-50 mcg IV.

Dexmedetomidine can also be used in this setting. It can be used as the sole anesthetic or in combination with other anesthetics. With α-2 agonism, it provides dose-dependent sedation, anxiolysis, and analgesia without respiratory depression, but it can cause hypotension and bradycardia. It is administered with a slow intravenous loading dose of 0.2 to 1.0 mcg/kg over 10 minutes followed by a continuous infusion of 0.2 to 1.0 mcg/kg/h that is titrated to effect.

Several other anesthetic techniques for awake craniotomy have been used. For example, fentanyl in combination with the antiemetic droperidol (once formulated as Innovar) has been used in neurosurgical procedures where endotracheal intubation was avoided to allow the patient to verbalize responses.[21] Other combinations include sufentanil with propofol and nitrous oxide[24] and alfentanil with droperidol and nitrous oxide.[25] All of these techniques keep patients comfortable for long procedures and allow them to cooperate during cortical mapping, but the

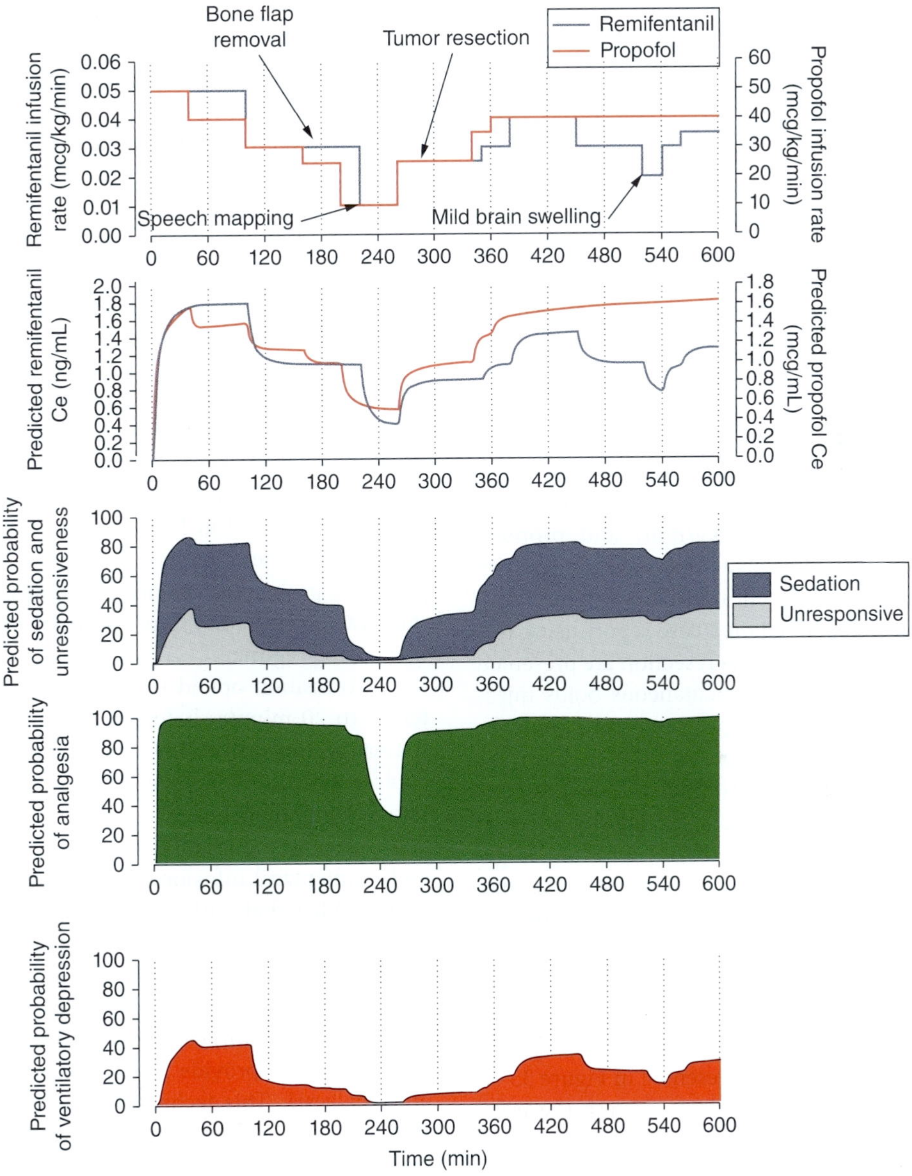

FIGURE 35–3 Infusion rates and simulation of predicted propofol and remifentanil effect-site concentrations and selected drug effects for a published case report using these drugs for an awake craniotomy.[20] Predictions of drug effect-site concentration (Ce) levels and drug effects were based on published pharmacokinetic and pharmacodynamic models.[11-13,19,22,23] The top plot presents the infusion rates, the second plot presents the predicted propofol and remifentanil Ce levels, and the bottom 3 plots present the predicted probability of loss of responsiveness,[19] sedation defined as the probability of responsiveness to name with tactile stimuli (Modified Observer's Assessment of Alertness and Sedation score of 3),[19] analgesia defined as a loss of response to a moderately painful pressure on the anterior tibia,[18] and intolerable ventilatory depression defined as the probability of a respiratory rate of less than 4 breaths per minute in an unstimulated state.[23] Time points within the procedure are labeled in the top plot. Of note, the remifentanil infusion was decreased in response to increased brain swelling. With the decrease in the remifentanil infusion, the swelling abated.

subtle advantage of one neuroleptanalgesic technique over another is difficult to define.[26]

Sample Propofol–Remifentanil Dosing Regimen for Awake Craniotomy

As mentioned above, both propofol and remifentanil have desirable features that make them an attractive choice for an awake craniotomy. Both are considered to be *soft* anesthetic drugs, or drugs that are designed to be safer with an increased therapeutic index and a rapid predictable metabolism to inactive metabolites.[27]

After preoxygenation with 100% oxygen, a 50-mg propofol bolus is administered for placement of a nasopharyngeal airway and bladder catheter. A remifentanil (0.05 mcg.kg/min) and propofol (50 mcg/kg/min) infusions are started during patient positioning and placement in the head frame. Infusion rate changes, based on a case report using this technique for a glioblastoma resection are presented in Figure 35–3.[20] Small subcutaneous bolus injections (1–3 mL) of 0.5% bupivacaine with epinephrine 1:200,000 are administered just before insertion of the 3-pin head frame. Additional bupivacaine is injected along the intended craniotomy incision site. During the initial phase of the procedure, target effects are analgesia to blunt response to bone flap removal and moderate sedation to provide comfort yet permit arousal when prompted.

During cortical speech mapping, the propofol and remifentanil infusions are decreased to 10 and 0.01 mcg/kg/min, respectively. Predicted drug concentrations and effects are presented in Figure 35–3. Simulations predict that with decreasing the infusion rates, a patient should rapidly become alert and cooperative (ie, within 2–5 minutes) to participate and perform tasks to assist the neurosurgical team in identifying the language centers in the cerebral cortex before initiating tumor resection.

With speech mapping completed, the remifentanil and propofol infusions are increased and maintained for tumor resection. The target effects again are adequate analgesia for tumor resection and sedation to provide patient comfort yet permit arousal. Although highly variable among patients presenting for an awake craniotomy, arterial blood gas measurements obtained at hourly intervals during this phase of the anesthetic in 1 patient revealed pH levels of 7.343 to 7.382, partial pressure of carbon dioxide of 45.5 to 51.7 mm Hg, and partial pressure of oxygen levels of 85 to 112 mm Hg.[20]

A potential drawback to this technique is mild to moderate ventilatory depression, leading to increased cortical tissue swelling, which makes it difficult to replace the bone flap. A reduction in the remifentanil infusion may increase the respiratory rate and decrease cortical swelling (see Figure 35–3). This issue raises an important point. As long as the patient is responsive, the patient is able to self-rescue with prompting. If the patient is unresponsive, then intervention may be required to maintain adequate oxygenation and ventilation. As illustrated in Figure 35–3, there are periods (turning the bone flap and closure) where the predicted probability of both unresponsiveness and intolerable ventilatory depression are present with this dosing regimen.

A transition opioid is appropriate to administer 15 to 20 minutes before procedure completion to treat postoperative pain. Typical transition opioid choices and doses include intravenous hydromorphone 1 mg, morphine 5 mg, or fentanyl 150 mcg. After closure and head pin removal, the propofol and remifentanil infusions are terminated. Simulations predict that within 3 minutes, a patient will have a 95% probability of being awake.

Overall, these simulations illustrate how remifentanil (0.01–0.1 mcg/kg/min) and propofol (10–50 mcg/kg/min) can be titrated within a therapeutic range to provide robust control of sedation and analgesia. This technique can respond to the rapid changes in surgical stimuli and allow for rapid reversal of narcosis and patient cooperation to identify speech and motor areas of the cerebral cortex when appropriate.

REFERENCES

1. Wijdicks EF, Ropper AH, Hunnicutt EJ, Richardson GS, Nathanson JA. Atrial natriuretic factor and salt wasting after aneurysmal subarachnoid hemorrhage. *Stroke*. 1991;22(12):1519-1524.
2. Linn FH, Rinkel GJ, Algra A, van Gijn J. Headache characteristics in subarachnoid haemorrhage and

benign thunderclap headache. *J Neurol Neurosurg Psychiatry*. 1998;65(5):791-793.
3. Priebe HJ. Aneurysmal subarachnoid haemorrhage and the anaesthetist. *Br J Anaesth*. 2007;99(1):102-118.
4. Chang HS, Hongo K, Nakagawa H. Adverse effects of limited hypotensive anesthesia on the outcome of patients with subarachnoid hemorrhage. *J Neurosurg*. 2000;92(6):971-975.
5. Hunt WE, Hess RM. Surgical risk as related to time of intervention in the repair of intracranial aneurysms. *J Neurosurg*. 1968;28(1):14-20.
6. Teasdale GM, Drake CG, Hunt W, et al. A universal subarachnoid hemorrhage scale: report of a committee of the World Federation of Neurosurgical Societies. *J Neurol Neurosurg Psychiatry*. 1988;51(11):1457.
7. Bloomfield R, Noble DW. Etomidate and fatal outcome—even a single bolus dose may be detrimental for some patients. *Br J Anaesth*. 2006;97(1):116-117.
8. Wagner CE, Bick JS, Johnson D, et al. Etomidate use and postoperative outcomes among cardiac surgery patients. *Anesthesiology*. 2014;120(3):579-589.
9. Albrecht S, Ihmsen H, Hering W, et al. The effect of age on the pharmacokinetics and pharmacodynamics of midazolam. *Clin Pharmacol Ther*. 1999;65(6):630-639.
10. Bouillon TW, Bruhn J, Radulescu L, et al. Pharmacodynamic interaction between propofol and remifentanil regarding hypnosis, tolerance of laryngoscopy, bispectral index, and electroencephalographic approximate entropy. *Anesthesiology*. 2004;100(6):1353-1372.
11. Minto CF, Schnider TW, Egan TD, et al. Influence of age and gender on the pharmacokinetics and pharmacodynamics of remifentanil. I. Model development. *Anesthesiology*. 1997;86(1):10-23.
12. Minto CF, Schnider TW, Shafer SL. Pharmacokinetics and pharmacodynamics of remifentanil. II. Model application. *Anesthesiology*. 1997;86(1):24-33.
13. Schnider TW, Minto CF, Shafer SL, et al. The influence of age on propofol pharmacodynamics. *Anesthesiology*. 1999;90(6):1502-1516.
14. Shafer SL, Varvel JR, Aziz N, Scott JC. Pharmacokinetics of fentanyl administered by computer-controlled infusion pump. *Anesthesiology*. 1990;73(6):1091-1102.
15. Coda B, Tanaka A, Jacobson RC, Donaldson G, Chapman CR. Hydromorphone analgesia after intravenous bolus administration. *Pain*. 1997;71(1):41-48.
16. Coda BA, O'Sullivan B, Donaldson G, Bohl S, Chapman CR, Shen DD. Comparative efficacy of patient-controlled administration of morphine, hydromorphone, or sufentanil for the treatment of oral mucositis pain following bone marrow transplantation. *Pain*. 1997;72(3):333-346.
17. Drover DR, Angst MS, Valle M, et al. Input characteristics and bioavailability after administration of immediate and a new extended-release formulation of hydromorphone in healthy volunteers. *Anesthesiology*. 2002;97(4):827-836.
18. Johnson KB, Syroid ND, Gupta DK, et al. An evaluation of remifentanil propofol response surfaces for loss of responsiveness, loss of response to surrogates of painful stimuli and laryngoscopy in patients undergoing elective surgery. *Anesth Analg*. 2008;106(2):471-479.
19. Kern SE, Xie G, White JL, Egan TD. A response surface analysis of propofol-remifentanil pharmacodynamic interaction in volunteers. *Anesthesiology*. 2004;100(6):1373-1381.
20. Johnson KB, Egan TD. Remifentanil and propofol combination for awake craniotomy: case report with pharmacokinetic simulations. *J Neurosurg Anesthesiol*. 1998;10(1):25-9.
21. Manninen P, Contreras J. Anesthetic considerations for craniotomy in awake patients. *Int Anesthesiol Clin*. 1986;24(3):157-174.
22. LaPierre CD, Johnson KB, Randall BR, Egan TD. A simulation study of common propofol and propofol-opioid dosing regimens for upper endoscopy: implications on the time course of recovery. *Anesthesiology*. 2012;117(2):252-262.
23. LaPierre CD, Johnson KB, Randall BR, White JL, Egan TD. An exploration of remifentanil-propofol combinations that lead to a loss of response to esophageal instrumentation, a loss of responsiveness, and/or onset of intolerable ventilatory depression. *Anesth Analg*. 2011;113(3):490-499.
24. Weiss FR, Schwartz R. Anaesthesia for awake craniotomy. *Can J Anaesth*. 1993;40(10):1003.
25. Welling EC, Donegan J. Neuroleptanalgesia using alfentanil for awake craniotomy. *Anesth Analg*. 1989;68(1):57-60.
26. Gignac E, Manninen PH, Gelb AW. Comparison of fentanyl, sufentanil and alfentanil during awake craniotomy for epilepsy. *Can J Anaesth*. 1993;40(5 pt 1):421-424.
27. Bodor N, Buchwald P. Soft drug design: general principles and recent applications. *Med Res Rev*. 2000;20(1):58-101.

CHAPTER

36

Anesthesia for Cervical Spine Surgery

Clint Christensen, MD

INTRODUCTION

Several patient management goals influence anesthetic drug selection in patients undergoing cervical spine surgery for severe cervical spine disease. Two of these are anesthetic choice and dosing technique to facilitate awake airway management and dosing techniques to optimize spinal cord monitoring. This chapter will briefly review some of the techniques, among many, that can be used to achieve these goals.

CASE DISCUSSION

A 56-year-old, 80-kg (176 lb), 165-cm (5′5″) female with bilateral hand numbness and arm pain is recently diagnosed with 2 cervical herniated discs is scheduled for C5-6, C6-7 anterior cervical discectomy and fusion. Neck and arm pain are exacerbated with neck extension. An awake fiberoptic bronchoscopy is planned for endotracheal tube placement.

PREMEDICATION

Analgesia and Sedation for Awake Fiberoptic Intubation

Attaining optimal intubating conditions for an awake fiberoptic intubation in a patient with a known or suspected unstable cervical spine is a challenge. There are several, sometimes conflicting, goals that include good patient cooperation, adequate analgesia during intubation, minimal cervical spine movement, and adequate cardiopulmonary function. Several pharmacologic options are available to the anesthesiologist to assist in achieving these goals. Selected agents are presented in Table 36–1.

The mainstay of analgesia for an awake fiberoptic bronchoscopy is topicalization of cranial nerves IX and X with a local anesthetic. Topicalization works best in a dry mouth and when there is adequate time for the local anesthetics to take effect (up to 20–30 minutes). Common local anesthetics include lidocaine and benzocaine spray.

For topical administration, 5% lidocaine ointment can be applied to a tongue depressor. Patients are asked to suck in the tongue depressor as they would with a lollipop. This approach helps abolish the oral gag reflex. To ablate the periglottic cough, 1 to 2 mL of 4% lidocaine can be administered to the posterior pharynx and supraglottic structures via a microatomizer device. The subglottic cough is ablated via an additionally 2 to 3 mL of 4% lidocaine injected transtracheally or through the fiberoptic scope upon visualization of the vocal cords. When using lidocaine, special care should be taken to avoid local anesthetic toxicity, given that the cranial nerves are near vascular structures and the choice of using high-concentration lidocaine preparations and the possibility of exceeding maximal dosing recommendations (ie, 5 mg/kg of lidocaine without epinephrine).

Benzocaine (Cetacaine) spray is an effective combination drug used for topicalization. It consists of 14% benzocaine, 2% tetracaine, and 2% butamben. It has a rapid onset of action and can last 30 to 60 minutes. Recommended dosing is up to 3 sprays for a total spray time of 2 seconds. With each second of spray, approximately 28 mg of benzocaine is administered. Benzocaine is most worrisome because it can lead to methemoglobinemia with prolonged exposure. This can be a rare, potentially life-threatening, complication in debilitated and young (< 2 years) patients.

TABLE 36–1 Selected topical anesthetics, sedatives, and analgesics for an awake fiberoptic intubation.

Agent	Dose	Comments
Topical anesthetics		
Lidocaine	5% paste 2% or 4% liquid preparation for topical spray or nebulizer	Maximal dose: 5 mg/kg
Benzocaine	2-second spray	Excessive dosing may cause methemoglobinemia.
Opioids		
Remifentanil	0.05 mcg/kg/min Consider 0.25–0.5 mcg/kg bolus to speed onset of effect	Requires up to 15 minutes to reach pseudo–steady state if dosed only as a continuous infusion
Fentanyl	0.5–1.0 mcg/kg	
Sedatives		
Midazolam	0.5–2.0 mg	Requires up to 5–8 minutes to reach peak effect
Dexmedetomidine	0.2–0.7 mcg/kg/h Consider 0.5-mcg/kg bolus to speed onset of effect	May cause hypotension
Ketamine	10–20 mg	May increase secretions Potent analgesia
Adjuncts		
Glycopyrrolate	0.2–0.4 mg	Antisialagogue
Atropine	0.1–0.5 mg	Antisialagogue

Several intravenous sedatives and hypnotics can be used as adjuncts to topicalization for awake fiberoptic bronchoscopy and tracheal intubation. For example, additional analgesia can be achieved with a remifentanil infusion. Opioids are useful in blunting the gag response but can also produce unwanted respiratory depression at higher doses. Figure 36–1 presents a set of simulations of a remifentanil infusion (0.05–0.1 mcg/kg/min) with the resultant effect-site concentrations and predicted analgesic, sedative, and ventilatory depression effects. (See also Table 36–2.)

Of note, once a remifentanil infusion is started, it can require a longer than expected to reach a near–steady state. As illustrated in the figure, the time required to reach 90% of the effect-site concentration is more than 20 minutes for the continuous infusion. Infusion rate changes prior to reaching near–steady state (also called pseudo–steady state) may result in excessive or inadequate dosing. To mitigate this delay, clinicians can (1) start the infusion early (ie, during topicalization with local anesthetic) so that at the time of fiber optic bronchoscopy, the effect from remifentanil has been established or (2) administer a small bolus (ie, 0.5 mcg/kg) to quickly achieve a desired effect. In this simulation, with a small bolus, the time required to reach 90% of the end effect site concentration is less than 1 minute (see Figure 36–1).

These simulations also predict that a remifentanil infusion, as dosed, will likely not produce significant sedation but pose a risk of ventilatory

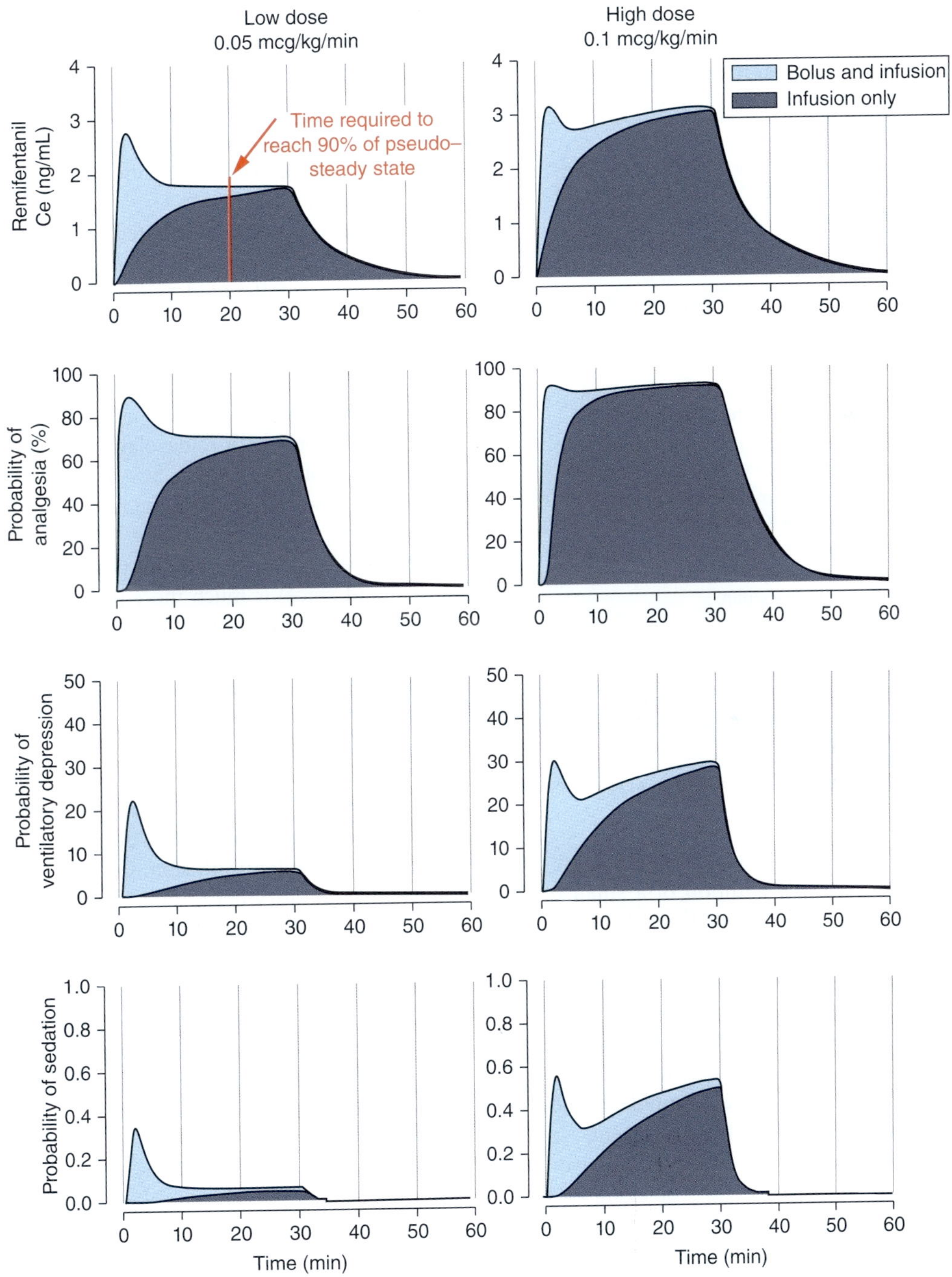

FIGURE 36–1 Simulations of selected remifentanil infusions with and without a bolus dose. The upper 2 plots present the predicted effect-site concentration (Ce) levels that result from infusion rates of 0.05 and 0.1 mcg/kg/min with and without a bolus dose of 0.5 mcg/kg. The lower plots present the predicted analgesic, ventilatory depressant, and sedation effects. Predictions of remifentanil concentrations and effects are based on published pharmacokinetic and pharmacodynamic models.[1-3] Assumptions of model predictions are presented in Table 36–2.

TABLE 36–2 Definitions, assumptions, and limitations of drug concentration and effect predictions presented in figures 36–1 and 36–2.

Definitions
Ventilatory depression is defined as the probability of a respiratory rate of less than 4 breaths/min in an unstimulated state.[4]
Sedation is defined as the probability of responsiveness to name with tactile stimuli (MOAAS score of 3).[5]
Analgesia is defined as a loss of response to a moderately painful pressure on the anterior tibia.[1]
Assumptions
Pharmacokinetic predictions assume the patient demographics described in the Case Discussion.
The interaction between midazolam and propofol is additive for sedation (Chapter 3).
The interaction between midazolam and opioids is synergistic for analgesia (Chapter 3).
When simulating inhalation agents, the assumptions include normal pulmonary function and blood flow and a minute volume of 6 liters/min.
Limitations
Predictions do not account for severe cardiac (ie, low cardiac output), hepatic, renal, or pulmonary disease.
Predictions do not account for or opioid or benzodiazepine tolerance.

MOAAS, Modified Observers Assessment of Alertness and Sedation Score.[6]

depression with higher infusion rates (ie, > 0.05 mcg/kg/min). With the addition of a small bolus, sedation is again unlikely, but the risk of ventilatory depression is substantially increased. Special care should be used when dosing remifentanil in this fashion. Remifentanil has a rapid onset of effect. It can quickly suppress ventilatory function before carbon dioxide accumulates in blood. With slower onset opioids, carbon dioxide accumulates and can offset ventilatory depression to some extent.

Midazolam is as an effective sedative and amnestic and can be used alone or along with an analgesic. A common dose for fiberoptic intubation is 0.5 to 2.0 mg. Special care should be taken when using midazolam combined with remifentanil. Both drugs will potentiate the effects of one another. Figure 36–2 illustrates the kinetic profile of a midazolam bolus (2 mg in an 80-kg individual) administered with remifentanil. Of note is the time required for midazolam to achieve maximal effect (6–9 minutes). This is of clinical relevance since anesthesiologists are accustomed to a rapid onset of effect with bolus dosing (within 90 seconds), and if no effect is observed, they may be tempted to administer additional midazolam before it reaches peak concentrations.

Several key points illustrated in Figures 36–1 and 36–2 merit discussion. The analgesic effect of the low-dose remifentanil infusion is more pronounced with midazolam (see Figure 36–2; second plot from top) than without it (see Figure 36–1; left column, second plot from top). Not only is the effect of the midazolam more pronounced, but its onset is more rapid. Thus, with midazolam, the problem of a slow onset of effect with a low-dose remifentanil infusion is resolved, making the remifentanil bolus unnecessary.

Sedation (defined as a responsive to tactile stimuli and voice) is much more pronounced when midazolam is administered with the remifentanil. Remifentanil accentuates midazolam's sedating effect. In the absence of remifentanil, this midazolam dose provides anxiolysis but is not likely to produce sedation as defined above.

Ventilatory depression is also increased. With 2 mg of midazolam, the probability of ventilatory depression rises from 6% to 11% during a 30-minute low-dose remifentanil infusion. Of note, the probability of respiratory depression is much less using a combination of midazolam and remifentanil than using a higher remifentanil infusion rate (reaching near 30% probability of ventilatory depression) or a small remifentanil bolus (reaching over 20% probability of ventilatory depression). In patients suspected to be sensitive to opioids and benzodiazepines, a lower dose of midazolam (0.5–1.0 mg) is prudent.

These figures illustrate how combining drugs that interact with the central nervous system via different mechanisms (ie, opioid versus γ-aminobutyric acid receptors) may be more beneficial than using a single drug and escalating the dose to achieve a desired effect. Small doses of combined therapy allow maximizing desirable effects (in this case sedation and analgesia) while minimizing adverse effects (ventilatory depression).

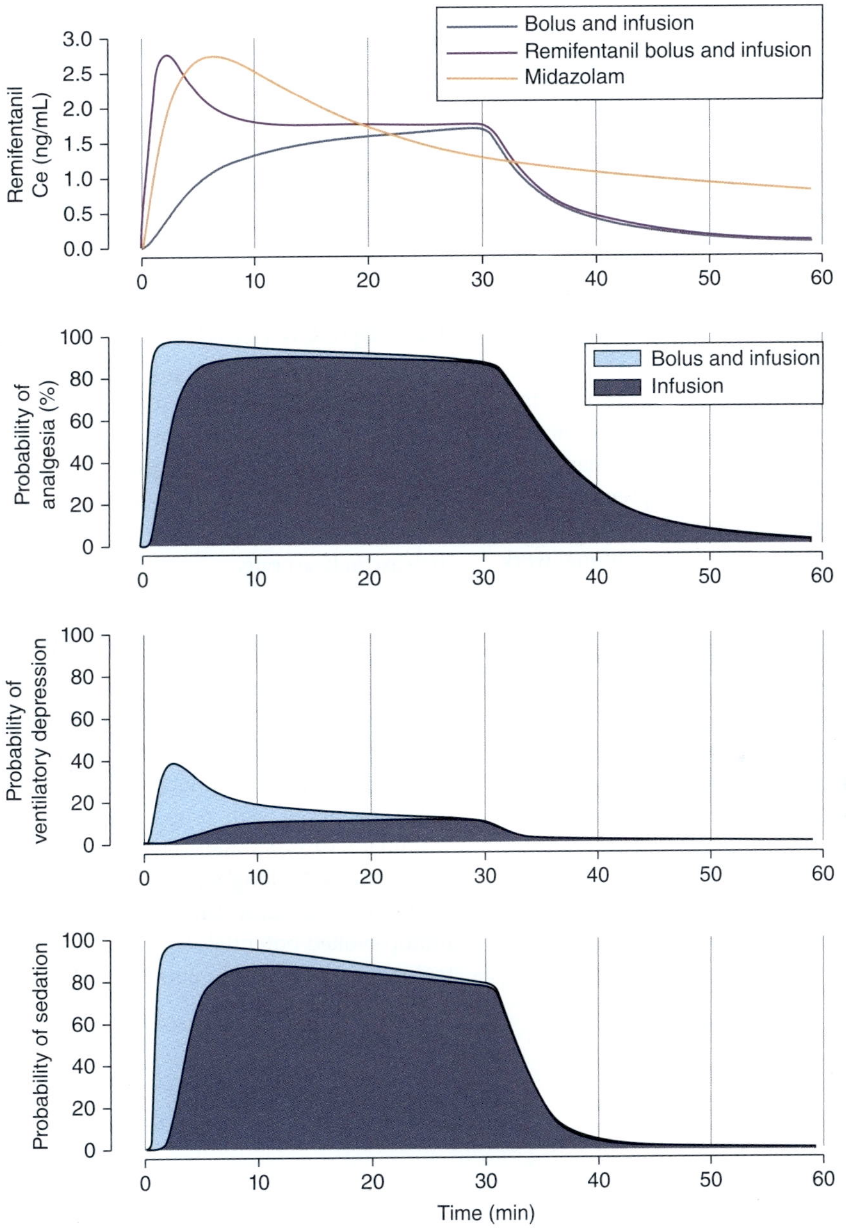

FIGURE 36–2 Simulations of a 2-mg midazolam bolus added to the remifentanil infusion (0.05 mcg/kg/min) with and without a bolus (0.5 mcg/kg) (presented in Figure 36–1). The top plot presents the effect-site concentration (Ce) levels for each drug. The lower plots present the analgesic, ventilatory depression, and sedating effects in the presence of one another. Predictions of drug concentrations and effects are based on published pharmacokinetic and pharmacodynamic models.[1-3,7,8]

Ketamine is an effective sedative and analgesic. A common dose is 10 to 20 mg administered a few minutes prior to fiber-optic intubation. Ketamine provides amnesia and intense analgesia while maintaining upper airway tone and respiratory drive. If administered too early, ketamine can increase oral secretions. Adverse side effects include dysphoria with hallucinations and excessive secretion. Hallucinations are limited with concomitant use of midazolam and secretions are limited with an antisialagogue. When administered as a bolus, plasma concentrations exhibit a slow climb to reach the peak effect-site concentration and a slow decrement, suggesting that it may last the duration of an awake intubation process (Figure 36–3). Given that ketamine has active metabolites and in some countries is prepared as an enantiomer (both S and L ketamine), it is difficult to study or predict its behavior. As such, minimal work has been done exploring how ketamine interacts with other anesthetics, and its effects may be variable.

Dexmedetomidine is an effective sedative that is administered as a continuous infusion. Like remifentanil, it is slow to achieve pseudo–steady state (Figure 36–4). A major advantage to dexmedetomidine is that it causes minimal respiratory depression, yet it may cause bradycardia and hypotension. If a bolus is used to achieve a therapeutic effect quickly, the bolus should be administered slowly (ie, over 10 minutes) which helps to reduce the adverse hemodynamic effects of bradycardia and hypotension.[11] Unlike most other sedatives, dexmedetomidine, when administered for a prolonged period, will have a persistent effect long after the infusion is terminated. Like ketamine, dexmedetomidine's interaction with other analgesics and sedatives is not well described. Thus, in the presence of a dexmedetomidine infusion or a ketamine bolus, dosing additional opioid or sedative drugs should be done with careful titration.

Adjuncts to Anesthesia for Awake Fiberoptic Intubation

To manage secretions, an antisialagogue such as glycopyrrolate (0.2–0.4 mg) or atropine (0.1–0.5 mg) can be used. They are effective but should be administered 20–30 minutes prior to initiating airway instrumentation. Special care should be taken in patients with known cardiac disease, who may not tolerate an increase in heart rate.

INDUCTION OF ANESTHESIA

Once endotracheal tube placement has been confirmed, some clinicians may choose to perform a brief neurologic examination demonstrating upper extremity function prior to inducing anesthesia. Induction can be achieved with propofol (0.5–2.0 mg/kg) or etomidate (0.1–0.3 mg/kg) to render the patient unconscious. No long acting paralytics are warranted at this time because they can disrupt monitoring motor-evoked potentials (MEPs). Neurologic monitoring teams will likely obtain MEP measurements

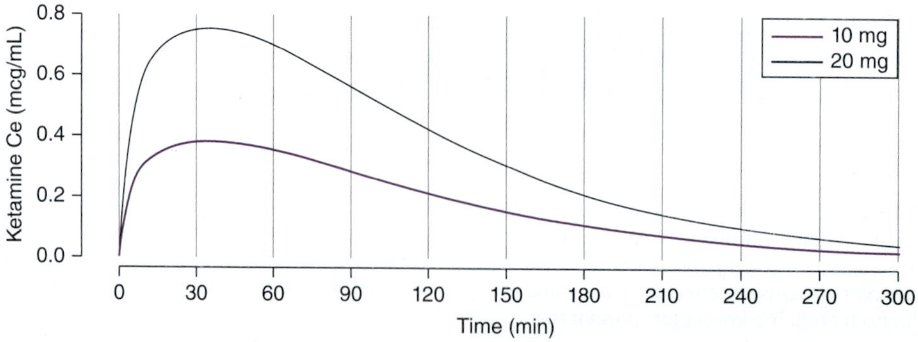

FIGURE 36–3 Simulation of 2 ketamine boluses—10 and 20 mg. Predictions of drug concentrations are based on a published pharmacokinetic and pharmacodynamic models.[9,10] The time required to reach the predicted peak effect-site concentration (Ce) is 30 minutes. The decrement time required for the predicted Ce to drop to 10% of the peak value is approximately 4.5 hours.

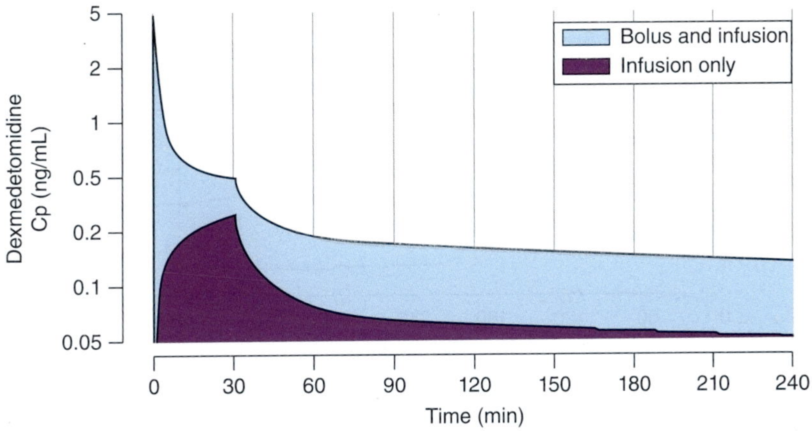

FIGURE 36–4 Simulation of a dexmedetomidine infusion (0.5 mcg/kg/h) with and without a slow bolus (0.5 mcg/kg) administered over 5 minutes. Predictions of drug concentrations are based on published pharmacokinetic models.[11,12] The decrement time required for the predicted plasma concentrations to drop to 10% of the concentrations at the end of the 30-minute drug administration period is 9.5 hours for the continuous infusion and more than 15 hours for the bolus and continuous infusion. Caution should be used in interpreting these time estimates, given that they simply describe the decrement time in plasma concentration but do not predict the duration of any effect (ie, sedation, analgesia, or vasodilation).

shortly after induction prior to surgery to establish a baseline.

MAINTENANCE OF ANESTHESIA

The neuroanesthesiologist is often called upon to administer an anesthetic that will provide adequate analgesia and sedation yet allow monitoring of both MEPs and somatosensory evoked potentials (SSEPs) to continually assess the function of the spinal cord throughout the surgical period. Sedatives and analgesics are primarily used to meet anesthetic needs to include patient immobility.

Opioids

Anesthesiologists often rely on high-dose opioid techniques to provide patient akinesia during surgery yet allow MEP monitoring. Sufentanil, fentanyl, and remifentanil can all be used to achieve this effect. They are best administered as continuous infusions rather than intermittent boluses because this way they have a more consistent profile in analgesic effect and provide better conditions for MEP monitoring.

All of the fentanyl congeners are capable of achieving and maintaining profound analgesia during surgery, but they have quite different profiles once their administration is terminated at the end of surgery. Consider a simulation of effect-site concentrations for fentanyl, remifentanil, and sufentanil infusions for a 3-hour spine surgery presented in Figure 36–5. The infusion rates were selected based on their ability to produce a near-equivalent opioid effect, namely a greater than 95% probability of analgesia (defined as a loss of response to tibial pressure).

Once the infusions are terminated, the decrement in effect-site concentration is quite different for each drug. Because of the rapid decline in drug effect, remifentanil will require a transition opioid such as hydromorphone, fentanyl, or morphine to provide analgesia during emergence. In contrast, fentanyl and sufentanil have a prolonged opioid effect. This may provide analgesia but prolong emergence and be associated with unwanted respiratory depression. Between fentanyl and sufentanil, sufentanil has a faster kinetic profile. Once the infusion is terminated, it has a concentration decrement that is much slower than remifentanil but faster than fentanyl.

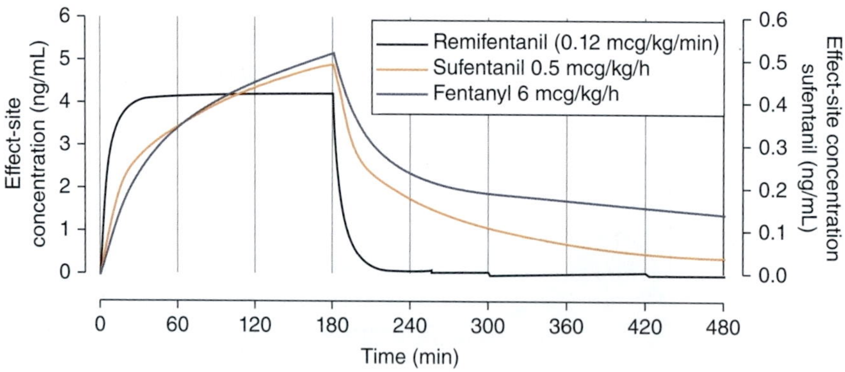

FIGURE 36–5 Simulations of effect-site concentrations for near-equipotent 3-hour infusions of sufentanil (0.5 mcg/kg/h), remifentanil (0.12 mcg/kg/min), and fentanyl (6 mcg/kg/h). Predictions of drug concentrations are based on published pharmacokinetic models.[1-3,13-15] Predictions of the effect-site 50% decrement times (time required for the effect-site concentration to drop by 50% from what it was when the infusions were turned off) were 4, 27, and 47 minutes for remifentanil, sufentanil, and fentanyl infusions, respectively.

A history of chronic opioid consumption is useful to consider when selecting which opioid to use for infusion. Sufentanil or fentanyl is appropriate in patients who chronically consume large quantities of opioids. Opioid-naive patients can be well managed with remifentanil followed by a transition opioid. Of note, postoperative pain management requirements are less for the anterior approach than the posterior approach to the cervical spine.

Potent Inhaled Agents

Inhalational anesthetics have a profound dose-dependent depressive effect on evoked potential responses, with MEP's being depressed more than SSEP's. Therefore, in order to obtain adequate evoked potential responses, inhalation agents should be dosed to keep end-tidal concentrations at or below 0.5 minimum alveolar concentration (MAC). To meet the anesthetic requirements, opioids are frequently added. The unique features of remifentanil make it potentially very useful in this setting. It can be dosed to achieve a profound level of analgesia, even with only 0.5 MAC, without any consequence of prolonged infusions.

Figure 36–6 presents a simulation of selected anesthetic effects for a 3-hour combined technique using 0.5 MAC of desflurane (4.2%) and an opioid infusion (remifentanil 0.2 mcg/kg/min, sufentanil 0.7 mcg/kg/h, or fentanyl 6 mcg/kg/h). The simulated effects include loss of responsiveness, analgesia, and ventilatory depression. Given that fentanyl and sufentanil have a prolonged effect with infusions, they were terminated 45 minutes prior to the end of the procedure.

Key points from this simulation are:

- As dosed, desflurane in combination with remifentanil provided a high probability of unresponsiveness despite only 0.5 MAC during the 3-hour procedure. As dosed, fentanyl and sufentanil in combination with desflurane provided between 85% and 95% probability of unresponsiveness. For all opioids, the effect quickly dissipated once the desflurane and opioid infusions were shut off.
- Once the procedure ended, the time required for the probability of analgesia to drop below 50% was more than 2 hours for fentanyl and 1.5 hours for sufentanil but only 16 minutes for remifentanil. This simulation again illustrates the need for a transition opioid for remifentanil to maintain an analgesic effect shortly after the infusion is turned off.
- If the sufentanil or fentanyl infusion is turned off 45 minutes prior to the estimated end of surgery after infusing for more than 2 hours, the analgesic effect slowly declines likely providing analgesia during emergence and for the immediate postoperative period.

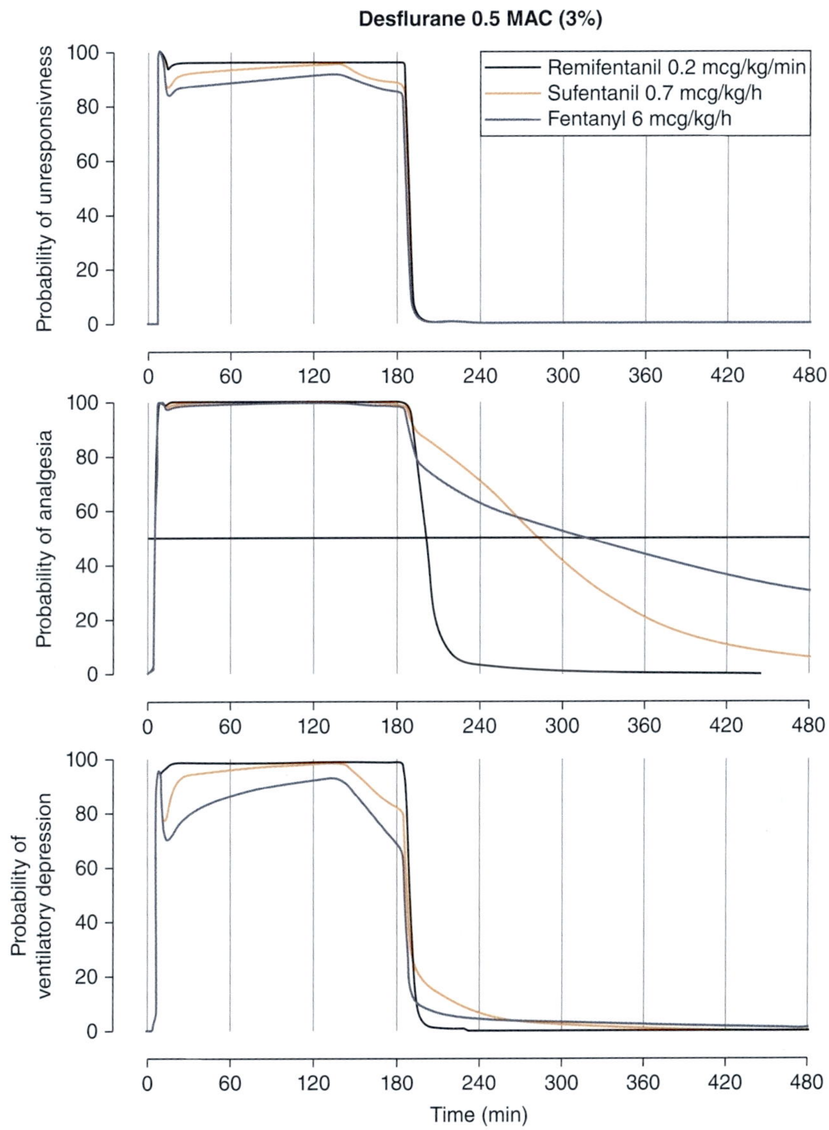

FIGURE 36–6 Simulation of selected anesthetic effects following a 3-hour combined desflurane–opioid anesthetic. Induction consisted of propofol 2 mg/kg and fentanyl 150 mcg. Desflurane was maintained at 0.7 minimum alveolar concentration (MAC) (4.2%) for 3 hours. The opioid infusions were sufentanil 0.7 mcg/kg/h, remifentanil 0.2 mcg/kg/min, and fentanyl 6 mcg/kg/h. The fentanyl and sufentanil infusions were terminated 45 minutes prior to the end of the 3-hour procedure, whereas the remifentanil infusion was maintained for the duration of the entire procedure. Predictions of drug concentrations and effects were based on published pharmacokinetic and drug interaction pharmacodynamic models.[14-20] Predicted drug effects include loss of responsiveness, defined as unresponsive to verbal and painful tactile stimuli (top plot); analgesia defined as a loss of response to painful tibial pressure (middle plot), and intolerable ventilatory depression defined as a respiratory rate less than 4 breaths per minute in an unstimulated state (bottom plot).

- As dosed, the probability of intolerable ventilatory depression quickly dissipates once anesthetic delivery is terminated. Within 10 minutes, the probability is less than 20% for all 3 opioids and reaches less than 5% in 13, 45, and 70 minutes for remifentanil, sufentanil, and fentanyl, respectively.

Intravenous Sedative Hypnotics

In contrast, propofol affects evoked potentials less than volatile anesthetics.[21] For example, SSEPs are usually adequate even when propofol is administered in doses that produce burst suppression. For a total intravenous anesthesia (TIVA) technique, propofol in combination with remifentanil infusions can be initially dosed at 100 and 0.1 to 0.2 mcg/kg/min, respectively, and subsequently titrated based on hemodynamic responses and/or patient movement in response to surgical stimuli. If evoked potential monitoring becomes inadequate in the presence of potent inhaled agents, consideration should be given to converting the anesthetic to a TIVA technique.

Figure 36–7 presents a simulation of selected anesthetic effects for a 3-hour combined technique using propofol 100 mcg/kg/min and an opioid infusion (remifentanil 0.2 mcg/kg/min, sufentanil 0.7 mcg/kg/h, or fentanyl 6 mcg/kg/h). As before, the opioid infusions were dosed to achieve near-equivalent high probability of analgesic effect, and the fentanyl and sufentanil were terminated 45 minutes prior to the end of the procedure.

Key points from this simulation are:

- One potential concern with TIVA is the risk of intraoperative awareness. As dosed, propofol in combination with remifentanil leads to a predicted high probability of unresponsiveness. The opioid effect from remifentanil is significantly enhanced by propofol, providing profound analgesia and similarly, the sedation effect from propofol is somewhat enhanced by remifentanil. Higher remifentanil infusion rates or supplemental opioid administration may be warranted in patients with substantial opioid tolerance from prolonged exposure.
- Propofol in combination with sufentanil or fentanyl as dosed leads to a predicted probability of unresponsiveness that is somewhat lower than propofol combined with remifentanil. To compensate, a higher propofol infusion rate may be warranted.

Some clinicians advocate the use of processed electroencephalographic monitoring when using TIVA in conjunction with neuromuscular blockade. This is done to identify changes in patient response to painful stimuli that would normally lead to patient movement. Of note, neuromuscular blockade will not influence any hemodynamic response to painful stimuli such that heart rate and blood pressure are still useful as surrogates of response to surgical stimuli. That said, when administering a TIVA, constant monitoring of the intravenous catheter is warranted to ensure continuous administration of the anesthetic.

It is notoriously difficult to obtain adequate evoked potentials in patients with preexisting neurologic dysfunction. A minimally depressive TIVA may be needed for optimal neurologic monitoring in patients with preoperative neurologic findings.[22]

To achieve this goal, other sedatives to consider may include ketamine and dexmedetomidine. In instances when opioid-based anesthetics make obtaining SSEP signals difficult, clinical experience suggests that replacing the opioid with ketamine may improve SSEP monitoring.[23-25] Dosing is not well defined; some authors advocate generous dosing (0.4–0.6 mg/kg/h) to avoid the use of propofol,[26] whereas others recommend low-dose ketamine infusions (0.05–0.1 mg/kg/h) or intermittent ketamine boluses (10 mg/h) as an adjunct to an anesthetic, minimizing the dose of other agents. Ketamine may be especially useful in patients who have persistent intraoperative hypotension that is exacerbated with additional opioid.

One caveat with ketamine should be considered if the agent is dosed as a bolus at the beginning of a procedure. As the ketamine concentration declines, and the associated increase in evoked potential amplitude also declines, the result can be misinterpreted as nerve injury from surgery rather than a dissipating effect from a pharmacologic agent.

Dexmedetomidine (0.2–1.0 mcg/kg/h) is a useful adjunct, especially in patients with persistent hypertension, despite presumed adequate opioid dosing. Judicious dosing of dexmedetomidine has been found

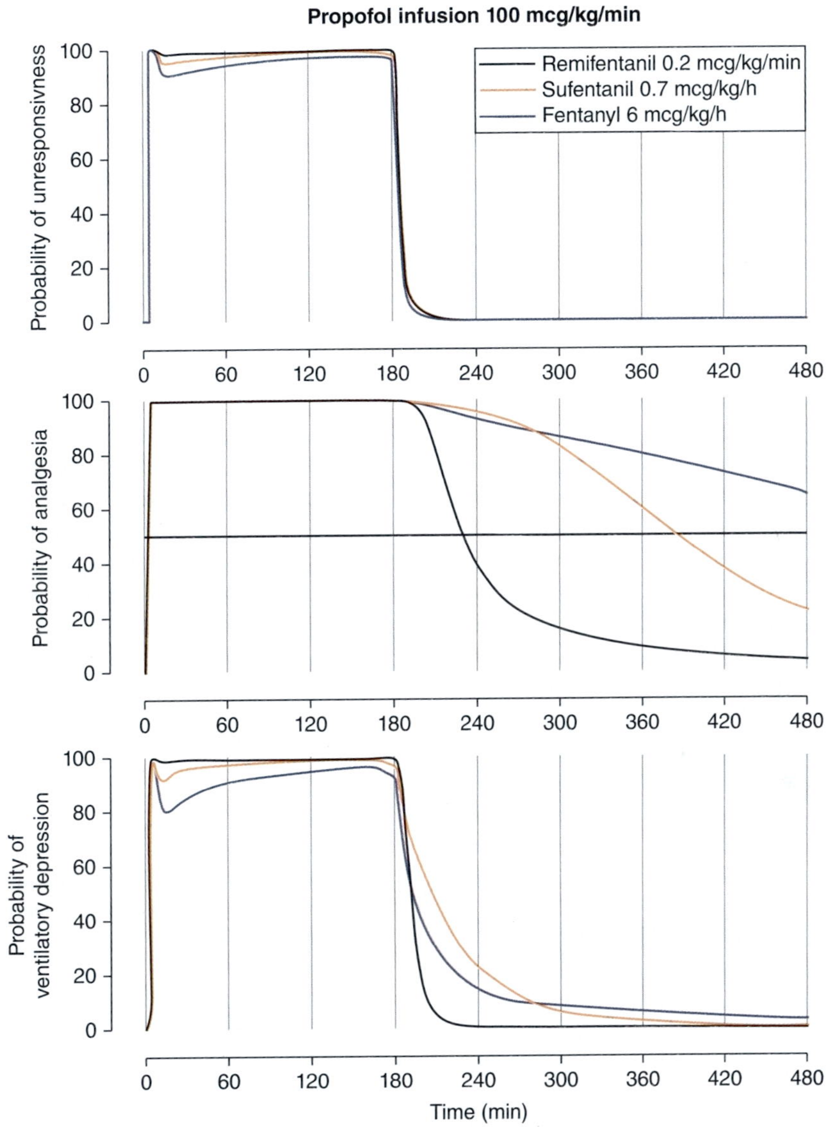

FIGURE 36–7 Simulation of selected anesthetic effects following a 3-hour combined propofol–opioid anesthetic. Induction consisted of propofol 2 mg/kg and fentanyl 150 mcg. Propofol was maintained at 100 mcg/kg/min for 3 hours. The opioid infusions were sufentanil 0.7 mcg/kg/h, remifentanil 0.2 mcg/kg/min, and fentanyl 6 mcg/kg/h. The fentanyl and sufentanil infusions were terminated 45 minutes prior to the end of the 3-hour procedure, whereas the remifentanil infusion was maintained for the duration of the entire procedure. Predictions of drug concentrations and effects were based on published pharmacokinetic and drug interaction pharmacodynamic models.[1-3,14,15,20] Predicted drug effects include loss of responsiveness (top plot), analgesia (middle plot), and intolerable ventilatory depression (bottom plot).

to have minimal impact on SSEPs but may adversely affect the amplitude of MEPs at higher doses.[27] For TIVA using propofol and remifentanil in a pediatric population, the addition of dexmedetomidine was found to have a dose-dependent suppression of MEP amplitude that was not clinically significant[28] for lower doses. Dosing that achieved predicted plasma concentrations of 6 to 8 ng/mL led to changes in MEP amplitude that required lower dexmedetomidine dosing.[28] Similar findings have been found with adults when TIVA[29,30] or desflurane combined with remifentanil are used.[31] Caution should be used in prolonged infusions, as it can delay emergence with its profound sedating effect.

An additional adjunct anesthetic to consider in patients who require evoked potential monitoring is lidocaine. When combined with propofol and sufentanil, lidocaine was found to not have any detrimental affect on SSEPs or MEPs[32] and can significantly reduce propofol requirements. A suggested dosing regimen is 1.5 mg/kg/h, with a maximal infusion rate of 120 mg/h, stopping the infusion 45 minutes prior to the anticipated end of the surgical procedure (to coincide with the termination of the sufentanil infusion).[32]

When considering the use of any new combination of anesthetic drugs, it is prudent to discuss their use with the neuromonitoring team to assess their real-time influence on evoked potential monitoring.

Neuromuscular Blocking Agents

MEPs, but not SSEPs, are sensitive to neuromuscular blocking drugs. As such, neuromuscular blockers, in general, should not be used for procedures that require MEP monitoring. Small doses of neuromuscular blockers may be used for patient positioning just prior to surgery, but they should be dosed such that their effect dissipates prior to surgical dissection near the spinal cord. On the other hand, for SSEPs, neuromuscular blocking agents may minimize artifact from muscle movement and improve signal acquisition.

EMERGENCE

Major goals for emergence are (1) a smooth emergence with minimal coughing and bucking, so as to decrease the risk of neck hematoma, and (2) a rapid emergence, to facilitate a timely postoperative neurologic examination in the operating room prior to transfer to the recovery room. To minimize coughing, one approach is to maintain an analgesic effect through emergence. If using remifentanil, a transition opioid should be used. Either a fentanyl (1–3 mcg/kg) or hydromorphone (3–7 mcg/kg) bolus is a useful transition opioid. The transition opioid should be administered within 10 to 15 minutes of the end of the procedure (see Figure 36–7). If using sufentanil, consider terminating the infusion at the beginning of closure. With a fairly quick closure (15–20 minutes), sufentanil effect-site concentrations will be on the decline but provide analgesia through emergence and extubation.

Other adjuncts useful in minimizing the risk of developing a neck hematoma from coughing and retching during emergence include lidocaine and antiemetics. Lidocaine, administered as a bolus (1–2 mg/kg) can blunt the gag response to endotracheal tube removal. Antiemetics are useful in minimizing postoperative nausea and vomiting, which may also increase the risk of a neck hematoma.

REFERENCES

1. Johnson KB, Syroid ND, Gupta DK, et al. An evaluation of remifentanil propofol response surfaces for loss of responsiveness, loss of response to surrogates of painful stimuli and laryngoscopy in patients undergoing elective surgery. *Anesth Analg.* 2008;106(2):471-479.
2. Minto CF, Schnider TW, Egan TD, et al. Influence of age and gender on the pharmacokinetics and pharmacodynamics of remifentanil. I. Model development. *Anesthesiology.* 1997;86(1):10-23.
3. Minto CF, Schnider TW, Shafer SL. Pharmacokinetics and pharmacodynamics of remifentanil. II. Model application. *Anesthesiology.* 1997;86(1):24-33.
4. LaPierre CD, Johnson KB, Randall BR, White JL, Egan TD. An exploration of remifentanil-propofol combinations that lead to a loss of response to esophageal instrumentation, a loss of responsiveness, and/or onset of intolerable ventilatory depression. *Anesth Analg.* 2011; 113(3):490-499.
5. Kern SE, Xie G, White JL, Egan TD. A response surface analysis of propofol-remifentanil pharmacodynamic interaction in volunteers. *Anesthesiology.* 2004;100(6): 1373-1381.
6. Chernick DA, Gillings D, Laine H, Hendler J, Silver JM, Davidson AB. Validity and reliability of the Observer's

Assessment of Alertness/Sedation Scale: study with intravenous midazolam. *J Clin Psychopharmacol.* 1990; 10(4):244-251.

7. Albrecht S, Ihmsen H, Hering W, et al. The effect of age on the pharmacokinetics and pharmacodynamics of midazolam. *Clin Pharmacol Ther.* 1999;65(6):630-639.
8. Fidler M, Kern SE. Flexible interaction model for complex interactions of multiple anesthetics. *Anesthesiology.* 2006;105(2):286-296.
9. Ihmsen H, Geisslinger G, Schuttler J. Stereoselective pharmacokinetics of ketamine: R(−)-ketamine inhibits the elimination of S(+)-ketamine. *Clin Pharmacol Ther.* 2001;70(5):431-438.
10. Satori V, Zanderigo E, Kvasnica M, Morari M. Optimal infusion policy of intravenous morphine and ketamine—a mixed-integer linear programming application. *Conf Proc IEEE Eng Med Biol Soc.* 2005;3:2363-2366.
11. Dyck JB, Maze M, Haack C, Vuorilehto L, Shafer SL. The pharmacokinetics and hemodynamic effects of intravenous and intramuscular dexmedetomidine hydrochloride in adult human volunteers. *Anesthesiology.* 1993;78(5):813-820.
12. Dyck JB, Maze M, Haack C, Azarnoff DL, Vuorilehto L, Shafer SL. Computer-controlled infusion of intravenous dexmedetomidine hydrochloride in adult human volunteers. *Anesthesiology.* 1993;78(5):821-828.
13. Gepts E, Shafer SL, Camu F, et al. Linearity of pharmacokinetics and model estimation of sufentanil. *Anesthesiology.* 1995;83(6):1194-1204.
14. Shafer SL, Varvel JR, Aziz N, Scott JC. Pharmacokinetics of fentanyl administered by computer-controlled infusion pump. *Anesthesiology.* 1990;73(6):1091-1102.
15. Syroid ND, Johnson KB, Pace NL, et al. Response surface model predictions of emergence and response to pain in the recovery room: an evaluation of patients emerging from an isoflurane and fentanyl anesthetic. *Anesth Analg.* 2010;111(2):380-386.
16. Johnson KB, Syroid ND, Gupta DK, et al. An evaluation of remifentanil-sevoflurane response surface models in patients emerging from anesthesia: model improvement using effect-site sevoflurane concentrations. *Anesth Analg.* 2010;111(2):387-394.
17. Lerou JG, Booij LH. Model-based administration of inhalation anaesthesia. 3. Validating the system model. *Br J Anaesth.* 2002;88(1):24-37.
18. Lerou JG, Dirksen R, Beneken Kolmer HH, Booij LH, Borm GF. A system model for closed-circuit inhalation anesthesia. II. Clinical validation. *Anesthesiology.* 1991; 75(2):230-237.
19. Manyam SC, Gupta DK, Johnson KB, et al. Opioid-volatile anesthetic synergy: a response surface model with remifentanil and sevoflurane as prototypes. *Anesthesiology.* 2006;105(2):267-278.
20. Schnider TW, Minto CF, Shafer SL, et al. The influence of age on propofol pharmacodynamics. *Anesthesiology.* 1999;90(6):1502-1516.
21. Liu EH, Wong HK, Chia CP, Lim HJ, Chen ZY, Lee TL. Effects of isoflurane and propofol on cortical somatosensory evoked potentials during comparable depth of anaesthesia as guided by bispectral index. *Br J Anaesth.* 2005;94(2):193-197.
22. Hermanns H, Lipfert P, Meier S, Jetzek-Zader M, Krauspe R, Stevens MF. Cortical somatosensory-evoked potentials during spine surgery in patients with neuromuscular and idiopathic scoliosis under propofol-remifentanil anaesthesia. *Br J Anaesth.* 2007; 98(3):362-365.
23. Agarwal R, Roitman KJ, Stokes M. Improvement of intraoperative somatosensory evoked potentials by ketamine. *Paediatr Anaesth.* 1998;8(3):263-266.
24. Erb TO, Ryhult SE, Duitmann E, Hasler C, Luetschg J, Frei FJ. Improvement of motor-evoked potentials by ketamine and spatial facilitation during spinal surgery in a young child. *Anesth Analg.* 2005;100(6): 1634-1636.
25. Ubags LH, Kalkman CJ, Been HD, Porsius M, Drummond JC. The use of ketamine or etomidate to supplement sufentanil/N2O anesthesia does not disrupt monitoring of myogenic transcranial motor evoked responses. *J Neurosurg Anesthesiol.* 1997;9(3): 228-233.
26. Penney R. Use of dexmedetomidine and ketamine infusions during scoliosis repair surgery with somatosensory and motor-evoked potential monitoring: a case report. *AANA J.* 2010;78(6):446-450.
27. Brennen K, Konig M, Mahmoud M. Use of dexmedetomidine and ketamine infusions during scoliosis repair surgery with somatosensory and motor-evoked potential monitoring: a case report. *AANA J.* 2011;79(2):89; author reply 90.
28. Tobias JD, Goble TJ, Bates G, Anderson JT, Hoernschemeyer DG. Effects of dexmedetomidine on intraoperative motor and somatosensory evoked potential monitoring during spinal surgery in adolescents. *Paediatr Anaesth.* 2008;18(11): 1082-1088.
29. Anschel DJ, Aherne A, Soto RG, et al. Successful intraoperative spinal cord monitoring during scoliosis surgery using a total intravenous anesthetic regimen including dexmedetomidine. *J Clin Neurophysiol.* 2008;25(1):56-61.
30. Mahmoud M, Sadhasivam S, Salisbury S, et al. Susceptibility of transcranial electric motor-evoked

potentials to varying targeted blood levels of dexmedetomidine during spine surgery. *Anesthesiology.* 2010;112(6):1364-1373.

31. Bala E, Sessler DI, Nair DR, McLain R, Dalton JE, Farag E. Motor and somatosensory evoked potentials are well maintained in patients given dexmedetomidine during spine surgery. *Anesthesiology.* 2008;109(3):417-425.

32. Sloan TB, Mongan P, Lyda C, Koht A. Lidocaine infusion adjunct to total intravenous anesthesia reduces the total dose of propofol during intraoperative neurophysiological monitoring. *J Clin Monit Comput.* 2014;28(2):139-147.

CHAPTER 37

General Anesthesia for Emergency Cesarean Delivery: A Look at Pharmacokinetics and Pharmacodynamics in the Parturient

Zuzana Stehlikova, MD

INTRODUCTION

Cesarean delivery is one of the most common surgical procedures. In the United States, more than 1 million cesarean sections are performed each year, accounting for more than 30% of births. The majority of these procedures are performed using a regional technique; general anesthesia is reserved for patients who have a contraindication to a regional block or for emergencies, when there is not enough time for a regional block. Consequently, general anesthesia for cesarean delivery is relatively rare, and providers may be less comfortable administering it to parturients. Their discomfort is warranted. Although straightforward, general anesthetic for cesarean section is fraught with adverse events, including an increased risk of awareness, aspiration, difficult airway with hypoxia, drug-related uterine atony, and neonatal respiratory depression.

Numerous studies have characterized how physiologic changes of pregnancy alter the distribution, metabolism, and concentration-effect relationship of anesthetic drugs. Unfortunately, for most anesthetics, this body of knowledge has not transferred into dosing recommendations specific to the parturient. Anesthesiologists are left to rely on experience and careful titration to achieve unconsciousness and analgesia while avoiding adverse effects.

The purpose of this chapter is to review how physiologic changes associated with pregnancy influence kinetic and dynamic behavior of anesthetic drugs when used for general anesthesia under emergency conditions and explore through simulation how dosing technique may contribute to worrisome adverse effects.

PHARMACOKINETIC CONSIDERATIONS IN PREGNANCY

Intravenous Agents

A summary of physiologic changes that influence intravenous anesthetic drug kinetics is presented in Table 37–1. Volume of distribution increases for most drugs due to a 40% to 45% increase in blood volume as well as an increase in body fat and total body water during pregnancy.[1] Protein binding is reduced secondary to a 25% decline in albumin levels toward the end of pregnancy. Although levels of α-1-acid glycoprotein can decline in pregnancy, as an acute phase protein, levels exhibit a variable pattern. In some studies, third-trimester levels did not differ significantly from those obtained from nonpregnant women of childbearing age.[2] Accelerated redistribution of intravenous anesthetics can be expected secondary to a 40% increase in cardiac output.[1]

Elimination and metabolism are significantly altered during pregnancy. Hepatic blood flow does not appreciably change; however, some enzymatic activity is decreased (CYP1A2, CYP2C19) and some

TABLE 37–1 Physiologic changes in pregnancy that influence anesthetic drug kinetics.

Drug distribution	
Cardiac output	⇑
Body fat	⇑
Blood volume	⇑
Total body water	⇑
Drug protein binding To albumin To α-1-acid glycoprotein	 ⇓ ⇓⇑ or no change
Metabolism	
Hepatic blood flow	No change
Cytochrome P450 activity CYP1A2, 2C19 CYP3A4, 2D6, 2C9, UGT	 ⇓ ⇑
Pseudocholinesterase	⇓
Elimination	
Biliary	⇓⇑ or no change
Renal	⇑

increased (CYP3A4, CYP2D6, CYP2C9, UGT).[3] Therefore, hepatic clearance for a particular drug will be highly dependent on the exact metabolism and may increase (as can be expected for benzodiazepines and propofol that are metabolized by CYP, or morphine, which is metabolized by UGT), decrease (eg, caffeine, which is metabolized by CYP1A2) or remain unchanged.[2,3] Renal clearance during pregnancy is increased. The glomerular filtration rate increases 50% above prepregnancy levels.[2,3] Possible changes of tubular secretion and reabsorption of drugs are not well defined. Activity of pseudocholinesterase is diminished by 25%; however, succinylcholine recovery is not prolonged in pregnant patients.[4]

Inhalation Agents

Pharmacokinetics of inhaled anesthetics is also altered in pregnancy. When altering the concentration of inhaled anesthetics, alveolar concentration will rise more rapidly as a result of decreased functional residual capacity and increased minute ventilation; however, this is partially offset by increased cardiac output.

PHARMACODYNAMIC CONSIDERATIONS IN PREGNANCY

Intravenous Agents

The data on potency of intravenous anesthetic drugs in pregnancy are limited. Studies with propofol suggest that there is little or no change during the first trimester. Mongardon et al examined 57 patients at 11 weeks' gestation. Although the researchers found a statistically significant difference in mean propofol dose required for loss of consciousness in comparison to a nonpregnant control group, the difference was clinically negligible (1.8 versus 1.9 mg/kg), with predicted propofol effect-site concentration of 4.6 versus 5.0 mcg/mL.[5] Higuchi et al studied 36 patients at 6 to 12 weeks' gestation and concluded that venous propofol concentration at the time of loss of consciousness did not differ from the nonpregnant group.[6] Studies exploring propofol necessary for loss of consciousness later in pregnancy (ie, second or third trimester) when the influence of physiologic changes associated with pregnancy are perhaps more pronounced are not available.

Potency of other induction agents has not been directly evaluated. Common practice is to use induction doses that do not differ from nonpregnant patients: thiopental 4 mg/kg, etomidate 0.3 mg/kg, propofol 2 mg/kg, and ketamine 1 mg/kg.[7]

Inhalation Agents

Multiple studies by Chen et al provide solid evidence of 30% reduction of minimum alveolar concentration (MAC) of all volatile anesthetics as early as 8 weeks' gestation.[8,9] It was observed that MAC remains reduced for 24 to 36 hours postpartum with normalization to prepregnancy levels by 72 hours after delivery.[10] Although progesterone is likely responsible for decreased MAC in pregnancy, a simple linear correlation has not been demonstrated; the exact mechanism is unclear.[10]

CLINICAL RELEVANCE OF PHARMACOKINETIC AND PHARMACODYNAMIC CHANGES IN PREGNANCY

Overall, predictions of intravenous drug behavior in pregnant patients are near impossible to make. For example, following an intravenous bolus of an anesthetic drug, plasma concentrations may be higher or lower because of several competing physiologic changes. Plasma concentrations may be less due to an increased volume of distribution. The amount of free drug available to exert an effect should increase due to a decrease in plasma protein that normally binds up most of the circulating drug. Peak concentrations decline faster due to rapid redistribution. Hepatic metabolism will vary by drug and its associated enzymatic pathway. Drugs that are removed unchanged by the kidney may have increased clearance.

There is a paucity of literature exploring anesthetic drugs in late pregnancy. From what information is available, Table 37–2 presents pharmacokinetic changes for selected anesthetics. One group has explored propofol pharmacokinetics in pregnancy and reported a similar volume of distribution yet more rapid clearance compared to nonpregnant females in several studies.[11,12]

The majority of work describing the pharmacokinetics of thiopental in pregnancy was done 40 years ago. The data are conflicting. Some investigators reported an increase in the volume of distribution, whereas others reported an increased in clearance.[13-15] Interestingly, 10% of the thiopental induction dose was still detected in maternal blood 12 hours after induction.[16]

Pharmacokinetic assessment of ketamine suggested reduced clearance in pregnancy.[17] There are no studies evaluating pharmacokinetics of etomidate in pregnancy. Higher clearance, shorter half-life, and unchanged volume of distribution were observed for morphine.[18]

TABLE 37–2 Pharmacokinetic changes for selected intravenous anesthetics.

	Volume of Distribution	Clearance
Propofol	Unchanged	⇑
Etomidate	Not known	Not known
Thiopental	Conflicting data	Conflicting data
Ketamine	Conflicting data	⇓
Morphine	Unchanged	⇑

ANESTHETIC CONSIDERATIONS FOR CESAREAN DELIVERY

There are several competing goals and concerns (Table 37–3) when using general anesthetic for cesarean delivery that make up the "dilemma of obstetric anesthesia and analgesia." It is necessary to provide adequate anesthetic depth to ensure maternal comfort, limit fetal drug transmission, provide hemodynamic stability in the face of impending blood loss, and avoid uterolytic effects of volatile anesthetics.[19]

Historically, induction of general anesthesia was performed with thiopental and

TABLE 37–3 Selected concerns with general anesthesia in the parturient.

Induction
Adequate to blunt the response to laryngoscopy? Ensure loss of consciousness?
With an unanticipated "can't intubate, can't ventilate," will patients emerge from anesthesia prior to becoming hypoxic?
Immediately following induction
How quickly do inhaled agents achieve therapeutic effect following induction? Is it fast enough to avoid awareness?
With unanticipated delays between induction and delivery of the fetus, does the risk of awareness increase?
Once the fetus has been delivered
With increased sensitivity to anesthetics, can the dose of inhaled agents be reduced to minimize uterine atony and still avoid awareness?
Any advantage to total intravenous anesthesia over inhaled agents for maintenance of anesthesia once the fetus is delivered?

succinylcholine followed by nitrous oxide and an inhalational anesthetic. Although this is still regarded as a standard, with more modern drugs available, induction techniques may vary. In fact, induction drugs vary on how they meet the induction goals described above.

Neonatal Depression

A main goal is to minimize neonate anesthetic effects. Anesthetic drugs are highly lipophilic and rapidly cross the placentofetal barrier. A measure of drug crossover to the neonate is the umbilical artery–to–umbilical vein ratio. This ratio is 0.87 for thiopental, 0.70 for propofol, and 0.5 for etomidate.

Propofol has been faulted for higher incidence of neonatal depression. This was based on a single publication from 1989 where parturients were induced with 2.8 mg/kg propofol or 5 mg/kg of thiopental. Twenty-five percent of the neonates born to mothers who had received propofol had lower Apgar scores than those who received thiopental (7.7 versus 8.2).[20] In contrast, several other studies showed comparable Apgar scores in propofol versus thiopental induction.[12,21-23] Data on the effect of maintenance propofol infusion on neonatal depression are inconclusive. Gin et al noted decreased neurobehavioral scores in infants delivered after 2-mg/kg propofol bolus followed by a 150-mcg/kg/min, but not a 100-mcg/kg/min, propofol infusion.[11] Similarly, a 1.5- to 2.5-mg/kg induction bolus of propofol followed by a 200-mcg/kg/min propofol infusion,[24] a 2.5-mg/kg bolus followed by an 83-mcg/kg/min propofol infusion,[25] and a 2-mg/kg bolus followed by a 100-mcg/kg/min infusion[26] did not cause any appreciable difference in Apgar scores or neurobehavioral assessment. No correlation between neonatal propofol levels and Apgar or neurobehavioral scores was found.

There are limited data regarding the effect of ketamine on the neonates. It has been shown that ketamine can increase uterine tone.[27] However, it seems that it does not cause significant neonatal depression at induction doses of 1 mg/kg.[28] At higher doses (1.5 and 2 mg/kg), low Apgar scores and muscular hypertonicity have been reported.[17,29]

A similar lack of data applies to etomidate. Few studies reported comparable Apgar scores after a 0.3-mg/kg induction dose,[30] and one study observed slightly decreased base excess on umbilical blood gas analysis but similar Apgar scores in comparison to thiopental 5-mg/kg induction in the control group.[31] Temporary suppression of cortisol concentration in infants that peaked at 2 hours and normalized 6 hours after delivery has also been reported.[30,32] Clinical relevance of this finding was not defined, but given the short-lived effect and no reports of adverse outcomes, it is likely not significant.

All inhalational agents equilibrate very quickly in fetal tissues and can cause neonatal depression. All of them, including sevoflurane and desflurane, are in clinically applicable concentrations considered equally safe for the fetus.[33]

Addition of a small remifentanil bolus to induction agents (0.5 and 1 mcg/kg) was evaluated for cesarean delivery in several studies. All consistently observed transitory, yet clinically significant neonatal respiratory depression, in 10% to 14% of infants.[34-37] Umbilical cord blood gas at delivery was not different from the control group.

From the perspective of the fetus, all induction agents are considered safe in the recommended induction doses, whereas higher doses can potentially lead to neonatal depression. Reduction of the induction–delivery and the uterine incision–delivery intervals to a minimum as well as maintenance of stable maternal hemodynamics to optimize placental blood flow and fetal oxygenation would probably have larger impact on the fetus than the choice of an induction agent. Addition of a remifentanil bolus to standard induction is not recommended.

Hemodynamic Stability

Several publications addressed hemodynamic stability after different induction agents in cesarean delivery. Not surprisingly, etomidate induction offered the most stable hemodynamics. Propofol 2.0 to 2.5 mg/kg was observed to cause hypotension after induction. Although mean blood pressure was significantly lower in comparison to thiopental in several studies,[22,38] some studies demonstrated comparable hemodynamic stability[23,24,39] and a few found even better stability in comparison to thiopental.[40] Ketamine uniformly showed significantly higher blood pressure and heart rate after induction of general anesthetic for cesarean delivery.[41,42] Addition of a 1.0-mcg/kg (but not 0.5-mcg/kg) remifentanil bolus to induction agents led to significant attenuation of sympathomimetic response to laryngoscopy.[35,37] However, although hemodynamics remained stable in healthy parturients, blood pressure was lower and required treatment in 2 of 21 preeclamptic patients.[36]

In conclusion, hemodynamic effects of all induction agents in standard doses were of limited clinical significance. If hypotension occurred, it was easily treated with ephedrine or phenylephrine.

Uterolytic Effect

Intravenous anesthetics, opioids, or muscle relaxants have no effect on uterine tone. In contrast, the dose-dependent uterolytic effect of all volatile agents has been well recognized. Although complete uterine unresponsiveness to oxytocin will follow administration of greater than 2 MAC of volatile anesthetic, the uterus will remain responsive to oxytocin with MAC less than 0.8 to1.0.[43]

Awareness

Providing adequate depth of anesthesia is the most challenging part of general anesthetic for cesarean delivery. Suggested techniques for preventing awareness are listed in Table 37–4. Unfortunately, incidence of awareness after general anesthesia for cesarean delivery is still alarmingly high—0.1% to 0.9%—significantly higher than in the general population.[19] A proportion of patients experiencing awareness may develop serious psychological sequelae, including post-traumatic stress disorder.[44]

TABLE 37–4 Techniques to prevent awareness during cesarean delivery.

Avoid drug errors
Give induction-dose propofol 2 mg/kg, thiopental 4 mg/kg, or etomidate 0.3 mg/kg.
Use desflurane or sevoflurane and focus on achieving end-tidal 0.7 minimum alveolar concentration rapidly.
Add 50% nitrous oxide after induction (some advocate highest concentration of nitrous oxide compatible with maternal and fetal oxygenation).
Consider adding ketamine.
Give opioid after delivery.
Consider benzodiazepine after fetal delivery.
Consider Bispectral Index Scale monitoring.

Why is awareness seen more often after cesarean section, despite decreased MAC and faster update of inhalational anesthetics? Several studies suggest that awareness during cesarean section is caused by reluctance to use adequate doses of intravenous anesthetics and inhalational agents because of concerns of neonatal drug exposure and their effects on uterine tone.[19,45] Some authors go even further suggesting that all cases of awareness are due to underdosing unless there is convincing, verifiable evidence to the contrary.[46] Others accept the possibility of awareness even with standard doses of anesthetic.[47] For example, standard induction doses with propofol and succinylcholine may lead to periods of inadequate anesthesia, especially with prolonged airway management as illustrated with simulation in Figure 37–1.

CASE DISCUSSION

A 68.2-kg (150-lb), 165-cm (5′5″) female needs an emergency cesarean section. Her respiratory rate is 12 breaths per minute and her tidal volume is 500 mL/breath. Induction dosing includes a 2-mg/kg propofol bolus followed 15 seconds later by a 1-mg/kg succinylcholine bolus. Laryngoscopy and skin incision occur 3 and 4 minutes after propofol administration, respectively. Maintenance of anesthesia is with 2% sevoflurane in oxygen started 4 minutes after the propofol bolus. Fresh gas flow is set to 2 L/min. Eleven minutes after incision, the fetus is delivered, and a 2-mcg/kg fentanyl bolus is administered. The procedure ends after 60 minutes. (Assumptions made and limitations of these simulations are presented in Table 37–5.)

In this simulation, 2 key points emerge. (1) Induction agents have a rapid onset of effect, achieving peak effect-site concentrations within 2 minutes (see Figure 37–1A). The onset of unresponsiveness is rapid but of short duration (< 5 minutes). The onset of paralysis is equally rapid but lasts up to 10 minutes. With difficult airway management, there

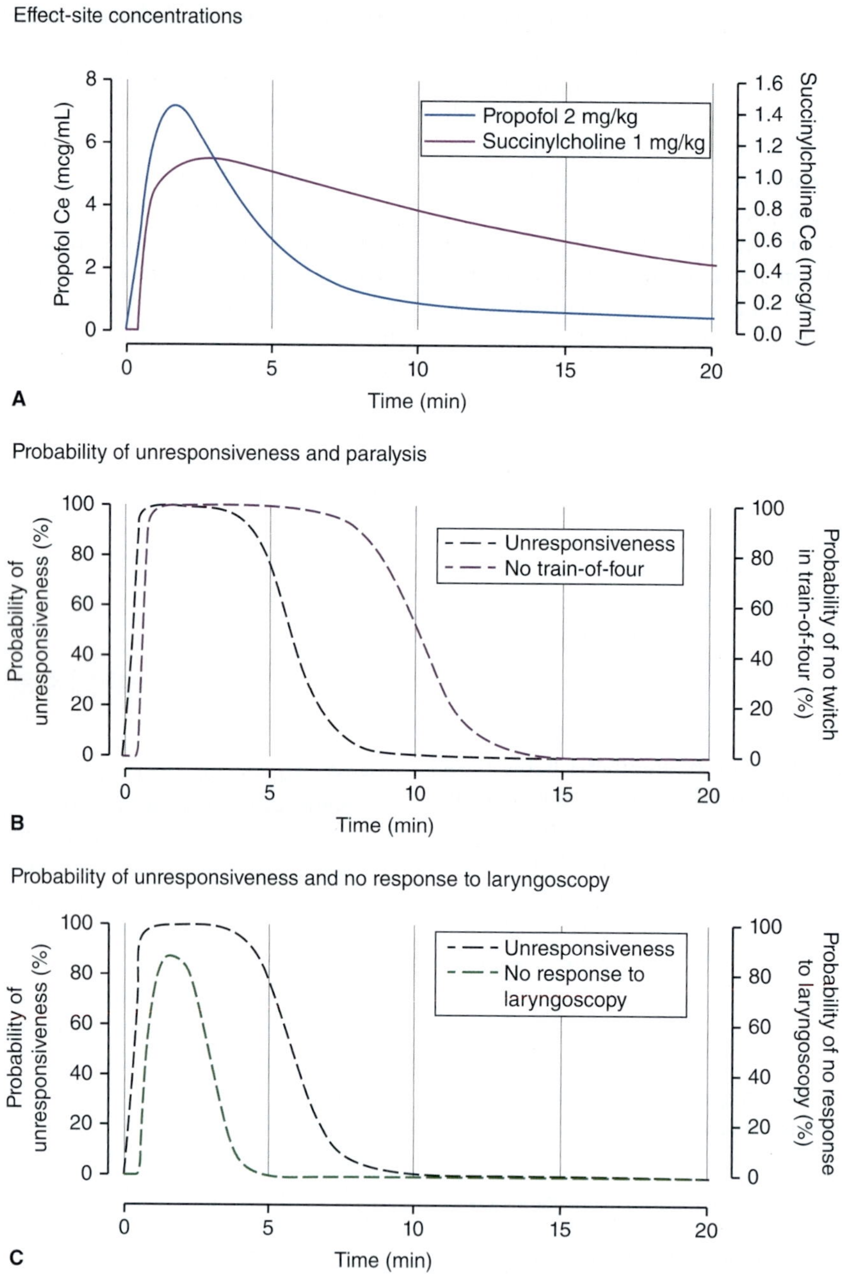

FIGURE 37–1 Simulations of effect-site concentration (Ce) levels and drug effects for induction drugs only. The propofol and succinylcholine reach peak concentrations in 1.5 and 2.5 minutes, respectively (A). The probability of unconsciousness and muscle paralysis remains above 90% for 4 and 7 minutes, respectively (B). The probability of no response to laryngoscopy remains above 80% for just over 1 minute (C).

TABLE 37–5 Limitations and assumptions of simulations presented in Figures 37–1, 37–2, and 37–3.

Limitations
Simulations assume a 30% reduction in inhalation agent dose to achieve an equivalent effect but make no assumptions for intravenous agents.
Models that predict unresponsiveness have been created in the presence of a mild stimuli. More anesthetic is likely required to ensure unresponsiveness in the presence of moderate to severe stimuli.
No model of consciousness or awareness exists—only models of responsiveness. Patients may be unresponsive but still be conscious or aware, although this is unlikely in the presence of a painful stimulus and no paralytic. By contrast, patients may be responsive but have no memory of an event. Although not identical, unresponsiveness is the best available surrogate of unconsciousness.
Assumptions
Minute ventilation and cardiac output remain stable throughout the cesarean section.
The parturient has no comorbidities (eg, preeclampsia, obesity, or opioid tolerance).
Blood loss is not excessive.

may be a delay in administering a volatile anesthetic, and it is possible that patients would be responsive but still paralyzed. (2) Laryngoscopy is one of the most painful stimuli encountered during a cesarean section. Rendering a parturient completely unresponsive (no heart rate or blood pressure change, or no movement if no paralytic is used) requires large doses of anesthetic and may not be tolerated (ie, worrisome hypotension or fetal depression). A conventional dose of propofol by itself provides only a brief period of unresponsiveness to laryngoscopy.

The critical period for awareness in cesarean delivery is the time from skin incision to delivery of the neonate. Benzodiazepines and opioids are withheld prior to delivery to prevent neonatal respiratory depression. Especially in the setting of emergency cesarean delivery, there is limited time to reach adequate end-tidal concentration of inhalational agents before incision, as illustrated in simulations presented in Figures 37–2 and 37–3. These simulations illustrate 2 key points: (1) although the end-tidal inhalation agent levels may quickly rise, there is a substantial lag in the rise of the effect-site concentration (up to 10 minutes) and associated analgesic and sedative effects (see Figure 37–2A). (2) A delay in administering inhalation agent of longer than 3 to 4 minutes after the induction dose of propofol leads to a brief period around incision where the probability of unresponsiveness drops below 50% (see Figure 37–3A).

Some methods proved to cause unacceptably high incidence of awareness (up to 40%) with a 2.5-mg/kg propofol bolus followed by 0.25% to 0.5% halothane and 50% nitrous oxide,[25] or 9% incidence of awareness with a 2.5-mg/kg propofol bolus followed by a propofol infusion 83 mcg/kg/min with 50% nitrous oxide.[25]. An approach advocated in the past—0.5 MAC of inhalational agent with 50% nitrous oxide administered before delivery—carries about a 1.3% incidence of awareness. A simulation of 0.5 MAC sevoflurane (1%) with and without nitrous oxide is presented in Figure 37–3C. Although nitrous oxide improves the probability of unresponsiveness from incision to delivery, model predictions suggest that up to 20% of patients may not be unresponsive for brief periods of time.

How can we assess the required dose of anesthetic that will reliably prevent awareness? An isolated forearm test was used to assess the depth of anesthesia in the past. This test is very sensitive, and many patients with a positive response to verbal instruction will not develop postoperative awareness. As many as 52% of patients who received thiopental 4 mg/kg for induction followed by 0.5% halothane and 50% nitrous oxide responded to verbal instruction in the period between induction and delivery of the fetus; all these patients denied awareness postoperatively.[48] In a study by Baraka, 72% of patients had a positive isolated forearm test after 4-mg/kg thiopental followed by 0.5% halothane, and only 10% of patients reported awareness.[42] The clinical significance of a positive isolated forearm test on implicit memory is unknown.

Evaluation of the Bispectral Index Scale (BIS) was more recently used; however, there are limitations of BIS in predicting postoperative awareness. It has been demonstrated that 0.5 MAC with 50% nitrous oxide of isoflurane[49] and sevoflurane[50] do not reliably achieve a BIS less than 60. On the contrary, 0.7 MAC of sevoflurane with 50% nitrous oxide[50] produced BIS values less than 60. Most recently, Chin evaluated MAC of sevoflurane needed to

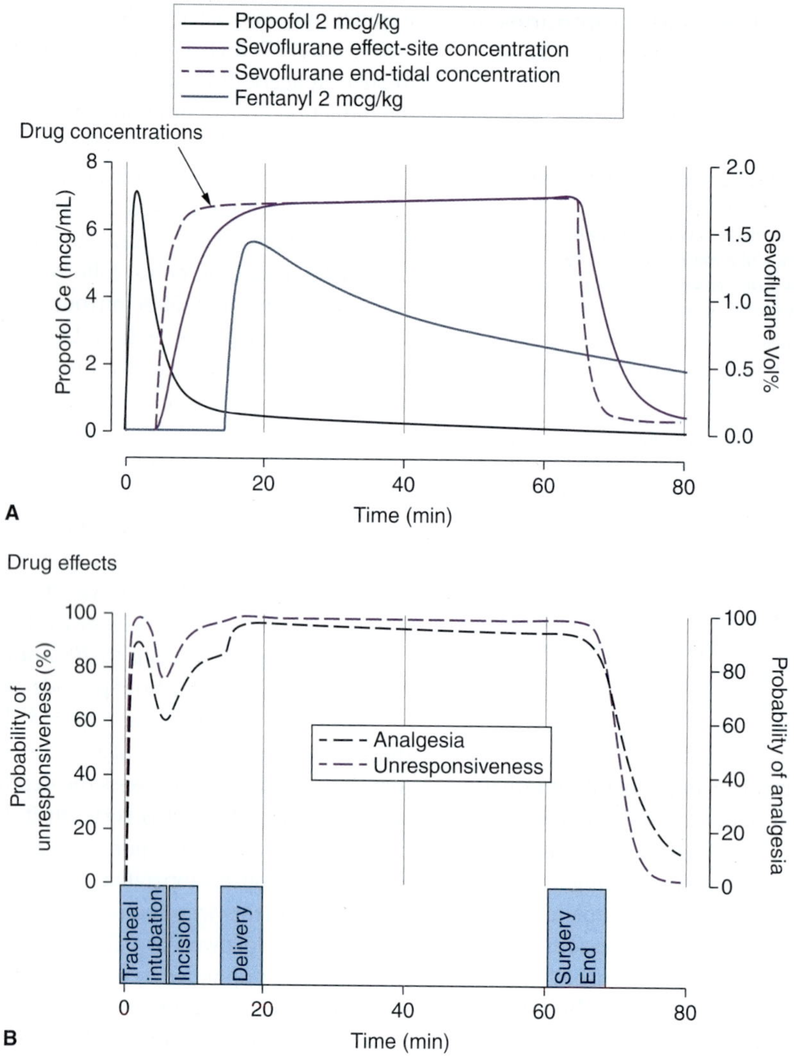

FIGURE 37–2 Simulations of effect-site concentration (Ce) levels and drug effects for induction and maintenance drugs. The Ce lags behind the end-tidal concentration for sevoflurane. For example, following induction, the Ce and end-tidal concentration reach near–steady state (within 10% of the highest concentration) at 4 and 15 minutes, respectively (arrow). The fentanyl bolus reaches peak Ce within 5 minutes of administration and then declines to 45% of its peak by the end of the procedure (A). The probability of unresponsiveness from propofol and sevoflurane remains above 95% for the entire procedure, except between 4 and 15 minutes following the propofol bolus, where it drops as low as 78%. The probability of analgesia to a moderate noxious stimulus peaks with the propofol at 1.5 minutes and then quickly drops to below 35% until fentanyl is administered. Once the fentanyl reaches peak effect, the probability of analgesia from fentanyl combined with sevoflurane remains at 99% or higher throughout the procedure (B).

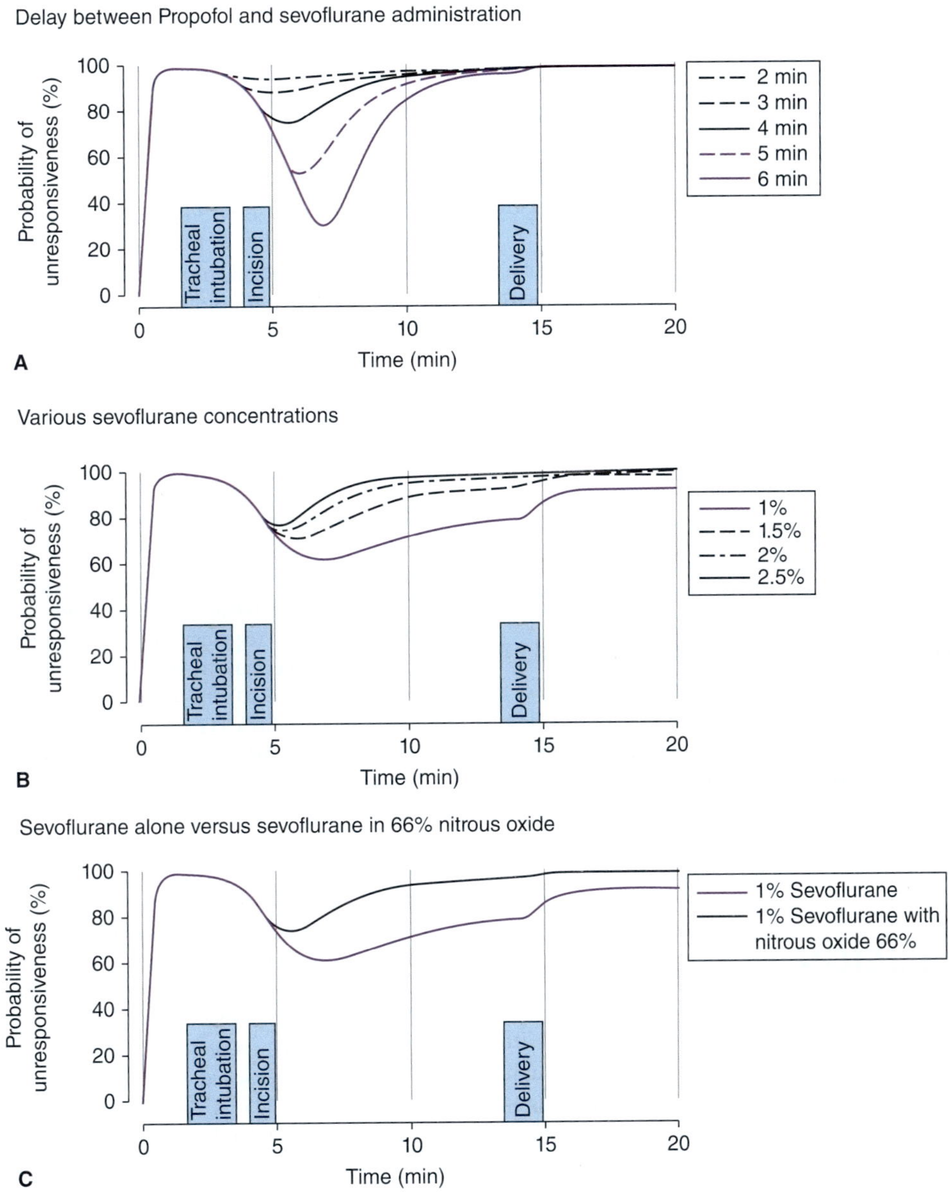

FIGURE 37–3 Simulations of the delay between propofol and sevoflurane administration (A), various sevoflurane concentrations for maintenance (B), and sevoflurane in 66% nitrous oxide (C). For delays between the propofol bolus and starting sevoflurane of 3 minutes or less, the probability of unresponsiveness remains high (> 85%). For delays longer than 4 minutes, the probability drops to 51 and 23% for 5- and 6-minute delays, respectively. With lower doses of sevoflurane (< 2%), the probability of unresponsiveness can remain between 55% and 75% for the 10 minutes following incision (B). Adding 66% nitrous oxide increases the probability of unresponsiveness. The probability of unresponsiveness is between 67% and 95% for the 10 minutes following incision for 1% sevoflurane in 66% nitrous oxide (C).

achieve BIS less than 60. When used with 50% nitrous oxide, 0.61 MAC led to BIS less than 60 in 50% of patients, and 0.75 MAC led to BIS less than 60 in 95% of patients undergoing cesarean delivery.[49]

Auditory evoked potential index used in a study by Allahyary et al suggested that 0.6% end-tidal isoflurane concentration with 50% nitrous oxide provided inadequate depth of anesthesia.[51]

A few studies suggest that ketamine, either as sole induction agent or as adjunct, can decrease risk of awareness.[42] Ketamine 1 mg/kg was compared to thiopental 3 mg/kg (both followed by 60% nitrous oxide), and the observed awareness was 2% versus 32%.[28] Similarly, ketamine 1 mg/kg was superior to thiopental 4 mg/kg in abolishing an isolated forearm test performed prior to delivery.[48] Of note, 2 studies demonstrated better postoperative pain control after cesarean delivery in groups that used ketamine—both as a sole induction agent[52] and as an adjunct.[41] Unfortunately, associated hallucinations and unpleasant dreams, albeit seen less often in obstetrics,[52] limit widespread use of ketamine.

It has not been studied whether benzodiazepines administered after delivery decrease risk of awareness prior to delivery. However, addition of benzodiazepine after fetal delivery could increase the depth of anesthesia and have an impact on awareness in the later stage of cesarean delivery.

CONCLUSION

In conclusion, parturients have risks for awareness. They are young females and receive anesthesia with neuromuscular blocking agents.[53] It seems, though, that the majority of reported cases of awareness in obstetrics were related to low doses of anesthetic agents. Some alteration of awareness risk can be achieved with adequate doses of induction agents or with addition of ketamine. However, it appears that the main focus should be aimed at reaching a minimum 0.7 MAC of an inhalational agent as fast as possible following the induction.[54] Desflurane and sevoflurane offer faster uptake and therefore are preferable to isoflurane. Fifty percent nitrous oxide is still recommended prior to delivery of the fetus and should be increased to 70% after delivery. Currently, there is no consensus on monitoring of the depth of anesthesia during general anesthesia for cesarean delivery, but it is clear that hemodynamic parameters as an indicator of awareness are unreliable in emergent cesarean delivery.

In summary, general anesthesia for emergent cesarean delivery presents complex and challenging tasks for an anesthesiologist. The stress of an emergent procedure that is infrequently performed and possible medicolegal implications make this procedure even more demanding.

REFERENCES

1. Little BB. Pharmacokinetics during pregnancy: evidence-based maternal dose formulation. *Obstet Gynecol.* 1999;93(5 pt 2):858-868.
2. Larsson A, Palm M, Hansson LO, Basu S, Axelsson O. Reference values for alpha1-acid glycoprotein, alpha1-antitrypsin, albumin, haptoglobin, C-reactive protein, IgA, IgG and IgM during pregnancy. *Acta Obstet Gynecol Scand.* 2008;87(10):1084-1088.
3. Anderson GD. Pregnancy-induced changes in pharmacokinetics: a mechanistic-based approach. *Clin Pharmacokinet.* 2005;44(10):989-1008.
4. Leighton BL, Cheek TG, Gross JB, et al. Succinylcholine pharmacodynamics in peripartum patients. *Anesthesiology.* 1986;64(2):202-205.
5. Mongardon N, Servin F, Perrin M, et al. Predicted propofol effect-site concentration for induction and emergence of anesthesia during early pregnancy. *Anesth Analg.* 2009;109(1):90-95.
6. Higuchi H, Adachi Y, Arimura S, Kanno M, Satoh T. Early pregnancy does not reduce the C(50) of propofol for loss of consciousness. *Anesth Analg.* 2001;93(6):1565-1569.
7. Chestnut DH. *Chestnut's Obstetric Anesthesia: Principles and Practice.* 4th ed. Philadelphia: Mosby/Elsevier; 2009: 545-547.
8. Chan MT, Mainland P, Gin T. Minimum alveolar concentration of halothane and enflurane are decreased in early pregnancy. *Anesthesiology.* 1996; 85(4):782-786.
9. Gin T, Chan MT. Decreased minimum alveolar concentration of isoflurane in pregnant humans. *Anesthesiology.* 1994;81(4):829-832.
10. Chan MT, Gin T. Postpartum changes in the minimum alveolar concentration of isoflurane. *Anesthesiology.* 1995;82(6):1360-1363.
11. Gin T, Yau G, Chan K, Gregory MA, Oh TE. Disposition of propofol infusions for caesarean section. *Can J Anaesth.* 1991;38(1):31-36.

12. Gin T, Gregory MA, Chan K, Buckley T, Oh TE. Pharmacokinetics of propofol in women undergoing elective caesarean section. *Br J Anaesth.* 1990;64(2): 148-153.
13. Finster M, Mark LC. Thiobarbiturates in obstetric anesthesia. *Clin Anesth.* 1974;10(2):163-172.
14. Kosaka Y, Takahashi T, Mark LC. Intravenous thiobarbiturate anesthesia for cesarean section. *Anesthesiology.* 1969;31(6):489-506.
15. Finster M, Morishima HO, Mark LC, Perel JM, Dayton PG, James LS. Tissue thiopental concentrations in the fetus and newborn. *Anesthesiology.* 1972;36(2):155-158.
16. Esener Z, Sarihasan B, Güven H, Ustün E. Thiopentone and etomidate concentrations in maternal and umbilical plasma, and in colostrum. *Br J Anaesth.* 1992;69(6):586-588.
17. Little B, Chang T, Chucot L, et al. Study of ketamine as an obstetric anesthetic agent. *Am J Obstet Gynecol.* 1972;113(2):247-260.
18. Gerdin E, Salmonson T, Lindberg B, Rane A. Maternal kinetics of morphine during labour. *J Perinat Med.* 1990;18(6):479-487.
19. Robins K, Lyons G. Intraoperative awareness during general anesthesia for cesarean delivery. *Anesth Analg.* 2009;109(3):886-890.
20. Celleno D, Capogna G, Tomassetti M, Costantino P, Di Feo G, Nisini R. Neurobehavioural effects of propofol on the neonate following elective caesarean section. *Br J Anaesth.* 1989;62(6):649-654.
21. Gin T, Gregory MA, Chan K, Oh TE. Maternal and fetal levels of propofol at caesarean section. *Anaesth Intensive Care.* 1990;18(2):180-184.
22. Moore J, Bill KM, Flynn RJ, McKeating KT, Howard PJ. A comparison between propofol and thiopentone as induction agents in obstetric anaesthesia. *Anaesthesia.* 1989;44(9):753-757.
23. Valtonen M, Kanto J, Rosenberg P. Comparison of propofol and thiopentone for induction of anaesthesia for elective caesarean section. *Anaesthesia.* 1989; 44(9):758-762.
24. Abboud TK, Zhu J, Richardson M, Peres Da Silva E, Donovan M. Intravenous propofol vs thiamylal-isoflurane for caesarean section, comparative maternal and neonatal effects. *Acta Anaesthesiol Scand.* 1995; 39(2):205-209.
25. Dailland P, Cockshott ID, Lirzin JD, et al. Intravenous propofol during cesarean section: placental transfer, concentrations in breast milk, and neonatal effects. A preliminary study. *Anesthesiology.* 1989;71(6):827-834.
26. Yau G, Gin T, Ewart MC, Kotur CF, Leung RK, Oh TE. Propofol for induction and maintenance of anaesthesia at caesarean section. A comparison with thiopentone/enflurane. *Anaesthesia.* 1991;46(1):20-23.
27. Oats JN, Vasey DP, Waldron BA. Effects of ketamine on the pregnant uterus. *Br J Anaesth.* 1979;51(12): 1163-1166.
28. Peltz B, Sinclair DM. Induction agents for Caesarean section. A comparison of thiopentone and ketamine. *Anaesthesia.* 1973;28(1):37-42.
29. Downing JW, Mahomedy MC, Jeal DE, Allen PJ. Anaesthesia for Caesarean section with ketamine. *Anaesthesia.* 1976;31(7):883-892.
30. Crozier TA, Flamm C, Speer CP, et al. Effects of etomidate on the adrenocortical and metabolic adaptation of the neonate. *Br J Anaesth.* 1993;70(1):47-53.
31. Downing JW, Buley RJ, Brock-Utne JG, Houlton PC. Etomidate for induction of anaesthesia at caesarean section: comparison with thiopentone. *Br J Anaesth.* 1979;51(2):135-140.
32. Reddy BK, Pizer B, Bull PT. Neonatal serum cortisol suppression by etomidate compared with thiopentone, for elective caesarean section. *Eur J Anaesthesiol.* 1988;5(3):171-176.
33. Abboud TK, Zhu J, Richardson M, Peres da Silva E, Donovan M. Desflurane: a new volatile anesthetic for cesarean section. Maternal and neonatal effects. *Acta Anaesthesiol Scand.* 1995;39(6):723-726.
34. Van de Velde M, Teunkens A, Kuypers M, Dewinter T, Vandermeersch E. General anaesthesia with target controlled infusion of propofol for planned caesarean section: maternal and neonatal effects of a remifentanil-based technique. *Int J Obstet Anesth.* 2004;13(3):153-158.
35. Ngan Kee WD, Khaw KS, Ma KC, Wong AS, Lee BB, Ng FF. Maternal and neonatal effects of remifentanil at induction of general anesthesia for cesarean delivery: a randomized, double-blind, controlled trial. *Anesthesiology.* 2006;104(1):14-20.
36. Yoo KY, Jeong CW, Park BY, et al. Effects of remifentanil on cardiovascular and bispectral index responses to endotracheal intubation in severe pre-eclamptic patients undergoing Caesarean delivery under general anaesthesia. *Br J Anaesth.* 2009;102(6):812-819.
37. Draisci G, Valente A, Suppa E, et al. Remifentanil for cesarean section under general anesthesia: effects on maternal stress hormone secretion and neonatal well-being: a randomized trial. *Int J Obstet Anesth.* 2008; 17(2):130-136.
38. Grounds RM, Twigley AJ, Carli F, Whitwam JG, Morgan M. The haemodynamic effects of intravenous induction. Comparison of the effects of thiopentone and propofol. *Anaesthesia.* 1985;40(8):735-740.

39. Gregory MA, Gin T, Yau G, Leung RK, Chan K, Oh TE. Propofol infusion anaesthesia for caesarean section. *Can J Anaesth.* 1990;37(5):514-520.
40. Gin T, Gregory MA, Oh TE. The haemodynamic effects of propofol and thiopentone for induction of caesarean section. *Anaesth Intensive Care.* 1990;18(2):175-179.
41. Nayar R, Sahajanand H. Does anesthetic induction for Cesarean section with a combination of ketamine and thiopentone confer any benefits over thiopentone or ketamine alone? A prospective randomized study. *Minerva Anestesiol.* 2009;75(4):185-190.
42. Baraka A, Louis F, Dalleh R. Maternal awareness and neonatal outcome after ketamine induction of anaesthesia for Caesarean section. *Can J Anaesth.* 1990;37(6):641-644.
43. Dogru K, Yildiz K, Dalgiç H, Sezer Z, Yaba G, Madenoglu H. Inhibitory effects of desflurane and sevoflurane on contractions of isolated gravid rat myometrium under oxytocin stimulation. *Acta Anaesthesiol Scand.* 2003;47(4):472-474.
44. Aaen AM, Moller K. Through and beyond anaesthesia awareness. *BMJ.* 2010;341:c3669.
45. Paech MJ, Scott KL, Clavisi O, Chua S, McDonnell N; ANZCA Trials Group. A prospective study of awareness and recall associated with general anaesthesia for caesarean section. *Int J Obstet Anesth.* 2008;17(4):298-303.
46. Nickalls RW, Mahajan RP. Awareness and anaesthesia: think dose, think data. *Br J Anaesth.* 2010;104(1):1-2.
47. Hull CJ. Awareness is due to negligence during general anaesthesia for caesarean section. *Int J Obstet Anesth.* 1997;6(3):178-180.
48. Gaitini L, Vaida S, Collins G, Somri M, Sabo E. Awareness detection during caesarean section under general anaesthesia using EEG spectrum analysis. *Can J Anaesth.* 1995;42(5 pt 1):377-3.
49. Chin KJ, Yeo SW. A BIS-guided study of sevoflurane requirements for adequate depth of anaesthesia in Caesarean section. *Anaesthesia.* 2004;59(11):1064-1068.
50. Chin KJ, Yeo SW. Bispectral index values at sevoflurane concentrations of 1% and 1.5% in lower segment cesarean delivery. *Anesth Analg.* 2004;98(4):1140-1144.
51. Allahyary E, Zand F, Tabatabaee HR. Evaluation of the adequacy of general anesthesia in cesarean section by auditory evoked potential index: an observational study. *Acta Anaesthesiol Taiwan.* 2008;46(1):16-24.
52. Ngan Kee WD, Khaw KS, Ma ML, Mainland PA, Gin T. Postoperative analgesic requirement after cesarean section: a comparison of anesthetic induction with ketamine or thiopental. *Anesth Analg.* 1997;85(6): 1294-1298.
53. Ghoneim MM, Block RI, Haffarnan M, Mathews MJ. Awareness during anesthesia: risk factors, causes and sequelae: a review of reported cases in the literature. *Anesth Analg.* 2009;108(2):527-535.
54. McCrirrick A, Evans GH, Thomas TA. Overpressure isoflurane at caesarean section: a study of arterial isoflurane concentrations. *Br J Anaesth.* 1994;72(1): 122-124.

Index

Page numbers followed by italic *f* or *t* denote figures or tables, respectively.

D

E

F

I

Q

R

T